Fourth edition

PHARMACOLOGY and MEDICINES MANAGEMENT for Nurses

George Downie MSc FRPharmS HonFCPP
Director of Pharmacy and Medicines Management,
NHS Grampian, Aberdeen, Scotland, UK

Jean Mackenzie BA(Open) RGN SCM
DipN(Lond) RCT RNT
Formerly Lecturer, School of Nursing and Midwifery,
The Robert Gordon University, Aberdeen, Scotland, UK

Arthur Williams OBE FRPharmS
Formerly Chief Administrative Pharmaceutical Officer,
Grampian, Orkney, Shetland and Tayside Health Boards,
Scotland, UK

In association with
Caroline Hind PhD BPharm MRPharmS
Pharmacist Facilitator, Pharmacy Medicines Unit,
NHS Grampian, Aberdeen, Scotland, UK

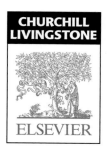

CHURCHILL
LIVINGSTONE

ELSEVIER

Edinburgh London New York Oxford Philadelphia St Louis Sydney Toronto 2008

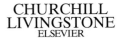

First edition 1995
Second edition 1999
Third edition 2003
Fourth edition 2008

ISBN-13: 9780443103315

British Library Cataloguing in Publication Data
A catalogue record for this book is available from the British Library

Library of Congress Cataloging in Publication Data
A catalog record for this book is available from the Library of Congress

 your source for books, journals and multimedia in the health sciences

www.elsevierhealth.com

Working together to grow
libraries in developing countries

www.elsevier.com | www.bookaid.org | www.sabre.org

ELSEVIER   BOOK AID International   Sabre Foundation

The Publisher's policy is to use **paper manufactured from sustainable forests**

Printed in China

Contents

Preface

In this fourth edition, every effort has been made to reflect current practice in the management of medicines.

In Section 1, the basic principles of the control and handling of medicines have been strengthened. Nurse prescribing has also been updated along with other measures designed to improve patients' access to medicines. Nurses are increasingly involved in making decisions about the planning and delivery of drug therapy. Effective drug therapy requires a partnership between patient and carer; this relationship is explored in Chapter 7.

Section 2 gives a concise introduction to the clinical pharmacology that underpins the therapeutic use of drugs.

In Section 3, the main drugs acting on organ systems are described, together with their indications, side-effects and benefits to patients.

Self-assessment exercises are included for the first time. These are presented in a variety of formats designed to challenge and stimulate the reader. The self-assessment questions and answers have been formulated to help readers assess their understanding of pharmacology and medicines management. A wide range of questions has been included, which can be answered by using the text. Readers are invited to contact the authors, via the publishers, on any issues arising from the questions (or any other part of the text).

Readers' comments on previous editions are always appreciated and have been taken into account. Illustrations have been increased and enhanced by the use of colour.

Unlike other publications in this field, we have sought to produce a text that links the management of medicines to their therapeutic use against a background of clinical pharmacology. We consider that this approach will provide a basis for those working in adult nursing to develop the skills needed to ensure that patients in hospital and the community benefit from modern medicines.

George Downie
Jean Mackenzie
Aberdeen 2008   **Arthur Williams**
Caroline Hind

Acknowledgements

A book of this size and diversity could not have been written without the help of a number of colleagues. We are deeply indebted to them for sparing time and energy to contribute to and review material within their own areas of interest and expertise.

Our grateful thanks go to each one of them; Lesley Anderson (for secretarial services), Airlie Bryce, Eileen Grant, Jill Kettle, Jane Mair, Carol Noble, Karen Watson (for the section on Intensive Care).

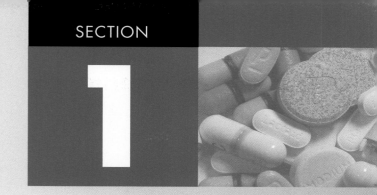

MEDICINES
MANAGEMENT

Medicines in society today and tomorrow

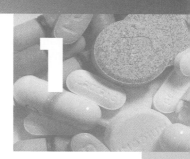

Medicines have an impact on the lives of people of all ages. In the main, the impact is beneficial, enhancing lifestyles and prolonging, and often saving, lives. However, in developing countries neither the benefits nor the hazards of modern drug therapy are experienced. Thanks to the innovative work of the global pharmaceutical industry, prescribers and their patients have access to a range of effective drugs and delivery systems that could scarcely be imagined when the NHS was established in 1948. The therapeutic explosion comes, however, with a hefty price tag for both the industry and the consumer. In developing a new drug, thousands of compounds are screened for therapeutic activity and safety. To bring a new drug to the market requires massive expenditure over a period of many years. The importance of the research and development effort involved to the global economy is vast. Pharmaceutical companies target their research efforts to those therapeutic areas in which the returns are likely to be profitable. One major drug can generate sales of billions of pounds per annum. The problem of research priorities remains unresolved, but the ultimate aim is to develop medicines designed to meet the needs of individual patients. Few resources can be diverted to finding treatments for very rare diseases, because of the low returns (profits) generated. Orphan drugs need to be adopted. Prescription medicines are vitally important, but it should not be forgotten that over-the-counter medicines play an important role in self-care, thus releasing resources for the NHS. By making some potent medicines available without prescription, access to medicines has been improved for those who can afford them. It is important that this deregulation is carried out within carefully defined conditions. Medicines are not just commodities; they are potent therapeutic agents that should be treated with the respect they merit.

Despite the progress made in the development of new drugs, massive problems remain, especially in addressing the needs of the developing world. New pandemics threaten the world, in particular avian influenza. The availability of effective antiviral drugs and new vaccines should not cause complacency.

In confronting the unmet needs in the treatment of cancer, the AIDS crisis, tuberculosis, tropical diseases, Alzheimer's disease, respiratory and cardiovascular diseases, and diabetes, innovative global research programs will be required. The problems of resistance to antibiotic therapy, especially in hospitals, require constant vigilance, as does the need to reduce the side-effects of drug treatment.

Not only will appropriate drug treatment make people feel better, but also links between ill health and poverty will, in time, be broken. In the UK and other countries, drug costs have long been a cause for concern for politicians. There are no signs that the financial and other tensions created by the introduction of new drugs will abate. In some ways, this is to be welcomed because it is a sign that there is a dynamic research environment producing valuable drugs. The establishment of bodies charged with the assessment of new drugs (the National Institute for Health and Clinical Excellence) has brought into sharp focus the need to manage the introduction of new drugs on an equitable basis. 'Postcode prescribing' is an evil that must be eliminated.

Controversy will always be associated with the development and introduction of new drugs. The actions of the pharmaceutical companies in aggressive marketing, price fixing, profiteering (alleged), and the use of uninformed human volunteers and laboratory animals in drug testing are often criticised (and worse). It is beyond any doubt that the benefits of modern drugs in both the treatment and the prevention of disease are here to stay. Safety issues relating to the introduction of new drugs remain a cause for concern, as recent events relating to the withdrawal of rofecoxib illustrate. There are real possibilities that some drugs may be replaced by treatments such as stem cells (regenerative medicine), organ transplantation, and even using organs grown in the laboratory. In time, the present research methods, like some of our drugs, will become redundant. Several important drugs in use today are derived from plants. This source of effective medicines is by no means exhausted.

Information technology will play an even more important role in both the discovery and the management of medicines. Electronic prescribing, automation and improved communications will all help to ensure that the benefits of modern drug therapy will be available to more people than ever before. Evidence-based prescribing decisions are increasingly being supported by IT. Delays in introducing an NHS-wide IT system are currently a cause for concern, as are the escalating costs of the system.

Healthcare professionals are adapting their practice to meet the higher expectations of patients and those who pay for health services. Greater specialisation, increased responsibilities and improved joint working will all develop in the years ahead. Along with these increased responsibilities (such as prescribing) will go the need for continuing professional development, further education and participation in research programmes. The need to maintain the highest professional, ethical standards during times of great change both in society and in the clinical environment cannot be overemphasised. Worries about possible litigation should be responded to by ensuring compliance with current standards and being aware of the need to be accountable for one's actions. Ethical dilemmas such as the issue of assisted dying may arise in the context of drug therapy. As the boundaries of practice expand, ethical issues will be ever present. In the 1990s, a policy decision by the Crown Prosecution Service has led to an increasing number of doctors being prosecuted for gross negligence or recklessness at work.

Since the publication of the Shipman report (2005), GPs in small practices have expressed their concerns regarding the administration of powerful narcotics to patients in terminal care. If the 'Shipman effect' has an adverse impact on patient care, this is to be deplored.

There is more attention given in the media to issues relating to drug use (legal and otherwise) than ever before. Bad news is reported more often than good. Newspapers have always been a source of information on drugs and medical research (Fig. 1.1). If the story involves sex, it is more likely to be reported than a story involving the overuse of vitamins.

As the delivery of healthcare changes and NHS reorganisations proceed apace, the challenges faced by those charged with delivering safe and effective drug therapy in hospitals and the community will increase. Patients need to be given help in making decisions regarding their care, including the use of medicines and other healthcare products. It is widely accepted that there is a need to improve patient compliance with

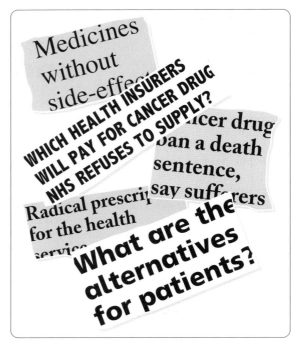

Fig. 1.1 Medicines are in the news almost every day.

drug therapy. The concept of concordance is replacing the rather simplistic approach to non-compliance. Issues of safety are of significance in the broader public health debate. Patient choice has to be provided when practicable and worthwhile. Abuse of both prescribed and other medicines must be dealt with but, owing to the covert nature of this activity, difficulties may arise. Increasingly, people are using complementary and alternative therapies despite the limited research that supports the use of such treatments. The expert patient and the expert carer will both play an increasing role in the achievement of safer drug therapy. Patients are better informed than ever before, but this may be seen as a threat by some health professionals.

Patient safety remains a key consideration. The National Patient Safety Agency is responsible for issuing patient safety alerts. Following a prioritisation process (based on feedback from practitioners), topics are selected for a safety alert. Current safety issues include the safer use of the oral anticoagulant warfarin. Patients with disabilities must be given the help they need in using medicines. This is a requirement of law in the UK.

The impact of globalisation on health is ever present. The greatly increased access to air travel generates thousands of potentially infectious contacts each day. All practitioners need to be aware of this risk.

The prevention of disease by the use of well-managed vaccination programmes, population screening for individuals at high risk, and emphasis on the links between poor diet and ill health are all being given high priority. Smoking cessation campaigns are also being conducted. Despite all these efforts, the incidence of preventable diseases remains unacceptably high. In the developed world, patients' expectations of their healthcare services are high and will continue to be so despite the prevalence of unhealthy lifestyles.

For the foreseeable future, patients will continue to depend on the availability of safe and effective medicines, especially in the final years of their lives. All those involved in delivering therapy with modern drugs bear a heavy responsibility to ensure that the undoubted benefits of modern medicines are fully realised.

FURTHER READING AND RESOURCES

THE PHARMACEUTICAL INDUSTRY

Association of the British Pharmaceutical Industry (http://www.abpi.org.uk) (A representative body that provides a wide range of information relating to the structure and function of the pharmaceutical industry.)

RESEARCH INTO PERSONALISED MEDICINE

[Anonymous] 2006 Translational medicine research collaboration between four Scottish Universities, NHS Scotland and Scottish Enterprise [editorial]. Pharmaceutical Journal 276:411

Hutton N 2005 Diversify or die: what long-term future for the pharmaceutical industry? Pharmaceutical Journal 274:363–364

Kayne S 2006 Secretive, partisan and unaccountable authorities work against patient welfare. Pharmaceutical Journal 276:139–140

Moberly T 2005 Rationing and access to orphan drugs. Pharmaceutical Journal 275:569–570

Wootton D 2006 Bad medicine: doctors doing harm since Hippocrates. Oxford University Press, Oxford

MEDICINES TODAY

MedicinesComplete (http://www.medicinescomplete.com/mc/) (Information on drugs. Subscription service.)

National Prescribing Centre (http://www.npc.nhs.uk) (Information on drugs. Access restricted to NHS staff with prescribing budget responsibilities.)

UK Medicines Information (http://www.ukmi.nhs.uk) (Information on drugs.)

US Centers for Disease Control and Prevention (http://www.cdc.gov./travel) (Travellers' health risks.)

OTHER AGENCIES

Medicines and Healthcare products Regulatory Agency (http://www.mhra.gov.uk)

National Institute for Health and Clinical Excellence (http://www.nice.org.uk/)

Scottish Executive Health Department 2002 The right medicine: a strategy for pharmaceutical care in Scotland. SEHD, Edinburgh

Scottish Medicines Consortium (http://www.scottishmedicines.org.uk/)

DEREGULATION

Bayliss E, Rutter P 2004 General practitioners' views on recent and proposed medicine switches from PoM to P. Pharmaceutical Journal 273:819–821

Highfield R 2006 Medicines without side-effects. Daily Telegraph 25 April 2006

THE NHS

Information Centre for Health and Social Care (http://www.ic.nhs.uk)

Johnson L 2006 A radical prescription for the health service. Sunday Telegraph 7 May, p B4

Moberly T 2006 Healthcare moves into the community [news feature]. Pharmaceutical Journal 276

Office of Health Economics (http://www.ohe.org) (Full range of health statistics from the Office of Health Economics.)

Office of Health Economics 2006 Compendium of health statistics 2006. Population and health trends in the UK and NHS structural changes and finance. OHE, London

DRUGS AND THE MEDIA

Bartlett C, Sterne J, Egger M 2002 What is newsworthy? Longitudinal study of the reporting of medical research in two Bristol newspapers. British Medical Journal 325:81–84 (This article has many useful references.)

THE FUTURE OF DRUG THERAPY

Holland S, Lebacqz K, Zoloth L (eds) 2001 The human embryonic stem cell debate: science, ethics and public policy. MIT Press, Cambridge

Jell G, Bonzani I, Stevens M 2005 Stem cells in regenerative medicine. Pharmaceutical Journal 275:695–698

INFORMATION TECHNOLOGY

McWilliam S 2005 How mobiles and pharmacy are set to revolutionise chronic disease treatment. Pharmaceutical Journal 276:7–8

National Health Service 2005 Electronic Prescription Service. An introduction for health professionals. NHS, London

ROLE OF THE HEALTHCARE PROFESSIONAL

Nursing and Midwifery Council (http://www.nmc-uk.org)

Nursing and Midwifery Council 2004 The NMC code of professional conduct: standards for conduct, performance and ethics. NMC, London

Royal College of Physicians (http://www.rcplondon.ac.uk)

Royal College of Physicians 2005 Doctors in society: medical professionalisation in a changing world. Report of a working party. RCP, London

PUBLIC HEALTH

Maguire T 2005 Irrational humans and public health. Pharmaceutical Journal 274:174

Marteau TM, Kinmonth AL 2002 Screening for cardiovascular risk: public health imperative or matter for individual informed choices? British Medical Journal 235:78–80

Wishart A 2006 One in three. Profile, London

THE PATIENT

TravelHealth.co.uk (http://www.travelhealth.co.uk) (General travel health advice to the public.)

World Health Organization (http://www.who.int/ith/index.html) (Information on disease outbreaks and general advice on travel.)

PATIENT SAFETY

Central Office of Information 2005 The final report of the Shipman Inquiry. Online. Available: http://www.the-shipman-inquiry.org.uk

Doll R, Bradford Hill A 1992 The progress of medical science. British Medical Journal 305:521–526

Doll R, Peto R 1981 The causes of cancer. Oxford University Press, Oxford

Fletcher C 1984 First clinical use of penicillin. British Medical Journal 289:1721–1723

Macfarlane G 1984 Alexander Fleming: the man and the myth. Chatto and Windus, London

National Patient Safety Agency (http://www.npsa.nhs.uk)

Saferhealthcare (http://www.saferhealthcare.org.uk) (Knowledge and innovation for safer health care.)

Shorter E 1997 A history of psychiatry. Wiley, Chichester

Waksman SA 1940 The soil as a source of microorganisms antagonistic to disease-producing bacteria. Journal of Bacteriology 40:581–600

Waksman SA 1958 My life with microbes. Robert Hale, London

Control of medicines in hospital and community

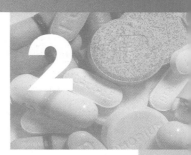

2

CHAPTER CONTENTS

KEY OBJECTIVES

After reading this chapter, you should be able to:

- name the key legislation that underpins the control of medicines
- identify the particulars that are considered standard requirements on all medicine labels
- describe the storage requirements for *all* medicinal products in hospital and list the additional storage requirements for controlled drugs (CDs) in hospital
- describe the procedure for selecting, checking, administering and recording a CD.

INTRODUCTION

On the establishment of the NHS in 1948, the range of safe and effective medicines available to the prescriber was very limited indeed. Most of the drugs that are now taken for granted were not even a gleam in the eye of the molecular chemist in 1948. Safe and effective cardiovascular drugs, anticancer agents, oral diuretics and psychoactive drugs did not exist. In the 1940s and early 1950s, simple, although not always harmless, inorganic and organic chemicals and products of very dubious composition, derived from naturally occurring products, were still widely prescribed. Natural products remain a very important source of valuable medicines, but today we have sophisticated methods of extraction, purification and standardisation that, in the case of licensed medicines, guarantee consistency of quality. Methods of drug delivery were also very basic indeed, with oral solid dosage forms adequate but crude by today's standards. Simple oral liquid preparations were often poorly formulated, foul-tasting and inconvenient to use. Although some quality assurance procedures were in

Table 2.1   Development of medicines over 80 years

Decade	Drug(s) developed
1920s	Insulin
1940s	Penicillin and streptomycin
1950s	Chlorpromazine, corticosteroids and thiazide diuretics
1960s	Benzodiazepines, ampicillin, vinblastine, melphalan, propranolol and cytarabine
1970s	Cefalexin, enflurane, doxorubicin, clotrimazole, naproxen, streptokinase and cimetidine
1980s	Clozapine, salmeterol, lisinopril, goserelin, erythropoietin and ranitidine
1990s	Monoclonal antibodies, colfosceril and lamotrigine, third-generation cephalosporins, anticancer agents, and products such as insulin lispro produced by recombinant techniques using sophisticated biological methods
2000s	Gene therapy, more drugs from natural sources, more emphasis on chemoprevention, cell/organ transplantation; safer drugs

place, these were aimed at testing the final product rather than controlling the whole manufacturing process.

The Medicines Act of 1968 marked a new beginning in the control of all aspects of the production, testing and marketing of medicines. Some idea of the progress made in the development of medicines over the past 80 years can be gained from the summary shown in Table 2.1. The need for effective control systems has developed accordingly. In 2005, the Commission on Human Medicines (CHM) replaced the Committee on Safety of Medicines and the Medicines Commission. The duties of the CHM are based on the need of ministers for advice on major policy matters relating to medicines.

Standards of pharmaceutical production and quality assurance are very high indeed. Before a product can be given a product licence and marketed, safety and efficacy must be established, although neither proof of a therapeutic advance over existing products in the UK nor evidence of cost-effectiveness is required.

Medicines are subject to a range of control in terms of legislation as well as local policies. This is necessary to ensure that:

- medicines are manufactured to the highest standards
- medicines are tested and evaluated before being licensed

- the potential for abuse is minimised
- medicines are stored securely under appropriate conditions
- medicines are used in such a way as to minimise risk to both patient and donor
- medicines are administered appropriately to enable the best possible therapeutic outcome to be achieved
- the safety of patients is always the prime consideration.

The manufacture, packaging and distribution of medicines depend on the expertise of the pharmaceutical industry. At local level, the pharmaceutical service provides a comprehensive service designed to meet the needs of patients and those providing nursing care. The objectives of achieving successful patient care depend on the integrity and security of all stages of the supply chain from manufacturer to patient. All those involved in using medicines for diagnosis, treatment or palliation must be aware of the need to ensure compliance with their legal, ethical and professional responsibilities.

LEGAL CLASSIFICATION OF MEDICINAL PRODUCTS

The supply, storage and use of all medicinal products are controlled by the Medicines Act 1968. Three classes of products are defined in the Act; these are shown in Box 2.1. Legislation for controlled drugs (CDs) is provided by the Misuse of Drugs Act 1971. The Medicines Act is concerned primarily with regulating the legitimate use of medicines; the Misuse of Drugs Act is mainly concerned with the prevention of the abuse of CDs.

Certain legal requirements apply to the sale, supply, dispensing and labelling of each class of medicinal product. These requirements are applicable mainly in the community, for example sale/supply of medicines by community pharmacists and others. In hospital practice, all medicines are treated in the same way, no distinction being made between the different classes listed in Box 2.1. However, CDs are subject to additional security and recording requirements. The key elements of the legislation that affect practice directly or indirectly are described below.

PRESCRIPTION-ONLY MEDICINES

There are three classes of prescription-only medicines (PoM):

- medicinal products containing listed substances
- medicinal products containing a drug controlled under the Misuse of Drugs Act 1971
- medicinal products for parenteral use (there are some specific exemptions).

The Medicines Act provides that no one may administer a PoM otherwise than to him- or herself, unless they are a practitioner (registered doctor, dentist or supplementary prescriber) or acting in accordance with the directions of a practitioner. Certain exemptions to this rule are made in the case of life-saving drugs, for example adrenaline (epinephrine),

certain antihistamines and antidotes; normally, this exemption would not apply in hospitals.

The administration of medicines in hospitals is normally covered by a health authority policy statement that permits administration of medicines only in accordance with the written prescription of a medical, dental or nurse practitioner. The only exception to this rule is when a patient group direction has been set up (see p. 87).

PRESCRIBING OF POMS

In hospital practice, the in-patient prescription includes directions to the nurse for administration of the medicine. If a prescription is written for an outpatient, more details of the patient are required than would be the case for an in-patient, for example address of patient, quantity of medicine to be supplied and directions for use. In the community, a prescription from the patient's GP is required.

EMERGENCY SUPPLY OF POMS

In hospital practice, situations under which medicines can be supplied without a prescription will be defined in the local code of practice for medicine management. A community pharmacist can, under specified conditions, supply PoMs in an emergency without a prescription on the request of a doctor, a supplementary prescriber, a nurse prescriber or an individual patient.

EXEMPTIONS FROM CONTROLS

Special arrangements apply to particular classes of persons, for example midwives, chiropodists (podiatrists), optometrists, ambulance paramedics and masters of ships, and other named organisations (consult specialist literature for details).

LABELLING OF MEDICINAL PRODUCTS

Standard labelling requirements are described in the Act. This is a matter for the pharmacist or manufacturer to comply with (Figs 2.1 and 2.2). The main particulars included on a label of a medicinal product are listed below; it is important to note that the information on the label must be clear, legible, comprehensible and in English.

- The name of the product (this may be an approved name and/or a proprietary name).
- The pharmaceutical form (e.g. tablets, capsules).
- The strength of the product, distinguishing between active and non-active ingredients (excipients). All excipients must be given in the case of injectable, topical and eye preparations.

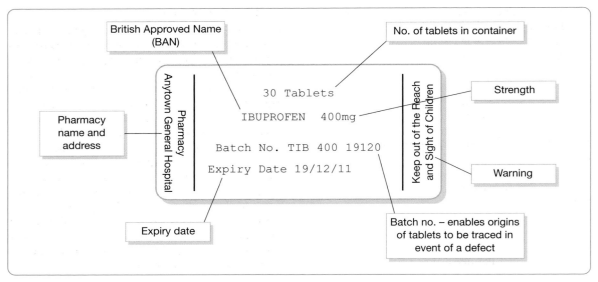

Fig. 2.1 Example of a pharmacy-generated label.

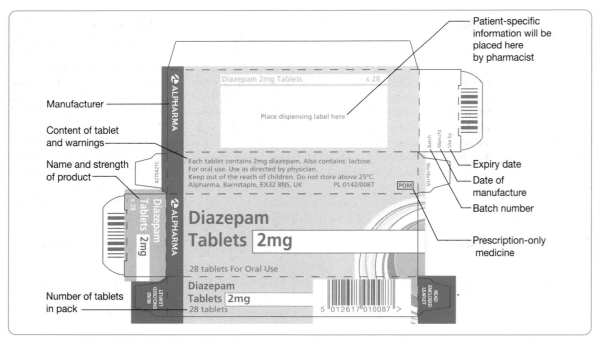

Fig. 2.2 Example of information on a manufacturer's original pack.

- The quantity in the container, expressed in appropriate terms; for example, in the case of tablets the number of dosage units, in the case of an ointment the weight contained in the pack.
- List of excipients known to have a recognisable action.

- Any special storage instructions, including a warning to keep out of the reach and sight of children.
- Method/route of administration.
- A date after which the product should not be used (expiry date).

- Any special warnings required by the marketing authorisation for the product.
- Name and address of the holder of the marketing authorisation and number of this authorisation.
- Batch reference number.
- Instructions for use if for self-medication.
- Special precautions for disposal.

Additional labelling requirements apply to dispensed medicines. It is common practice for the pharmacist to add further information to labels, such as presentational changes to the product (e.g. colour change of tablet).

Nurses should expect to be supplied with pharmaceutical products that are labelled in accordance with their needs. Pharmacists will always be willing to discuss any particular needs or concerns.

STORAGE OF MEDICINAL PRODUCTS IN HOSPITAL

Although different classes of drugs are defined under the Medicines Act, in hospital and community practice all medicinal products are treated in the same way, i.e. secure storage in locked cupboards. In many instances, the controls applied to the different types of medicine in hospitals exceed legal requirements. This is necessary to ensure the protection and safety of both patients and staff. Health authorities have a duty to ensure that regulations are drawn up and applied to all aspects of the use of medicines.

Separate locked cupboards are required for the following:

- internal medicines
- external medicines
- disinfectants/antiseptics
- clinical reagents.

A lockable drug refrigerator is also required. Separate sections will be required within a cupboard or refrigerator, for example to segregate oral preparations from injections. Other storage facilities are provided for larger volume products.

SELF-ADMINISTRATION SYSTEMS (IN HOSPITALS)

When it is considered appropriate for a patient to self-administer her or his medicines, an individual locked patient medication cabinet will be required (see p. 116).

PATIENTS' OWN DRUGS

On admission to hospital, patients are encouraged to bring with them their current medicines. This enables current therapy to be validated, and, if appropriate, the medicines can be used. There appear to be a number of advantages in using patients' own drugs in hospital, although there may be risks involved (Fradgley and Pryce 2002). To avoid these risks, a quality checklist for assessment of patients' own drugs should be used (Fradgley and Pryce 2002). If it is decided to use patients' own drugs, suitable arrangements must be made for safe storage of the drugs. Separate storage in a locked individual patient medication cabinet may be appropriate, especially if the patient is to self-administer medicines. It should be remembered that the medicines brought in by patients are the patients' property, and permission should be sought either to use them or to dispose of them.

CONTROLLED DRUGS

Drugs of addiction that produce dependence (see Ch. 14), such as diamorphine and pethidine, require special controls. The Misuse of Drugs Act 1971 and the Misuse of Drugs Regulations 2001 regulate the importation, export, supply and use of such drugs. Offences involving CDs are dealt with taking into account all circumstances, including the harmful nature of the drug that is misused and the quantities involved. The debate on how such offences should be dealt with in the community continues. In general, a more relaxed attitude to 'minor' offences appears to prevail. In the realm of clinical practice, however, offences involving CDs are always treated as major incidents.

Controlled drugs are classified according to their potential to cause harm if abused. Drugs in class A are the most harmful.

- Class A examples: cocaine, diamorphine, methadone and morphine.
- Class B examples: oral amphetamines, barbiturates and codeine.
- Class C examples: buprenorphine, most benzodiazepines, cannabis and clenbuterol.

Within the regulations, five schedules are defined. The details in the schedules are not of great practical interest to nurses, but aspects of supply, possession, prescribing and record keeping are important. Most drugs used in clinical practice are subject to schedule 2 requirements. Schedule 3 includes barbiturates and temazepam. Strictly according to the law, records are not required to be kept of temazepam, but in view of the great potential for abuse CD records are made.

The use of CDs in medicine is permitted by the Misuse of Drugs Regulations 2001 (as amended). Different levels of control are applied within the regulations. The main controls are as follows.

- A licence is needed to import or export.
- Compounding/manufacturing is permitted by a practitioner or pharmacist.
- A pharmacist may supply to a patient on the prescription of an appropriate practitioner.
- These drugs may be administered to a patient by a person acting in accordance with the instructions of a doctor or dentist.
- Safe custody and record keeping are required.
- The following persons are also authorised to be in possession of and to supply CDs:
  — medical or dental practitioner
  — matron or acting matron of a hospital or nursing home
  — the sister or acting sister for the time being in charge of a ward, theatre or other department.
- Certain CDs may be administered or supplied under a patient group direction (see p. 87).

The authority is limited to obtaining ward stocks from no other source than the pharmacist responsible for the dispensing of medicines in the particular hospital. In some situations, when there is no on-site pharmacy, the hospital pharmacy normally providing the pharmaceutical service is regarded as being within this provision. Limitations are applied to the authorisations, in that they apply only so far as is necessary for the practice or exercise of their profession. A sister or acting sister in charge of a ward, theatre or department may not supply any CD other than for administration to a patient in accordance with the prescription of a doctor (or dentist). It should be noted that, apart from healthcare personnel, other groups of workers are permitted to possess/supply CDs, for example the master of a ship, person in charge of a recognised laboratory and manager of an offshore installation.

Certain barbiturates and appetite suppressants (e.g. diethylpropion) are also classed as CDs. Most of the requirements for prescription writing, ordering, recording and storing CDs apply to the following drugs:

- amobarbital
- butobarbital
- phenobarbital
- secobarbital.

Because of its use in the treatment of epilepsy, the regulations covering phenobarbital are not so comprehensive, in that neither the handwriting requirements (see below) nor the storage and recording requirements for CDs apply.

PRESCRIPTION OF CDS FOR THE TREATMENT OF MISUSERS (WITHIN THE NHS)

Special regulations are applicable to the supply of CDs to persons who are dependent on such drugs. For example, only a doctor who holds a licence issued by the Secretary of State may prescribe certain CDs (e.g. diamorphine, dipipanone) for a dependent person. (Any doctor may prescribe CDs to an opioid-dependent person for the treatment of pain.) A special prescription form is used to enable people dependent on opioids to receive daily supplies of methadone for consumption under supervision. This procedure is designed to limit the diversion of methadone for illegal purposes. Prescribers in drug treatment centres may be given exemption to 'own handwriting' requirements. This allows the use of rubber stamps for prescribing.

CONTROLLED DRUGS IN HOSPITAL

Certain of the legal requirements concerning drug control do not strictly apply in hospitals. However, health authorities are required to institute safe procedures in accordance with official circulars, reports and professional standards. Failure to institute or comply with these procedures would leave the health authorities or individuals liable to legal action. In practice, a positive attitude to all aspects of safe use of medicines will benefit patients and safeguard healthcare workers.

LEGISLATION AND RESPONSIBILITY OF STAFF

Procedures involved in the handling of CDs are drawn up by health authorities against the background of the legal and professional responsibilities defined in the documents listed below, and may be supplemented when necessary in accordance with local requirements.

- The Misuse of Drugs Act 1971.
- Misuse of Drugs Regulations 2001 and amendments.
- The Aitken Report: Control of Dangerous Drugs and Poisons in Hospitals 1958.
- The Roxburgh Report: Control of Medicines in Hospital Wards and Departments 1972.

- The Duthie Report: Guidelines for the Safe and Secure Handling of Medicines (Department of Health 1988).
- Safer management of CDs.
- Private CD prescriptions and changes to NHS prescriptions.

PRESCRIBING WITHIN THE NHS

Preparations that are subject to the prescription requirements of the Misuse of Drugs Regulations 2001 are distinguished throughout the British National Formulary (BNF) by the symbol CD. A CD may be prescribed only by a doctor or dentist who is registered or provisionally registered. CDs in schedules 2 and 3 must never be prescribed by telephone or by fax.

In-patient prescriptions are normally written on a standard prescription sheet. For outpatients (or patients on discharge from hospital), detailed information is required. It is not lawful for a practitioner to issue a prescription for a CD (included in schedule 2 or 3), or for a pharmacist to dispense it, unless it complies with the following requirements. The prescription must:

- be in writing in ink or otherwise so as to be indelible, and signed by the person issuing it with her or his usual signature and be dated by her or him (computer-generated prescriptions are acceptable, apart from the signature, which must be handwritten)
- specify the address of the person issuing it
- have written on it, if issued by a dentist, the words 'for dental treatment only'
- specify (in the handwriting of the person issuing the prescription) the name and address of the person for whose treatment it is issued
- specify (again in the prescriber's own handwriting or in computer-generated form) the dose to be taken, the form of the medicine and, where appropriate, the strength of the preparation, and either the total quantity (in both words and figures) of the preparation or the number (in both words and figures) of dosage units to be supplied.

The following regulations also apply in the community.

- Prescriptions for CDs are valid for 28 days from the date signed by the practitioner (or from a specified start date).
- The quantity prescribed should be restricted to meet the clinical need of patients up to a maximum of a 30-day quantity. (If the prescriber considers a 30-day quantity insufficient to meet the patient's needs, this should be recorded in the patient's notes.)

- Instalment dispensing (28-day period) is permitted.
- Prescription stationery must be kept secure and never be presigned. Loss of prescription stationery must be reported to the fraud liaison officer as soon as the loss or theft is discovered.
- Prescriptions for self or close family should be dealt with in accordance with legal requirements and professional codes of practice.
- Returned dispensed medicines should not be reissued.

PRESCRIBING CDS OUTWITH THE NHS (SCHEDULE 2 AND 3 CDS)

In general, all the above provisions apply. Special prescription forms must be used, and the prescriber must be registered to prescribe privately. Information will be collected centrally by the NHS so that private prescribing of CDs can be monitored as with NHS prescriptions.

- Healthcare professionals collecting CDs on behalf of patients should provide evidence of identity.
- A signature is required (on the prescription form) of the person collecting the drug. Patient confidentiality must be safeguarded in seeking to establish the identity of the person.
- GP computer prescribing systems are being modified to aid in the identification of prescriptions for CDs.

ORDERING

Supplies of CDs for hospital wards and departments may be ordered only by a sister or an acting sister. Although the Misuse of Drugs Act/Regulations use this precise terminology, today this would be interpreted as the nurse in charge of the ward or his or her deputy. Using the order book (reference no. 90-500) provided for the purpose, the following details must be provided for each product.

- The name of the preparation (in block letters); modified-release preparations should normally be entered using the brand name, although when there is no doubt regarding bioequivalence between brands, a generic description may be used.
- The formulation.
- The strength (in figures and words).
- The total quantity (in figures and words).

A separate page should be used for each product (Fig. 2.3). The nurse signs and dates the order, adding her or his designation. Unless the order has all the necessary detail written in the correct manner, the pharmacist cannot supply the drug.

Name of preparation	Strength	Quantity
MORPHINE SULPHATE SLOW-RELEASE TABLETS	10mg (TEN)	30 TAB. (THIRTY)

(Each preparation to be ordered on a separate page)

Ordered by   *G. Clark*   Date 9/9/08
(Signature of Sister or Acting Sister)

Supplied by   *Rachel Sangster*   Date 9/9/08
(Pharmacist's Signature)

Accepted for delivery   Date 09/09/08
(Signature of messenger)

TO BE RETAINED IN THE PHARMACEUTICAL DEPARTMENT

Fig. 2.3 Order form for controlled drugs.

The whole order book is sent to the pharmacy department where the pharmacist prepares the order and signs the requisition. The person acting as messenger for the return of drugs to the ward or department also signs the requisition. The original requisition is then retained in the pharmaceutical department. In situations in which supply of a CD is required outwith normal working hours and there is no pharmacy on site, the order may be faxed to the central pharmacy department, followed by confirmation by telephone. In rural hospitals, it may be necessary to have two CD order books, because one may be in transit between the hospital and the pharmacy department.

If an order that has been written is incorrect or no longer requires to be supplied to the ward or department, it must be clearly cancelled by writing cancelled diagonally across the order between two parallel lines, and the cancellation must be signed by the nurse. The cancellation must appear on both the white original and the pink copy of the order book. At no time should any entry be obliterated. Cancelled orders should not be torn out.

Order books should be stored in the CDs cupboard whenever possible. Replacement order books are obtained from pharmacy departments.

DELIVERY AND RECEIPT TO WARDS AND DEPARTMENTS

Delivery of CDs may be made in a locked box or by a designated messenger. If CDs are collected from the pharmacy, the appropriate section should be completed by the messenger. Careful consideration should be given as to persons suitable to act as messengers carrying CDs.

On receipt of supplies of a CD and the order book by a ward or department, two nurses – one of whom is a registered nurse – should check the drugs against the copy requisition. If all is found to be correct, the copy requisition is signed (Fig. 2.4) and the order book retained in the ward or department. If there is any discrepancy, the pharmacy should be notified at once.

An entry is then made in the ward CDs record book (reference no. 90-501), with details of the new supply, keeping records of the different forms and strengths of each preparation in separate sections or pages (Fig. 2.5A). The page is headed with the name of the preparation (in block letters), its form and strength. The columns are filled appropriately to include the number of tablets or vials, or the volume of liquid received, the date and the serial number of the requisition. When there is continuity of use of a page or section, the existing stock balance is added to the new supply. When it is necessary to start a new section or page, the index is amended accordingly.

STORAGE

Controlled drugs are required to be stored in a separate locked cupboard constructed and maintained to prevent unauthorised access to the drugs. It is customary for this cupboard to be within another locked cupboard. Preferably, the cupboard should be sited where it is visible to nursing staff on duty. With this recommendation, however, there is the disadvantage that 'visible' cupboards are also often in

Name of preparation	Strength	Quantity
MORPHINE SULPHATE SLOW-RELEASE TABLETS	10 mg (TEN)	30 TAB. (THIRTY)

(Each preparation to be ordered on a separate page)

Ordered by	*G. Leart* (Signature of Sister or Acting Sister)	Date 9/9/08
Supplied by	*Rachel Sangster* (Pharmacist's Signature)	Date 9/9/08
Accepted for delivery	(Signature of messenger)	Date 09/09/08
Received by	*C. Bowden* (To be signed in the ward in the presence of the Messenger)	Date 9/9/08

TO BE RETAINED BY THE SISTER

Fig. 2.4   Copy order for controlled drugs.

the busiest parts of a ward, for example at the nurses' station or within the patient area of a Nightingale-type ward. These locations are not conducive to a clear, uninterrupted environment in which to concentrate on checking drugs, and so extra care is essential. A warning light indicating when the cupboard is open is normally provided. The locked compartment in the cupboard must not be used for the storage of any other items.

The key to the CDs cupboard must be kept separate from other keys and held in the possession of the designated nurse in charge of the ward.

Spare keys for CDs cupboards may be kept in the hospital pharmacy. If there is no pharmacy on site, local arrangements are usually made for spare keys to be held in the safe keeping of the senior nurse manager concerned. In departments in which CDs are stored but which do not have 24-h supervisory cover – such as outpatient clinics – arrangements must be made for the safe keeping of the key(s) to the CDs cupboard out of working hours.

Loss or suspected loss of keys should be reported in the first instance to the senior nurse manager on duty, whose duty it is to inform a senior member of the pharmacy staff and, if necessary, the security officer for the hospital.

As with all other drugs, CDs should not be transferred to other containers but must be retained in the original container, which should not be defaced in any way.

From autumn 2006, all healthcare providers who hold stocks of CDs must have an approved standard operating procedure.

ADMINISTRATION IN HOSPITALS

The basic procedure for giving any medication applies also to the giving of a CD. Instructions relating specifically to CDs are as follows.

- Two persons must be involved in the administration of a CD, one of whom must be a registered nurse or a registered doctor.
- The keys to the CDs cupboard are obtained from the nurse in charge.
- The stock amount of the drug to be used is checked against the last entry in the CDs record book.
- After the dose is selected, the remaining stock is returned to the cupboard, which is then locked.
- The date, the name of the patient, the amount of the drug to be given and the stock balance are entered in the record book (Fig. 2.5B).
- Both persons involved take the prepared drug to the patient – one to administer the drug, the other to act as witness.
- The time of administration and the signatures of the two persons are entered in the record book.
- The keys of the CDs cupboard are returned to the nurse in charge.

In order to prevent diversion of drugs, it has been suggested that two people should always be involved

NAME, FORM OF PREPARATION AND STRENGTH ...... DIAMORPHINE INJECTION 10 mg ......

AMOUNT(S) OBTAINED			AMOUNTS ADMINISTERED						
Amount	Date received	Serial no. of requisition	Date	Time	Patient's name	Amount given	Given by (signature)	Witnessed by (signature)	STOCK BALANCE
20 AMP	7/9/07	07							20 AMP
			9/9/07	7.10am	A. PATIENT	10 mg	J. Milne	G. Bennett	19 AMP
			9/9/07	11.35am	A. PATIENT	20 mg	J. Milne	M. Edgar	17 AMP
			10/9/07	–	STOCK CHECKED AND FOUND CORRECT S.Smith SISTER				17 AMP
10 AMP	16/9/07	08							

(a)

NAME, FORM OF PREPARATION AND STRENGTH ...... MORPHINE IN CHLOROFORM WATER 20mg in 5ml

AMOUNT(S) OBTAINED			AMOUNTS ADMINISTERED						
Amount	Date received	Serial no. of requisition	Date	Time	Patient's name	Amount given	Given by (signature)	Witnessed by (signature)	STOCK BALANCE
200 ml	16/8/07	06							200 mL
			8/8/07	3.20pm	A. PATIENT	10 mL	J. Milne	M. Duncan	190 mL
			18/8/07	6.40pm	B. PATIENT	5 mL	L. Cowie	M. Stewart	185 mL
			↓	↓	↓	↓	↓	↓	✱ 60 mL
200 ml	23/8/07	11							260 mL
			25/8/07	5.30am	A. Patient	10 mL	Laura Luther	J. Riddel	250 mL

THE ABOVE PROCEDURE TO BE ADOPTED IF THERE IS CONTINUITY OF USE AND AN ACCURATE BALANCE
ALTERNATIVE PROCEDURES WHERE THEORETICAL BALANCE DOES NOT EQUAL ACTUAL BALANCE

									170 mL
			19/9/07	9am	F. BROWN	10 mL	L. Armstrong	C. Conner	160 mL
									40 mL
			23/9/07	STOCK CHECKED J. Murray SISTER LOSSES IN MEASURING					30 mL
			23/9/07	BALANCE RETURNED TO PHARMACY J. Murray					NIL
200 ml	23/9/07	14	23/9/07						200 mL

OR

IF THERE IS CONTINUITY OF USE THE CORRECTED BALANCE SHOULD BE ADDED TO NEW SUPPLY
WHERE LOSSES APPEAR EXCESSIVE PHARMACY SHOULD BE NOTIFIED

(b)

Fig. 2.5 Extract from ward controlled drugs record book.

in the administration of a CD in the community. This is clearly impracticable in many situations.

KEEPING WARD OR DEPARTMENT CDS RECORD BOOKS

The sister or acting sister is required to keep a drug register. The record book must be kept in accordance with the guidance given on page 16. At no time should any entry be obliterated. Replacement ward CDs record books are available from the pharmacy department.

When CDs are dispensed by the pharmacy for a named individual in-patient, each supply should be recorded in a separate section of the ward CDs record book.

When arriving at a stock balance of liquid oral medicines, it may not always be possible to obtain exactly the theoretical number of doses from each container. Accordingly, records may be made as illustrated in Figure 2.5B.

CHECKING STOCK AND STOCK BALANCES

By nurses. This is undertaken in accordance with locally agreed procedures. Regular checks are part of ward drug management. The intervals vary from on a shift basis, daily to weekly.

By pharmacists. These checks are made at least at 3-monthly intervals but may be required more frequently. A written record of the check is made in the ward CDs record book by the pharmacist carrying out the check.

Other agencies. The Healthcare Commission, the police and the Commission for Social Care Inspection have wide-ranging powers of entry and inspection to premises where CDs are stored.

PROCEDURE TO BE ADOPTED IF (A) THE CDS ORDER BOOK AND/OR WARD CDS RECORD BOOK AND/OR (B) CDS ARE MISSING

In the event of loss or suspected loss of these items, the nurse in charge of the ward or department should contact the senior nurse manager on duty, who will inform the senior pharmacy manager if this becomes necessary.

DISPOSAL

An individual dose or part dose of a CD that is prepared and is unsuitable for taking back into stock should be disposed of in the ward or department, and a record made in the ward CDs record book. The destruction must be witnessed by a registered nurse. The same procedure should be adopted when only part of the contents of an ampoule is required for administration. Any accidental breakage should be dealt with in the same way.

In all cases of disposal or loss of small amounts of a CD, the amount should be recorded beside the entry in the CDs record book. Similarly, if after a dose is removed from its original container the patient refuses the medicine, it should be flushed down the sink with running water. An entry recording refusal by the patient should be made and signed by two nurses, one of whom is a registered nurse. If the contents of a syringe used in a syringe driver are only partly used, a similar procedure is followed. Spills and breakages should be similarly accounted for, and the pharmacist should be contacted to correct any imbalance in stock. Used fentanyl patches may contain a small amount of fentanyl and so should be disposed of by removing the backing, folding the patch in half so that it sticks to itself and placing it in a special medicines waste collection. No record of the disposal is required.

DESTRUCTION

It is illegal to destroy CDs (and other medicinal products) by means of the public sewerage system. Although it is acceptable to dispose of part of an ampoule or unit dose vial or unused dose at ward level by flushing down a sink with running water, quantities in excess of this should be returned to the pharmacy for supervised destruction. The pharmacist will arrange for safe destruction within the professional and legal requirements. The guiding principle of destruction is that the active drug should be rendered irretrievable and should not pollute the environment. CD denaturing kits are available.

CDS BROUGHT IN BY PATIENTS ON ADMISSION

Some problems can arise at ward level with CDs brought in by patients on admission. These will have been obtained by the patient on prescription. Technically, it is illegal for the ward sister to receive these drugs from the patient. However, in such situations the pharmacist may lawfully accept such drugs for destruction. On rare occasions, a patient may be in possession of illicit CDs. This is obviously a very delicate matter and is dealt with having regard to all clinical and legal considerations. At the present time, it is illegal for the pharmacist to receive such drugs, and it may be necessary to call in the police to deal with the matter. In such situations, medical confidentiality will be observed unless there are compelling reasons to the contrary.

UNWANTED OR TIME-EXPIRED CDS HELD AT WARD/DEPARTMENTAL LEVEL

These should be returned to the pharmacy, having made suitable records in the ward CDs record book.

RETENTION OF RECORDS

All CDs order books and record books must be retained for 2 years after the date of the last entry. After this time, such documents should be destroyed by burning or shredding.

OTHER ASPECTS OF THE CONTROL OF MEDICINES

While legal aspects of the control of medicines remain central to all hospital medicine policies, it is important to recognise the changes that are occurring that make an impact on the way medicines are controlled. Computerised medicine management systems and automated dispensing systems provide the opportunity to follow the movement of medicines from the manufacturer through to the administration of a dose to the patient. Although security must be maintained throughout all transactions involving medicines, it is also vitally important to provide information to the users of medicines as to costs and compliance with formulary recommendations.

CONTROLLED STATIONERY

The term *controlled stationery* refers to any stationery that, in the wrong hands, could be used to obtain medicines fraudulently. All medicine order books and stationery of this kind must be kept in a secure place so as to reduce the likelihood of misuse.

SAMPLES AND CLINICAL TRIAL MATERIALS

It is essential to ensure that all such materials are received from the pharmaceutical department and not directly from a manufacturer.

MEDICINES LIABLE TO DIVERSION

The security of all medicines is vitally important, as is the security of medicines that may be especially attractive to the drug user (e.g. temazepam). Such drugs should be subject to checks as agreed with senior nurse and pharmacy managers.

BORROWING OF MEDICINES

Legislation to remove Crown Immunity (Medicines Control Agency 1992) means that the practice of borrowing medicines between wards is no longer acceptable.

COMMUNITY CLINICS AND FAMILY PLANNING CLINICS

Just as with wards and departments in hospitals, clear guidance is needed for all staff working in clinic settings. Responsibilities must be defined at all stages from ordering to use of the medicine.

MANAGEMENT OF MEDICINES IN DAY HOSPITALS

The day hospital aims to provide facilities for assessment, diagnosis and rehabilitation of patients who do not require hospital admission, as well as to maintain the level of rehabilitation achieved by patients discharged from in-patient care. Such departments are an accepted component of healthcare for elderly people and also for psychiatric patients. Day hospitals operate during daylight hours and cater for the needs of appropriately selected patients, allowing them to remain in the community.

The management of medicines in a day hospital is many-sided, as elderly patients present a wide range of conditions that require to be assessed and treated. On the first visit to the day hospital, patients are asked to bring all their medicines with them. The medicines are examined by the doctor, and patients asked in detail what each is being taken for, the number to be taken, the frequency and so on. At this time, patients are also asked if they are able to gain access to the medicines or if they are experiencing any other difficulties with them. If there is any doubt about a patient's ability to cope with the medicines at home, appropriate action should be taken. This may involve contacting a relative of the patient, the GP, the district nurse or the community pharmacist. The use of a suitable compliance aid should be considered. If necessary, the liaison health visitor will be asked to visit the patient at home to try to assist with the problem. Because patients attending a day hospital are outpatients under the care of their GP, the geriatrician does not normally prescribe medicines for them. The geriatrician may, however, withdraw medication immediately from a patient for a suspected adverse reaction; suggest to the GP the need for a medicine or a change in prescription; and, in response to laboratory results or the severity of symptoms, prescribe a course of antibiotics, for example when otherwise there might be an unacceptable delay in written advice reaching the patient's own doctor.

On subsequent visits, the patient is normally required to bring only those medicines that have to be taken during the period of the visit. It is tempting for the patient to transfer to smaller containers only those medicines that will be required, but this practice is to be discouraged.

Some of the patients attending the day hospital may be capable of remembering to take their medicines as well as undertaking the procedure involved. Others, who normally are supervised or assisted in taking their medicines by relatives or a neighbour, will need this support maintained by the day hospital staff. The nurse is in an ideal position to supervise patients taking their medicines. It is important to be alert to the possibility of unwanted side effects, which can have serious consequences, especially in older people.

Small amounts of medicines for the relief of unexpected discomfort in patients may be held in the day hospital; these include simple analgesics and antacids. Supplies of certain medicines that must never be omitted should also be kept. These may include antibiotics, oral antidiabetic drugs and antihypertensives.

Apart from medicines, other nursing procedures involving pharmaceutical products may have to be carried out. These may include urine testing, catheter irrigation, stoma care and surgical dressings. Resuscitative measures may have to be instigated if a patient collapses, and so the nurse must ensure that relevant and updated emergency medicines are available. The importance of keeping accurate records of medicines that patients attending the day hospital are taking, and of maintaining good lines of communication between all personnel involved, cannot be overemphasised. The principles and practice of medicine management apply to day hospitals as much as in other situations. The notable feature of the day hospital in this context, however, is that the patients form a mobile and ever-changing group – making patient identification and staff stability of the utmost importance.

DISPOSAL OF TIME-EXPIRED AND UNWANTED MEDICINES

Under the Environmental Protection Act 1990, a duty of care requirement was introduced. The effect of this legislation was to place very clear responsibilities on healthcare staff to ensure that time-expired and unwanted medicines (and in some cases containers) are safely disposed of. Both community and hospital pharmacists must provide the necessary disposal services within the legal framework, ensuring avoidance of environmental hazard. Nurses need to be aware of the provisions of the legislation so that in their own practice, and in giving advice to patients and carers, they can be confident of working within the law. The duty of care requirements also apply to the disposal of other clinical waste such as used syringes and needles.

CONTROL OF SUBSTANCES HAZARDOUS TO HEALTH

The Control of Substances Hazardous to Health (COSHH) Regulations 1988 (Health and Safety Executive 1988) are designed to provide a framework of control within which all substances hazardous to health can be used safely. Many substances used in healthcare and healthcare settings are hazardous to health. The administration of cytotoxic drugs presents particular hazards to staff. These are discussed in more detail elsewhere (see p. 381). Key elements of the COSHH Regulations are listed below.

- Responsibility for ensuring compliance with the regulations lies with the employer.
- In practice, responsibility is delegated to the manager of a department or a safety officer.
- Known health hazards must be given high priority.
- Microbiological hazards are included.
- Having determined that a substance is hazardous, the following actions must be taken:
  — assess the risk in the particular setting in which the product is used
  — control the risk
  — produce data sheets (on procedures to be followed) for guidance of staff
  — introduce and monitor compliance with data sheet requirements
  — carry out review of procedures and health surveillance of staff involved.

The assessment of risk should take the form of a written statement and should be carried out in a systematic way. All the controls introduced are designed to either avoid exposure to the hazardous substance or limit the exposure to an accepted safe level. Control methods range from the use of protective clothing to the use of mechanical ventilation systems. An outline of the contents of a COSHH data sheet is given in Box 2.2.

As with all procedures, it is essential to monitor compliance with the controls and to ensure that any equipment used to contain the risk is maintained in good order. All staff share the responsibility of achieving and maintaining safe working practices within the COSHH Regulations. In seeking to improve the health of patients, every effort must be made to avoid damaging the health of those caring for them. Risks to patients from administered medicines are outside the scope of the COSHH Regulations.

> **Box 2.2** Contents of control of substances hazardous to health data sheet
>
> - Name of substance
> - Chemical formula
> - Occupational exposure limit
> - Form of product
> - Uses of product
> - Specific health hazards
> - Sensitisation
> - Other harmful effects
> - Specific hazards
> - Dealing with spillages
> - Disposal of surplus material
> - First aid

HAZARD WARNINGS AND DRUG WITHDRAWALS

Every precaution is taken by manufacturers and distributors of medicines to ensure that all medicines comply with the relevant standards and are safe for their intended use. However, mistakes do occasionally occur in the manufacturing, packaging or labelling. In order to avoid any risk to patients or staff, it is the responsibility of the health departments to issue any hazard notification without delay. This is normally done through health service channels on a 24 h/day basis. Nurses would be provided with written information on the particular hazard by the pharmacist. It may be necessary to check ward stocks and withdraw the affected product from use. On occasion, when there is a risk to public health, warnings regarding a particular product will be communicated via the news media.

Following the receipt and evaluation of clinical data regarding hitherto unknown clinical hazards, the Medicines Control Agency may withdraw a product licence. The effect of this is to remove the product from use.

PRODUCT LICENCES

All products marketed for human use in the UK must have a product licence. Normally, licensed products are used for the indications defined in the licence. On occasion, doctors may need to prescribe a drug for a non-licensed indication or may prescribe a non-licensed drug on a named-patient basis. Pharmacists will advise their professional colleagues on the implications of prescribing outwith the product licence arrangements. Some drugs are restricted to prescribing by hospital specialists, owing to potentially dangerous side effects (e.g. with phenylbutazone).

CONTROL OF MEDICINES IN HER MAJESTY'S PRISONS

Special precautions are applicable to the control of medicines in Her Majesty's Prisons (Pike 2005).

PHARMACEUTICAL SERVICES

THE PHARMACIST'S ROLE

Safe and effective management of drug therapy depends on many factors, not least of which is the availability of a comprehensive pharmaceutical service.

The pharmacist has an important role in advising on the prescribing of medication as part of the multidisciplinary team providing patient care. Safety, efficacy and cost-effectiveness are key elements. The role includes the provision of advice on the choice of therapy to the prescriber and information to the patient. This information is provided verbally and reinforced with a patient information sheet. Technical services designed to contribute to the achievement of optimal drug therapy include dispensing, the compounding of sterile preparations for parenteral administration, and the provision of a radiopharmaceutical service. These specialist services are generally provided by highly trained technicians working under the direction of a pharmacist. The role of the pharmacist continues to expand as the focus is increasingly on issues that relate directly to patient care rather than the actual pharmaceutical product. However, suitability of the product for its intended purpose remains a key responsibility.

CLINICAL PHARMACY

The use of highly structured documentation for recording the prescribing and administration of medicines has made it possible for pharmacists to discharge their professional responsibilities at ward level. By visiting the ward and attending ward rounds, they are able to obtain detailed information on the medicines prescribed for each patient. They are able to contribute their professional skills on all facets of the use of medicines. Ideally, the pharmacist will be a member of a clinical team and advise on all aspects of the prescribing and use of medicines. Interpretation of prescriptions, checking dosage levels and monitoring prescriptions for possible drug interactions are a vital part of the pharmacist's

Box 2.3 Key elements of a clinical pharmacy service

- Review of prescriptions:
  — dosage
  — route of administration
  — adverse drug reactions
  — drug interactions.
- Rapid response to changing needs for medicines
- Advice on formulation/presentation of medicines to meet the needs of individual patients
- Formulary management systems: development and monitoring
- Advice on aids to patient compliance

role but, working at ward level, the pharmacist has access to more information on the patient's clinical condition, special problems, etc. than would be the case if working solely within the pharmaceutical department. As electronic links between clinical areas and the pharmaceutical department are developed, the pharmacist's role is being enhanced. Decentralisation of pharmaceutical services will also contribute to improved pharmaceutical care.

Clinical pharmacists with specialist skills are integral members of directorate teams. They undertake such roles as medication review, drug history taking, discharge planning, education and training, and formulary management (see Box 2.3). Pharmacist-led clinics (anticoagulant and pain control) are becoming well established. Consultant pharmacists are being appointed in NHS hospitals in such specialities as cardiovascular medicine and oncology.

PHARMACEUTICAL CARE

The concept of pharmaceutical care developed in the USA is being adapted for UK practice. It refers to the pharmaceutical contribution to direct patient care resulting from the practice of clinical pharmacy. In effect, it involves helping patients to get the most benefit from their medicines. In practical terms, the provision of pharmaceutical care follows a problem-solving approach with several key elements that are familiar to nurses:

- assessment of the patient's drug-related needs
- determination of the patient's actual or potential problems
- development with other health professionals of a pharmaceutical care plan designed to deal with problems identified
- implementation and monitoring of the plan.

The rate and extent to which pharmaceutical care will be further developed in the UK depends on many factors, in particular the availability of resources. Nevertheless, with increasing emphasis on care in the community, plans are needed for patients receiving complex therapy in their own homes. Cooperative working between pharmacists and community healthcare staff (especially nurses) is essential if effective pharmaceutical care is to be implemented successfully.

Significant benefits can be achieved for individual patients in introducing a system whereby the pharmacist prepares a pharmaceutical care plan. As with clinical pharmacy services, the overall objective is to utilise the skills of the pharmacist so that the benefits of drug treatment are fully realised for the patient. Table 2.2 outlines the process by which a pharmaceutical care plan may be established.

MEDICINES MANAGEMENT

In an attempt to prevent avoidable ill health from the use of medicines, reduce NHS waste and help patients get the most from their treatment, a government initiative known as medicines management is being implemented in both primary and secondary care organisations throughout the UK. Medicines management is a system of processes and behaviours that determines how medicines are used by patients and by the NHS. Medicines management services provide patient-focused care based on need, and include all aspects of supply and use of medicines from the level of an individual patient to that of the organisation. The services include:

- reviewing prescriptions
- monitoring medication
- managing repeat prescribing
- providing services for nursing and residential homes
- educating patients about their medicines.

Improving working relationships across the primary–secondary care interface is seen as important to the success of this initiative. A uniform approach to prescribing using an agreed formulary must be encouraged.

The greatest impact on nursing staff will be the utilisation of patients' own drugs while in hospital. Newly prescribed medicines and medicines issued on discharge will be supplied increasingly in patient packs. It is anticipated that original pack dispensing will lead to greater efficiency overall through a reduction not only in waste but also in the need for hospital dispensing and the delays associated with the discharge process. A further benefit of the system

Table 2.2 Development of a pharmaceutical care plan

Stage	Action by pharmacist	Notes
1	Establish contact with the patient	The need for a good professional working relationship cannot be overstated.
2	Collect and interpret information on patient's condition and drug history (including use of non-prescription medicines)	Aspects that will require particular attention include: • non-compliance of the patient • practical problems with medicine use • drug interactions • incidence of side effects • poor medicine hygiene/storage.
3	List patient's problems in priority order	It will be important to establish the degree of risk involved in order to prioritise the problems.
4	Establish whenever possible the desired *outcome* of each problem identified	In some situations, the outcome may be very easy to define, for example improve the storage of medicines. Thereafter, outcomes may be less easy to define, but every effort must be made to do so.
5	Examine alternatives available and choose the best in particular circumstances	As with all stages, the needs of the *individual patient* will be the paramount consideration.
6	Design and implement a monitoring plan based on patient's needs	The plan should focus on outcomes that can be measured.
7	Implement plan	Effective communication within the healthcare team is vital, especially between community nursing staff and the pharmacist.
8	Follow-up to *determine* overall success of the plan	It is emphasised that pharmaceutical care plans have an overall requirement of a long-term commitment to the patient.

includes facilitation of the self-administration of medicines (see Box 2.4).

SUPPLEMENTARY PRESCRIBING BY PHARMACISTS

Suitably trained community pharmacists may prescribe within agreed clinical management plans for individual patients. The schemes are intended to enhance patient care by providing quicker and more efficient access to healthcare through an increased and flexible use of pharmacists' skills. This form of prescribing is classed as supplementary prescribing, i.e. the responsibility for clinical management of a specified patient will be passed to the pharmacist *once a diagnosis has been established or a treatment plan has been prepared* (Department of Health 1999). The management plan will specify in detail the dose, frequency and formulation of the medicine. In hospital practice, pharmacists are often involved in managing prescribing for patients on discharge into the community.

DISTRIBUTION OF MEDICINES AND PHARMACEUTICAL PRODUCTS

DISTRIBUTION TO HOSPITAL WARDS

Several different methods are used to supply medicines to wards. Depending on circumstances, the system of medicine distribution used is a product of many factors, including availability of resources, clinical need, local geography and overall strategy of the hospital being served.

The overall aim of any medicine distribution system is to ensure that the necessary medicines of the appropriate quality are available when required in quantities that reflect both current and to some extent future usage. Increasingly automated/computer-

Box 2.4 Advantages of original pack dispensing

Patient aspects
- Greater acceptability
- Improved convenience
- More focused on patient's need
- Improved information about the medicine
- Fewer changes to the medication
- Increased opportunity to take responsibility for own medicines and their administration
- Reduction in delays at time of discharge from hospital
- Improved compliance

Safety
- Increased security
- Child resistance
- More hygienic
- Better labelling
- Reduction in medication and dispensing errors
- Reduction in prescription fraud

Economic aspects
- Reduction in wastage of medicines
- Stock control
- Reduction in dispensing time

controlled systems of medicine distribution are being developed, with the joint aims of reducing labour costs and increasing patient safety.

Significant quantities of medicines and related products that are not routinely prescribed are supplied for use in wards. These can be considered broadly as described below.

Resuscitation packs. These are supplied by the pharmacy in accordance with local policy. The packaging and presentation of drugs will be a matter for the pharmaceutical service. It is vital to ensure that the contents are presented for quick access and replenished immediately following an emergency, and that regular checks are made to ensure the products are not allowed to pass their expiry date.

Nursing care products. In order to avoid multiplicity of products in use for nursing care procedures such as catheter care, skin care and eye bathing, a formulary of nursing care products is a possible approach. Such a formulary contains monographs on the products that are available for use by nurses without medical prescription.

Diagnostic agents. Clinical reagents are normally supplied on a routine stock basis. Other more specialised agents are supplied on request.

Disinfectants, antiseptics, skin cleansers, etc. It is now standard practice for wards (and departments) to use a range of products as agreed by the control of infection committee. The disinfection policy will contain information on the use of products, together with supporting technical information. The products are supplied on a routine indenting or topping-up basis. A brief discussion of the properties and uses of disinfectants appears in Chapter 25. In view of the limitations of chemical agents, physical means of disinfection are preferred, but in view of concerns regarding the great risks of cross-infection the use of alcohol-based hand rubs is vitally important.

DISTRIBUTION TO HOSPITAL DEPARTMENTS

The distribution of medicines and related products to departments (e.g. to operating theatres) often involves considerable bulk, but the product range is less extensive than is supplied to wards. However, it is still important to achieve standardisation, because duplication of products is costly and may cause confusion. Computer generated drug orders facilitate the introduction and maintenance of a standard range of products. Specialised clinical pharmacy services are also required in hospital departments.

Special arrangements are often required in accident and emergency departments, such as the provision of patient-ready packs of analgesics and antibiotics, which can be issued to patients without nurses having to undertake 'dispensing'. Such packs issued to patients should be accompanied by patient information leaflets.

TECHNICAL SUPPORT SERVICES

The drug distribution arrangements previously described are supplemented by specialist technical support services. These are dispensing services that require pharmaceutical expertise and special environmental conditions such as those provided in an aseptic suite. These central, pharmacy-based services have been developed in response to the growing complexity of drug therapy and the need to provide the highest possible standards of patient care.

Central intravenous additive services. The addition of drugs to intravenous fluids is best performed in an aseptic dispensing suite rather than a clinical area where full aseptic standards may be impossible to achieve. By providing these services centrally, nurses are relieved of time-consuming manipulative tasks and are able to concentrate on clinical care. On occasion, it will be necessary to make an addition to an intravenous fluid at ward or departmental level, but this should be undertaken only when there is no alternative.

Parenteral nutrition services (see also p. 423). The administration of nutrients, vitamins and minerals in combination in a single container presented ready for use represents a far safer method of administration than that provided by using a series of separate containers. Containers of suitable volume are prepared under strict aseptic conditions within the pharmacy. This reduces the risk of infection and helps to ensure accuracy of the therapy.

Cytotoxic reconstitution services (see also p. 391). The risks inherent in reconstituting cytotoxic drugs without due attention to the safety of the doctor or nurse undertaking this task are well recognised. Full protection of operator and product can be achieved only within a specialised unit having all the necessary facilities, such as vertical laminar airflow cabinets, air-conditioning and facilities for staff to change into sterile protective clothing. As with the other specialist services, the medicine is provided as an accurately compounded, fully labelled, ready to use sterile product. Although this greatly reduces hazards, care is required when administering the medicine so as to avoid aerosol formation or spillage, which may contaminate the environment and thus any persons in the immediate vicinity.

Radiopharmaceuticals. Major hospital pharmaceutical departments provide a supply service of sterile radioisotope injections for use in specialised diagnostic procedures. The injections are formulated in order to accumulate in a particular organ or part of the body, for example phosphate injection becomes concentrated in bone and thiosulphate in the liver, and albumin microspheres are temporarily trapped in the lung capillaries. These chemicals are labelled with a short-acting radionuclide such as technetium-99m (half-life 8 h), which rapidly decays. A camera that is sensitive to the radioactive particles emitted by the technetium scans the organ or part of the body. This illustrates different concentrations within a particular organ, and in this way abnormalities can be located.

MEDICINE INFORMATION SERVICES

The provision of information on many aspects of the use of medicines and properties of drugs is an integral part of pharmaceutical services. The organisation of this service and method of provision will vary considerably, depending on circumstances. In larger acute hospitals, a department under the control of a full-time specialist pharmacist will provide the service on a local, regional or national basis. The clinical pharmacist will also be a source of information on drugs. Information pharmacists work closely with their clinical colleagues when the nature of the query requires highly specialised information that can be obtained only by a literature search. Pharmaceutical manufacturers are an important source of product information, and professional bodies such as the Royal Pharmaceutical Society of Great Britain provide invaluable technical information to practising pharmacists.

All specialist drug information services are available to health professionals but are not normally available directly to members of the public. With the rapid development of information technology (the Internet), drug information is widely available to health professionals and the general public. In accessing information via the Internet, it is important to validate the original sources.

An important part of the practising pharmacist's work is also to provide patients with the necessary information to enable them to use their medicines in the most effective way (see Ch. 7).

COMMUNITY PHARMACY SERVICES

Community pharmacists are responsible for the supply of medicines and provision of pharmaceutical care to patients in the community (Bryce et al. 2004). In addition, they are responsible for the provision of a wide range of healthcare products, surgical appliances, dressings, etc.

Medicines are supplied on prescription and, where legislation permits, are also sold over the counter. In many instances, an individual will seek the pharmacist's advice and guidance on a particular health problem. This may result in a medicine being recommended and sold to the client, or the pharmacist may suggest self-referral to the GP. In July 2006, community pharmacists in Scotland can offer, as part of the NHS, advice on minor ailments that may lead to the supply of a medicine. There is considerable and increasing use of proprietary medicines by the public, and this should always be borne in mind by healthcare staff in both community and hospital practice. Members of the public often regard purchased medicines as being little more than ordinary household commodities. As a result, important information on the patient's full current medications may not be readily ascertained. Community pharmacists will provide information on the use of medicines to community healthcare staff and give invaluable support and guidance to their clients.

For many years, community pharmacists have played a vital part in healthcare provision. There is great potential to extend further the contribution that they can make, not only in the treatment of illness but also in aspects of public health such as dental health, skin care, safer sex and smoking cessation. With the growing emphasis on self-care for the treatment of self-limiting conditions, more people are seeking the professional advice of the pharmacist for the treatment of minor ailments. Such advice is provided within the context of locally agreed protocols.

The use of computer technology enables the pharmacist to exercise a monitoring role (e.g. on repeat prescriptions) by maintaining patient medication records, including information on allergies to specific drugs. The development of an electronic prescription service will link the GP directly with the community pharmacist.

The provision of information on the use of medicines is of growing importance. The pharmacist is well placed to provide the necessary information in the most suitable form for patients and their carers.

As more patients are cared for in their own homes and in the community, the community pharmacist's services are becoming ever more important. In addition to providing services to patients in care homes, the community pharmacist provides a range of services to patients with special needs, such as people who misuse drugs.

DEVELOPMENT OF FORMULARIES

It is widely accepted that a drug formulary is an essential element in the drive to achieve safe and rational prescribing while at the same time controlling costs. Table 2.3 outlines the stages in formulary development that would be followed by a drug and therapeutics committee in hospital with a multidisciplinary membership of doctors, pharmacists, nurses and other specialists.

The method of presentation of the formulary varies from a simple listing of products to a compendium giving full details of the formulations, actions and uses of each drug, side-effects, dosage levels and costs. Presentation of the information is increasingly by means of computerised systems that also facilitate monitoring of formulary compliance. The choice of drug for inclusion in the formulary is based on safety, efficacy, cost and advice provided centrally. The classification system used by the BNF is generally adopted in local formularies.

Government policy has strongly encouraged the development of drug formularies throughout the NHS. Drug formularies have significant advantages for patient care, especially when linked electronically

Table 2.3 Stages in formulary development in the hospital setting

Stage	Definition
1	Request for inclusion of product by consultant(s)
2	Consideration by drug and therapeutics committee
3	Inclusion in formulary (or rejection or suggestion of alternative)
4	Publication of information on product to prescribers
5	Monitoring of impact, cost and benefits
6	Depending on outcome, use of drug extended, curtailed or discontinued

Box 2.5 Advantages and disadvantages of drug formularies

Advantages
- Lower prescribing costs
- Encourage generic prescribing
- Improve drug safety
- Improve patient care (by linking with prescribing systems)
- Reduce range of products to be stored
- Facilitate drug purchasing in hospitals
- Educational value
- Provide opportunity for multidisciplinary working
- Improve continuity of care, especially when a joint hospital–community formulary is in place

Disadvantages
- Restrict clinical freedom
- Inhibit introduction of new products:
  — reduce research efforts
  — stifle innovation by pharmaceutical industry.
- Restrict the patient's choice
- Reduce treatment options

with prescribing systems. Some of the advantages and disadvantages are summarised in Box 2.5.

Although opponents of drug formularies may still be heard, there can be little doubt that, as the range of drugs available to the prescriber continues to expand and costs continue to escalate, formularies will become even more important.

Effective multidisciplinary working methods and consultation can do much to reduce the difficulties outlined above. Collaborative effort leading to ownership is a key element of formulary development. On the advice of government departments, health authorities have been given the responsibility to develop joint formularies in which agreement is reached between primary and secondary care regarding which drugs should be prescribed.

The nurse plays an increasingly important role in both formulary development (as a member of the drug and therapeutics committee) and formulary management. Devolved drug budgets are an incentive to nurses in achieving and monitoring formulary compliance. To carry out this important task, the need for accurate, up to date information on the usage of medicines is vital. Pharmaceutical services are provided in such a way that staff who are responsible for the use of medicines receive regular feedback on levels of use of both formulary and non-formulary drugs. The introduction of a formulary system may create problems for nurses when patients receiving a non-formulary medicine are admitted for in-patient care. The approach to this problem will vary depending on local arrangements. For example, patients may continue to be given the medicine(s) using supplies they have brought in on admission. This approach needs the support and advice of the clinical pharmacist (and/or prescriber) to ensure that the medicine(s) are suitable for use. When the prescriber considers it to be appropriate, another medicine may be substituted. In such situations, nurses can help to explain to patients the reasons for any change in therapy. On the other hand, the nurse may become the patient's advocate and ask that the patient be maintained on the original therapy when, in the nurse's professional view, it would be disadvantageous to change the patient's therapy.

Nurse prescribing is now well established and is supported by a Nurse Prescribers' Formulary that is included in the BNF.

PATIENT PROTOCOLS

SHARED-CARE PROTOCOLS

Doctors in general practice and hospitals are developing shared-care protocols for the care of patients suffering from chronic illnesses such as asthma, diabetes and hypertension. Patient protocols have strong links with drug formularies, because protocols contain details of drug treatment regimens. Shared-care protocols represent an agreement between consultant, GP and patient on the approach to diagnosis and treatment of

---

Box 2.6 Outline of a shared-care protocol

- Brief introduction to condition dealt with in protocol
- Objectives of protocol
- Responsibilities of consultant, for example:
  - communication between consultant, patient and GP
  - source of supply of medicines
  - treatment regimen (drug, dose, route, etc.).
- Responsibilities of GP, for example prescribing (and administration) of the drug(s)
- Responsibilities of patient, for example attendance at clinic(s)
- Contact telephone numbers, etc.

---

a particular illness. The purpose of the protocol is to standardise treatment and to help ensure continuity of care and involvement of the patient. An outline of a shared-care protocol is given in Box 2.6.

Computerisation of the management of patient care greatly assists in the introduction, monitoring and audit of the benefits (or otherwise) achieved by use of the protocol. Shared-care protocols also provide a framework within which the patient can become fully involved in the treatment plan.

Nurses will normally be involved in drawing up shared-care protocols, especially those nurses working in close liaison with their colleagues in the community.

In addition to shared-care protocols, GPs are adopting protocols for use within their own practices on the treatment of such conditions as urinary tract infection, intractable pain and chronic bronchitis.

Protocols may be seen by some doctors as limiting clinical freedom and as a potential threat to innovation. There are also legal implications and concerns that patient protocols may be unduly influenced by cost factors. Advantages claimed for patient protocols include improved patient care, elimination of the wide variation in diagnosis and treatment, and opportunities for the introduction of clinical audit. A protocol for the treatment of urinary tract infection in general practice contained the following elements:

- Organisation of care, for example:
  - assessment and treatment of the patient
  - problem solving and follow-up.
- Patient checklist.
- Practice audit.

As protocols are developed, there will be many opportunities for nurses to contribute to their development.

LOCAL POLICIES

In small hospitals with no resident doctor, in specialist units and in some community settings, the strict criteria laid down by the Nursing and Midwifery Council (2004) with respect to the administration of medicines either cannot be applied or, if applied, could introduce dangerous delay with consequent risks to patients. In these situations, an agreed local policy may be drawn up for use by nurses. When a policy of this kind applies, it must clearly state:

- the circumstances in which particular PoMs may be administered in advance of examination by a doctor
- the form, route and dosage range of the medicines so authorised
- which nurse(s) are allowed to be involved in the administration of these medicines.

THE FUTURE OF FORMULARIES

There can be no doubt that the financial pressures arising from the introduction of new drugs will continue to mount. Nurses and their colleagues have great opportunities to contribute to the achievement of safe and cost-effective drug treatment through the development of formularies.

One approach that may provide a framework for future development is the management of medicines in patient-focused care. This concept, developed in the USA, seeks to address the fragmentation that so often is seen in the provision of patient care. Key aspects of patient-focused care are:

- improving continuity of care
- decentralisation of services within the hospital
- introduction of total quality management
- establishing critical care pathways/protocols.

The excellent cooperative working between nurses and clinical pharmacists augurs well for the future.

SELF-ASSESSMENT QUESTIONS

SECTION A

All nurses and midwives, both pre- and postregistration, should be able to complete the following statements (only one response is correct).

1. The policy and procedures for the control of medicines in hospital are set by:
   a. the ward consultant
   b. the health authority
   c. the ward pharmacist
   d. the hospital
   e. the ward sister or charge nurse.

2. The secure, safe and proper storage of medicines in a hospital ward is the ultimate responsibility of:
   a. the ward pharmacist
   b. the ward sister or charge nurse
   c. all staff on the ward
   d. the ward consultant.

3. In a ward, you would expect to find inhalers stored in:
   a. the drug refrigerator
   b. the controlled drugs cupboard
   c. the internal medicines cupboard
   d. the external medicines cupboard.

4. Controlled drugs are so called because they are:
   a. palliative
   b. dangerous
   c. a cause of dependence
   d. expensive.

SECTION B

Any registered nurse or midwife working in a *ward* should be able to answer the following questions.

1. You are approached by the ward consultant, who asks you for the drug cupboard keys. What should you do?

2. The nurses making a routine check of the ward's controlled drug stock report that a tablet of morphine sulphate is missing. There should be 18.
   a. What advice should you give them?
   b. What action should you take?

3. What is the local policy for transcribing prescribed medicines?

4. How long should controlled drugs order books and record books be retained after the date of the last entry?

5. How should a fentanyl patch be disposed of?

6. At what points in the handling of medicines could they be misappropriated?

7. What does the Nursing and Midwifery Council say you must do in relation to the label on a medicine?

8. Is a student nurse permitted to check the selection and administration of a controlled drug?

SECTION C

Any nurses or midwives working in the *community* should be able to answer the following questions in their area of work. These questions are for reflection – no answers are given.

1. What controls are in place for the safe storage of medicines in your sphere of practice?

2. What precautions do you take to ensure maximum security of medicines in your day-to-day work?

3. How should you advise a patient or relative to dispose of a pack of tablets, a liquid medicine and several syringes?
4. What provision is made in your area for patients who are unable to collect their prescriptions from the pharmacy?
5. Are community nurses and midwives permitted to carry controlled drugs?

REFERENCES

Bryce A, Downie G, Hind C 2004 Implementation of pharmaceutical care model schemes in Grampian. Pharmaceutical Journal 273:690–691

Department of Health 1988 Guidelines for the safe and secure handling of medicines (Duthie Report). Department of Health, London

Department of Health 1999 A review of prescribing, supply and administration of medicines (Crown Report 2). Department of Health, London

Fradgley S, Pryce A 2002 An investigation into the clinical risks in the use of patients' own drugs on surgical wards. Pharmaceutical Journal 268:63–67

Health and Safety Executive 1988 Control of Substances Hazardous to Health Regulations 1988. Statutory instrument no. 1657. HMSO, London

Medicines Control Agency 1992 Guidance to the NHS on the licensing requirements of the Medicines Act 1968. MCA, London

Nursing and Midwifery Council 2004 Guidelines on the administration of medicines. NMC, London

Pike H 2005 Helping prisons give most patients responsibility for their own medicines. Pharmaceutical Journal 275:221–223

FURTHER READING AND RESOURCES

[Anonymous] 1968 Medicines Act 1968. HMSO, London

[Anonymous] 1971 Misuse of Drugs Act 1971. HMSO, London

[Anonymous] 1985 Misuse of Drugs Regulations 1985. Statutory instrument no. 2066. HMSO, London

[Anonymous] 1990 Environmental Protection Act 1990. HMSO, London

[Anonymous] 1997 Prescription Only Medicines (Human Use) Order 1997. Statutory instrument no. 1830. HMSO, London

[Anonymous] 2001 Guide to the Misuse of Drugs Act 2001 and the Misuse of Drugs Regulations. HMSO, London

[Anonymous] 2002 Consultation starts on supplementary prescribing by pharmacists and nurses [editorial]. Pharmaceutical Journal 268:521

Audit Commission 2001 A spoonful of sugar. Medicines management in NHS hospitals. Audit Commission, London

Bellingham C 2002 Pharmacists who prescribe: the reality. Pharmaceutical Journal 268:238–239

Burton SS, Duffus PRS 1995 An exploration of the role of the clinical pharmacist in general practice medicine. Pharmaceutical Journal 254:91–93

Central Office of Information 2005 The final report of the Shipman Inquiry. Online. Available: http://www.the-shipman-inquiry.org.uk

Department of Health 2002 Proposals for supplementary prescribing by nurses and pharmacists and proposed amendments to the Prescription Only Medicines (Human Use) Order 1997. Department of Health, London

Hassell K, Whittington Z 2001 Managing demand: transfer of management of self limiting conditions from general practice to community pharmacies. British Medical Journal 323:146–147

Royal Pharmaceutical Society of Great Britain 2006 Medicines, ethics and practice: a guide for pharmacists. RPSGB, London

Scottish Executive Health Department of Primary and Community Care 2006 HDL (2006) 27 Safer management of controlled drugs (CDs); private CD prescriptions and changes to NHS prescriptions. SEHDPCC, Edinburgh

The role of the nurse in drug therapy

3

KEY OBJECTIVES

After reading this chapter, you should be able to:

- identify the key elements of the role of the nurse in drug therapy
- assess, plan, implement and evaluate prescribed drug therapy
- name appropriate reference sources to assist in the administration of medicines
- summarise the role of the nurse in primary care in relation to drug therapy.

INTRODUCTION

From the earliest days of their career, all nurses are involved to some extent in the management of medicines. Although responsibilities increase and change with time, the safe and effective management of medicines remains a high priority for all practising nurses. The importance of establishing a firm basis of learning during preregistration training is well recognised, as is the need to progress to wider aspects as part of professional development. Thus, nurses build on the knowledge and skills acquired to prepare themselves for the particular responsibilities and duties in their chosen speciality. As with all health professionals, nurses have a responsibility to keep up to date and to make their contribution to professional issues of the day.

THE ROLE OF THE NURSE IN DRUG THERAPY

REQUISITES FOR THE ROLE

PHARMACOLOGY AND PHYSIOLOGY

To be safe in the administration of medicines and to be able to advise patients appropriately, the nurse requires an understanding of basic pharmacology, which includes:

- drug absorption mechanisms (see p. 125)
- the metabolic action of the liver (see p. 128)
- the method by which substances are transported in the bloodstream (see p. 126)
- the excretory function of the kidneys (see also Ch. 18).

Without an appreciation of the relevant physiology, a nurse's understanding of how drugs act in the body is incomplete, and therefore safety and effectiveness in practice is open to question. A lack of specialist knowledge of the physiology of extremes of age may hazard the very young or very old patient, who is often more at risk from adverse drug reactions than patients in other age groups.

In a study by King (2004), one group of nurses identified the need for more pharmacology knowledge in practice. It claimed that improved pharmacology teaching might increase nurses' confidence in performing drug administration, patient education and nurse prescribing.

LEGAL AND PROFESSIONAL RESPONSIBILITIES

The standards expected of each individual registered nurse, midwife and health visitor with respect to medicines are made explicit by the Nursing and Midwifery Council (2004a). To meet such standards, the expectation is that nurses are personally accountable for their practice and, in so doing, act at all times to promote and safeguard the interests and well-being of patients and clients. This requirement applies to all persons on the Council's register, irrespective of the part on which their name appears.

Each health authority is required to establish policies and procedures that set out in detail instruction and guidance on the administration and storage of medicines. These policies are derived from statutory sources and government health circulars of guidance issued by the Department of Health. Local policies that relate to a functional unit such as a hospital or ward may also exist within this wider context. Copies of relevant policies should be readily accessible. It is incumbent on nurses to become fully conversant with them and to adhere to them at all times.

The clauses of the Code of Professional Conduct apply as much to the management of medicines as to any other aspect of nursing practice. The major tenets of the Code are:

- respect for patient/client
- consent for treatment/care
- cooperation with others in the team
- protection of patient confidentiality
- maintenance of professional knowledge and competence
- trustworthiness
- minimisation of risk (Nursing and Midwifery Council 2004a).

ETHICAL ISSUES

A range of ethical issues arise which are associated with the management of medicines and with which the nurse should be familiar. They are mentioned here for completeness but offer no right or wrong answers,

because there are none. Indeed, there are probably even more questions raised than are answered. They are also included in the relevant chapter, although a detailed discussion of each is beyond the scope of this book.

Much discussion takes place over the allocation of resources. Monies ring-fenced for active treatment, or for care for those who will not get better and are entitled to maximum quality of life, may be better spent on prevention of disease. A hot topic is 'postcode prescribing', in which treatment is available in one part of the country but not in another. Such a situation flies in the face of the ethos of the NHS, in which the intention is to provide equality of care for all at the point of delivery.

The question arises of withholding treatment from those who persist with unhealthy disease-forming habits. The human rights lobby for individual freedoms arises with such issues as the right to refuse treatment, euthanasia and the beliefs of faith groups. Consideration of the staff's rights must also be included in any discussion and include topics such as the right not to participate in termination of pregnancy (Conscience Clause, Abortion Act 1967, 1990) and also their right to withdraw from the care of someone to whom they are related or know as a neighbour or friend. Nurses' rights will be meaningful to them, although it should be remembered that those left to carry on with the duties may not approve or be sympathetic. All healthcare personnel, whatever their individual standpoint, have a duty of care.

In the event of an error, greater respect will be granted to the nurse who owns up rather than conceals it. Although every effort must be made to minimise them, errors will always occur and in their own way provide opportunities for learning (see p. 104).

There may also be the rare occasion when nurses witness an incident or practice that they believe is unprofessional and their conscience tells them that it is the time to 'whistle blow'. Full investigation by the nurse manager will be required.

THE MEDICINES

A working knowledge of medicines in common use should be developed, which includes:

- range of presentation of medicines
- ordering/requisitioning procedures
- storage of medicines and disposal of unwanted medicines
- legislation and health authority policies
- prescribing/recording procedures
- dosage levels

- routes/methods of administration
- rationale for the particular therapy
- safe handling of drugs known to be hazardous
- methods of promoting effectiveness of and/or reducing the need for drug therapy.

A bank of knowledge/understanding of the following aspects should be acquired on a continual basis:

- mode of action of drugs
- recognition of side effects and methods of minimising/dealing with unavoidable side effects
- signs and symptoms of drug toxicity
- methods of dealing with effects of drug toxicity
- drug–drug interactions
- drug–food interactions
- effects of disease states on drug therapy
- potential dangers of self-medication
- use of clinical reagents
- use of drugs in diagnostic tests
- aspects of research into drugs
- methods of achieving/improving patient concordance.

Acquiring and using knowledge contribute to safety in the administration of medicines, and by understanding the theory behind the administration of medicines nurses can act with confidence. In the exercise of professional accountability, however, nurses must be prepared to acknowledge any limitations to their knowledge or practice. It is important, too, to recognise that information about medicines and their management keeps changing, and that practising nurses have a responsibility to keep pace with new developments. Up-to-date knowledge, of course, is not in itself sufficient to guarantee safe practice.

OBSERVATION

By continual observation, a nurse assesses the patient's condition before and after drug treatment and, in so doing, helps to establish when treatment is indicated and whether it is being beneficial or otherwise. Nurses routinely measure and record indices such as blood pressure, pulse rate and weight, but it is the ability to note (and report) significant changes in these recordings that is important.

Observable changes in a patient receiving specific forms of drug therapy may include:

- allergic reaction, ranging from skin rash to anaphylaxis
- muscular weakness arising from potassium loss in diuretic therapy

- bruising or overt bleeding arising from too high a dose of an anticoagulant
- euphoria associated with corticosteroid therapy
- depression associated with antihypertensive drug therapy
- anorexia in patients receiving digoxin therapy
- breakdown of oral mucosa in patients receiving cytotoxic drugs
- signs of hypoglycaemia in a patient who has received insulin without adequate food.

COMMUNICATION

From the moment people become patients, their continued well-being (and eventual restoration to health) depends on effective communication between nurse and patient and among healthcare personnel. Nowhere is this more important than with all aspects of drug therapy.

If patients are unable to communicate, information about a medical condition and/or drug therapy may be found on a medical pendant or bracelet, or on a medication card on their person.

An equally important part of the communication process is a willingness to listen. Patients are often happy to talk about their illnesses and treatments, and by appropriate questioning and astute follow-up of cues, it is possible to assess how much patients understand their disorder and which problems are most real to them. A patient's gesture, facial expression or mood can convey, respectively, the nature or location of pain, the like or dislike of taking a medicine, and the likelihood of taking the medicines.

Particular opportunities for communication between nurse and patient arise at the time that medicines are being administered. For example, when applying a preparation to an area of broken skin, the nurse may help to ease pain by engaging the patient in some topic of conversation so as to divert attention from the procedure. It is not always appropriate, however, to deal with detailed questions at the time of administration, as this may cause too much delay or increase the risk of error in the procedure itself. Nevertheless, patients are entitled to know:

- the name of the medicine
- why it is being given
- the dose they are to have
- how often it is to be taken
- if known, the length of the course of treatment
- any likely side effects, as appropriate.

If questions cannot be dealt with fully at the time of administration, patients should be assured that a more detailed explanation will be given later. Patients may need additional explanation and reassurance when a new treatment is to be begun or when a medicine is changed or discontinued. If requested or considered desirable, a family member should be included in discussions. Wherever possible, instructions should be provided in written form.

The nurse should also be willing to learn from the patient (see Ch. 7). Many patients, especially those suffering from chronic conditions such as dermatological conditions, asthma, myasthenia gravis or Parkinson's disease, will almost certainly have far more practical experience than the nurse in managing their condition. For example, such patients are likely to know, by personal experience, the optimum time for administration of their medicine.

PRACTICAL SKILLS

Apart from the situations in which patients manage their own drug therapy, medicines are administered by nurses using skills acquired through learning and practice. Improvements in drug presentation, such as prefilled syringes and aseptic dispensing services, continue to assist the safety of drug administration. Application of modern technology in clinical areas and the development of certain procedures hitherto carried out by doctors, however, have placed additional demands on nurses' skills and technical abilities. The use of electronically controlled drug delivery systems, pumps and other devices requires quite different skills from those traditionally associated with nursing. Against this background, it is important that the traditional practical skills of the nurse are not neglected.

The degree of skill required in the administration of medicines varies considerably depending on the dosage form used, the route/method of administration, and the extent to which the patient cooperates or is able to cooperate. For example:

- the giving of a tablet to a relatively well, intelligent and cooperative adult presents few problems
- administering a small volume of a liquid medicine from a dropper to a severely disabled child presents a greater challenge
- to succeed in administering an intramuscular injection to a very agitated and uncooperative patient demands experience, skill and tenacity.

The motor skills required include manual dexterity and coordination of hand and eye, coupled with lightness and delicacy of touch. Specialised situations, such as those met with in dermatology and ophthalmology, call for skills acquired only through repeated practice.

COMMITMENT

The least tangible part of the nursing role is the nurse's overall attitude to patients and the management of their medicines. Relevant skills and knowledge are vital if nurses are to discharge their basic responsibilities. However, without an informed respect for drugs generally, the full benefits of drug therapy will not be achieved and drug therapy may fail.

On a professional level, the nurse should have an awareness of the place of all medicines in the care of the patient. It is vital to recognise the reasons for the need to be systematic in adherence to both national (legal) and local standards. This recognition should be based on a broad understanding of the principles involved and not merely the mechanical following of a set of rules. An overall sense of the need for security in its widest sense is required, coupled with an appreciation of economic factors. An enquiring attitude of mind, associated with a knowledgeable, well-informed approach, will give the nurse confidence to play a full part in ensuring safe and effective drug therapy.

It is also important to consider those attitudes that are, to a large extent, linked with personal qualities. These include powers of observation and the ability to keep calm and work under pressure. Being selective in dealing with interruptions during procedures involving medicines calls for judgement, patience and occasionally a sense of humour. The nurse must exercise judgement, because a degree of flexibility may be called for on occasion; firmness, linked with tact, is a prerequisite. The balanced assessment of one's own knowledge, or lack of it, is important, as is the willingness to ask and seek advice.

Nurses have a duty to encourage patients (without causing anxiety) to regard all medicines with respect. In exercising the necessary skills and demonstrating the correct attitude, nurses set an example for patients to follow. Special emphasis on certain aspects, such as the need for safe storage of medicines, can be reinforced by the attitude adopted by nurses and the care and concern they show. A patient may be reluctant to take the medicines and/or unable to see the need for them. This demands patience and perseverance by the nurse. Often, the problem arises with those in greatest need of the treatment. With a responsibility to act as a role model in health education, the nurse should respect medicines at all times, on both a professional and a personal level.

THE ROLE OF THE NURSE (IN SUMMARY)

Although it is recognised that the emphasis will vary depending on the speciality in which the nurse works, the role of the nurse in drug therapy can be broadly summarised under the following headings:

- to ensure that the correct dosage is given at the correct time and by the correct route, observing any special requirements
- to observe/report any side effects and consequences of drug interactions
- to take action to alleviate unavoidable side effects
- to observe and assess the patient so that medical and nursing decisions can be made
- to participate in education and guidance of patients (and in some cases their relatives) with regard to their drug therapy
- to take action to promote patient compliance and the achievement of therapeutic objectives
- to provide nursing care to help reduce, or obviate, the need for drug therapy
- to follow recognised procedures for the control of medicines and pharmaceutical products
- to contribute to the evaluation, research and development of new treatments, and/or the reassessment of existing treatments
- to contribute to the development of medicine management in a changing environment.

The discharge of every aspect of the nurse's role in drug therapy is essential for the well-being of the patient.

Many changes and developments continue to take place within healthcare and the health professions. A number of them are having, and will continue to have, an increasing impact on the practising nurse, whether in hospital or community. Some of the areas of significant development are as follows:

- provision of healthcare in the primary care sector
- complexity of drug therapy in both hospitals and the community
- specialisation in the use of drugs
- new drug delivery systems
- drug presentation, packaging and drug distribution systems
- side effects of drug treatment
- interest in alternative medicine
- the need to use resources effectively
- the need to ensure that whoever is administering the drugs is not harmed by them
- the need to ensure the safe and effective use of medicines by older people
- the use of computers in clinical practice, both in hospitals and in the community
- self-care
- access by the general public to technological information about medical conditions and their treatment

- clinical pharmacy services
- reduction in junior hospital doctors' hours and changes in GPs' contract
- professional aspirations of healthcare workers.

The practising nurse cannot fail to be aware of the great benefits as well as the potential dangers of drug therapy. As nurses are accountable for their clinical actions, it is essential that well-founded confidence is acquired in whatever is undertaken. This confidence is achieved through the acquisition of practical skills supported by the necessary theoretical knowledge. No matter how careful and expert the prescriber or dispensing pharmacist, the consequences for patients may be disastrous if nurses are ill equipped to discharge their vital role to the full.

The nurse's role is much more than a mechanical achievement of objectives. It is a professional role requiring knowledge, skills, judgement and commitment.

ASSESSING PATIENTS AND THEIR MEDICINES

Whether the patient has been newly referred to the community nurse or has been admitted to hospital, it is essential that the nurse is aware of the relevant details of the person who is to receive the medication. In hospital, the patient's name, date of birth *and* unit number are required to correctly identify the patient. Understanding patients' medical diagnoses and awareness of their physical capabilities and mental capacity are essential in achieving safe and effective drug treatment. Dietary, cultural and economic influences should also be noted, as well as availability of family support.

Patients should be asked if they are taking medicines of any kind – prescribed or non-prescribed – and whether they are experiencing any difficulty with them. The patient may reveal a belief in alternative medicine or some form of lay medicine, and this should never be discounted. The effect that individual drugs are having, or may be suspected of having, on the activities of living should be considered. For example:

- the constipating effect of some analgesics may affect elimination
- the nauseating effect of an antibiotic may interfere with eating and drinking
- a sedative drug may make communication difficult.

An examination of medicines brought into hospital by the patient may reveal patient non-compliance. Through observation and/or questioning, the nurse may be the first to discover that the patient is hyper-sensitive to a medicine.

PLANNING DRUG THERAPY

Medicines are prescribed by those qualified to do so, taking into account the patient's age and other factors including body mass, physical and mental condition, concurrent illness and, in some instances, the patient's specific requests or beliefs. The nurse can assist in suggesting times of administration that will fit in with other activities in which the patient is involved. When the presentation of the medicine (e.g. a large tablet) is likely to pose a problem, the nurse can draw the prescriber's attention to the patient's difficulty. In this situation, the clinical pharmacist can be of particular assistance. When an intravenous infusion is to be begun, it may be possible to take into account the patient's preference of arm to use. Here, the nurse can act as the patient's advocate. With the expanding role of the nurse in hospital and community, including the increasing introduction of nurse-led units, nurses are in an excellent position to represent their patients and speak up on their behalf regarding their medication requirements.

INTERPRETING THE PRESCRIPTION

Responsibility rests with the prescriber to provide the statutory components of a prescription, clearly and indelibly written or computer-generated, authorising the administration of any medicine(s) irrespective of whether the prescriber or another person is going to administer the medicine(s). Unless provided for in a specific protocol, or in very exceptional circumstances, instruction by telephone to administer a previously unprescribed substance is not acceptable (Royal Pharmaceutical Society of Great Britain 2005). On occasion, in community hospitals, there may be no alternative to a prescription being ordered by telephone. In such cases, locally agreed procedures should be followed. A registered nurse, in all situations, must take the message, repeating it to the doctor to ensure accuracy. Where possible, a second nurse should also take the message, again repeating it to the doctor to ensure accuracy. An entry should be made by the nurse(s) taking the message on the appropriate prescription sheet. The prescribing doctor should sign the entry at the earliest possible opportunity. Local policy will demand that, in any event, the prescription is signed within a set period of time, for example 24 h (Nursing and Midwifery Council 2004b). New prescriptions for controlled drugs (CDs) must never be ordered by telephone.

An alternative to telephoning prescriptions is using facsimile transmission (fax). Computerised prescribing systems are being developed for use in hospitals. In primary care, most GPs use computers for both acute and repeat prescribing. Whatever the method used, where the new prescription replaces an earlier one the latter must be clearly cancelled and the cancellation signed and dated by a registered practitioner.

Transcribing is the substitution by a registrant of the Nursing and Midwifery Council of an original order written by an independent prescriber (Nursing and Midwifery Council 2003). The Nursing and Midwifery Council states that there is no legal barrier to transcribing. Registrants, however, because there is considerable room for error and they are accountable for their actions, are strongly advised to check on local policy in such instances.

All prescriptions must bear:

- the full name of the patient
- the patient's address if at home or, in the case of an in-patient, the hospital and ward
- the patient's age/date of birth and unit number.

Six items must be present as part of the actual prescription before administration can take place.

1. The *date* (including day, month and year) of prescribing of each individual medicine, which should be coincidental with the date of commencement. As far as possible, medicines should not be prescribed prospectively, although it is recognised that, for practical purposes, preoperative medicines and diagnostic agents may have to be prescribed in this way.
2. The *name* of the medicine prescribed, written in full in block letters using the approved (generic) name for single-ingredient preparations. If the product is a compound formulation (i.e. contains more than one active component), the name of a proprietary (trade) product may be used. In some instances, the name will include the strength of the medicine to be used (e.g. glucose 5%) or, in the case of a compound, the ratio of strength of the components (e.g. co-amilofruse 2.5/20).
3. The *dosage* of the medicine to be given each time, prescribed using the metric system. Substitutes for actual dosage (e.g. one tab instead of 250 mg, one vial instead of 100 mg) must be avoided, except in the case of multi-ingredient formulations. Decimal fractions should be avoided (e.g. 250 micrograms and not 0.25 mg). When writing prescriptions, micrograms or nanograms should be written in full and not abbreviated.
4. The *route* (method) of administration, which may be abbreviated as follows:

— SL: sublingual
— PR: per rectum
— PV: per vaginam
— TOP: topical
— INHAL: inhalation
— SC: subcutaneous
— IM: intramuscular
— IV: intravenous
— ID: intradermal.

Oral and other forms of administration should be written in full using block letters. 'O' for oral is not a recognised abbreviation, as it may lead to error if linked to the dose prescribed. Further requirements for giving the medicine may have to be stated specifically. For example:

— ORAL after food
— TOP to both eyes
— INHAL via mask: 24% at 2 L/min.

A list of internationally recognised abbreviations and symbols is included inside the cover of the British National Formulary (BNF). Some of these are used in prescription writing, such as e/c (enteric-coated) and s/c (sugar-coated) (see also p. 534). Instructions of any length will require to extend to the next prescription line. When using the documents of the Aberdeen system of prescribing and recording medicines, the code letter opposite the name of the medicine is (as always) the one that is used (Crooks et al. 1965).

5. The *time(s)*, ticked or entered in writing. The prescription must specify the time of administration, with the exception of 'as required' prescriptions. In this situation, the prescribing instructions must be written in English, stating the symptom(s) to be relieved and the maximum frequency (e.g. 'As required for headache every 4 h'). For once-only prescriptions, the actual time should be indicated. A term such as *monthly* can lead to inaccuracies or omissions and is better written as 'four-weekly' or 'every 28 days'. When a specific number of doses, or number of days, a medicine is to be given, instructions to this effect must be clearly written. In an outpatient or a community setting, the duration of the course of treatment before review should also be stated on the prescription.

6. The full *signature* of a registered (or provisionally registered) practitioner for *each* individual prescription. Bracketing a number of prescriptions under one signature is not acceptable because, if one drug is discontinued, the signature for all the others is rendered invalid. Initials do not suffice, and an unsigned prescription has no validity.

Additional information may be provided in conjunction with the prescription. For example, if it has been agreed to allow the patient to keep a particular medicine within reach, the doctor should enter this on the prescription. A registered nurse may enter a specific preference of the patient in relation to the medicines, such as 'takes with a biscuit'. Some prescriptions may state that the medicine must be stored in the refrigerator.

The monitoring of prescriptions by the clinical pharmacist and/or pharmacy technician working at ward level provides additional safeguards for the patient.

Irrespective of who the prescriber is, the nurse administering the medicine is accountable for his or her actions (and inactions). *If any part of the prescription is unclear, absent or, in the nurse's view, incorrect, the nurse must seek clarification before administering the medicine.* When two nurses are involved in the administration of a medicine, each takes full responsibility for every step of the procedure, i.e. reading the prescription, selecting the medicine and witnessing its administration. Nevertheless, it is the nurse who administers the medicine who remains accountable (Department of Health 2004).

Nurses have to accept that when they move from place to place, they will be faced with styles of prescription sheet of many sorts. Certification to administer, for example, intravenous drugs in one authority does not confer permission in another. New authorisation must be obtained.

MINIMISING CROSS-INFECTION

Prior to any procedure involving medicines, the hands should be at least socially clean. If the procedure involves an aseptic technique, then an antiseptic handwash is required.

As far as possible, the hands should not come into contact with the medicine. Tablets and capsules should either be pushed through the foil side of a blister pack or tipped out into the cap of a medicine container before being placed in a medicine measure or spoon. Gloves should be used when applying creams or ointments, although the main reason for this is to protect the donor from receiving an unwanted dose of the active drug. Medicine trays should be washed after use and sticky medicine bottles wiped before being returned to the trolley or cupboard. All storage and preparation areas should be kept clean.

CHECKING THE PRODUCT

The label and/or packaging nearest to the product must be checked before administration. It is not sufficient to check the outer box or packet in which a blister pack, bottle or ampoule is contained. If there is any doubt about the legibility of the container information, the medicine must not be used and the container with its contents returned to the pharmacy.

Medicines should remain in their original container until required for use. They should not be transferred to another container.

Pharmaceutical products should be used only if they are in date and their colour, appearance/consistency and smell are unaltered. Unsuitable medicines should be returned to the pharmacy and the advice of the pharmacy technician and/or clinical pharmacist sought.

CALCULATING THE DOSE TO BE GIVEN

With the increasing potency and specificity of modern drugs, it is even more vital to ensure accuracy when administering medicines. Guidance on calculating medicine dosages is given in Chapter 4.

IDENTIFYING THE PATIENT

The patient must be identified correctly. In acute settings, all patients should wear a wristband (identity band). The checking of patients' wristbands is the only method available to correctly identify patients and match the details on the band to their care (National Patient Safety Agency 2005). Patients should still be addressed by name or possibly asked to state their name. A check may also be made of the name on the bed label or chart kept at the bedside. Factors contributing to ease of identification include knowing the patients in your care, checking medicines with a second nurse, and making proper use of wristbands and/or photographs.

Shift work, staff shortages, movement of staff from ward to ward or from team to team, and a high turnover of patients can create difficulties in knowing patients well. Not all disciplines like their patients to be 'labelled' (i.e. using identity bands) or can expect patients to state their name. Encouragement of patients to be more mobile and to socialise away from the bedside in day rooms can add to the problems, while deafness and confusion can compound them.

Not uncommonly, patients with the same name appear in a ward. It is vital that the nurse in charge draws the attention of the patients concerned and all staff to this occurrence. Checking each patient's hospital unit number *and* date of birth is the only safe means of distinguishing patients in this situation.

POSITIONING THE PATIENT

For safety and comfort, patients should be suitably positioned in advance of being given a medicine. For example:

- an upright position will assist the swallowing of a medicine (great care must be taken to avoid inhalation when administering medicines to patients who have to be nursed in the prone or recumbent position)
- when giving an injection, bladder irrigation or rectal medicine, only the area involved should be uncovered
- to facilitate the administration of an injection or a rectal medicine, the nurse should encourage the patient to relax.

SELECTING, CHECKING AND ADMINISTERING THE MEDICINE

Medicines should be administered by permanent staff on the ward who are more likely to be familiar with the patients (and the medicines most often used there), although it is recognised that this is not always possible. There are many other tasks that may be assigned to relief staff, which are potentially much less hazardous.

An essential part of the administration of medicines is the carrying out of a series of checks. Checking a medicine is an *active* process. The guiding principles of the checks involved are listed in Box 3.1.

Before any medicine is administered, it is essential to check on the recording sheet that it has not already been given and that there is no known drug or medicine sensitivity. The prescription is then carefully read and the appropriate form of the medicine identified. These two are *compared* and any calculation of dose carried out. The medicine is removed from its container and the label *rechecked* before the container is returned to trolley or cupboard. When two nurses are involved, *each* nurse must read both the prescription sheet *and* the details on the container. The medicine is finally made ready for administration and the patient identified. There is thus a series of checks to be made on every occasion. In the event of another member of staff or the patient questioning any aspect of the medication, the nurse must be willing to make further checks.

Although medicines require to be administered according to the prescription, they are often linked to other aspects of the patient's care. It falls to the nurse to integrate the administration of a patient's medicines with nursing care, investigations and other treatments without departing from the general instructions

Box 3.1 Guiding principles of checking

Work from the assumption that something may be wrong rather than presuming that most things are likely to be right. Checking involves *comparing* two things, for example product against prescription, identification bracelet against prescription.

Read on *prescription*:
- name of medicine
- strength to be used
- dose to be given
- route to be used
- additional information
- drug not already given.

Read on *product*:
- name of medicine
- strength available
- dose available
- route medicine intended for
- any specific instructions
- expiry date.

Check details on outer wrapper *and* inner container (e.g. ampoule, blister pack).

Read on *prescription*:
- patient's name
- date of birth
- hospital unit number.

Read on *identification bracelet*:
- patient's name
- date of birth
- hospital unit number.

If necessary, seek clarification from:
- nurse in charge
- medical staff
- ward pharmacist

- British National Formulary, MIMS, Data Sheet Compendium
- medicines information department.

If in doubt, STOP, CHECK, ASK and ASK AGAIN.
Stand back; ask yourself, 'Is this reasonable?'
Never be reluctant to get things checked.

Two persons, one of whom is registered, *should* be involved when administering:
- insulin
- heparin
- high doses (e.g. corticosteroids)
- cytotoxic chemotherapy (intravenous)
- any other medication locally stipulated.

Controlled drugs *must* be checked by two persons, at least one of whom is registered.

When two persons are involved:
- stand side by side
- *both* persons must be able to see both prescription *and* product
- use finger as pointer
- *read out* details one by one first on prescription, then on product, then recheck prescription
- stress each syllable (e.g. flu-o-cin-o-lone)
- make calculation of what is to be given independently, and then compare answers
- do not hesitate to use pen and paper to work out dose.

Do NOT proceed without further checking if:
- the number (e.g. of tablets, ampoules) or the volume to be given appears excessive
- the dose prescribed is outwith the normal range.

contained in the prescription. To achieve an optimal outcome, nurses must base their decisions on a sound knowledge of the purpose of the medication. Some medicines do not need to be given at a specific time of day but do need to be given in conjunction with a nursing procedure. For example, topical medicines may need to be applied in association with bathing, a surgical dressing or oral hygiene.

USING PROFESSIONAL JUDGEMENT

The nurse must be alert to those occasions when it would be unsafe to proceed in giving a medicine exactly as prescribed. For example:

- particularly in atrial fibrillation, digoxin is not administered unless the pulse rate is 60 beats/ min or above
- depending on the patient's baseline blood pressure and the severity of pain, it may be inappropriate to administer narcotic analgesics in the early postoperative period
- permission to use an alternative route of administration should be sought following an upper endoscopy when the throat has been anaesthetised or when a patient is being fasted.

When a dose has to be omitted or reduced (or the medicine is refused by the patient or not immediately obtainable), a record of the fact must be made, giving the reason, and initialled by the member(s) of staff involved.

TEACHING THE PATIENT

Through explanation and demonstration, the nurse gradually builds up patients' knowledge of, expertise in handling, and respect for their medicines. Every opportunity should be taken to teach hospital patients and/or their relatives about the medicines that will require to be continued following discharge. A period of self-administration of medicines prior to discharge has been shown to be worthwhile (see p. 116).

It may be important, for example, for patients to increase their fluid intake while taking a particular medicine. Instruction in the proper technique to use is essential for patients who have to use an inhaler. Teaching newly diagnosed diabetic patients how to self-administer insulin calls on the nurse's ability to demonstrate the procedure and to provide the necessary encouragement and supervision. Patient information leaflets, videos, etc. concerning their condition are useful adjuncts.

By alerting patients to potentially harmful situations (e.g. taking aspirin when receiving warfarin therapy), nurses can contribute significantly to patients' continued well-being. Increased understanding may also help patients in complying with the prescribed therapy.

Teaching is an essential part of the treatment of patients, and time must be found for it despite other pressures. Much of what we learn results from copying others, and so nurses must display a high level of precision and professionalism in all aspects of the management of medicines. In so doing, they teach by example. Individual factors do, however, influence learning and consequently the approach to teaching. These include the patient's:

- level of intelligence and maturity
- knowledge
- past experience
- physical ability
- motivation.

When a patient is unable to acquire the necessary skill, the nurse may have to teach a relative or friend.

PROMOTING THE EFFECTIVENESS OF MEDICINES

Knowing how medicines act (along with thoughtful prescribing) allows the nurse to play a considerable part in improving efficacy of the drugs the patient is receiving.

- The absorption of some antibiotics (e.g. flucloxacillin) taken by mouth is decreased by the presence of food in the gut, and so it is advisable to give the medicine at least half an hour before a main meal.
- By restricting salt in the diet of those patients receiving diuretic therapy, there is less sodium to be reabsorbed by the renal tubules. Less water will be absorbed and thus more urine produced.
- In the terminal stages of a painful illness, when comfort has become the prime consideration, careful attention to timing of the giving of analgesics is essential to obtain complete pain relief. If this is done, the medicine can relieve pain just as it is due to break through, the only drawback being that this may mean wakening the patient.

MONITORING THE EFFECT OF MEDICINES

Indices recorded by nurses that reflect the effect of commonly used groups of medicines are referred to in Table 3.1.

Although nurses are greatly assisted in monitoring the effect of medicines by these recordings, there is no substitute for using general powers of observation. Nurses are ideally placed to get to know their patients well and, although they may not always fully understand what process is developing, often know intuitively when even the most minor change in the patient's condition is taking place.

Laboratory tests are also used as a basis for making adjustments to doses/frequency of administration of certain medicines.

Prothrombin times. These (reported as international normalised ratio) indicate the capacity of the blood to clot and are used to monitor the effect of anticoagulant drugs. Daily dosages are calculated according to the prothrombin time. While maximum anticoagulation is the aim in the prevention of thrombus formation, extreme caution is required to prevent overanticoagulation and subsequent bleeding.

White blood cell count. This reflects the patient's resistance to infection. Frequent checks of the white blood cell count (in particular the neutrophil count) are carried out on patients receiving immunosuppressant or cytotoxic therapy, as these drugs can reduce the count to a dangerously low level and hence lower the patient's resistance to infection.

Therapeutic drug monitoring. Laboratory techniques are used to determine the level of a particular drug in the plasma. Doses are adjusted to achieve or maintain the desired therapeutic level of drug in the patient's blood. Such monitoring is commonly used

Table 3.1   The effect of medicines on the patient's vital signs and other indices

Index	Effect
Temperature	Body temperature will be *reduced* when: • an appropriate antibiotic is given for bacterial infection • an antipyretic is used to control disturbance of the heat-regulating centre • an antithyroid drug is used to treat hyperthyroidism.
Pulse	The heart rate is *slowed*, *steadied* and *strengthened* by: • cardiac glycosides. (The radial and apical rates may require to be measured by two nurses simultaneously.) The pulse is *increased* by: • antimuscarinic drugs • thyroxine.
Respiration	The rate and pattern of breathing are likely to be *improved* by: • diuretics • bronchodilators • antibiotics. (The forced expiratory volume may require to be estimated using a peak flow meter before and after inhaling bronchodilators.) Analgesics, by relieving pain, may make breathing more comfortable but in high doses may *depress* respiration to a dangerous level.
Blood pressure	The blood pressure can be *raised* by: • corticosteroids. High blood pressure is treated with: • antihypertensives. (They may cause the blood pressure to fall sharply when the patient stands up, and therefore close monitoring, including records of lying and standing blood pressure, is essential.) The blood pressure can be *lowered* when using: • strong analgesics. (Extreme caution is needed in states of shock and following anaesthetic.)
Weight	Weight loss (or lack of it) may reflect the beneficial (or otherwise) effect of a high-dose diuretic. (A careful record of the patient's weight taken at the same time each day in the same clothing should be kept when high doses of diuretic are being given.)
Urinary output	Urine formation is *increased* with diuretics. Retention of fluid in the tissues with subsequent *oliguria* occurs with corticosteroids. (A record of both intake and output of fluid helps monitor fluid balance.)
Glycosuria	The blood glucose level and consequent presence of glucose in the urine are *lowered* by: • insulin • sulphonylureas and *raised* by: • corticosteroids • thiazide diuretics. (Monitoring of diabetes is now largely done by testing a sample of capillary blood taken from the thumb or earlobe several times per day. Patients receiving high doses of corticosteroids or thiazide diuretics may have their urine tested for glucose at regular intervals.)

in the management of epilepsy and certain psychiatric conditions.

Serum concentrations. These should be monitored in all patients receiving aminoglycosides (e.g. gentamicin) to avoid toxicity and ensure efficacy. Older people, the obese, those with cystic fibrosis or those with renal impairment *must* have serum concentrations monitored.

As technology advances, analysis of, for example, blood gas determination can be carried out at ward level, obviating the need for samples to be sent to a central laboratory.

MAINTAINING THE COMFORT OF THE PATIENT

Nursing measures alone are not always sufficient to achieve maximum functioning of body systems and therefore comfort. Nevertheless, it is always better to try simple remedies in non-emergency situations before resorting to the use of medicines. Moreover, the start of a course of drug therapy does not indicate the discontinuation of these measures. In other words, medicines do not *replace* nursing care. Some examples of nursing interventions may be cited.

- Pain may be relieved with or without analgesics by:
  — maintaining good communication
  — giving the patient reassurance
  — careful positioning
  — promoting sleep
  — applying local heat or massage.
- Constipation may be relieved with or without laxatives by:
  — increasing fluid intake
  — providing high-fibre foods
  — encouraging mobility
  — maximising the gastrocolic reflex
  — providing privacy for toilet purposes.
- Insomnia may be relieved with or without hypnotics by:
  — creating peace of mind
  — avoiding caffeine-containing drinks late at night
  — making a comfortable bed
  — ensuring a quiet, undisturbed environment.

In some patients, unavoidable side effects arise as the result of taking medicines, and precautions have to be taken to minimise these effects. Certain groups of drugs are predictable in the nature of the effects they produce.

Strong analgesics. Opioids such as diamorphine make patients feel sick, and this can be especially distressing postoperatively or, for example, following myocardial infarction when stress should be kept to a minimum. It is common practice for an antiemetic to be prescribed in conjunction with an opioid.

Sedatives. Patients may become disoriented as well as drowsy. It may be necessary to erect cot sides (with permission) and advisable to position the patient's bed within view of the nursing staff, especially at night. Outpatients should be advised to avoid alcohol and not to drive or operate machinery.

Diuretics. These are given early in the morning so that urinary frequency has worn off by the middle of the day, allowing freedom of activity for the remainder of the day. Incontinence of urine can be precipitated (as can falling) in an attempt to reach the toilet in time. When applicable, patients should be told what to expect, should be shown some means of summoning assistance, and should have their bed positioned close to the toilet or have a commode placed at the bedside. Some form of padded protection may be needed.

Oral iron preparations. These colour the stools black, and the patient should be warned accordingly. This can be especially alarming to a patient who has a history of passing blood in the stools and mistakes the discoloration for a recurrence of bleeding.

Many patients, despite having serious conditions and receiving powerful medication, remain relatively well. Their appearance, however, may be deceptive, and nurses must be forever vigilant in detecting the onset of an adverse reaction.

DISPOSAL OF TIME-EXPIRED AND UNWANTED MEDICINES

In general, doses of medicines removed from their original container for administration to a patient should not be returned to that container. An unopened ampoule may be returned to the box, but great care should be taken to ensure that the ampoule is replaced in the correct box.

The disposal of unwanted medicines must comply with the duty of care legislation (see p. 19). The clinical pharmacist and community pharmacist will advise and help to ensure compliance with local policies. The disposal of cytotoxic drugs requires particular care (see p. 392), as does the disposal of CDs (see p. 17). The contents of partially used ampoules should be flushed down a sink with running water.

KEEPING RECORDS

A prescription sheet and recording sheet should be raised for all in-patients and, on discharge or transfer, filed with the patient's case records whether or not entries have been made. In hospital, all medicines must be entered on the patient's prescription sheet, including any lay medicines the doctor has authorised the patient to continue to receive. On each occasion a medicine is administered, a record to this effect is made and signed or initialled as appropriate by those involved. When a medicine that is due is not given, for whatever reason, or a medicine is given earlier than prescribed or only part of the dose is given, the appropriate recording should be made.

EVALUATING AND REPORTING BACK

Maintaining effective drug therapy cannot be ensured without some form of feedback by the nurse to the prescriber. A medicine may make the patient feel nauseated every time it is taken, or a patient may report gaining little benefit from it. It is equally important to note that a patient is, for example, sleeping better or breathing more easily as the result of medication. Observing and reporting *any* new clinical features following the start of a course of drug therapy are an essential part of the nurse's role. As the result of the evaluative process, the medicine may be discontinued, exchanged for another, continued as before, or continued with some alteration to the prescription.

THE ROLE OF THE NURSE IN PRIMARY CARE

Over and above the role in drug therapy described for all nurses, there are duties and responsibilities for nurses and midwives working in the community.

THE COMMUNITY NURSE

With the continuation of the trend towards care in the community, the role of the community nurse in relation to drug therapy continues to expand. Early discharge from hospital, an ageing population, and (as a consequence of modern medicine) the increase in the number of people surviving chronic disease and disability have all contributed to this expanded role. Whether urban or rural, community nurses throughout the UK provide a daytime nursing service and an on-call system at night that ensure there is equity of care for all. The nurse plays a key role in the community, alongside GPs and allied health professionals. Information technology is of major assistance in meeting the flow of interprofessional and intraprofessional information regarding drug therapy.

The vast majority of people taking medicines at home take complete responsibility, with no involvement of the community nurse. When the community nurse, for whatever reason, is asked to make a home visit, certain key principles with regard

> **Box 3.2** Sample of an over-75s medication review
>
> - Is the patient able to read the labels?
> - Can the patient open all the containers?
> - Are the medicines being taken as prescribed?
> - Does the patient understand the reason for taking the medication?
> - Is the patient managing the medication with regard to constipation, nausea, difficulty swallowing and drowsiness?
> - Are any over-the-counter medicines being taken on a regular basis? If so, what are they?
> - Are the medicines suitably stored?
> - Does the patient have a compliance device? If so, is it being used correctly?
> - Has the patient acceptable quantities of current medicines?
> - Have all discontinued medicines been returned to the pharmacy or GP?

to drug therapy must be adhered to. Assessment is a vitally important responsibility. When there is physical or mental impairment, the nurse's powers of observation must constantly be used to spot clues suggestive of non-compliance. Checks are made on most visits to ensure that medicines are being taken as prescribed and that there are no obvious drug interactions or side effects. Checks should be made that capsules are not being opened, and that enteric-coated or slow-release tablets are not being crushed (see p. 49). Assessment also includes observing if medicines are being managed safely and effectively in all respects. In the over-75 age group, the use of a checklist may assist this process (see Box 3.2).

Older people may be found to be having difficulty as the result of stiff, weak or shaky hands, or because their short-term memory is failing. In such cases, assessment may have to extend to establishing whether a family member, home carer or neighbour is able to assist. Home care assistants often have to help to prompt, encourage and facilitate the taking of a medicine. They may also administer the medicines from a compartmentalised dosage system if required. With the introduction of more blister packs, further assistance may be needed.

Community nurses get to know their patients especially well and, as a result, are in a good position to assist in the monitoring of all drug therapy. The nurse must have a keen awareness at all times of possible side effects or drug interactions that may arise from the prescribed drug therapy and take appropriate action. If there is any uncertainty whatsoever, reference should be made to the BNF. The occurrence of side effects should be documented and reported to the prescriber so that, if necessary, changes in therapy can be made.

Patients may receive conflicting advice about their medicines from the media and from well-meaning neighbours, relatives and friends, which may cause confusion in their minds, leading to non-compliance. Patients should be encouraged and, if need be, helped to read the manufacturer's instructions. Community nurses are often able to give the patient suitable guidance, with the help of the GP and community pharmacist when necessary. Making simple written lists of the medicines, using laypersons' terms such as 'bowel tablet' instead of laxative, often helps both the patient and carer. These terms may also be written on the container. Care must be taken when there is altered vision. One study found that 37.5% could not differentiate blue, green and lavender (Griffiths et al. 2004). 'Take the blue tablet at breakfast and the green one at lunchtime' could lead to confusion.

As part of the assessment process, the nurse should be aware also of the possibility that the patient may be taking over-the-counter medicines. Some patients may purchase proprietary medicines that conflict with prescribed medicines. For example, aspirin-containing preparations potentiate the effect of oral anticoagulants and should therefore be avoided by patients receiving this therapy. Normally, the GP and community pharmacist will give the patient guidance, but the patient may be unaware of the presence of aspirin in a proprietary product. The BNF contains lists of products (in therapeutic groups) that cannot be prescribed on the NHS. However, these products may be purchased from a pharmacy. Whenever possible, it is advisable for patients to obtain their medicines from the same outlet. Pharmacists get to know their clients well, which provides an ideal opportunity to spot discrepancies in prescribing practice. They also have a key role in offering advice, filtering out those who need to consult their GP and supporting self-care (Jones et al. 2004).

Patients may use a lay (unorthodox) remedy or some form of complementary medicine. Unless there are specific difficulties, the patient's wishes in the matter should be respected.

Increasingly, community nurses, provided that they have undertaken the relevant training, are involved in prescribing certain medicines in certain situations. This calls for in-depth understanding of pharmacology and the increased responsibilities involved (see Ch. 5).

Essentially, the community nurse has the same responsibilities with regard to the administering and recording of medicines as the hospital nurse. Naturally, there is a difference in emphasis, but the principles are the same. The patient's consent must always be obtained. The detailed guidelines given in Chapter 4 apply equally to the community nurse but, of course, a second nurse will not be present to carry out the checking procedure. Where appropriate, relatives may be asked to check drugs, helping them to feel part of the caring team instead of being simply bystanders. Full records of medicines administered by the nurse, normally only parenteral forms, are kept in the patient's home and maintained and signed by the community nurse. Listing the current drug therapy in the nursing notes assists members of the primary team visiting and facilitates continuity of care.

In an emergency, a medicine may be administered on the authority of a verbal message or facsimile but must be confirmed in writing by the medical practitioner within 24 h. CDs will be prescribed by the patient's GP and supplied by the community pharmacist. Community nurses, unlike hospital nurses, do not keep stocks of CDs. The drugs are the patient's property and are kept in the patient's home along with formal written authorisation from the GP for the nurse to administer the medicine. The nurse has a responsibility to check that medicines are prescribed in appropriate doses. In palliative care, for example, when the patient's need for pain relief may change, and although the GP has prescribed the medicine, the nurse has a responsibility to know the safe limits of dosage of the particular medicine. The community nurse keeps a record in the home of parenteral doses administered, together with the balance remaining.

Normally, community nurses do not carry any medicines other than those required for the treatment of anaphylaxis. It is their responsibility to know the current treatment and dosages of medicines used for anaphylaxis and to check that expiry dates are not exceeded.

Theft from cars is a major concern for the community nurse. Medicinal products should always be out of sight and the vehicle locked. Once the nurse gets to know clients and their families, it may at times be necessary to weigh up what is the best action – to take the bag when calling on the patient or leave it in the car.

In very exceptional cases, a nurse may collect dispensed medicines for delivery to a patient if in the nurse's professional opinion the patient's safety and/or comfort would otherwise be in jeopardy. The nurse must balance the risk of contravening the law and professional guidance with a duty of care to the patient. If the drug is a CD, proof of identity and a signature on the prescription form will be required. Security must be maintained throughout the time that the medicines are in the nurse's possession.

The safekeeping and correct storage of medicines in the home are aspects of the role in which advice may be sought from the patient or family or offered by the nurse. Prescribed medicines are the property of the patient and should always be regarded as such. If there are any concerns about leaving medicines (or equipment associated with the use of medicines) in the patient's home, the nurse manager or patient's GP should be consulted. When there is drug misuse in the home, CDs such as temazepam may need to be kept locked. Patients should be advised to store all medicines in a cool, dry and safe (although not necessarily locked) place out of the reach and sight of children. The need for special storage requirements (e.g. refrigeration for insulin and for certain eye drops) and the importance of noting and responding to expiry dates (e.g. eye drops must not be used beyond 4 weeks of opening) should also be emphasised.

Because the GP prescribes the vast majority of all medicines, it follows that the scope for improving patient compliance in the community is considerable. Many of the strategies for improving compliance by the patient, discussed in Chapter 7, can be used by the community nurse.

When a controlled dosage system ('tablet box') is to be introduced, the community pharmacist will provide this service. This includes dispensing the medicines into the compliance aid, labelling it and sealing it. Regular assessment of the patient's ability to use the aid safely and of the continued suitability of the aid in use should be made. When it is not possible to get a compliance aid filled by the pharmacist and nurses choose in the patient's interests to place the dispensed medicines into the compliance aid, they must ensure the same level of accuracy and be aware that they are accountable for their actions (Nursing and Midwifery Council 2004b). Despite strenuous and ingenious efforts by the nurse, family, neighbours and home care team, the severely confused patient may be beyond immediate help, and alternative arrangements such as admission for long-term care may be required in the patient's best interests.

The scale of unused medicines in the community is now being fully recognised. Wasteful though it may seem, it is too dangerous to recycle even completely unopened packages and containers. Many patients, when a medicine is no longer required, do nothing about disposing of it. Others hang on to medicines in the belief that they may find a use for them on some future occasion and, besides, do not want to see them wasted. While doctors are being urged to prescribe realistic quantities of medicines, nurses need to encourage patients, relatives and carers of the need for safe disposal of unwanted medicines via the community pharmacist or GP/chemist. The Environmental Protection Act 1990 demands the safe disposal of pharmaceutical products. It is not acceptable to flush away unwanted medicines. Specialist advice should be sought when necessary from the community pharmacist, especially when larger quantities are to be disposed of.

Sharps containers should be supplied when necessary and advice given regarding safe disposal of sharps, storage of such containers in the home and arrangements for their ultimate removal.

THE PRACTICE NURSE

With the number of procedures previously undertaken in hospital outpatient departments now being carried out in GP practices and health centres, the role of the practice nurse (PN) has taken on increasing importance. As well as having either a community nursing qualification or a PN qualification, PNs are trained to carry out a range of procedures that extend beyond those required of a registered nurse. The majority of PNs work in a treatment room within the practice, although some also do home visits. A variety of clinics and domiciliary services (asthma, blood pressure, cardiac, diabetes, respiratory, stoma care, well woman, wart removal, weight reduction, smoking cessation, etc.) are PN-led or led by specialist practitioners. Dressings, ear syringing and administration of injections (e.g. hydroxocobalamin for pernicious anaemia, flupentixol for mental health problems, parenteral progestogen-only contraception) are routinely performed.

An especially busy time for the PN is from October to December, when much time is taken up with the annual administration of influenza vaccine. The vaccine is recommended for everyone over the age of 65 and for those in long-stay facilities. People of any age with a chronic condition of the lungs, heart or kidneys, or who have diabetes or are immunocompromised, are also given the vaccine. Immunisation may be recommended for healthcare staff in years when the risk is considered to be higher than usual. Pneumococcal vaccine is also provided for those over 65 years and at risk patients such as those with chronic conditions, asplenia or immune deficiency.

With the increase in world travel all the year round and to far-flung regions, the PN has a wide variety of travel immunisations to attend to. The relevant vaccine(s) for the geographical region being visited, the vaccination programme, the storage instructions and any particular advice can be accessed by the PN on an Internet database.

New patient medical checks, blood pressure checks for hypertensive patients and venepunctures required by the GPs are all done by the PN. First aid, treatment of minor injuries and assisting with minor surgery add to the many skills required.

Only those PNs who have undergone the nurse prescribing course and gained authorisation to do so are permitted to prescribe. Patient group directions are drawn up by some practices.

The PN is responsible for the ordering and safe storage of medicines held in the treatment room. Of special importance is ensuring that medicines are in date, that all medicines including CDs are appropriately stored, and that vaccines are stored at the correct temperature in a locked refrigerator.

THE COMMUNITY MIDWIFE

The general principles of prescribing, administering and recording of medicines apply similarly in relation to community midwifery. All medicines being taken by the mother and any medicines administered to her during labour and to the baby must be recorded. Community midwives who also work in a hospital maternity unit may be permitted, without a medical prescription, to administer certain drugs that are listed on agreed standing orders previously signed by the doctor. The list is likely to include the following.

- For the mother:
  - a narcotic analgesic, intramuscularly (morphine, diamorphine, pentazocine)
  - a local anaesthetic (for infiltrating the perineum prior to episiotomy) (lignocaine [lidocaine])
  - an antiemetic, intramuscularly (promazine)
  - ergometrine and oxytocin (Syntometrine), intramuscularly (to prevent haemorrhage in third stage of labour)
  - a mild analgesic, oral
  - an antacid
  - a mild laxative
  - cream/suppositories (to soothe haemorrhoids).

In addition, a dose of ergometrine and a dose of naloxone may be listed for administration to the mother in the event of haemorrhage and opioid-induced respiratory depression, respectively.

- For the baby:
  - phytomenadione (vitamin K_1), intramuscularly (see BNF caution)
  - naloxone, intramuscularly (to reverse depressant effect of opioids).

For a planned home confinement, the drugs required may be either obtained (and stored) by the patient from the community pharmacy on production of a GP's prescription, or provided by the GP for use by the community midwife and stored in the community hospital until required by the patient. The drugs required will be similar to those previously mentioned in the standing orders. Requisitions for medical gases can also be made by the community midwife.

In remote areas, special arrangements for the management of medicines need to be made to cover the wide range of duties undertaken by the triple-duty nurse.

It is customary for vaccinations to be administered by health visitors in clinics. The administration of immunological agents by nurses can be facilitated by a patient group direction.

SPECIALISED DRUG THERAPY IN THE HOME

In addition to haemodialysis and peritoneal dialysis, several forms of therapy more usually associated with in-patient care are carried out in the patient's home. The number of patients involved is not large, but this trend is steadily increasing. There are many benefits to treatment at home:

- less time in hospital
- less risk of infection
- care at home
- greater autonomy
- ability to return to work
- best option for those living in remote rural areas
- frees up beds
- saves money.

The extent to which the community nurse is involved in the therapy will depend on several factors. In a number of situations, patients will be taught to carry out procedures themselves but will need support and guidance from the nurse, who will also carry out periodic checks on the patient's technique. Technical support services (e.g. equipment maintenance) will also be required.

HOME PARENTERAL THERAPY

Intravenous therapy may be continued at home using a centrally placed access device, such as the Hickman catheter or the Port-a-Cath, inserted in hospital when treatment was initiated.

Three main groups of patients may be taught to self-administer intravenous medication by one of these methods.

1. Patients suffering from cystic fibrosis, advanced bronchiectasis or cytomegalovirus retinitis (in immunocompromised patients) are taught to administer intravenous antibiotics. The specific benefit for these patients is the reduced risk of developing nosocomial infections.
2. Home parenteral nutrition (see also p. 426) is used for patients with severe intestinal failure. In most instances, the therapy is required in the short term when the condition is reversible, but in some patients therapy must be continued for life.
3. Oncology patients may receive intravenous cytotoxic therapy at home or intermittently attend a hospital clinic for repeat pulses of chemotherapy.

In each case, the community nurse may be involved in the maintenance of the line and in providing ongoing support for the patient and carer(s).

Continuous intravenous administration of drugs using a syringe pump is available for use in the patient's home for pain control and antiemetic treatment in terminal care (see Ch. 26) and other specialised forms of therapy, such as insulin. A battery-operated syringe pump is also available for the intravenous injection of drugs in boluses at regular but infrequent intervals.

The subcutaneous route using a syringe driver may also be used in the domiciliary setting for the continuous infusion of drugs used in palliative care.

HOME NEBULISER THERAPY/OXYGEN THERAPY

Nebulisers are occasionally prescribed for asthmatic patients who have been found to be unresponsive to conventional treatment. Dangers associated with this form of treatment have been identified, particularly when the nebuliser in use has not been prescribed.

Home oxygen is prescribed by the GP and is supplied in England and Wales by regional pharmacy contractors and in Scotland by pharmacists registered to do so; the nurse oversees its use and advises the patient or carer.

The forms of home therapy briefly described above have a number of advantages, the greatest being that many patients are able to resume a reasonably normal lifestyle. Care in patient selection for any form of sophisticated home therapy is extremely important, as is the need for training and continuing support. In certain situations, the community nurse will need special instruction in the techniques involved, which

can best be provided in the ward where the treatment is initiated. Community nurses, in responding to this technological revolution, are working to ensure that their patients receive maximum therapeutic benefit.

SELF-ASSESSMENT QUESTIONS

SECTION A

For all nurses.

1. Who is accountable for the safe administration of a medicine?
2. What are the key principles surrounding the administration of medicines?
3. Is it permissible to administer a medicine on a telephone instruction?
4. What methods may be used to identify a hospital patient prior to the administration of a medicine?
5. Which age group is more likely to develop an adverse drug reaction?
6. What aspects of their drug treatment are patients entitled to know?
7. What factors does a nurse have to take into consideration when assessing patients' ability to take their medicines safely?
8. How should unused medicines be disposed of?
9. What indices may give the nurse a clue as to what to expect or what is happening to a patient receiving medication?
10. What should a nurse do if the patient requests a medicine before the due time?

SECTION B

For primary care nurses. For reflection – no answers given.

1. You are caring for a terminally ill patient who is receiving oral morphine. Her daughter is a drug abuser.
   a. What are the foreseeable dangers?
   b. How may the mother and daughter relationship be affected?
   c. What are the ways round this problem?
2. District nurses are visiting a known drug abuser to dress wounds. He is continually asking for stronger pain relief.
   a. How can this be assessed?
   b. Are there safety issues for the nurses?
3. An elderly patient is unable to use her controlled dosage system correctly. She takes any quota of tablets at a time. What are the implications of this practice?

4. You find that one of your patients has not been taking his analgesia as recommended. He has been taking it on a 'when I'm sore' basis rather than round the clock. What should you do?

REFERENCES

[Anonymous] 1967 Abortion Act 1967 (amended 1990). HMSO, London

[Anonymous] 1990 Environmental Protection Act 1990. HMSO, London

Crooks J, Clark CE, Caie HB et al. 1965 Prescribing and administration of drugs in hospital. Lancet i:373

Department of Health 2004 Building a safer NHS for patients: improving medication safety. Report from the Chief Pharmaceutical Officer. Department of Health, London

Griffiths R, Johnson M, Piper M et al. 2004 A nursing intervention for the quality use of medicines by elderly community clients. International Journal of Nursing Practice 10:166–176

Jones R, Britten N, Culpepper L et al. 2004 Oxford textbook of primary medical care. Oxford University Press, Oxford

King RL 2004 Nurses' perceptions of their pharmacology educational needs. Journal of Advanced Nursing 45:392–400

National Patient Safety Agency 2005 Wristbands for hospital inpatients improves safety. NHS safer practice notice 11. NPSA, London

Nursing and Midwifery Council 2003 Competent consent and record transcribing. NMC News. NMC, London, p. 13

Nursing and Midwifery Council 2004a The code of professional conduct: standards for conduct, performance and ethics. NMC, London

Nursing and Midwifery Council 2004b Guidelines for the administration of medicines. NMC, London, pp. 5 and 8

Royal Pharmaceutical Society of Great Britain 2005 The safe and secure handling of medicines: a team approach. A revision of the Duthie Report 1988. RPSGB, London

FURTHER READING AND RESOURCES

[Anonymous] 1974 Health and Safety at Work Act 1974. HMSO, London

Department of Health 1988 Guidelines for the safe and secure handling of medicines (Duthie Report). Department of Health, London

Jones R, Britten N, Culpepper L et al. 2004 Oxford textbook of primary medical care. Oxford University Press, Oxford

Nursing and Midwifery Council (http://www.nmc-uk.org)

Royal College of Nursing (http://www.rcn.org.uk)

Administration of medicines

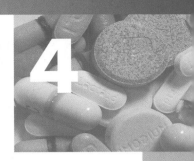

4

KEY OBJECTIVES

After reading this chapter, you should be able to:

- outline the procedure for administering an oral medicine
- demonstrate how to fill a syringe in preparation for administration of an injection
- plot the sites for the administration of subcutaneous and intramuscular injections on a blank model
- list the hazards associated with the administration of injections and describe how they may be minimised
- outline the advice you would give to a patient being discharged using glyceryl trinitrate patches for the first time

- be able to interpret the prescription for an oral (or other non-injectable) preparation
- be able to calculate an oral (or other non-injectable) dose
- be able to interpret a standard label for an oral (or other non-injectable) preparation
- be able to interpret and calculate as above for a parenteral dose.

INTRODUCTION

Many conditions are treated systemically using medicines administered either by mouth or by injection. The procedural details are highly relevant

Table 4.1 Advantages and disadvantages of different routes of medicine administration[a]

Route	Advantages	Disadvantages
Oral	Cheap, easy, no special equipment. Acceptable to most people. Suitable for self-medication.	May be compromised by irritant effects/presence of food. Enzyme action may limit effectiveness.
Sublingual	Drug absorption through buccal or sublingual mucosa avoids gut enzymes. Rapid action.	Taste of drug may be a problem.
Transdermal	Easy to use. Long action can be achieved. Avoids adverse effects of gastrointestinal tract enzymes.	Relatively high cost. Drug may build up in skin so that action continues when patch removed.
Inhalation	Rapid action (inhaled anaesthetics). Limits systemic absorption. Avoids gut enzymes.	Needs specialised drug delivery system. Loss of dose – patient swallows most of drug. Technique needs to be taught.
Intranasal	Similar to inhalation.	May irritate nasal mucosa. Needs special drug delivery system. Absorption may vary.
Subcutaneous	Rapid absorption. Bypasses gastrointestinal tract. Patients may be taught to use this method.	Absorption may be too rapid.
Intramuscular	Good absorption. Bypasses gastrointestinal tract.	Local irritancy. May be painful. Hazard of nerve damage. Skill involved.
Intravenous	Rapid action can control rate of administration. Suitable for large volumes and drugs that would be irritant intramuscularly.	Relatively high cost. Skills involved. Extravasation risk. Specialist drug delivery system needed.
Rectal	Suitable for drugs that may irritate the upper gut. Fairly rapid action.	May not be acceptable to some people. Variable absorption.

[a]It is important to note that many factors affect drug absorption. The chemical properties of the drug and physiological variables (e.g. blood flow) all influence the rate at which a drug is absorbed.

to all nurses, because by far the majority of medicines are given by these routes. The transdermal route is also included. The advantages and disadvantages of each route are given in Table 4.1. These routes are not specific to any system of the body, and so they have been grouped together in one chapter.

ADMINISTRATION OF MEDICINES BY MOUTH

For the majority of patients, the most convenient and acceptable method of receiving medication is by mouth. Most medicines taken by mouth are intended to be swallowed, and are referred to as *oral* medicines. Others, known as *sublingual*, are specifically for

dissolving under the tongue; some, known as *buccal*, are for holding against the mucous membranes of the cheek.

ORAL ADMINISTRATION

Tablets, capsules and liquid preparations are relatively easy to administer and are suitable delivery systems for drugs that are effective when given orally. If a tablet or capsule sticks in the oesophagus, it can cause irritation to the point of ulceration of the mucosa, especially with drugs such as ferrous salts. Small tablets are generally easy to swallow. Larger uncoated tablets may present problems; torpedo-shaped coated tablets are more patient-friendly. It is important that soluble tablets and effervescent tablets are completely dissolved in water prior to administration. To ensure complete transit from mouth to stomach, tablets and capsules should be swallowed with a large drink, ideally when standing. Where this is not possible, the patient should be in the sitting position (Channer 1985).

The disguising of medicines in food and drink without informed consent is a complex issue. Covert administration of medicines to patients in Norwegian nursing homes was revealed in a study of 243 patients, of whom 95% had their drugs mixed in food and beverages routinely (Kirkevold and Engedal 2005).

The principles involved are underpinned by the Human Rights Act 1998. Registered nurses need to be sure that what they are doing is in the best interests of the patient, and are reminded of their accountability in any decision they make regarding what may be seen as misleading the patient (Nursing and Midwifery Council 2006, pp. 7–8). The doctor and pharmacist are available to suggest alternatives and to provide professional support. Any duty of care argument should be supported by good record keeping (Nursing and Midwifery Council 2006, p. 8).

ADMINISTERING ORAL SOLID DOSAGE FORMS

Patients have their own preferences as to the order in which they take their medicines. For example, they may take unpleasant-tasting ones first or those that for some reason cause them a problem. Patients who have difficulty swallowing tablets may be assisted in a number of ways.

- A drink beforehand moistens the mouth and gets the swallowing process started.
- When the tablet is large and is scored, it may be split in two or even four. A specially designed tablet splitter may be helpful. Some tablets are not designed to be split, and attempts to do so could lead to an inaccurate dose being administered. If for any reason the tablet is unsuitable, the pharmacist should be asked to advise.
- In certain instances, the tablet may be crushed using a mortar and pestle or specially designed tablet crusher. Enteric-coated or sustained-release formulations must not be split or crushed, because this could destroy the properties of the tablet and cause gastric irritation or premature release of the drug into an incompatible pH. The crushing of a tablet or opening of a capsule not specifically designed for this purpose renders its use unlicensed (Nursing and Midwifery Council 2006, p. 6).
- Some patients find it helpful to place the tablet at the back of the tongue, take a draught of water and tilt the head back before swallowing. This stimulates the back of the tongue and produces a swallowing reflex.

- For those who cannot swallow tablets or capsules, a liquid form of the medicine may be available.
- For dysphagic patients, consideration of the viscosity of an oral liquid medicine is important. Patients with swallowing difficulties may be more able to swallow a more viscous preparation than a very mobile liquid.

Whenever possible, patients should put the tablet or capsule into the mouth themselves. By observing patients attempting to take a tablet and assessing their capabilities generally, the nurse can decide how best to present further medicines. The methods employed are:

- taking directly from a spoon or medicine measure
- transferring from spoon or measure into the palm of the hand
- picking up using the thumb and forefinger.

However, some difficulties are encountered with each of these methods. For example:

- a spoon is not advisable for patients with any degree of tremor
- medicine measures are not designed with the size of an adult's nose in mind
- unless the medicine measure is completely dry, tablets can adhere to the measure and may be lost
- tablets or capsules may be dropped or may stick to the hand if moist
- intention tremor and stiff joints may make picking up difficult or impossible.

In general, patients who are elderly, frail, poorly sighted or confused are helped if the tablets are placed in a row on the medicine tray, accompanied by a glass of water or a suitable beverage. In this way, they are more likely to see what they are to take: the colour of the tablets and the number. They can then safely pick each one up themselves and so retain some degree of independence. Hemiplegic patients find this a helpful method, especially when more than one tablet has to be taken. Using the unaffected hand, they require to break down the process. For example:

- pick up glass, take drink, lay down glass
- pick up first tablet, place in mouth
- pick up glass, take drink, lay down glass
- pick up next tablet ... and so on.

White tablets may be overlooked when they are laid out on a white tray, and so care must be taken to ensure that none has been missed. If the tray is used in this way, it must be washed before and after use.

Care must be taken, particularly when there is facial paralysis, to ensure that the tablets are swallowed and not retained in the side of the mouth. Patients who do not want to take their tablets are sometimes known to retain the tablet between the gum and cheek until the staff are out of sight and then reject the tablet, often into the bed.

An adequate volume of fluid, for example at least 100 mL, ensures transport into the gastrointestinal tract. Apart from personal tastes and preferences, the choice and volume of liquid to be used will depend on a number of factors. Clearly, for patients on restricted fluids the volume may be critical. Milk may inhibit the absorption of some drugs, and acidic fruit cordials tend to cause capsules to swell, which may make swallowing more difficult. Improved formulations are a help in disguising the taste of many drugs, but children of all ages may welcome the traditional 'spoonful of sugar'.

Severely breathless patients may find swallowing difficult, and very drowsy patients may be unable to cooperate in taking medicines, with a risk of accidental inhalation. In such cases, other routes may have to be used.

If a patient rejects part of a dose or vomits after swallowing a dose of medicine, the doctor should be informed of this along with the time lapse between drug administration and emesis or rejection. Vomitus should be retained for examination of drug content.

ADMINISTERING ORAL LIQUID DOSAGE FORMS

- All liquid medicines should be thoroughly shaken before use and measured at eye level in a good light using a suitably designed measure, i.e. a measure with clear graduations that is convenient to pour into.
- When pouring a liquid medicine, the bottle is held with the label uppermost so that any drips will not deface the label.
- Viscous suspensions, syrups, etc. can be more completely administered if taken from a suitable graduated spoon rather than from a medicine measure. A standard 5-mL spoon should normally be used. However, medicine spoons of different designs are available, the choice depending mainly on acceptability to the patient. Care should be taken not to overfill a medicine spoon when administering a viscous preparation.
- The formulation of liquid medicines presents many problems, not least of which is to achieve an acceptable taste. If particular problems are experienced, the clinical pharmacist should be consulted, as dilution or an alternative formulation may be available.
- It is necessary to ensure that soluble (effervescent) tablets are completely dissolved prior to

administration, but an excessive volume should not be used because this could make the resulting solution less acceptable to the patient.
- When the medicine is presented in powder form to be reconstituted (e.g. unstable antibiotics), the date of reconstitution or expiry should be marked on the bottle. The diluent and volume to be used will be specified on the label. If further dilution of the reconstituted medicine is required, this should be undertaken only in the pharmacy.
- Reconstituted medicines will normally require storage in a refrigerator, and it is very important to shake the bottle well prior to administration.
- When liquids are being instilled in the mouth from a dropper, a separate bottle and dropper are used for each patient.
- In some instances, a specially designed oral syringe may be useful, for example for severely disabled people or when specially potent oral liquid medicines are in use. Graduated droppers are supplied for use with high-dose oral morphine preparations.
- The bottle should be wiped clean after use to reduce the build up of bacteria and make for safer handling.

The administration of oral medicines is summarised in Box 4.1.

Box 4.1 Administration of oral medicines

Documentation
- Prescribing and recording sheet

The medicine
- Oral solids (tablet, capsule, lozenge, granules)
- Oral liquids (mixture, suspension, emulsion, linctus)

The nurse and the patient
- Identification of patient
- Explanation given to patient

Technique
- The nurse's hands should be socially clean
- Whenever possible, the patient should be in an upright position
- Whenever possible, patients should put the medicine into the mouth themselves
- The nurse should witness the medicine being taken
- If required, any fluid taken should be recorded on the patient's fluid balance chart
- Any medicines rejected should be retained

Problems
- Irritation of gastrointestinal tract
- Aspiration of the medicine
- Staining of teeth and lips

SUBLINGUAL ADMINISTRATION

First-pass metabolism is avoided when drugs are given by the sublingual route (i.e. under the tongue), because the drug passes directly into the general blood circulation via the blood vessels on the undersurface of the tongue. Sublingual tablets are uncoated, ready for absorption. Once the tablet has been placed under the tongue, the patient should keep the mouth closed and refrain from swallowing saliva for as long as possible, as this contains the drug that will be absorbed. As absorption through the oral mucosa is rapid, the effects of the drug become apparent within a minute or two.

Tablets to be given by this route must be prescribed as such. The method of administration is simple, requiring no liquid and demanding little effort from the patient. The cooperation of the patient is necessary, however, and a clear explanation of this method of administration should be given. Although no harm will ensue if the tablet is swallowed, the patient will benefit from the drug *only* if it is taken sublingually.

The ease with which drugs can be given by this route can be used to advantage in pre- and postoperative patients and in those who are terminally ill, in whom swallowing of tablets can be a problem.

The sublingual route is also useful when there is risk of symptoms arising unexpectedly and when a rapid effect is wanted, such as in angina. Patients who are prescribed glyceryl trinitrate tablets for *prevention* of anginal attacks should be advised to carry with them a small supply of the tablets at all times. The expiry date (8 weeks after *opening*) should be carefully noted on the label of the container. Once individual patients realise which activities tend to precipitate an attack, they should get into the habit of placing the tablet under the tongue just before embarking on any of these activities. When the tablet is used to *alleviate* an anginal attack, it should be taken immediately the pain is experienced and retained under the tongue until the pain is relieved, after which any of the tablet remaining is spat out. This may help to prevent headache caused by cerebral vasodilatation, which often follows administration of this drug. Sublingual glyceryl trinitrate may also be administered in the form of an aerosol spray.

BUCCAL ADMINISTRATION

When a tablet is to be held in the mouth against the mucous membranes, the method of administration is described as buccal. This specific route appears on the packaging and on the prescription. It refers to the area high up between the upper lip and the gum where

---

Box 4.2 Medicine round

Documentation
- Kardex system or individual prescribing and recording sheet at each patient's bedside or in document trolley

The medicine
- Mainly oral medicines (possibly medicines for inhalation also)
- Stored in alphabetical order according to approved name
- Individual locked medicine cabinet or trolley locked to wall when not in use
- Unlocked trolley never left unattended
- Sufficient spoons, medicine measures, oral syringes, etc. available

The environment
- So far as possible, uninterrupted

The nurse and the patient
- Each patient greeted and accurately identified

Technique
- Nurse works systematically according to local circumstances
- After use, non-disposable items washed, sticky bottles wiped and trolley/individual cabinet restocked as appropriate

Hazards
- Medicine(s) given to wrong patient
- Interruptions leading to error
- Medicines given too soon or much later than the time prescribed
- Misappropriation of medicines from unsupervised trolley/individual cabinet

---

the dosage form is left to dissolve. Tablets for buccal administration are uncoated to facilitate absorption. Glyceryl trinitrate and prochlorperazine maleate are available as buccal tablets. The site chosen should be varied to reduce the risk of dental caries.

MEDICINE ROUNDS

Despite an increase in self-administration, the majority of medicines in hospital are still administered consecutively to groups of patients in the form of a medicine round (Box 4.2). A medicine trolley or an individual medicine cabinet may be used.

Table 4.2 Hazards associated with injections

Risk/cause	Possible outcome	Prevention
Contamination		
Dirty preparation area	Infection	Keep preparation areas clear and clean.
Unwashed hands	Septicaemia, especially if patient is immunocompromised	Wash hands using chlorhexidine gluconate handwash before and after preparing injection.
Unswabbed vial tops	–	Swab rubber-capped vials using alcohol swab and allow to dry.
Aerosolisation		
Spraying the atmosphere with injection solution	Reduced sensitivity to the medication	Inject equivalent volume of air to volume of injection required. Attach sheathed needle to syringe when expelling air from syringe.
Needlestick injury		
Resheathing needles	Hepatitis B HIV	NEVER replace sheath on needle.
Incorrect disposal of needle	Localised infection	Always use sharps receptacle for disposal of needles. Do NOT overfill sharps receptacle.
Nerve damage Improper siting of injection	Paralysis of a limb	Select appropriate site avoiding large nerve(s).

ADMINISTRATION OF MEDICINES BY INJECTION

Medicines should be administered by injection only when no other route is suitable, because of their hazardous nature (Clinical Resource and Audit Group of NHS Scotland 2002). When there is no alternative but to use this method, every precaution must be taken to minimise the risks involved (see Table 4.2). In the interests of safety, staff training in the preparation and administration of intravenous injections should be supported by a standard operating procedure (Millar et al. 2006). There are a number of reasons why some medicines require to be administered by this method. For example:

- they may not be absorbed when given by mouth (e.g. gentamicin)
- they may be destroyed in the stomach (e.g. insulin)
- rapid first-pass metabolism may be extensive (e.g. lignocaine [lidocaine])
- a fast onset of action may be required in an emergency
- very precise control over dosage may be needed
- because the patient is unable, for whatever reason, to take the medicine by mouth
- to achieve high drug plasma levels.

Because the routes used for administering injections do not involve the gastrointestinal (enteral) tract, drugs prepared for injection are often described as for *parenteral* use.

PRESENTATION AND PREPARATION OF SMALL-VOLUME INJECTIONS

Small-volume injections are presented in the form of an ampoule or a rubber-capped vial.

AMPOULES

Ampoules are mostly made of glass (an inert material) of special quality that does not react with the contents. Plastic ampoules are now used for certain products. Sizes range from 0.25–50 mL. Ampoules normally

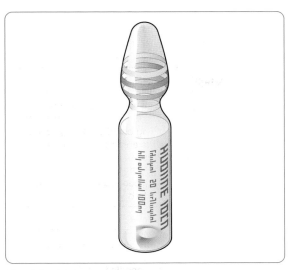

Fig. 4.1 Ampoule.

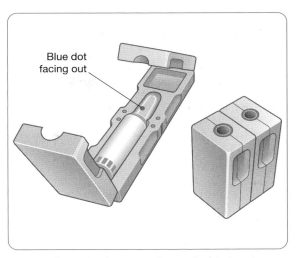

Blue dot facing out

Fig. 4.2 Example of an ampoule-opening device.

contain solutions ready for use but may contain a sterile powder for reconstitution.

An ampoule has a body containing the drug, a top, and a narrow constriction in between referred to as the neck (Fig. 4.1). The neck may be marked with a white ring, or the top may have a coloured spot. These indicate where the ampoule is to be snapped off to enable the contents to be accessed. Some ampoules have coloured rings on the neck that help in avoiding mix-ups. These rings must not be used to identify the product.

Ampoule-opening devices of various designs are available (Fig. 4.2). Plastic ampoules are accessed by twisting off a tab on the neck or by direct penetration with a needle at a site indicated on the ampoule. Ampoules whose tops have been removed cannot be resealed and are therefore for single use only. Any unwanted contents must be discarded.

After shaking down any solution that has entered the neck, the neck is wiped with an alcohol swab to remove any surface contamination and the top snapped off using an ampoule sleeve to protect the fingers from glass spicules and/or any sharp edges. Less commonly, it may be necessary to make a scratch on the ampoule using a small file.

VIALS

Rubber-capped vials are used for solutions for injection and sterile powders for reconstitution (Fig. 4.3). They are squat glass containers closed with a rubber plug that is held in place by a metal ring. The exposed rubber surface is generally covered with a protective pull-off metal or plastic disc.

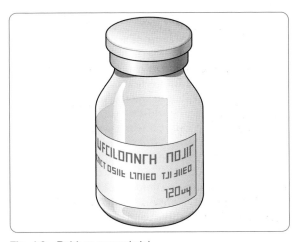

Fig. 4.3 Rubber-capped vial.

Rubber-capped vials are capable of being used as multidose containers, because the rubber plug is self-sealing if correctly used. They should, however, be used as such only if the stability of the contents permits and there is a suitable antimicrobial preservative present in the formulation.

The disc is removed and the exposed surface swabbed with an alcohol swab and *allowed to dry*, prior to puncturing the centre of the rubber plug with a needle. To facilitate withdrawal of fluid, the plunger of the syringe is first withdrawn and air injected, the volume of air being the same as the volume of fluid to be withdrawn. The required dose is removed or the required volume of the appropriate reconstitution fluid is added prior to the removal of the dose. Great care is essential in calculating what portion of the total volume is required from multidose vials. It is vitally important to follow the instructions regarding reconstitution and to ensure that the powder is dissolved before withdrawing the dose.

The needle is then changed after drawing up the injection and before injecting the patient, in case particles of rubber are retained inside the needle. Another good reason is that when a needle is inserted through the rubber cap, it may become dulled or the needle coating that helps it glide through the skin may be removed (Beyea and Nicoll 1996). Besides, because of the high risk of needlestick injury when resheathing a needle, the practice of using a new needle for administering the injection to the patient is obligatory (Royal College of Nursing 2006).

RECONSTITUTION OF MEDICINES FOR INJECTION

Where there are problems of stability, the drug may be presented in powder form, which requires reconstitution with a diluent. Reconstitution is most often done using water for injections, although in certain instances special diluents may be required. It should be recognised that the addition of 1 mL of diluent to 250 mg of a drug will produce a volume in excess of 1 mL. Normally this is of little consequence, but it may be important if a fraction of the total content of the vial is to be administered. For emaciated patients, the volume of reconstituting fluid should be the minimum compatible with the physical and other properties of the drug such as solubility, and any possible local irritancy should be taken into account. Once the contents of a multidose vial have been reconstituted, the vial must be dated and stored in the refrigerator.

On occasion, it may be desirable to combine two drugs in the same injection. This may present problems such as the physical/chemical incompatibility in the syringe and in the management of any subsequent drug reaction. The prime considerations here should be the safety and comfort of the patient. Comfort of the patient, however, should not be allowed to detract from safety in drug therapy. The advice of the prescriber and clinical pharmacist will often be helpful in resolving these difficult situations.

ROUTES OF ADMINISTRATION

The routes most commonly used for administering injections are:

- subcutaneous (SC; into the fatty layer beneath the skin)
- intramuscular (IM; into skeletal muscle)
- intravenous (IV; into a vein).

Intravenous medicines given by direct venepuncture are administered only by a doctor. A nurse who has undertaken specific training and is in possession of authorisation to do so may administer intravenous medication when venous access has already been established (Clinical Resource and Audit Group of NHS Scotland 2002). In clinical practice, there is widespread use of the intravenous route for the administration of drugs such as antibiotics and diuretics. However, some drugs still require to be given by either the subcutaneous or intramuscular route, and therefore nurses must maintain the skills involved.

The subcutaneous route is generally used for administering small doses of non-irritating, water-soluble substances. Drugs commonly given subcutaneously include:

- insulin
- heparin
- hyoscine
- vaccines.

Patients receiving outpatient treatment for certain ongoing conditions are encouraged to self-administer subcutaneous medication when possible. Examples include the administration of insulin, heparin, interferon and granulocyte-colony stimulating factor. Alternatively, a family member may be taught to do this.

The intramuscular route is used for administering formulations such as aqueous solutions, oily solutions and aqueous suspensions. Drugs commonly given intramuscularly include:

- analgesics
- sex hormones
- corticosteroids.

RATE OF ABSORPTION

The rates at which drugs are absorbed and take effect after subcutaneous or intramuscular injection depend on two factors. These are the local blood circulation and the nature of the drug solution or suspension. Subcutaneous absorption occurs chiefly through the capillaries and is much faster compared with absorption following oral medication but usually slower than intramuscular absorption because of muscle tissue's excellent blood supply.

Absorption following intramuscular injection may be speeded up by massaging the area of injection.

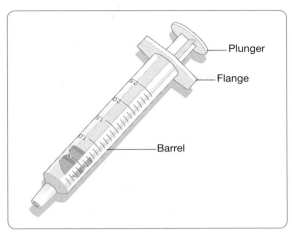

Fig. 4.4 Syringe.

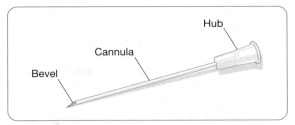

Fig. 4.5 Needle.

However, insulin-dependent diabetics are discouraged from massaging the site vigorously, in an attempt to preserve the state of the capillaries. An inflamed or oedematous site should be avoided when administering subcutaneous or intramuscular injections, so as to prevent a worsening of the inflammation/oedema and consequently a delay in absorption. In states of shock, blood flow to the skin and superficial muscle may be greatly reduced, thus reducing the absorption of drugs from these sites. In this case, intravenous injection should be used.

SYRINGES

A syringe consists of a barrel and a plunger (Fig. 4.4). The barrel is graduated. The plunger has a rubber stopper attached. Syringes are available in various sizes (e.g. 1, 2, 5, 10 and 20 mL). The choice of syringe is made according to the volume of medication to be injected. It should be noted, however, that insulin must always be measured using an insulin syringe. The tip of a syringe can vary, with the *concentric* Luer tip being the one used for subcutaneous and intramuscular injections. It is also used for introducing medication via an already sited intravenous cannula. For direct intravenous injections, the *eccentric* Luer tip is used to allow the needle to lie within the vein wall without puncturing the distal wall. The Luer tips of syringes interlock to an international standard with needle hubs.

Disposable syringes are made of a plastic material that is compatible with most substances to be injected. There are one or two exceptions, however. Paraldehyde, for example, should be administered using a glass syringe, because it dissolves plastic and rubber on prolonged contact. Syringes are individually sealed in a sterile pack. Before use, a check should be made that the seal has not been broken. Once a syringe has been removed from its pack, the utmost care is required to prevent contamination of the tip of the syringe.

NEEDLES

A needle consists of a hub and a cannula (Fig. 4.5). The cannula is hollow and is made of strong flexible steel that has been siliconised to assist penetration. For the same reason, the tip of the cannula is bevelled. Different types of needle have a different bevel. A shorter bevel encourages minimal penetration, as is required in an intradermal injection (see p. 63). A longer bevel allows easier deep penetration, as needed for an intramuscular injection (see p. 56). The gauge of the cannula is an indication of its diameter. The higher the gauge, the finer the bore. Higher gauges are used for 'watery' solutions and make for less painful injections. Low gauges are essential for injecting viscous (syrupy) solutions.

Needle lengths also vary. Selection of length depends on the route of the injection as well as the patient's age and physical build. A study by Chan showed that only 32% of patients received the correct dose of intramuscular injection, the reason being that needles could not penetrate the muscle due to excessive fat in patients' buttocks caused by obesity (Anonymous 2005).

Each needle is enclosed in a removable guard and individually sealed in a sterile pack. Before use, a check should be made to ensure that the pack has not been damaged. Once a guard is removed, the needle should be in one of three places only: in the ampoule or vial containing the medication, in the patient or in the sharps container.

For *drawing up any injection* from a glass ampoule, it is important to use a needle with a bore that is 21-gauge or smaller to filter out any shards of glass that may have entered the ampoule (Shaw and Lyall 1985).

For *administering* subcutaneous injections, a short fine-bore needle is used. For adults, this may be $\frac{1}{2}$ inch

(13 mm) or $\frac{5}{8}$ inch (16 mm), 25-gauge or 26-gauge; $\frac{1}{2}$ inch (13 mm), 26-gauge; or $\frac{3}{8}$ inch (10 mm), 27 gauge.

For *administering* intramuscular injections, the needle used has to be sufficiently long to reach deep into the muscle so as to increase the speed of effect and to reduce the likelihood of the drug seeping back along the needle track. For adults, a $1\frac{1}{2}$-inch (40 mm), 21-gauge (0.8 mm) needle is normally used. In severely emaciated adults, a 1-inch (25 mm), 23-gauge (0.6 mm) needle may be used.

When drawing up and injecting drugs with a known potential to cause sensitivity reactions, disposable gloves should be worn to prevent possible contact with the skin and the development of a sensitivity reaction. The special precautions that require to be taken when handling cytotoxic drugs are given in Chapter 19.

VOLUME

When preparing an injection, the nurse should give consideration to the volume that may be effectively accommodated in one site. Apart from the route to be used, the patient's age and physical build are factors that will influence the decision. Normally, the following would apply.

- For subcutaneous injections, no more than 2 mL should be injected at one site.
- For intramuscular injections, the volume injected at any one site should normally be no more than 3 mL. When a volume in excess of 3 mL is to be given, two separate sites may have to be used. No more than 1 mL should be given into the deltoid muscle.

SITE

The sites most commonly used for subcutaneous injections (Fig. 4.6) are as follows:

- middle outer aspect of the upper arm
- middle anterior aspect of the thigh
- anterior abdominal wall below the umbilicus.

(The back and lower loin may also be used.)

The sites most commonly used for intramuscular injections are as follows:

- upper outer quadrant of the buttock
- anterolateral aspect of the mid-thigh.

(The deltoid is used for hepatitis B and influenza vaccines.)

It is vital that the intramuscular injection is confined to the upper outer quadrant of the buttock or the anterolateral aspect of the mid-thigh so as to avoid damage to the sciatic nerve (Fig. 4.7) and to avoid penetrating a major blood vessel.

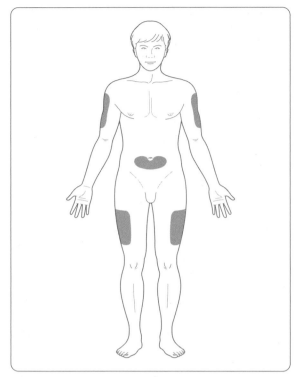

Fig. 4.6   Sites for administering subcutaneous injections.

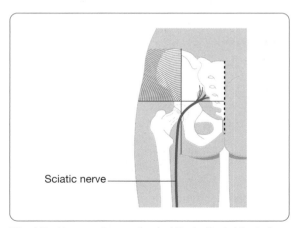

Fig. 4.7   Upper outer quadrant of the buttock (shaded area).

Rotation of the sites used for subcutaneous and intramuscular injections helps to reduce the likelihood of irritation and improves absorption. Rotation *within* the sites is also important. Patients who, for example, have to repeatedly self-administer subcutaneous injections may be taught to visualise a clock face on the site and systematically work round it. Where nurses are repeatedly administering injections, the site used on each occasion may be plotted on a diagram held at the bedside. Before administering any type of injection, the skin should be inspected on each occasion. Lesions, such as birthmarks, moles or scars, and inflamed or oedematous sites should be avoided.

SKIN PREPARATION

Despite now quite old research findings, old habits die hard. It is not considered necessary to use an alcohol swab to disinfect the skin prior to the administration of injections. Although there are inconsistencies in practice, the lack of skin preparation does not result in infections (Dann 1969, Koivisto and Felig 1978, Workman 1999). Torrance (1989) cites two studies that prove this point. One describes a series of 1078 injections given by all routes without any skin preparation, which resulted in no case of systemic or local infection. The second was a study of 7000 insulin injections given to a group of diabetic patients without skin cleansing, with no infection noted. Lipids in the epidermis provide an antibacterial barrier, so that removal of the lipids may encourage bacterial colonisation (Torrance 1989).

Clinical evidence suggests that no harm will be caused by pricking the skin *so long as it is socially clean*. Contaminated skin will need preparation to produce a low bacterial count. In this case, the site should first be made socially clean followed by a 30-s rub using an 'alcohol swab' (alcohol swabs contain 70% alcohol and a disinfectant such as chlorhexidine). The skin should then be allowed to dry for a further 30 s before proceeding to ensure that bacteria are rendered inactive (Cullen 2004) and so that the antiseptic does not cause irritation by being injected into the tissues. In immunosuppressed patients, the skin must be cleansed in this way, as this group of patients may become infected by inoculation of a relatively small number of pathogens.

ANGLE

The angles at which the needle is directed for subcutaneous and intramuscular injections are illustrated in Figure 4.8. It is common practice for subcutaneous injections of, for example, heparin or insulin to be given into the abdomen at an angle of 90° using a very short subcutaneous needle. An angle of between 45 and 90° may be used with a longer subcutaneous needle. Where the syringe and needle have been previously prepared in a pack (as for self-administration), the needle is usually very short and an angle of 90° is recommended.

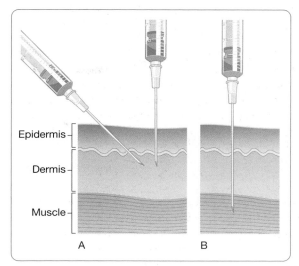

Fig. 4.8 Angles for the administration of (**A**) subcutaneous and (**B**) intramuscular injections.

IRRITANT OR STAINING SUBSTANCES

The injection may be known to irritate the tissues and stain the skin if it is allowed to seep along the needle track to the epidermis (e.g. iron sorbitol injection). To prevent this, several precautions should be taken. After the syringe is filled, the needle is changed so that the substance is contained in the syringe only and is less likely to drip from the tip of the needle as it penetrates the skin. To reduce pain as well as the risk of staining, the injection is made deep into the muscle of the upper outer quadrant of the buttock. The arm and thigh do not allow for the depth required and so should not be used.

A 21-gauge needle is normally suitable, but it is important that it is long enough to reach the muscle. As a rule of thumb, a $1\frac{1}{2}$-inch (40 mm) needle will do for most normal-sized adults. Obese patients (e.g. > 90 kg) will require a 2-inch needle. The so-called Z-track technique must be used. This technique involves displacement of the skin and subcutaneous tissue laterally prior to injection (Fig. 4.9). The injection is made slowly and steadily. Before withdrawing the needle, 10 s should be allowed to elapse so that the muscle mass can accommodate the volume of the injection. The site is not massaged, otherwise the medication may be forced into the subcutaneous tissue, causing irritation.

REDUCTION OF PAIN

For most people, the prospect of receiving an injection of any kind is not one that they relish. Pain caused

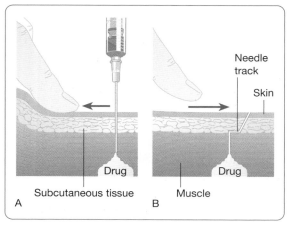

Fig. 4.9 Z-track technique: (**A**) Injection (**B**) Post-injection.

Box 4.3 Summary of methods for reducing pain associated with injections

- Use fine-bore needle where possible
- Do not exceed 3 mL of fluid at one site
- Rotate the sites
- Consider using skin coolant or local anaesthetic cream
- Consider using Z-track method for intramuscular injections
- Be prepared to listen to view of experienced patient
- Explain benefits of the injection
- Encourage patient to relax
- If appropriate, ask patient to turn foot inwards
- Insert needle *quickly*
- Inject medication *slowly*
- Withdraw needle *quickly*

---

by injections can be reduced in a number of different ways (Box 4.3). First, it is important to try to encourage patients to relax. This may be achieved by explaining to them what they should do. Patients should be positioned so that they are at ease. For example, for subcutaneous injections into the upper arm, the patient should be sitting with the hand resting on the iliac crest; for intramuscular injections, the patient should be lying *on*, as opposed to leaning over, a couch or bed.

When the buttock is the chosen site for intramuscular injection, administration may be made less painful by asking the patient to adopt the prone position and to point the feet inwards. Internal rotation of the femur helps to relax the gluteus maximus muscle. Alternatively, the patient may lie on one side with the lower leg extended and the upper leg flexed.

As a general rule, with intramuscular injections the needle should be inserted (and withdrawn) *quickly*. Subcutaneous injections require the needle to be steadily *pushed* through the skin into the tissues and then eased out gently on completion of the injection.

Fine-bore needles create less pain on puncturing the skin and necessitate slow injection of the fluid. Pain can result from injecting too large a volume of fluid at one site or injecting the drug too quickly, resulting in improper distribution of the drug. The medication should be injected using *slow, steady pressure* at a rate of about 10 s/mL (Beyea and Nicoll 1996).

The skin may be cooled using a volatile spray such as ethyl chloride. A further possibility is to use a local anaesthetic agent such as Emla (eutectic mixture of local anaesthetic) cream.

Subcutaneous administration may be carried out by means of a high-pressure jet of liquid, using an injector that delivers an accurate dose without the aid of a needle. This technique may be useful in mass inoculation programmes. There is a reduction in pain to the patient and no risk of needlestick injury. The risk of transmitting blood-borne infections by this method should be carefully considered.

Use of the Z-track technique (see p. 57) may also reduce the discomfort associated with intramuscular injections, because there is less likelihood of the medication leaking into the subcutaneous tissue by this method.

Needle phobia is a very real problem to those who suffer from it. Ten per cent of the population is said to be affected by it. Little is written about it. There have been instances of vasovagal reflex reaction (fainting) even resulting in death. Patients may need courage to admit they suffer from needle phobia, just as they need courage to admit they suffer from a painful condition. Physicians must learn how fearful the problem is to the individual concerned and that many appointments and opportunities are missed because of it, with consequent increase in morbidity. The development of microneedles that are 0.15–0.3 mm long will allow permeability of the skin without reaching pain receptors.

ADMINISTRATION

The process of checking a medicine for injection against the prescription is the same as for the administration of any medicine. This should be done immediately prior to the administration procedure. It

---

Box 4.4 Administration of subcutaneous injection

Documentation
- As for intramuscular injection

The medicine
- As for intramuscular injection

The environment
- Patient seated or in bed
- Privacy, warmth, comfort

The nurse and the patient
- Patient identified
- Explanation given to patient
- Patient assisted into supine position if abdomen is the chosen site
- Patient's skin cleanliness assessed

Technique (drawing up the injection)
- As for intramuscular injection (see Box 4.5)

Technique (administering the injection)
- Nurse ensures hands thoroughly washed

- Chosen site for injection exposed
- Skin pinched up between thumb and forefinger
- *For 90° angle*, syringe held in 'pencil grip'; *for 45° angle*, syringe 'cradled' across all four fingers and steadied with thumb
- *For 90° angle*, needle *pushed* through skin; *for 45° angle*, needle with bevel uppermost *pushed gently* through the skin
- Skin released slightly
- Fluid injected *slowly* and *steadily*
- Needle *gently* withdrawn
- Site gently compressed for a few seconds until any oozing stops
- Patient made comfortable
- Sharps carefully placed in disposal bin

Hazards
- Abscess formation

---

is not acceptable to prepare a substance for injection in advance of its immediate use or to administer a medication drawn into a syringe by another nurse without him or her being present (Nursing and Midwifery Council 2006, p. 5). Hands must be washed thoroughly using chlorhexidine gluconate solution at the start and finish of the procedure. Asepsis must be maintained throughout, because puncturing the integument provides easy access for pathogenic microorganisms. Every effort must be made to encourage the patient to relax and to minimise pain as far as possible. Extra support will be required for patients suffering from needle phobia. Careful disposal of syringes and needles is of great importance.

The procedure for administering a subcutaneous injection is outlined in Box 4.4. Patients may be taught to self-administer medication by this route. The procedure for administering an intramuscular injection is outlined in Box 4.5.

Patients with haematological conditions such as leukaemia, in which the platelet count is likely to be low, must never be given intramuscular injections, because of the high risk of bleeding into muscle tissue (because of its rich blood supply).

ADMINISTRATION OF SUBCUTANEOUS INSULIN

The needle that comes already attached to an insulin syringe is very short (5, 6 or 8 mm) and of fine bore (0.33 mm). It is essential to reach the correct layer of tissue, namely subcutaneous adipose tissue, on every occasion, and not to administer the insulin intramuscularly or by the intradermal route in error. Failure to reach the subcutaneous layer leads to altered rates of absorption and poor diabetic control (Peragallo-Dittko 1997). The recommended method is to pinch up the skin in order to raise the adipose tissue away from the underlying muscle. Using a gentle pushing technique, the insulin is injected at an angle of 90° (Burden 1994). Such advice is thought to be important in thin diabetic patients, especially men, who it has been found may have less depth of subcutaneous fat than the length of the needles in use, resulting in the administration of an intramuscular injection and not a subcutaneous one (Spraul et al. 1988, Peragallo-Dittko 1997).

ADMINISTRATION OF SUBCUTANEOUS DALTEPARIN

In order to reduce the great risk of bruising leading to pain and unsightliness, a modified injection technique is recommended for the administration of subcutaneous low molecular weight heparins (Conaghan 1993). Efforts are directed at minimising the physical trauma that can be caused before, during and after the giving of an injection. Dann (1969) has shown that, in most patients, there is no need to disinfect the skin with an antiseptic. Besides, the

Box 4.5 Administration of intramuscular injection

Documentation
- Prescribing and recording sheets

The medicine
- Ampoule or vial containing prescribed drug
- Ampoule of water for injections (or other diluent) if necessary for reconstitution

The environment
- Patient in bed or on couch
- Privacy, warmth, comfort

The nurse and the patient
- Patient identified
- Nurse explains the procedure and indicates how the patient may assist
- Patient assisted into lateral or prone position
- Patient's skin cleanliness assessed

Technique (drawing up the injection)
- Nurse ensures hands are thoroughly washed
- Contents collected into body of ampoule by flicking ampoule with fingers
- Neck of ampoule wiped with alcohol swab
- Ampoule snapped at constriction using swab to protect fingers (or by using a plastic sleeve)
- Syringe assembled; 21-gauge needle attached
- Care taken to prevent needle from touching anything unsterile
- Syringe filled
- New guarded needle attached
- Air bubbles expelled from syringe by:
  - holding it perpendicular at eye level in a good light
  - pulling plunger back slightly
  - tapping syringe with fingers to collect small bubbles into one
  - pushing plunger until liquid fills needle.
- Final volume checked

Technique (administering the injection)
- Nurse ensures hands are washed just prior to administration if involved in positioning patient, and on completion of procedure
- Nurse ensures sufficiently large area of patient's buttock exposed to allow selection of exact site for injection while maintaining maximum privacy
- Fold of skin and tissue stretched taut or tissues pulled to one side (Z track)
- Syringe held using 'pencil grip'
- Needle inserted *quickly*
- Plunger withdrawn slightly to verify that needle has not penetrated blood vessel (if blood appears, needle withdrawn and injection repeated at another site using fresh dose, syringe and needle)
- Fluid injected *slowly*
- Needle withdrawn *quickly*
- Site gently compressed for a few seconds until minor seepage stops
- Patient made comfortable
- Sharps carefully placed in disposal bin

Hazards
- Abscess formation
- Nerve damage
- Injecting medication into large blood vessel

use of an alcohol swab leads to vasodilatation and encourages bleeding. Vigorous rubbing or pinching of the skin may damage capillaries (Koivisto and Felig 1978). The preferred site is the abdomen, because of the greater depth of subcutaneous fat, although abdominal surgery may limit the available area. Brenner et al. (1981) claim that using an angle of 90° leads to fewer bruises. In addition, the amount of movement of the needle throughout the procedure should be kept to a minimum (McGowan and Wood 1989–1990). It is recommended that a roll of tissue be gently *lifted* before slowly inserting the needle. It is also generally thought that the plunger should *not* be withdrawn prior to injecting, as this can lead to negative pressure and the formation of a haematoma (Springhouse Corporation 1993). Once the needle has been removed, only light pressure over the injection site using cotton wool is necessary to stop any backflow of blood from the injection site.

INTRAVENOUS INJECTION
Administering a drug directly into a vein avoids all complications of drug absorption and, as a result, an effective blood level of the drug can be achieved in a matter of seconds. The intravenous route is used:

- in emergency situations such as shock and status asthmaticus
- to administer general anaesthetic agents (e.g. propofol)
- for larger volumes (e.g. 5–20 mL)
- when the preparation has irritant properties (e.g. cytotoxic drugs)

- when subcutaneous or intramuscular injections would cause intolerable pain (e.g. aminophylline).

Intravenous injections may, however, be associated with a number of complications, such as:

- a haematoma caused by puncturing through, instead of into, the vein
- necrosis caused by the drug escaping into the surrounding tissues when the needle slips out of the vein and is simply lying in the tissues
- phlebitis at the injection site, resulting from a high concentration of an irritant agent, repeated injections or prolonged administration
- because of rapidity of action, intoxication or death if an error is made when calculating or measuring the dose.

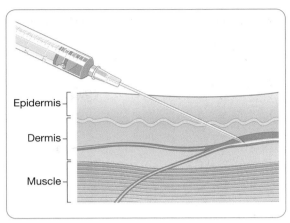

Fig. 4.10 Intravenous injection.

Those drugs recommended for administration intravenously by medical staff only will be made known within each trust.

It is important, however, that nurses understand how the procedure is carried out so that they can, if called on, play a supporting role. The standard approach to prescribing, administering and recording medicines is followed. To reduce the risk of introducing micro-organisms into the bloodstream, it is essential that the hands are washed, sterile equipment used and an aseptic technique practised. The patient should be given an explanation of what is to be done and should be in a comfortable position with the site to be used exposed. A vein in the elbow or the back of the hand is normally used. With the help of a tourniquet, the vein is distended to allow access. If indicated, the site of injection is swabbed with a suitable antiseptic and allowed to dry. A syringe with an eccentric nozzle and a 1-inch (25 mm) 20-gauge needle with an intravenous bevel are used for giving an intravenous injection. All air bubbles are expelled from the syringe and the needle filled with drug. Holding the syringe in line with the vein, the needle with the bevel up is pushed through the skin into the vein in the direction of the heart (Fig. 4.10). Before injecting, the position of the needle must be verified by gently pulling the plunger. If no blood is aspirated, the needle must then be withdrawn and another attempt made. After releasing the tourniquet and making an initial injection of 0.1 mL, there should be a pause of at least 30 s to observe the response before the remainder is slowly injected (up to 10 min). It is dangerous to give a rapid intravenous injection, as this exposes tissues and organs such as the heart and brain to high concentrations of a drug that has been poorly diluted with blood. A drug solution injected over 2 min will be 60 times more dilute than if injected over 2 s. After completing the injection, a sterile swab should be placed over the injection site, the needle slowly removed and gentle pressure maintained to avoid a haematoma.

Alternatively, intravenous drugs may be administered intermittently via the upper inlet of an indwelling intravenous cannula or into the administration set of an intravenous infusion by means of a three-way stopcock or multiple-inlet device. If there is not a continuous fluid infusion to keep the cannula patent, a dilute heparin solution should be injected before and after the drug is administered to prevent blood from clotting in its lumen.

A summary of common routes for injection is given in Table 4.3.

OTHER ROUTES OF INJECTION

Although parenteral administration is normally accomplished by subcutaneous, intramuscular or intravenous routes, occasionally other routes are used to deliver a drug to a particular tissue or organ.

Intra-arterial injection. This route is sometimes used to inject or infuse drugs into an artery supplying the affected organ if the drugs are rapidly metabolised or systemically toxic. Cytotoxic drugs for the treatment of local neoplasms or radio-opaque substances used in arteriography may be injected in this way.

Intra-articular injection. In inflammatory conditions of the joints, particularly rheumatoid arthritis, corticosteroids are given by intra-articular injection to relieve inflammation and increase joint mobility. Insoluble, long-acting compounds such as triamcinolone hexacetonide are used. Corticosteroids should not be injected into infected joints. Tissues or joints injected with corticosteroids have an increased

Table 4.3 Summary of common routes for injections

	Subcutaneous	Intramuscular	Intravenous
Definition	Fatty layer beneath the skin	Into muscle	Into a vein
Indications	Drug would be destroyed in stomach if taken orally Self-administration desirable	Oral medication cannot be tolerated/used	Emergency situations Irritant medication Anaesthetics
Contraindications	Shock Inflamed or oedematous site	Emaciation Inflamed or oedematous site Shock Low platelet count Irritant substance	Poor venous access Irritant substance
Who may administer	Registered nurse Student nurse under supervision of registered nurse	Registered nurse Student nurse under supervision of registered nurse	Registered nurse who has received specialist training Into already sited cannula
Relative rate of onset of action	Slow	Moderate	Rapid
Maximum volume at one site	2 mL	3 mL	20 mL
Sites (commonest)	Outer aspect of upper arm Anterior aspect of thigh Abdominal wall, i.e. below umbilicus	Upper outer quadrant of buttock Anterolateral aspect of mid-thigh	Forearm Back of hand Antecubital fossa at elbow

Needle
  Length
 	
  Gauge
	$\frac{1}{2}$ inch (13 mm) or $\frac{5}{8}$ inch (16 mm)
	25-gauge (26- or 27-gauge if abdomen used)
		$1\frac{1}{2}$ inch (40 mm)
		
		21-gauge
			1 inch (25 mm)
			
			20-gauge

Angle	45–90° to the skin	90° to the skin	As near to parallel to the skin as possible
Hazards	Abscess formation	Nerve damage Abscess formation Injecting into large blood vessel	Cardiac embarrassment caused by very rapid administration Haematoma Extravasation Phlebitis/thrombophlebitis Air or particle embolism Localised infection Septicaemia

susceptibility to infections. It is therefore essential to observe full aseptic precautions when making these injections.

Intradermal (intracutaneous) injection. Intradermal injections are small-volume injections of the order of 0.02–0.1 mL, given with a tuberculin syringe and a 16-mm, 26-gauge needle. The most common site used is the anterior aspect of the mid-forearm to allow for ease of inspection. The injection is given just under the skin, holding the syringe about parallel (about 10–15°) to the skin and with the bevel facing upwards. The needle is advanced, and while doing so is elevated under the skin. The technique is most commonly used for the administration of certain diagnostic agents such as tuberculin purified protein derivative and skin testing solutions in the diagnosis of allergy. As the potential allergen is slowly injected, a small weal forms. The needle is slowly withdrawn and the site is not massaged, in an effort to reduce interference with the formation of the weal.

In testing for allergy, a distinct benefit in *not* cleansing the skin beforehand is that there is no risk of causing irritation that could interfere with the interpretation of the result. The local reaction is assessed 24–72 h later by measuring its diameter.

Intrathecal injection. It is necessary to administer some drugs intrathecally if they have poor lipid solubility and, as a result, do not pass the blood–brain barrier. In the treatment of meningitis, water-soluble antibiotics are administered by the intrathecal route to achieve adequate concentrations in the cerebrospinal fluid. Drugs administered by this route include penicillins, the choice of which will depend on the results of bacteriological examination of the cerebrospinal fluid. Doses have to be very carefully calculated and are much smaller than would be given by intramuscular or intravenous injection because, in effect, the antibiotic is being introduced into a closed system. An example of an adult dose of an antibiotic given intrathecally is 1 mg daily of gentamicin increasing if necessary to 5 mg daily. However, the use of the intrathecal route for administering antibiotics appears to have diminished, e.g. benzylpenicillin is no longer recommended for intrathecal administration.

Methotrexate is administered intrathecally (15 mg at weekly intervals) to treat meningeal leukaemia. Antifungal agents, opioids, corticosteroids and radio-opaque substances, used in the diagnosis of spinal lesions, are sometimes administered by this route. A product specially prepared for the intrathecal route should be used. In many instances, intrathecal therapy is supported by a course of the drug given by intramuscular or intravenous injection.

Drugs for intrathecal injection are normally injected between lumbar vertebrae 3 and 4 into the subarachnoid space of the spinal cord as part of the procedure of lumbar puncture. The role of the nurse is directed towards careful positioning of the patient, assisting the doctor in maintaining an aseptic technique, and providing the patient with support and encouragement throughout the procedure.

It is vitally important to maintain full asepsis in this procedure, because of the risk of infection being introduced into the central nervous system. Great care has to be taken with all the procedures involved. In view of the potential hazards involved in the intrathecal injection of drugs, whenever possible the drug should be supplied in a form that is ready to use without further manipulation. In any event, the injection – as well as being sterile – must not contain particulate matter. A sterile, disposable bacterial filter (0.22 µm) must be used between the syringe and needle as a final safeguard for the patient.

Because drugs injected intrathecally come into immediate, direct contact with nervous tissue, the consequences of inadvertent injection of drugs intended for administration by other routes may be catastrophic for the patient.

USE OF SYRINGE DRIVERS

Medication may be administered via a syringe driver either intravenously or subcutaneously (see also Fig. 26.3). The subcutaneous route is the more common of these routes and is typically used for the administration of heparin, insulin and cytotoxic drugs, and in palliative care (for technique, see p. 520).

In palliative care, this route is used when the patient has difficulty in swallowing, is vomiting or may be semi-conscious or unconscious. The use of a syringe driver allows continuous subcutaneous infusion treatment to be delivered and a steady concentration of analgesia to be achieved without the need for repeated injections. Diamorphine can be given by syringe driver to maintain analgesia. Other drugs administered in this way include antiemetics, sedatives and antimuscarinics.

SUBCUTANEOUS INFUSION

Patients suffering from dehydration for whatever reason may be treated by the administration of fluids by subcutaneous infusion. The great advantage of this method is that the infusion may be commenced as required by community nursing staff or relatives. An infusion of 3 L should be run over a 12- or 24-h period. The administration of the enzyme hyaluronidase assists in the subcutaneous absorption of the fluid.

INTRAVENOUS INFUSION

When large volumes of fluid (50 mL upwards) require to be administered over a prolonged period, the most effective method is intravenous infusion. The indications for intravenous infusion are:

- when a patient cannot take oral medication
- when a rapid response is required
- to maintain or restore blood volume
- when a drug is inactivated in the gastrointestinal tract
- when there is a problem of absorption from the gut
- to supply electrolytes or nutrients
- when it is important to control plasma levels of a drug
- to administer irritant substances (e.g. cytotoxic agents)
- in life-threatening infections, when it is vital to establish high concentrations of antibiotics in the tissues.

Intravenous infusions are normally packed in plastic containers and delivered to the patient via an intravenous administration set (Fig. 4.11) attached to an intravenous cannula (Fig. 4.12) that has been inserted into the patient's vein. Because of the considerable risk of introducing infection directly into the bloodstream, the infusion fluid, all parts of the administration equipment and any dressings used must be sterile.

Introducing an intravenous cannula and establishing the free flow of the infusion are the doctor's responsibility. Registered nurses (and midwives) who are appropriately trained are permitted to prepare the prescribed medication and administer it into an already established cannula. The care of the patient before and after the procedure, and the satisfactory maintenance of the intravenous line, rests with the nurse assigned to the patient.

Before assembling an intravenous line, it is important to do the following.

- Read and carefully check the label of the infusion container against the fluid prescription. This should be carried out by a registered nurse or by a student nurse under the supervision of a registered nurse. Local policy may dictate that two members of staff are to be involved at all times.

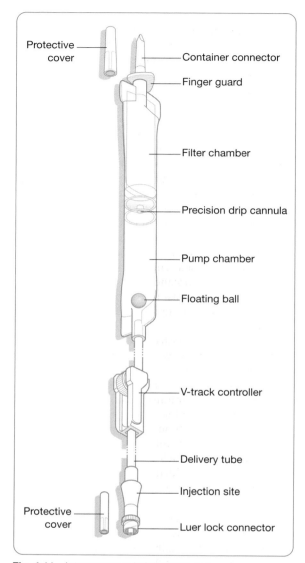

Fig. 4.11 Intravenous administration set.

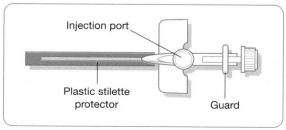

Fig. 4.12 Intravenous cannula.

- Check the expiry date.
- Record the batch number of each container so that, in the event of an adverse reaction to the infusion, the offending containers may be identified and withdrawn.
- Inspect the container to ensure that it has no flaws and that the fluid is clear and free from particulate matter.

The entry port of the container is pierced by the spike of the appropriate administration set, the filter chamber squeezed to fill the set with fluid, air removed from the tubing and the control clamp closed. The free end of the administration set is covered by its sheath until required for use. Once an infusion container is connected to an administration set, the risk of contamination through any of the points of entry should be recognised. The container is hung on an intravenous infusion stand that should be adjusted so that the container is just less than a metre above the cannula insertion site to achieve the optimum flow rate (Auty 1989).

The flow rate is adjusted by means of a roll clamp attached to the tubing. When accurate control of flow rate is essential, an automatic infusion system may be used that pumps solutions at a preset rate. As the fluid runs through the administration set, the container empties and, in so doing, collapses.

Adjuncts are sometimes used with this system, for example a calibrated burette may be incorporated in the system into which the infusion drips. One or more drugs can be added to the burette, and this is very useful, particularly in neonatal and intensive care units, for intermittent infusion of potent drugs in precise volumes. Drugs may be slowly injected through an additive port in the administration set or can be added to minibags usually containing either glucose 5% or sodium chloride 0.9% intravenous infusion. The contents of these secondary containers are infused using a Y-administration set, three-way tap or non-return valve. This method may be used to give a higher intermittent blood level of a particular drug than would be achieved if the drug were added to the larger primary container, or to avoid an incompatibility with a drug that may already be present in the primary container.

Drugs commonly given by intravenous infusion include antibiotics, lignocaine (lidocaine), heparin and potassium chloride. Cytotoxic drugs are frequently given by intravenous infusion. The infusion maintains a steady blood level of the drug over a prolonged period of time, and the patient is spared the pain of frequent injections. The addition of drugs to intravenous infusion fluids presents a number of hazards (e.g. resulting from interaction between the drug and the infusion fluid). Drugs should not be added to blood, plasma, lipid emulsions, saturated mannitol solutions, sodium bicarbonate solutions, amino acid solutions or dextran solutions, because these infusion fluids are particularly likely to be degraded.

In addition to interactions, the fluid infused can be contaminated by micro-organisms if admixtures are not carried out under strict aseptic conditions. Ideally, these additions should be made by pharmacy staff using laminar air flow cabinets in aseptic rooms and administered within 12–24 h. Complications such as thrombophlebitis (damage to the endothelium as the result of inflammation of the vein accompanied by formation of a blood clot) may arise at, and spread beyond, the site of cannula insertion. This results from physical or chemical irritation often related to the duration of the infusion or the type of fluid infused. Glucose is mildly acidic and, on autoclaving, a small quantity is broken down to hydroxymethylfurfural, and these two factors appear to cause a higher incidence of thrombophlebitis when glucose infusions are given. Blood for transfusion should never be mixed with any drug or solution other than sodium chloride 0.9%, because of the danger of interaction. If a unit of blood is preceded by a solution such as glucose, agglutination may result. To avoid this, the administration set should be flushed with sodium chloride 0.9% solution or changed.

The standard procedure for prescribing, checking and recording the administration of medicines similarly applies to intravenous infusions. The procedure should be explained to the patient in advance and the opportunity given to attend to toilet needs. A change into a garment with wider sleeves may be required to ensure that the infusion flow is unobstructed. If possible, whichever arm/hand will make things easier for the patient should be used. The patient should be comfortable, with the site of introduction of the infusion exposed and well lit. Some pain is usually experienced with the insertion of a needle, especially in the back of the hand, and patients appreciate having support and encouragement at this time.

The commonest sites of introduction are the forearm, the back of the hand and the antecubital fossa at the elbow. In an emergency, a vein in the foot or the external jugular vein may have to be used. A large straight vein, preferably at the junction of two veins and not running over a joint, is the one of choice.

The insertion of an intravenous cannula should be regarded as a minor surgical procedure. This, together with the fact that a cannula is to be lying in the vein for possibly several days, means that asepsis is an important objective. The prevention of microbial contamination begins with the appropriate handwashing technique. Careful preparation of the skin is important prior to insertion of the cannula. Although clipping extra-long hairs with scissors facilitates the subsequent removal of adhesive tape and is acceptable, shaving the skin is not recommended, because it produces tiny abrasions that may become infected. Any visible dirt is washed from the area with soap and water.

Before completing the preparation of the skin, the venous outflow is blocked and the vein distended by applying pressure above the site. This may be achieved in one of three ways:

- the use of a tourniquet
- the use of a sphygmomanometer cuff inflated to 100 mmHg
- with the help of an assistant, making sure not to apply too great pressure, as this may occlude the arterial supply.

The vein can also be made more prominent in different ways. For example:

- asking the patient to open and close the fist
- gently tapping the vein
- immersing the hand in hot water.

Increased venodilatation can also be achieved using glyceryl trinitrate applied in the form of a cream or transdermal patch (see p. 72) distal to the site of cannulation 20–30 min before venepuncture is performed.

Finally, the site is rubbed firmly for at least 30 s using a 70% alcohol swab and allowed to dry before puncturing the skin. Any further finger contact with the vein should be avoided.

Intravenous cannulae of different gauges are available. A small-gauge cannula (e.g. 19-gauge) is sufficient for the delivery of most therapy and limits both the size of the wound and the incidence of intra-vascular complications. When viscous fluids are to be administered, a large-gauge cannula (e.g. 18-gauge) is required. If a blood transfusion is likely to be required, the cannula introduced at the start of the infusion must be of large gauge (e.g. 16-gauge).

The cannula is checked to ensure that it is patent and has no obvious defects. With the bevelled edge uppermost, the cannula is firmly entered under the skin a short distance away from the vein, always pointing the cannula proximally towards the heart. It is then gently pushed into the vein, making sure to enter the plastic covering on the needle as well as the needle itself into the vein. Some types of cannula show a flash of blood at the hilt of the needle, indicating that the needle, but not necessarily the plastic cannula, is in the vein. The tourniquet is then removed and simultaneously the needle withdrawn and the plastic cannula gently advanced into the vein. A well-sited cannula should introduce with little or no resistance. The tubing of the administration set is quickly attached. Gentle pressure on the vein proximal to the cannula tip prevents a leakage of blood through the cannula.

When a small vein is used, the tubing may be attached earlier so that the cannula advances, while at the same time infusing fluid through it, thus displacing the walls of the vein. The control clamp is released and the flow rate observed. Subcutaneous swelling around the cannula indicates that it is not in the vein and must be removed.

The cannula is secured using an adhesive dressing designed for the purpose. The adjacent tubing is taped so as to prevent any pull on the cannula. A light conforming bandage promotes the patient's comfort. A splint may be applied and is essential if the cannula has been positioned over a joint.

On completion of the procedure, the patient should be made comfortable with the arm supported on a pillow, if required. Personal requirements such as a drink, tissues, sickness basin, reading material, etc. should be placed within reach. The call bell should also be to hand and instruction in its use given.

A regimen of fluids to be infused is prescribed by the doctor. The rate of flow required (i.e. the number of drops/min) can be calculated on the basis that, for solutions using a standard administration set, 1 mL equals 20 drops, that is:

$$\frac{\text{Volume of fluid (mL)} \times 20}{\text{Duration (min)}} \text{ drops/min.}$$

Thus, for 500 mL of fluid to be run through in 4 h the number of drops/min is:

$$\frac{500 \times 20}{240} = 41.66 \text{ rep.}$$

For working purposes, this figure may be regarded as 42.

To transfuse blood or blood components, a blood administration set is used that delivers 15 drops/mL.

Alternative methods of introducing an intravenous line are:

- surgically cutting down on a vein and introducing the cannula under direct vision (e.g. when no veins are visible or patent)

- by means of a central venous line (e.g. for prolonged feeding or for central venous pressure measurement).

Both these techniques are specialised procedures that are undertaken by experienced medical staff.

Throughout the ongoing administration of the infusion, the nurse's responsibilities are as follows.

OBSERVING THE PATIENT

Each time the patient is attended by the nurse, the patient's colour, respirations and general demeanour should be observed. An elevated temperature is noteworthy. Any apparent abnormality or change in the patient's condition should be reported to the nurse in charge or doctor.

OBSERVING THE INFUSION

A check is made that the infusion is running at the prescribed rate and that the container still has enough fluid in it. The nurse must anticipate the point when the container requires to be changed and estimate how much time will be required to get the next container checked and ready for use.

If the infusion is not running, a systematic list of checks should be made (Fig. 4.13).

When an infusion pump is in use, an alarm signals that the infusion is complete.

OBSERVING THE CANNULA SITE

The nurse must be alert to any:

- redness
- swelling
- leakage
- complaints from the patient of pain at or radiating from the cannula site.

KEEPING ACCURATE RECORDS

The following records must be maintained:

- fluid prescription sheet
- fluid balance chart
- nursing care plan and progress notes.

PROVIDING NURSING CARE

Even the most able patient requires some assistance when one limb is out of action. Indeed, patients are to be discouraged from trying to be too independent, as this can create movement of the cannula in the vein, especially one that crosses a joint, causing a mechanical phlebitis. Assistance with changing position, toileting, dressing, cutting up food, etc. will often be required.

REPORTING ABNORMALITIES

Although in most cases the infusion is established by doctors, doctors depend on nurses to notify them of any changes in the patient's condition, of either a localised or a generalised nature, and any difficulties encountered with the infusion. To reduce the risk of infection, it is normally recommended that administration sets be changed after 3 days (Band and Maki 1979, Josephson et al. 1985, Maki and Ringer 1987). However, sets should be changed directly following blood transfusion and, in the case of parenteral nutrition, daily.

The hazards associated with intravenous infusion may be localised or systemic and are potentially very dangerous.

Local hazards are:

- thrombophlebitis
- infection
- extravasation.

Systemic hazards are:

- septicaemia
- cardiac embarrassment caused by too rapid rate
- allergic reaction to fluid or drug
- air or particle embolism.

Consequently, checking procedures, asepsis, careful observation and prompt reporting are vitally important.

INFUSION SYSTEMS

Infusion systems are used to deliver fluids (including emulsions), electrolytes and drugs in solution by the intravenous (and subcutaneous) route. They have become increasingly sophisticated and widely used over the past 20 years. This trend will continue in the years ahead. In common with other drug delivery systems, infusion systems have all the key features outlined in Table 4.4.

The indications for the use of an infusion system include the need to maintain or restore blood volume, to deliver electrolytes and/or nutrients, and to administer drugs, especially those agents that are highly irritant and cannot be administered by other, more accessible routes. Infusion systems also provide the capability to control very accurately drug administration (e.g. cytotoxic therapy) over time, especially when a powered device is used.

INFUSION SYSTEMS RELYING ON GRAVITY

These infusion systems rely on gravity alone to provide the infusion pressure. It follows that the infusion container must be placed at a suitable height above

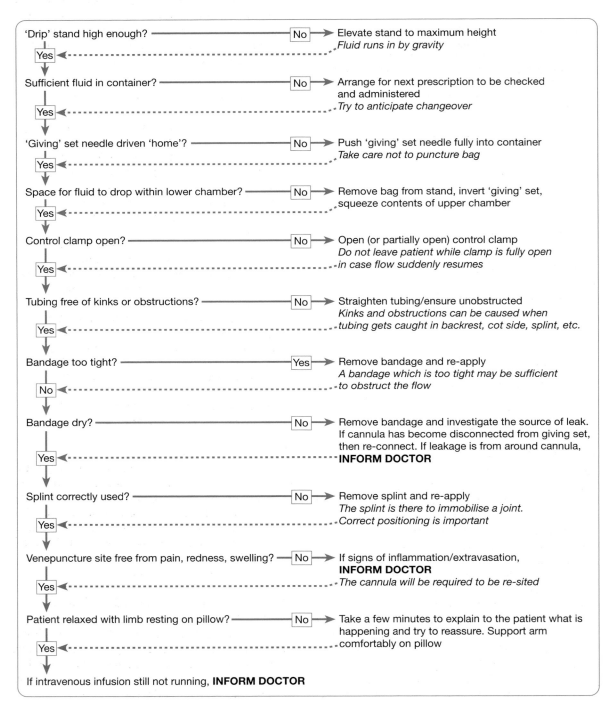

'Drip' stand high enough? ─────────── No ──→ Elevate stand to maximum height
  Yes ◄- *Fluid runs in by gravity*

Sufficient fluid in container? ─────────── No ──→ Arrange for next prescription to be checked
  Yes ◄- and administered
                                                              Try to anticipate changeover

'Giving' set needle driven 'home'? ─────────── No ──→ Push 'giving' set needle fully into container
  Yes ◄- *Take care not to puncture bag*

Space for fluid to drop within lower chamber? ─── No ──→ Remove bag from stand, invert 'giving' set,
  Yes ◄- squeeze contents of upper chamber

Control clamp open? ─────────── No ──→ Open (or partially open) control clamp
                                       Do not leave patient while clamp is fully open
  Yes ◄- *in case flow suddenly resumes*

Tubing free of kinks or obstructions? ─────────── No ──→ Straighten tubing/ensure unobstructed
                                                         Kinks and obstructions can be caused when
  Yes ◄- *tubing gets caught in backrest, cot side, splint, etc.*

Bandage too tight? ─────────── Yes ──→ Remove bandage and re-apply
                                       A bandage which is too tight may be sufficient
  No ◄- *to obstruct the flow*

Bandage dry? ─────────── No ──→ Remove bandage and investigate the source of leak.
                               If cannula has become disconnected from giving set,
                               then re-connect. If leakage is from around cannula,
  Yes ◄- **INFORM DOCTOR**

Splint correctly used? ─────────── No ──→ Remove splint and re-apply
                                          The splint is there to immobilise a joint.
  Yes ◄- *Correct positioning is important*

Venepuncture site free from pain, redness, swelling? ── No ──→ If signs of inflammation/extravasation,
                                                              INFORM DOCTOR
  Yes ◄- *The cannula will be required to be re-sited*

Patient relaxed with limb resting on pillow? ─── No ──→ Take a few minutes to explain to the patient what is
                                                       happening and try to reassure. Support arm
  Yes ◄- comfortably on pillow

If intravenous infusion still not running, **INFORM DOCTOR**

Fig. 4.13 What to do when an intravenous infusion stops.

Table 4.4 Key features of a drug delivery system

Structure	Containers, tubing, administration set, etc.
Energy source	Gravity or powered pump system
Control mechanism	Drip rate controller
Delivery port	Needle/cannula

the infusion site. Drip rate control is achieved by a simple mechanical clamp on the delivery tube. A drop sensor on the drip chamber monitors the rate of infusion. Such a device does not monitor resistance to infusion (leading to underinfusion), but overinfusion is effectively controlled. Drip rate controllers enable the flow rate to be selected in drops/min and controlled by identically powered valves. Such systems are acceptable in low-risk situations. A number of factors will influence the accuracy of drug delivery. Although the drop counting is accurate, the volume of delivery may not be (see p. 66). The use of volumetric controllers (calibrated in mL/h) avoids the need to carry out calculations on the drip rate.

POWERED INFUSION PUMPS

Infusion devices, such as infusion pumps and syringe drivers, are powered items of equipment that are capable of delivering fluids/drugs in a controlled manner in line with clinical requirements. Pumps have a number of advantages over gravity-powered systems. Notably, resistance to flow can be overcome by increasing delivery pressure. Safety mechanisms are normally provided if the entry port becomes blocked or displaced – normally referred to as occluded. Although the use of powered pumps does enable safe and accurate drug delivery to be achieved, the risks of malfunction must be recognised. The range of devices is summarised in Table 4.5.

Unfortunately, although giving great benefit to patients, the use of infusion systems is not without problems. Poor management procedures, lack of training and inadequate documentation have in many cases contributed to significant patient morbidity and mortality. Table 4.6 gives an indication of the range of problems that can arise.

SAFE MANAGEMENT OF INFUSION SYSTEMS

In order to achieve safe use of infusion systems, it is necessary to establish procedures that ensure that control is exercised at all stages from procurement of the equipment to use in patient care. A safe system will incorporate the following features.

- The structures and procedures established have the overall aim of reducing hazards to patients.
- Clear responsibilities for the choice of equipment and subsequent procurement are established, along with lines of accountability and responsibility. As few types of pump as possible should be used. They should be of the correct type and there should be adequate supplies of them. Extra sockets and cabling may have to be supplied. Operational manuals should always accompany items of equipment.
- A multidisciplinary committee is designated to oversee all aspects such as procurement, audit and monitoring, clinical/operational procedures and the effective communication of hazard warnings.
- Training needs are identified and met. Policy and procedure manuals should be readily available and kept up to date.
- Strong links are established with the local drug and therapeutics committee and other medicine management arrangements within the health authority. Infusion devices are used within the community, and so policies that recognise this dimension must also be established.

TECHNICAL SUPPORT

Technical staff play a vital role in carrying out a regular maintenance programme on all infusion devices. 'Imported' pumps, for example any that have been donated, should be checked before use. The functioning of all equipment sent for repair should be checked before its return to the clinical area. Technical staff also have an important advisory role in the day-to-day use of such equipment.

ROLE OF THE NURSE: INFUSION DEVICES

All clinical staff involved in the treatment of patients with an infusion device have specific responsibilities, but the responsibility for ongoing safety and comfort of the patient most definitely falls to the nurse. The potential for things to go wrong is very considerable, and the nurse's responsibilities are numerous. Knowledge of the principles involved is vital, and continuing evidence of clinical competence must be demonstrated. Attendance at in-service training sessions, as well as personal updating, is therefore imperative.

Table 4.5   Powered devices

Device	Notes
Drip rate pumps	Flow rate set in *drops/min*, peristaltic pump powers system. Such devices have few controls. The pressure of fluid in the line is not detected, and occlusion detection is very poor. As a result, these pumps are not recommended for use at present.
Volumetric pumps	Flow rate set in *mL/h*. Various safety features are present (e.g. alarm to signal empty infusion container, air in line, occlusion). These pumps are useful for medium and large flow rates and for large-volume infusions. They can employ many different methods for accurate delivery, and nurses must know the details for the pumps they will use.
Syringe pumps	A syringe containing the drug in solution is placed in a device that drives the plunger of the syringe at a predetermined rate. These devices are useful for low-volume/high-accuracy drug delivery. Syringes may be up to 60 mL. The volume is delivered in *mm/h* or *mm/24h*. Heparin, cancer chemotherapy and analgesia are commonly administered by this method. As with all devices, it is important to set up the equipment correctly (e.g. the correct size of syringe must be used and located securely in order to ensure accurate delivery). Miniature syringe pumps accepting syringes from 2 to 10 mL, which are battery-operated, can be used to achieve low rates of delivery (e.g. for insulin and for ambulatory patients).
Patient-controlled analgesia pumps	These devices provide for patient initiation of doses of a pain-relieving drug. Controls are built in to prevent overuse by the patient. Pumps for ambulatory use are similar but lighter for ease of carrying by the patient. A variety of programming options is available; loading dose, continuous infusion with or without bolus can be achieved. It is important to avoid free flow (siphonage) of solution, especially when patient supervision is minimal.
Other devices	
Pumps for the administration of anaesthetic agents	These pumps are designed for the specific purpose of administering anaesthetic agents.
Pumps using an elastomeric membrane	These disposable devices are 'powered' by an elastomeric membrane that contracts as a result of pressurisation caused by the filling process. They provide a simple method of administration especially suitable for home therapy.

Table 4.6   Examples of problems that can arise with infusion pumps

Type of error	Causes
Human error	Wrong rate/volume Failure to allow for priming volume Altered default settings Selection of inappropriate/wrong pump Incorrect loading (leading to occlusion or siphoning) Faulty pump in service Spillage of fluid (resulting in electric shock)
Equipment malfunction	Spontaneous failure Damage to equipment Flat battery Defect in set or bag Frequent alarms (staff start to ignore)
Other	Infiltration of tissues with fluid Patient or relative tampers with rate

The responsibilities of the nurse looking after patients with infusion devices may be summarised as follows.

- Being able to choose the most suitable pump by considering the following (Medical Devices Agency 2003).
    — Risk to the patient of:
        overinfusion
        underinfusion
        uneven flow
        high delivery pressure
        inadvertent bolus
        extravascular infusion.
    — Delivery parameters:
        infusion rate and volume required
        accuracy required (long and short term)
        alarms required
        ability to infuse into site chosen (venous, arterial, subcutaneous)
        suitability for infusing given drug (viscosity, half-life).
    — Environmental features:
        ease of operation
        frequency of observation and adjustment
        type of patient (e.g. very sick)
        mobility of patient (battery operation needed?).
- Using the administration set recommended by the pump manufacturer.
- Ensuring that all connections are tight but not overtight.
- Getting solutions, medications, rates and readings checked.
- Avoiding siphonage by positioning the device at the correct height.
- Keeping the alarm (when fitted) on and heeding it when it sounds.
- Ensuring that the medication is being administered.
- Checking the device every hour (in hospital) and on arrival at and departure from a home visit.
- Being observant at all times – of the patient, the infusion, the device and the documentation.
- Remembering that there is a patient attached to the infusion who requires reassurance.
- Keeping lines free from obstruction and, when more than one are in use, taping the lines (at both the pump end and the cannula end).
- Keeping all parts of the equipment clean (removing fluid from pump if spilled).
- Handling equipment carefully so as to avoid damage.
- Reporting abnormalities/discrepancies in rate at once.
- NEVER attempting to 'catch up' on the rate.

- Changing all components of the system every 24 h
- Recharging battery-operated devices by connecting to the mains supply.
- Labelling faulty equipment/reporting faults.
- Checking equipment on return from repair before next use.
- Instructing patients in the safe handling of portable equipment.

DISPOSAL OF SHARPS

Accidental inoculation with infected blood as a result of needlestick injury presents a major risk to the healthcare worker (Royal College of Nursing 2006). Despite the amount written about the prevention and management of sharps injury, many accidents still occur (May and Brewer 2001). Between July 1997 and June 2002, 1550 reports of blood-borne exposures in healthcare workers were reported, of whom 42% were nurses and midwives (Royal College of Nursing 2006). Sharps injuries can give rise to the transmission of HIV, the hepatitis B virus, hepatitis C and other blood-borne diseases. Injuries that do not involve contaminated blood, for example those that arise when drugs are being drawn up, carry with them fewer hazards but are nevertheless considered important because of the possible entry of infection through the punctured skin. Responsibility for safe practice rests with the employee through the Health and Safety at Work Act 1974 and the employer through the Control of Substances Hazardous to Health Regulations 1988.

One particularly important procedure in clinical practice is the disposal of needles. Resheathing of needles must not be attempted, and no attempt should be made to try to detach the needle from the syringe prior to disposal. The combined syringe and unsheathed needle should be carefully placed as a single unit in a rigid plastic sharps bin immediately after use. Needles should not be cut or bent, whether used or unused. It is the personal responsibility of the individual using the sharp to dispose of it safely (Royal College of Nursing 2006). Sharps containers should be sealed when two-thirds full. There should be a sufficient number of them to allow for replacement. In any case, no attempt should be made to press down the contents of a sharps container to create room for more. Sharps containers should be carried by their handles and placed in a secure place away from the public prior to ultimate disposal as medical waste by incineration or other high-temperature system. Although free sterile syringes and needles are available to people who abuse drugs, the risks of pilfering from sharps containers should not be overlooked. Access by patients and visitors (especially children) to sharps containers must be prevented. Staff should be aware of local inoculaton policy in the event of needlestick injury. The prospect of the availability of retractable syringes is good news.

TRANSDERMAL ADMINISTRATION

Although most preparations are applied topically to give a local effect, the topical route can also be used to achieve a systemic effect. This is the transdermal route of administration. Drugs administered in this way avoid first-pass metabolism by the liver (see p. 126). The best known is glyceryl trinitrate, used in the prophylaxis of angina. Where flexibility of dosage is required, this may be achieved with the application of an ointment containing 2% glyceryl trinitrate. Magnitude and duration of effect are directly related to the amount of ointment applied. It is therefore possible by this method to titrate the dosage against the clinical presentation of the patient. To obtain the optimum dosage, 12 mm (0.5 inch) of ointment is applied to the chest, arm or thigh on the first day, followed by 12-mm increments on each successive day until headache occurs; this length is then reduced by 12 mm. A graduated paper scale facilitates measurement of the dose. When applied to the skin, the ointment is covered with a simple dressing. It is not rubbed in. This is a messy procedure and therefore not commonly used.

A more sophisticated transdermal drug delivery system is the transdermal self-adhesive patch. Patches containing a reservoir of glyceryl trinitrate (see Fig. 4.14) are specially designed to achieve a prolonged and constant release of the drug. The main clinical indication for glyceryl trinitrate patches is in the prophylaxis of angina. The patches have also been used in the prophylactic treatment of phlebitis and extravasation, secondary to long-term venous cannulation.

Patches are available from which the average amount absorbed in 24 h is either 5 or 10 mg. One patch is applied every 24 h to a hairless area to ensure that it sticks well. The anterior or lateral chest wall is recommended, although the upper arm or shoulder is another suitable site. The site should have been washed and thoroughly dried, although not powdered, before applying the patch.

The sachet in which the patch is packaged should be torn rather than cut open, otherwise the patch might

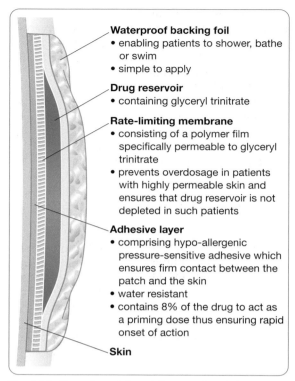

Waterproof backing foil
- enabling patients to shower, bathe or swim
- simple to apply

Drug reservoir
- containing glyceryl trinitrate

Rate-limiting membrane
- consisting of a polymer film specifically permeable to glyceryl trinitrate
- prevents overdosage in patients with highly permeable skin and ensures that drug reservoir is not depleted in such patients

Adhesive layer
- comprising hypo-allergenic pressure-sensitive adhesive which ensures firm contact between the patch and the skin
- water resistant
- contains 8% of the drug to act as a priming dose thus ensuring rapid onset of action

Skin

Fig. 4.14 Transdermal drug delivery system (rate-controlling membrane type).

be damaged. Without touching the sticky surface (which contains some medicament), the backing is removed and the patch applied, pressing firmly for about 5 s to ensure complete contact. The patch is then sealed to keep out air or water, by running the finger round its edge. A different area should be used each day to avoid skin irritation. Patients who are to be self-administering a transdermal drug for the first time should be counselled in its use. Tolerance to glyceryl trinitrate can develop, in which case the patch should be removed at bedtime and a fresh one attached next morning.

Several other drugs may be administered by this route. For example, a hyoscine patch to prevent motion sickness is placed behind the ear 5–6 h before travelling and replaced after 72 h, if necessary, by a patch behind the other ear; estradiol used in hormone replacement therapy is applied to unbroken areas below the waistline (not on or near the breasts or under the waistband) and is replaced after 3–4 days. Nicotine transdermal patches are available for weaning addicted smokers off their nicotine dependence. Fentanyl patches are widely used to relieve pain in palliative care.

The transdermal route of administration offers many advantages to the patient and the nurse, because it is non-invasive and convenient. However, the technology involved in developing and producing transdermal systems results in a relatively high-cost product. While the number of drugs that can be administered transdermally is gradually expanding, there are many problems to be overcome before a clinically effective product can be introduced. Not least of these problems is the efficient barrier to systemic absorption provided by the skin itself.

CALCULATIONS

With the development of clinical pharmacy services and the introduction of patient-specific medicines, the overall need for nurses to undertake calculations in connection with the administration of medicines and other pharmaceutical products has declined. Situations still arise, however, when nurses need to perform basic calculations, and these they must be able to do accurately and with confidence. Moreover, there is concern at the lack of numeracy among student nurses due to graduate (Hall 2006).

SI UNITS

In order to calculate how to obtain a particular dose for an individual patient, a sound understanding of Système International d'Unités (SI) units of mass (weight) and volume is essential.

The international system of units for mass and volume is as follows.

Mass:
1 kilogram (kg) = 1000 grams
1 gram (g) = 1000 milligrams
1 milligram (mg) = 1000 micrograms
1 microgram[a] = 1000 nanograms[a]
Volume:
1 litre (L) = 1000 millilitres
1 millilitre (mL) = 1000 microlitres (mL)

[a]It should be noted that these denominations must not be abbreviated in prescription writing, because of the possibility of confusion with other abbreviations.

UNITS OF ACTIVITY

The strength of some medicines obtained from natural products is expressed in units of activity per given volume, for example 100 units/1 mL (insulin), 5000 units/mL (heparin), 100 000 units/mL (nystatin). The abbreviation 'U' should not be used, because it has been mistaken for a zero, with disastrous consequences. The word 'units' must *always* be written in full.

PERCENTAGES

The strength of active ingredient in some pharmaceutical products may be expressed as a percentage, meaning parts per 100 parts. This is expressed in four ways.

- Percentage weight in volume (% w/v). The expression 5% w/v indicates that 5 g of active ingredient is present in 100 mL of product.
- Percentage weight in weight (% w/w). The expression 5% w/w indicates that 5 g of active ingredient is present in 100 g of product.
- Percentage volume in volume (% v/v). The expression 5% v/v indicates that 5 mL of active ingredient is present in 100 mL of product.
- Percentage volume in weight (% v/w). The expression 5% v/w indicates that 5 mL of active ingredient is contained in 100 g of product.

THE MOLE AND THE MILLIMOLE

The strength of a pharmaceutical preparation used in electrolyte replacement therapy is normally expressed in mmol/tablet or mmol/given volume f solution. In addition, the strength of a solution will be expressed as a percentage.

A mmol is one-thousandth of a mole, which is the molecular weight of a substance expressed in g. Nurses will not normally be expected to calculate mmol from first principles but may have to calculate how much of a given solution to measure to obtain a particular dose.

ARITHMETIC REQUIRED FOR CALCULATING MEDICINE DOSES

A prerequisite of safe practice is the need to abide by the principles of basic arithmetic.

An understanding of fractions, decimals and proportion is essential. For a variety of reasons, the subject of arithmetic has not always been understood or favoured by nurses (Wright 2006) prior to entering the profession, and so it is incumbent on those who lack confidence in their ability to do basic arithmetic or have simply forgotten the skills involved to seek help urgently. The use of a calculator to determine the quantity or volume of medication to be given 'should not act as a substitute for arithmetical knowledge and skill' (Nursing and Midwifery Council 2004, p. 7).

As a note of encouragement, the need to carry out complex calculations has been greatly reduced. Indeed, in many instances there is no need to make a calculation at all. The difficulties encountered are now being recognised, and help is available. What cannot be achieved, other than by the individual, is an acceptance that practice is needed in this area of study.

EXPRESSING THE STRENGTH OF ACTIVE INGREDIENT(S)

SOLID ORAL DOSE FORMS

In most cases, the strength of the active ingredient(s) present in each tablet or capsule will be expressed on the label of the product in g, mg or micrograms, for example amoxicillin 250 mg. Quantities of less than 1 g should always be expressed in mg, thus the expression 500 mg is used and not 0.5 g. Similarly, quantities of less than 1 mg should always be expressed in micrograms. This approach should always be followed when prescribing, recording the administration of and ordering or dispensing medicines. This reduces the need to use the decimal point, which, if incorrectly placed, can lead to massive errors in drug administration. The need for the decimal point to be used remains when doses such as 37.5 mg are required.

Products used for electrolyte replacement therapy, in addition to a strength of active ingredient being given in g or mg, will also have the strength quoted in mmol.

On some occasions, it is necessary to convert fractions of a mg into micrograms. This should rarely be required, because, for quantities less than 1 mg, the prescriber should use micrograms in writing the prescription and the label on the container should bear the strength of the product expressed in micrograms. Unfortunately, situations may arise when the dose is expressed in micrograms and the product available is labelled in mg, or vice versa.

Calculations involving solid dose forms will generally cause few problems, but as with all calculations the need for accuracy cannot be overstated. Sometimes, there will be no alternative but to subdivide a tablet (using a tablet splitter) or to give a number of tablets to obtain the prescribed dose. The medicine is transported to the patient on a medicine spoon or in a medicine measure.

An example of an oral solid calculation is given on p.75.

LIQUID ORAL DOSAGE FORMS

The amount of active ingredient per given volume is given for the strength of preparations such as antibiotic syrups. An ampicillin syrup will bear a label stating that the product contains 250 mg in 5 mL. It is in connection with the administration of liquids (oral and parenteral) that calculations are often required. A medicine measure, oral syringe or dropper will be used to measure and administer the medicine as appropriate.

Doses of liquid medicines (oral and parenteral) are calculated using the same principles.

LIQUID PARENTERAL DOSAGE FORMS
Small-volume injections

Two main approaches will be encountered, depending on the volume of the product.

- Small-volume injections will normally bear a label expressing the strength of the product in a manner similar to that used for oral liquids. For example, an injection will be shown to contain 25 mg per 1 mL, but care should be taken to note the volume contained in each ampoule because, if the ampoule contains 2 mL, the amount of active ingredient in 2 mL is 50 mg.
- The strength of injections of local anaesthetics such as lignocaine (lidocaine) is commonly expressed as a percentage w/v.

On the label of parenteral products for electrolyte replacement therapy (large or small volume), the strength is frequently expressed as a percentage, mass per given volume, and mmol per given volume.

The strength of adrenaline (epinephrine) injections is still frequently expressed as 1 in 1000. This indicates that 1 g of active ingredient is contained in 1000 mL of product. Of more value to the nurse is the fact that 1 mL of the injection contains 1 mg of adrenaline.

When a product is supplied in an ampoule or rubber-capped vial as a dry powder for reconstitution before use, the label will give the amount of dry powder contained in it. When reconstituting such products prior to injection, the total volume produced by adding the diluent to the powder must be known if part of the total dose contained in the ampoule or vial is to be administered.

The method used for calculating small-volume parenteral products is exactly the same as for oral dosage forms. Parenteral doses are measured using an appropriate size of syringe. Insulin must always be administered using a special syringe specifically calibrated for insulin units. Some products are prepacked in a syringe ready for use.

An example is given on p.76.

Large-volume parenteral products

Labels on containers of large-volume infusion solutions will generally give information on the strength of the product in percentage terms. For example, solutions of sodium chloride may contain 0.9% w/v, or a glucose infusion may contain 5% w/v. Solutions for electrolyte replacement therapy will also contain information on the number of mmol of given electrolytes per given volume.

Other pharmaceutical products

The strengths of products such as lotions, sterile topical solutions, ointments and antiseptic solutions will generally be expressed as a percentage, i.e. liquid preparations as a percentage w/v, solid or semisolid preparations as a percentage w/w. When very dilute antiseptic solutions are in use, the strength may be expressed as the number of parts of active ingredient in a given volume of solution (e.g. 1 in 5000, 1 in 2000). In the first example, 1 g of the active ingredient is contained in 5000 mL of product; in the second, 1 g is contained in 2000 mL of product.

MAKING A CALCULATION

Four steps are involved in making a calculation.

1. Check the validity of the prescription (see p. 34).
2. Check the details on the label or packaging (see p. 35).
3. Compare the details on the label with those of the prescription.
4. Provided that everything is in order, and only then, a calculation may be made.

Individuals have preferences in the way they make a calculation, but this does not matter as long as the correct answer is reached on every occasion. Two possible approaches are suggested here.

- *Using first principles.* This method is based on using the information available and can often be done mentally. It is frequently used for calculating oral medicines when the units in the prescription and on the label are the same. For example:
  — the patient is prescribed 10 mg of an oral drug
  — the label states that each tablet contains 5 mg of the drug
  — the patient should therefore receive two tablets.
- *Using a simple formula.* This method is based on simple proportion and is useful when calculating liquid doses and when the units in the prescription and on the label are different. Until experienced, the nurse may wish to make the calculation on paper. The formula is:

$$\text{dose required} = \left(\frac{\text{dose prescribed}}{\text{dose available}} \right) \times \text{volume containing available dose}$$

Put simply, and easier to remember, this reads as:

$$\left(\frac{\text{want}}{\text{got}} \right) \times \text{volume}$$

For example:
- the patient is prescribed 500 mg of a suspension
- the suspension is available as 250 mg of drug in 5 mL
- applying the formula,

$$\left(\frac{\text{want}}{\text{got}} \right) \times \text{volume}$$

$$= \left(\frac{500 \text{ mg}}{250 \text{ mg}} \right) \times 5 \text{ mL}$$

$$= 2 \times 5 \text{ mL}$$

$$= 10 \text{ mL}.$$

CALCULATIONS INVOLVING RECONSTITUTION OF INJECTIONS

When an injection has to be reconstituted from a powder before use, it should be noted that the resulting volume is in excess of the volume of diluent added, owing to the displacement effect of the powder. This must be taken into account if a dose less than that contained in the vial is required. An example follows.

- A vial contains 500 mg, but the dose required is 200 mg.
- The addition of 5 mL of diluent yields a volume of 5.25 mL when drawn into the syringe. This must be taken into account when using the formula.

DOSAGE CALCULATIONS INVOLVING BODY SURFACE AREA

In certain specialised forms of therapy (e.g. cytotoxic drug therapy), drug dosage is based on body surface area. The patient's body surface area is determined from a table (nomogram) using the patient's body weight and height.

CALCULATING DOSES SAFELY

Several key points should be uppermost in the mind of the nurse when making a calculation. These can be summarised as follows.

- Take great care when dealing with very small quantities (e.g. micrograms) and very large quantities (e.g. multiple tablets).
- Take great care with fractions of a mg. It is quite in order to ask the prescriber to change, for example, 0.25 mg to 250 micrograms.

Regular medicines – non-injectable

Date	MEDICINE (Block Letters)	DOSE	ROUTE OF ADMIN	TIMES OF ADMINISTRATION						SIGNATURE
				0800 hrs	1200 hrs	1400 hrs	1800 hrs	2200 hrs	Other Times	
Date	DILTIAZEM	360 mg	ORAL	✓						A. Prescriber

Label

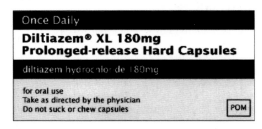

Once Daily

Diltiazem® XL 180mg
Prolonged-release Hard Capsules

diltiazem hydrochloride 180mg

for oral use
Take as directed by the physician
Do not suck or chew capsules

POM

Commentary

- A straightforward calculation
- Both prescription and label are in the same units

Workings

The prescribed dose is *more* than the amount contained in one capsule.

$$= \frac{\text{Dose required}}{\text{Strength available}}$$

$$= \frac{360 \text{ mg}}{180 \text{ mg}}$$

$$= \frac{36\cancel{0} \text{ mg}}{18\cancel{0} \text{ mg}}$$

$$= \frac{36}{18}$$

$$= \frac{6}{3}$$

$$= 2$$

The patient will be given:
2 capsules

Fig. 4.15 Example of calculation for a regular, non-injectable medicine. (From Downie G, Mackenzie J, Williams A 2006 Calculating drug doses safely: a handbook for nurses and midwives. Churchill Livingstone, Edinburgh. With permission of Elsevier.)

- Remember that you are *comparing* the label with the prescription.
- When two persons are calculating a dose, it is advisable to do so independently to increase accuracy.
- If in any doubt, do not proceed.
- If unsure about the dose, ask for clarification from the prescriber.
- Before administering a medicine, consider whether the quantity is reasonable.
- To ascertain availability of different strengths of a medicine, ask the pharmacist.

The examples in Figures 4.15 and 4.16 are included for demonstration purposes. More examples to practise may be found in the self-assessment exercises at the end of this chapter. For more detailed guidance on calculating drug doses and for up to date clinical examples to practise, refer to *Calculating drug doses safely* by Downie et al., published in 2006 by Churchill Livingstone.

INTENSIVE CARE

Intensive care is appropriate for patients requiring or likely to require advanced respiratory support, support of two or more organ systems or, in those with chronic impairment of one or more organ systems, additional support for an acute reversible failure of another organ.

Once-only medicines

Date	MEDICINE	DOSE	ROUTE OF ADMIN	TIME OF ADMIN	SIGNATURE
Date	PHYTOMENADIONE	1 mg	IM	1205 hrs	A. Prescriber

Label

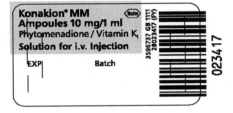

Konakion® MM
Ampoules 10 mg/1 ml
Phytomenadione / Vitamin K₁
Solution for i.v. Injection

EXP   Batch

3596737 GB 1111
2B023417 (FY)

023417

Commentary

- Take time when working with decimals
- If in doubt, use the formula
- Stick to the rules of arithmetic

Workings

The prescribed dose is *less* than the amount contained in 1 mL.

Applying the formula,

$$\frac{\text{Want}}{\text{Got}} \times \text{Volume}$$

$$= \frac{1\,\text{mg}}{10\,\text{mg}} \times 1\,\text{mL}$$

$$= \frac{1\,\text{mg}}{10\,\text{mg}} \times 1\,\text{mL}$$

$$= \frac{1}{10}\,\text{mL}$$

$$= 10\overline{)1.0}^{\,0.1}\,\text{mL}$$

$$= 0.1\,\text{mL}$$

The patient will be given:

0.1 mL IM injection

Fig. 4.16 Example of a calculation for a once-only medicine. (From Downie G, Mackenzie J, Williams A 2006 Calculating drug doses safely: a handbook for nurses and midwives. Churchill Livingstone, Edinburgh. With permission of Elsevier.)

Early referral is extremely important. Patients should be admitted to the intensive care unit (or intensive therapy unit, ITU) before their condition reaches a point from which recovery is impossible. Early referral improves the chances of recovery, reduces the potential for organ dysfunction, may reduce length of stay in the intensive care unit and hospital, and may subsequently reduce the costs of intensive care.

Admission criteria:

- severity of illness
- diagnosis
- age
- past medical history
- prognosis
- availability of suitable treatment
- recent cardiac event
- quality of life
- patient's wishes.

ORGAN SYSTEM MONITORING AND SUPPORT WITHIN THE ITU ENVIRONMENT

- Advanced respiratory support:
  — mechanical ventilation
  — possibility of a sudden deterioration in respiratory function requiring immediate endotracheal intubation and ventilation.
- Circulatory support:
  — need for vasoactive drugs to support arterial pressure or cardiac output
  — support for circulatory instability due to hypovolaemia
  — post cardiac arrest when intensive care is considered clinically appropriate
  — intra-aortic balloon pumping.
- Neurological support:
  — central nervous depression sufficient to prejudice the airway and reflexes
  — invasive neurological monitoring.
- Renal support:
  — haemodialysis, haemofiltration or haemodiafiltration.

FREQUENTLY SEEN CONDITIONS WITHIN THE ITU SETTING

SEPTIC SHOCK

Sepsis is the systemic response to an insult of proven or high likelihood of infection, compared with an infection that can be applied to a localised phenomenon. Sepsis can initiate a systemic inflammatory response syndrome and can affect other organs.

Criteria for systemic inflammatory response syndrome are:

- heart rate > 90 beats/min
- respiratory rate > 20 breaths/min
- temperature > 38°C or below 36°C
- leucocytes > 12 000 cells/mm^2 or < 4000.

The early twentieth century mortality rate from sepsis of 41% remains virtually unchanged today.

As inflammation becomes systemic, inflammatory responses throughout the body cause:

- body vasodilation
- increased intravascular space
- increased capillary permeability
- oedema
- hypovolaemia
- hypoperfusion with tissue hypoxia.

Treatment includes:

- empirical antibiotic therapy depending on the severity of the illness
- fluid resuscitation
- inotropes.

Cardiogenic, neurogenic and hypovolaemic shock, and toxic shock syndrome are also seen within the ITU setting.

NEUROLOGICAL INSULT

Neurological failure may occur after head injury, poisoning, cerebral vascular accident, cardiac arrest, metabolic encephalopathy (e.g. liver failure) or infections of the nervous system (meningitis or encephalitis). Loss of consciousness can lead to obstruction of airways and loss of protective airway reflexes that require mechanical ventilation.

Sustained high intracranial pressure can cause ischaemic brain damage and is usually fatal. Progressive cellular damage can cause:

- intracellular oedema and cell death
- hyperkalaemia
- capillary vasodilation
- seizures
- thermoregulatory issues.

Treatment for increased intracranial pressure while ventilated includes:

- bed 30° head-up tilt
- minimal endotracheal suction
- sedation, analgesia and possibly thiopentone
- titrating ventilation
- corticosteroids
- mannitol.

MAJOR TRAUMA

Such patients are admitted to the ITU for close observation and rigorous medical management. As well as experiencing multiple fractures, they may have suffered chest or heart injuries including diaphragmatic rupture; injuries to the aorta, pericardium, lungs and airways; and damage to other organs.

Treatment includes:

- restoration of adequate tissue perfusion and gas exchange
- analgesia
- correction of coagulopathy
- prompt attention to complications
- close monitoring
- adequate nutrition.

Spinal injuries, near drownings and burns are also seen in the ITU environment.

MULTIORGAN FAILURE

Multiorgan failure involves dysfunction of two or more organs and is one of the main causes of mortality in the ITU. Multiorgan failure can be used to describe two organ failure but is more often used when all organs are failing.

However caused, multiorgan failure represents a vicious downward spiral of gross ischaemia causing hypoxaemia and failure of most or all organs.

Treatment objectives include:

- oxygen saturations of 90–95%
- maintenance of cardiac output/oxygen delivery and blood pressure with adequate organ perfusion
- adequate metabolic and fluid homeostasis with intravascular filling, diuretics, vasoactive agents and/ or renal replacement therapy
- haemoglobin at > 9–10 g/dL
- careful infection control and antibiotics
- early nutrition (enteral or parenteral).

DRUGS USED IN THE ITU

SEDATION

Sedation is necessary for most ITU patients. It is used to ensure comfort for the critically ill, to help prevent patients 'fighting' the ventilator, and to help remove much psychological trauma that is associated with ITU admissions. However, most sedative drugs have severe respiratory and cardiovascular side effects as well as being cumulative.

Propofol is a commonly used sedative in the ITU environment. Advantages of propofol include a rapid onset of action and a rapid recovery even after prolonged infusion. It is administered as an emulsion in 10% Intralipid, and infusion volumes may contribute to the calorie load of the patient. This must be taken into account when enteral/parenteral feed is prescribed.

Dose. For continuous infusion: 4 mg/kg per h. It should be titrated to the required sedation level.

Benzodiazepines (diazepam and midazolam) are also used.

PARALYSING AGENTS

Paralysing agents, which are also known as muscle relaxants, are used in the ITU to help control acutely raised intracranial pressure and help to prevent surges in intracranial pressure in response to stimuli such as physiotherapy and endotracheal suctioning. They can also be used to facilitate ventilation.

Paralysing agents cannot cross the blood–brain barrier and therefore have no sedative or analgesic effects. For this reason, it is essential to accompany paralysing drugs with sedative/analgesic drugs in order to avoid the intolerable situation of a patient who is aware, often in pain, but unable to move.

Atracurium is the most popular paralysing agent used in the ITU environment. It is non-cumulative but can cause bradycardia and hypotension.

Dose. For continuous infusion: 200–400 micrograms/ kg per h.

ANALGESICS

Causes of acute pain in ITU patients can be obvious (e.g. surgery), but patients may also suffer from pre-existing chronic pain. Nursing and medical interventions can also cause pain (e.g. intubation, chest drain insertion/removal, endotracheal suctioning, dressing wounds and line insertion). Assessing pain, perceptions and needs can be difficult with ITU patients because of sedation, intubation and/or impaired psychomotor skills. However, comfort and pain relief are fundamental to nursing.

Alfentanil is 30 times more potent than morphine and of shorter duration than fentanyl, and is the usual drug of choice for a continuous analgesic infusion. Side effects include bradycardia, respiratory depression and urinary retention.

Dose. This is 1–5 mg/h (up to 1 microgram/kg per min).

Morphine, diclofenac, tramadol and paracetamol are also used.

INOTROPES

Conditions requiring the careful administration of inotropes include septic shock, cardiogenic shock and other low cardiac output states. Catecholamine inotropes (e.g. adrenaline [epinephrine], noradrenaline [norepinephrine] and dobutamine) are commonly used in the ITU setting. They increase the force of myocardial contraction and are usually given by a continuous infusion.

All inotropes should be titrated to the patient's weight. However, most critically ill patients need to be quickly commenced on a 'standard dose' until such time as the patient can be weighed.

Side effects include arrhythmias and myocardial ischaemia. Overdoses can cause life-threatening hypertension, necessitating careful titration and close monitoring with an arterial line, either invasive or non-invasive cardiac output monitoring and continuous electrocardiogram. Inotropes must NOT be attached to the central venous pressure monitoring line port, to prevent a surge of the drug being administered when flushing the line. They must also always be administered centrally, never peripherally, in order to prevent extravasation.

Dose. Standard starting concentration for adrenaline and noradrenaline: 30 micrograms/kg. For 70 kg: 30 micrograms × 70 = 2.1 mg of adrenaline or noradrenaline, usually made up to 50 mL of dextrose 5% to prevent oxidation.

However, the rate and concentration that may be doubled or tripled will depend on the patient's blood pressure. Isoprenaline and dopamine are also used.

ROUTES OF ADMINISTRATION

Intravenous drugs are usually administered centrally. Peripheral blood flow may be absent due to the patient's condition (e.g. shock or peripheral blood flow provides insufficient dilution).

Centrally administered drugs act more rapidly, and the patient must be closely monitored during and after administration. Residual particles of drugs in the lines may precipitate with subsequent drugs. Nurses must observe the lines during administration and flush them with sodium chloride 0.9% solution afterwards and between drugs.

Central lines may have single, double, triple or quadruple lumens and are commonly inserted into the internal jugular, femoral or subclavian vein. They allow continuous monitoring of the central venous pressure and the administration of multiple continuous infusions and boluses. Central line insertion can cause an air embolism, venous thrombosis, pneumothorax, infection, arrhythmias and arterial puncture.

- Intravenous drugs are the most common route for the critically ill. Total parenteral nutrition is often administered to the critically ill via a central line.
- Intramuscular drugs are seldom used, because of the increased risk of coagulopathy and unpredictable absorption due to varying cardiac output and blood flow.
- Subcutaneous heparin is commonly administered. However, absorption is variable.
- Oral administration includes nasogastric, nasoduodenal and nasojejunal feeding tubes. Surgical jejunostomy tubes are occasionally required. Drugs given by these routes should be in liquid form or finely crushed and dissolved in water. Varying splanchnic blood flow, inconsistent hepatic function and altered intestinal transit times make this an unreliable form of drug administration in the critically ill.
- Rectal absorption is also unpredictable.

CRITICAL CARE NURSING

Critically ill patients require close nursing supervision on a one-to-one basis. However, many patients are severely ill, requiring multiple interventions and have a dependency greater than one to one.

To be an effective critical care nurse, there is a need to meet the physical, psychological, spiritual and social needs of the patient as well as being a competent technician. While coping with the critical care environment, there is a risk of dehumanising patients.

Critical care nurses often work in stressful situations in which there are conflicting demands on their time from the patient, their significant others and the technology. Through training, education, experience and support, critical care nurses will learn how to meet all these demands while delivering the optimum level of care.

These specialist nurses need to maintain the safety, dignity and humanity of the patient while ensuring that the technology is functioning correctly. When critical care nurses become experts in their field, they are able to combine all the aforementioned functions while minimising the adverse effects of the technology.

SELF-ASSESSMENT QUESTIONS

SECTION A

All nurses and midwives, both pre- and postregistration, should be able to answer the following questions.

1. Apart from the patient's biographical details, what information *must* appear on every prescription?
2. What methods may be used to identify a hospital patient prior to the administration of a medicine?
3. How may a patient be assisted in taking an oral medicine?
4. How should you pour an oral liquid medicine?
5. Under what circumstances should a tablet be divided?
6. How should a tablet be divided?
7. List 10 locations on a ward where pharmaceutical products may be stored.
8. What should you do with a medicine container whose contents are time-expired?
9. What sources of reference are normally available to the nurse administering medicines?
10. You have just dispensed the patient's medicines when she asks you to take her to the toilet urgently. What should you do?

	Paracetamol	Prednisolone	Diamorphine
Class of drug			
Storage			
Formulations available			
Indications for use			
Contraindications			
Normal dose range			
Common side effects			

SECTION B

Using the British National Formulary if necessary, complete the above table.

SECTION C

1. Why must oral glyceryl trinitrate be given by the sublingual route?
2. Why must insulin be given by injection?
3. Why is the intravenous route used to administer drugs in an emergency?
4. Why should you never transfuse blood immediately following a glucose infusion?
5. Why should infusions containing potassium be administered and controlled via an infusion pump?
6. Why should the skin not be rubbed after injecting heparin?
7. Why is it crucial that intravenous drugs are never given by the intrathecal route?
8. Why should tablets or capsules be swallowed with a drink?
9. Why is the skin not cleansed when testing for allergens?
10. Why are intramuscular injections never prescribed for leukaemic patients?

SECTION D

1. Intramuscular injections are administered into the upper outer quadrant of the buttock so as to avoid:
   a. the vastus lateralis
   b. the gluteus maximus
   c. the sacroiliac joint
   d. the sciatic nerve.
2. After cleaning the top of a rubber-capped vial with an alcohol swab, you should wait:

a. 10 s
b. 30 s
c. 60 s
d. 15 s.

3. Place the following in order of speed of action from fastest to slowest:
   a. intramuscular
   b. oral
   c. transdermal
   d. subcutaneous
   e. intravenous.
4. The administration of medicines by injection is known as:
   a. paternal
   b. parenteral
   c. parental
   d. peritoneal.
5. The size of needle normally used for an adult receiving intramuscular injections is:
   a. 19-gauge
   b. 25-gauge
   c. 21-gauge
   d. 23-gauge.

SECTION E

Who would you inform if the following occurred?
1. Extravasation of a drug.
2. Faulty infusion pump.
3. Patient unable to swallow tablets.
4. Patient receiving intravenous infusion becomes breathless.
5. Patient has difficulty picking up tablets.
6. Pharmacy has supplied a change of formulation of a prescribed medicine.

81

SECTION F

1. Where are the gluteal muscles situated?
2. Where in the body is an intrathecal injection given?
3. Where is a buccal tablet placed?
4. Where can subcutaneous injections be given?
5. Where in the body are intravenous injections commonly given?
6. Where should reconstituted antibiotics normally be stored?
7. Where can you apply a transdermal patch?
8. Where on the body is allergy testing done?
9. Where should infusions with additives be prepared?
10. Where are drug prescription and recording sheets stored after a patient is discharged?

SECTION G

In the following examples, calculate what you would give to the patient.

1. See Figure 4.17.
2. See Figure 4.18.
3. See Figure 4.19.

SECTION H

In the examples on page 84, calculate what you would give to the patient.

Regular medicines − non-injectable

Date	MEDICINE (Block Letters)	DOSE	ROUTE OF ADMIN	TIMES OF ADMINISTRATION							SIGNATURE
				0800 hrs	1200 hrs	1400 hrs	1800 hrs	2200 hrs	Other Times		
Date	PROMAZINE	200 mg	ORAL	✓	✓		✓	✓			A. Prescriber

Label

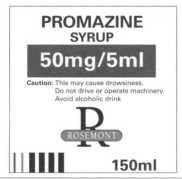

PROMAZINE
SYRUP
50mg/5ml

Caution: This may cause drowsiness. Do not drive or operate machinery. Avoid alcoholic drink

℞
ROSEMONT

150ml

Fig. 4.17 Calculation of a regular medicine: non-injectable. (From Downie G, Mackenzie J, Williams A 2006 Calculating drug doses safely: a handbook for nurses and midwives. Churchill Livingstone, Edinburgh. With permission of Elsevier.)

Regular medicines – non-injectable

Date	MEDICINE (Block Letters)	DOSE	ROUTE OF ADMIN	TIMES OF ADMINISTRATION						SIGNATURE
				0800 hrs	1200 hrs	1400 hrs	1800 hrs	2200 hrs	Other Times	
Date	OSELTAMIVIR	75 mg	ORAL	✓					2000	A. Prescriber

Label

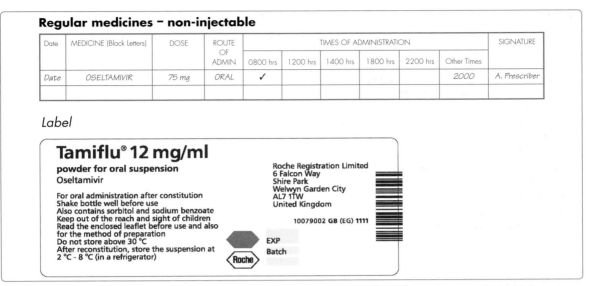

Fig. 4.18 Calculation of a regular medicine: non-injectable. (From Downie G, Mackenzie J, Williams A 2006 Calculating drug doses safely: a handbook for nurses and midwives. Churchill Livingstone, Edinburgh. With permission of Elsevier.)

Once-only medicines

Date	MEDICINE	DOSE	ROUTE OF ADMIN	TIME OF ADMIN	SIGNATURE
Date	FUROSEMIDE	2 mg	IV	2150 hrs	A. Prescriber

Label

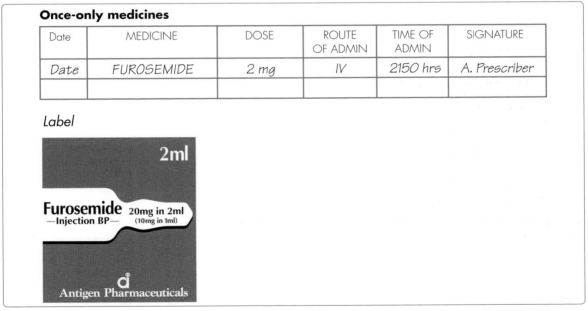

Fig. 4.19 Calculation of a once-only medicine. (From Downie G, Mackenzie J, Williams A 2006 Calculating drug doses safely: a handbook for nurses and midwives. Churchill Livingstone, Edinburgh. With permission of Elsevier.)

Dose prescribed	Dose available	What would you give?
1.5 g	300 mg/5 mL	mL
75 mg	25 mg/mL	mL
0.1 mg	0.05 mg	tablets
500 000 units	300 000 units/mL	mL
12 mg	4 mg	tablets
1 g	500 mg	tablets
60 mg	5 mg	tablets
15 mg	5 mg	tablets
24 mg	8 mg	tablets
125 micrograms	62.5 micrograms	tablets
100 mg	50 mg/mL	mL
0.5 g	250 mg/mL	tablets
100 mg	25 mg/mL	mL
0.4 mg	0.6 mg/mL	mL
62.5 mg	250 mg/mL	mL
175 micrograms	50 micrograms/mL	mL
1 g	250 mg	mL
20 000 units	5000 units/mL	mL
500 mg	250 mg	tablets
1.6 g	800 mg/3 mL	mL
3 mg	0.6 mg/mL	mL
125 micrograms	50 micrograms/mL	mL
12.5 mg	12.5 mg/2 mL	mL
50 micrograms	100 micrograms/mL	mL
1 million units	10 million units/mL	mL
0.5 g	500 mg	tablets
50 micrograms	100 micrograms/mL	mL
12 mg	15 mg/mL	mL
40 mg	80 mg/mL	mL
2.5 mg	10 mg/2 mL	mL

REFERENCES

[Anonymous] 1974 Health and Safety at Work Act. HMSO, London

[Anonymous] 2005 Big bottom may stop injections working effectively. Scotsman 29 November 2005

Auty B 1989 Choice for instrumentation for controlled IV infusion. Intensive Therapy and Clinical Monitoring 10:117–122

Band J, Maki D 1979 Safety of changing intravenous delivery systems at longer than 24-hour intervals. Annals of Internal Medicine 90:173–178

Beyea SC, Nicoll LH 1996 Administering IM injections the right way. American Journal of Nursing 96:34–35

Brenner LR, Wood KM, George D 1981 Effects of alternative techniques of low-dose heparin administration on haematoma formation. Heart Lung 10:657–660

Burden M 1994 A practical guide to insulin injections. Nursing Standard 8:25–29

Channer K 1985 Stand up and take your medicine. Nursing Times 81:41–42

Clinical Resource and Audit Group of NHS Scotland 2002 Good practice statement for the preparation of injections in near-patient areas, including clinical and home environments. CRAG, Edinburgh

Conaghan P 1993 Subcutaneous heparin injections – bruising. Surgical Nurse 6:25–27

Cullen B 2004 Skin disinfection prior to intradermal, subcutaneous and intramuscular injection administration. Online. Available: http://www.show.scot.nhs.uk/scieh/infectious/hai/infection_control/documents/Skin_Disinfection_Review_0800604.pdf

Dann TC 1969 Routine skin preparation before injection: an unnecessary procedure. Lancet ii:96–97

Downie G, Mackenzie J, Williams A 2006 Calculating drug doses safely: a handbook for nurses and midwives. Churchill Livingstone, Edinburgh

Hall J 2006 A third of new nurses fail simple English and maths test. Daily Telegraph 5 August 2006

Health and Safety Executive 1988 Control of Substances Hazardous to Health Regulations 1988. Statutory instrument no. 1657. HMSO, London

Josephson A, Gombert ME, Sierra MF et al. 1985 The relationship between intravenous fluid contamination and the frequency of tubing replacement. Infection Control 6:367–370

Kirkevold O, Engedal K 2005 Concealment of drugs in food and beverages in nursing homes: cross sectional study. In: John D 2005 Can we justify placebo use or covert drug administration? Pharmacy in Practice May:206–207

Koivisto VA, Felig P 1978 Is skin preparation necessary before insulin injection? Lancet i:1072–1073

Maki DG, Ringer M 1987 Evaluation of dressing regimens for prevention of infection with peripheral intravenous catheters. Journal of the American Medical Association 256:2396–2403

May D, Brewer S 2001 Sharps injury: prevention and management. Nursing Standard 15:45–52

McGowan S, Wood A 1989–1990 Administering heparin subcutaneously: an evaluation of techniques used and bruising at the injection site. Australian Journal of Advanced Nursing 72:30–39

Medical Devices Agency 2003 Infusion systems. Device Bulletin MDA DB 9503. Department of Health, London

Millar A, Hughes D, Kerr S 2006 The safe preparation of injections in near-patient areas. Hospital Pharmacist 13:128–130

Nursing and Midwifery Council 2004 Guidelines for the administration of medicines. NMC, London

Nursing and Midwifery Council 2006 Medicines management. A–Z advice sheet. NMC, London

Peragallo-Dittko V 1997 Rethinking subcutaneous injection technique. American Journal of Nursing 97:71–72

Royal College of Nursing 2006 Sharps injury. RCN, London

Shaw NJ, Lyall EGH 1985 Hazards of glass ampoules. British Medical Journal 291:1390

Spraul M, Chateleau E, Kovmovlidov J et al. 1988 Subcutaneous or nonsubcutaneous injection of insulin. Diabetes Care 11:733–736

Springhouse Corporation 1993 Medication administration and IV therapy manual, 2nd edn. Springhouse Corporation, Pennsylvania

Torrance C 1989 Intramuscular injection. Part 2. Surgical Nurse 2:24–27

Workman B 1999 Safe injection techniques. Nursing Standard 13:47–53

Wright K 2006 Barrier to accurate drug calculations. Nursing Standard 20:41–45

FURTHER READING AND RESOURCES

Gatford JD, Phillips N 2002 Nursing calculations, 6th edn. Churchill Livingstone, Edinburgh

King L 2003 Subcutaneous injection technique. Nursing Standard 17:45–52

Lapham R, Agar H 1995 Drug calculations for nurses: a step by step approach. Arnold, London

Lawson T 2002 Guide to simple and safe local steroid injections. Prescriber 13:48–55

Mallett J, Dougherty L (eds) 2000 The Royal Marsden Hospital manual of clinical nursing procedures, 5th edn. Blackwell Science, Oxford

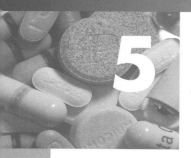

5 Nurse prescribing

CHAPTER CONTENTS

KEY OBJECTIVES

After reading this chapter, you should be able to:

- outline the rationale for the development of nurse prescribing
- list three of the features required in the development of a patient group direction
- detail the key points to consider before prescribing a medicine
- understand and discuss the responsibilities associated with prescribing rights.

INTRODUCTION

The prescribing of medicines by nurses is a significant development of their professional role. First recommended by the Royal College of Nursing in 1980 (Blatt 1997) and addressed in more detail in the Cumberlege Report (Department of Health and Social Security 1986), nurse prescribing evolved with the growing realisation that much of patients' and community nurses' time was being wasted in waiting to get prescriptions signed by a doctor when in many cases it was the nurse who had recommended the dressing or appliance in the first place. It was also apparent that community nurses were becoming increasingly skilled in managing pain relief for terminally ill patients (Humphries and Green 1999). Clarification of professional responsibilities was long overdue. The Crown Report (Department of Health 1989) took the matter further with the recommendation that suitably qualified nurses working in the community should be authorised to prescribe in defined circumstances from a limited list, i.e. a nurse prescribers' formulary. A further recommendation was that nurses should be able to supply medicines within group protocols. The legislation permitting nurse prescribing within the NHS received the royal assent in March 1992. This primary legislation was introduced to permit appropriately qualified nurses working in community practice who had had the recognised additional training to prescribe (within the NHS) medicines and appliances (surgical dressings, etc.) needed for the nursing care of their patients.

In 2000, further proposals to extend the range of prescription-only medicines that may be prescribed by independent nurse prescribers were issued for consideration. These wider prescribing powers were granted in 2001.

A joint Medicine and Healthcare Products Regulatory Agency and the Department of Health consultation was undertaken in 2005 to examine options for the future of independent nurse prescribing. This was in response to claims that the Nurse Prescribers' Extended Formulary (NPEF) was too complex, and that supplementary prescribing could not be used in all settings in which patients would benefit, such as emergency care, as the clinical management plan (CMP) must be prepared in advance. Experience had also shown that updating the formulary was difficult and resource-intensive. A working group of the Committee on Safety of Medicines first considered the responses to the consultations in September–October 2005, and decided to recommend that suitably trained and qualified nurses and pharmacists should be able to prescribe any licensed medicine for any medical condition, within their own competence.

LEVELS OF AUTHORISATION

For many years, nurses had access to a range of medicinal and nursing care products that were used without medical prescription. With the interests of patient need and the effectiveness and safety profile of the products in mind, written protocols were subsequently developed. Such protocols took the form of, for example, a formulary of nursing care products. Guidance included in the protocols was determined jointly by clinical staff.

The development of policies such as those for symptomatic relief provided a framework to allow the nurse to use a limited number of simple medications used in the treatment of minor ailments (e.g. simple analgesia, aperients and demulcents). Doctors initiated symptomatic relief for the individual patient by entering the words SYMPTOMATIC RELIEF on the prescription, along with their signature and the date. Nurses use their professional judgement in selecting the appropriate preparation and dose from the agreed limited list and then administer and record it. Provided the guidelines that accompany the symptomatic relief policy are adhered to by the nurse administering the medicine(s), it is the doctor who is accountable for the effects of the medicine(s). The policy provides benefit to patients, doctors and nurses by speeding up the process of relieving the patient's symptoms, reducing the number of times doctors are interrupted, and allowing nurses to exercise their professional role in order to meet the needs of patients. With the reduction in junior doctor working hours and the requirement for greater professional accountability, it is likely that the increasing use of patient group directions (PGDs) and of independent and supplementary prescribing will supersede patient-specific policies.

A number of levels of authorisation are currently in place that, depending on the training and accreditation the individual has received, allow nurses to utilise their knowledge of patients and make informed judgements of a patient's requirements. These include the use of PGDs, independent formulary prescribing and supplementary prescribing. With the extension of independent prescribing rights to include almost the full range of medicines in the British National Formulary (BNF), the role of the nurse in prescribing is becoming ever more important.

PATIENT GROUP DIRECTIONS

Following concerns about the legality of group protocols highlighted in the Crown Report 2 (Department of Health 1999), changes were made to the Medicines Act 1968 that allow the legal supply and administration of medicines under PGDs, replacing the term *group protocol*. PGDs are written instructions for groups of patients in specific situations who have not been individually identified before presentation for treatment (Department of Health 1999). They allow prescription-only medicines to be administered or supplied without the need for a patient-specific 'direction' of a doctor.

Patient group directions have been introduced in both hospital and community practice to reduce the time that patients have to wait for treatment. Increased use of the nurse's professional skills has resulted in more effective utilisation of resources. Those authorised to supply or administer medicines under PGDs include individually named registered nurses, midwives, health visitors, pharmacists, and a range of professionals allied to medicine who have undergone training and accreditation relevant to the clinical condition(s) to be treated and medicine(s) to be used. Each PGD is formally established by local professional advisory groups in wide consultation with senior representatives of the appropriate professional group. The legislation specifies that each PGD must contain the following information:

- the name of the business to which the direction applies
- the date the direction comes into force and the date it expires
- a description of the medicine(s) to which the direction applies
- the class of health professional who may supply or administer the medicine
- the signature of a doctor or dentist, as appropriate, and a pharmacist
- the signature by an appropriate health organisation
- the clinical condition or situation to which the direction applies
- a description of those patients excluded from treatment under the direction
- a description of the circumstances in which further advice should be sought from a doctor (or dentist, as appropriate) and arrangements for referral
- details of appropriate dosage and maximum total dosage, quantity, pharmaceutical form and strength, route and frequency of administration, and minimum and maximum period over which the medicine should be administered

- relevant warnings, including potential adverse reactions
- details of any necessary follow-up action and the circumstances
- a statement of the records to be kept for audit purposes.

All authorisations must be signed and dated. A senior nurse must sign the PGD when they relate to nurse supply or administration. Authorisation must be granted by the appropriate health authority or primary care organisation when PGDs are used within the NHS. Changes to the legislation in 2004 also enable private, charitable and voluntary healthcare providers to work under PGDs.

Staff participating in PGDs must have the approval of their professional manager and be provided with written authorisation to provide care within the specified direction. Examples of PGDs include:

- the administration of vaccines for childhood and adult immunisation programmes (such as administration of diphtheria, tetanus, acellular pertussis and inactivated polio vaccine [DTaP/IPV]; administration of hepatitis B vaccination)
- the administration of sodium chloride 0.9% injection for flushing intravenous catheters/cannulae
- the administration of tenecteplase in the management of myocardial infarction
- treatments for minor injuries
- treatments to support out-of-hours nurse practitioners
- administration of emergency hormonal contraception.

Many more have and are being developed.

All nurses supplying and/or administering medicines under a PGD must sign to confirm that they understand its contents and have received the appropriate training. A register of those nurses who have been authorised to supply/administer medicines under PGDs must be maintained by the senior nurse manager, and continuing education provided for those whose names are on it.

SUMMARY

The majority of patients receiving clinical care will continue to receive medicines that have been prescribed on an individual basis. In contrast, PGDs provide a system for authorising appropriately trained nurses and other healthcare professionals to supply and administer named medicines in identified clinical situations without the need for a separate, signed prescription for each individual patient. The benefits

of PGDs are significant and include the production of an evidence-based quality standard with improved response to anaphylaxis, earlier treatment and less administrative work (Jones 2001).

Responsibility rests with senior medical, pharmacy and nurse managers to ensure that PGDs are suitably prepared and that training is provided for those participating. Individual nurses, having been instructed on the bounds of professional responsibility, must not act beyond their professional competence. To do so would be in breach of the law.

NURSE PRESCRIBING

NURSE PRESCRIBERS' FORMULARY FOR COMMUNITY PRACTITIONERS

Nurse prescribing was introduced nationally for district nurses and health visitors in 1998. The Nurse Prescribers' Formulary for Community Practitioners (until 2005 called the Nurse Prescribers' Formulary for District Nurses and Health Visitors) enables community practitioner nurse prescribers to prescribe from a formulary of appliances, dressings and some medicines for patients in the community.

District nurses, health visitors and those practice nurses with a district nurse or health visitor qualification who had successfully completed a training programme in nurse prescribing were permitted to prescribe from a limited list. The necessary training to enable district nurses and health visitors to prescribe from this formulary is now integrated into university-based specialist practitioner programmes for new district nurses and health visitors. The formulary comprises a limited range of medicines, dressings and appliances suitable for use in community settings. The formulary is set out in the Drug Tariff and also in the BNF. Once qualified as prescribers, district nurses and health visitors can prescribe from this list using their own judgement and without consulting a doctor. They are legally accountable for their actions.

Community pharmacists are not able to dispense any prescriptions written by nurses with this qualification for products outwith the approved list. Products available for prescribing by nurses include laxatives, stoma care products, analgesics associated with minor trauma, bladder instillations, preparations for the treatment of simple skin and ear conditions, surgical dressings and treatments for head lice. It should be pointed out that treatments initiated by nurses should always be fully recorded and communicated to the patient's doctor as soon as possible.

Nurses are expected to have a suitable level of background knowledge of clinical pharmacology and therapeutics in order to be able to benefit fully from the training. Training programmes focus on the need for the nurse to be able to prescribe effectively from the Nurse Prescribers' Formulary. In addition to knowledge of the clinical pharmacology and therapeutics of the products included in the formulary, the nurse is required to demonstrate knowledge of the relevant legislation and to be fully aware of issues of accountability and professional responsibility. Training programmes also reinforce the principles, practices and procedures of nurse prescribing as well as providing an economic perspective. This prescribing qualification will still be valid even with the introduction of full independent nurse prescribing.

SUPPLEMENTARY PRESCRIBING

In April 2003, the Government enabled nurses and pharmacists to train to become supplementary prescribers. Supplementary prescribing is defined as a voluntary partnership between the independent prescriber (a doctor or dentist) and a supplementary prescriber to implement an agreed patient-specific CMP, with the patient's agreement. This enables qualified nurses to prescribe any medicine (including controlled drugs) within the framework of a patient-specific CMP agreed with a doctor or dentist. Such a partnership can be particularly helpful for patients with a long-term condition such as asthma or diabetes. The key principles that underpin supplementary prescribing include:

- the importance of communication between the prescribing partners, and the need for access to shared patient records
- that patients are treated as partners and are involved at all stages in decision making, including whether part of their care is delivered via supplementary prescribing.

The training for nurse supplementary prescribers was based on that for extended independent nurse prescribers, with an additional taught element relating to the nature, context and scope of supplementary prescribing.

Unlike district nurse, health visitor and extended nurse prescribing, there is no specific formulary or list of medicines for supplementary prescribing. Provided that medicines are prescribable by a doctor or dentist (an independent prescriber) at NHS expense, and that they are referred to in the patient's CMP, supplementary prescribers are able to prescribe all general sale list medicines, pharmacy medicines,

appliances and devices, foods and other borderline substances approved by the Advisory Committee on Borderline Substances and all prescription-only medicines. Exceptions are those drugs marked 'less suitable for prescribing' in the BNF. Amendments to the Misuse of Drugs Regulations 2001 to enable nurse and pharmacist supplementary prescribers to prescribe controlled drugs came into force in March 2005. As supplementary prescribers, nurses should not prescribe medicines that are not within their professional competence to do so.

The CMP is a lawful requirement that relates to an individual patient and enables the supplementary prescriber to manage the prescribing for that individual within agreed parameters. The CMP should contain enough detail to ensure patient safety and must:

- specify the range and circumstances within which the supplementary prescriber can vary the dosage, frequency and formulation of the medicines (or class of medicines) identified
- specify when to refer to the independent prescriber
- contain details of known sensitivities of the patient to particular medicines
- include arrangements for notification of adverse drug reactions
- contain the date of commencement of the arrangement and date for review (this is not normally longer than 1 year).

Supplementary prescribing involves a team approach, and it is important that there is clear understanding of individual roles and responsibilities, along with frequent communication between the prescribing partners, in order to ensure safe, effective prescribing. Even with the introduction of full independent nurse prescribing, supplementary prescribing may well still be the most appropriate mechanism for prescribing, for instance when a nurse or pharmacist is newly qualified as a prescriber or when a team approach to prescribing is clearly appropriate, or when a patient's CMP includes certain controlled drugs not allowable under full independent prescribing.

EXTENDED AND INDEPENDENT NURSE PRESCRIBING

In 1997, the Government set up the Review of Prescribing, Supply and Administration of Medicines (under the chairpersonship of Dr June Crown CBE). In 1999, the second report of the Review recognised the potential benefits to patients of extending prescribing responsibilities to healthcare professionals other than doctors, dentists and the then small number of district nurse and health visitor prescribers. As a result, following public consultation, the Department of Health introduced a wider formulary for (independent) nurse prescribing in 2002: the NPEF. Work to expand the NPEF took place from 2003 to 2005. By May 2005, the NPEF included a list of around 240 prescription-only medicines, together with all pharmacy and general sale list medicines prescribable by GPs for these medical conditions.

The extended prescribing of prescription-only medicines by independent nurse prescribers is intended to enhance patient care by:

- providing quicker and more efficient access to healthcare
- improving patient care without compromising patient safety
- making it easier for patients to get the medicines they need
- increasing patient choice in accessing medicines
- making better use of the skills of health professionals
- contributing to the introduction of more flexible team working across the NHS, allowing doctors more time to deal with more serious cases (Scottish Executive 2001).

To be legally eligible to prescribe from the NPEF, prescribers had to be a first-level registered nurse or registered midwife and their name held on the professional register of the Nursing and Midwifery Council with an annotation signifying that they had successfully completed the specific programme of training for extended formulary nurse prescribing. The standards for that training were approved by the Nursing and Midwifery Council. Following training, nurses prescribing from the NPEF were able to prescribe all general sale list and pharmacy medicines currently prescribable by GPs under the regulations, together with a list of prescription-only medicines for specified medical conditions.

In early 2005, the University of Southampton completed an evaluation of nurse prescribing for the Department of Health. The evaluation concluded that the limits of the extended formulary were in some cases restricting benefit to patients and efficient NHS practice. Experience had also shown that updating the extended formulary was a long and resource-intensive process, with proposed changes taking 12–17 months to put into effect. Furthermore, supplementary prescribing could not be used in all settings in which patients would benefit (e.g. emergency care and first-contact care), because it required the development of an individual CMP agreed with a doctor.

In October 2005, the Committee on Safety of Medicines, following an extensive consultation exercise, recommended to ministers that suitably trained and qualified nurses and pharmacists should be able to prescribe any licensed medicine for any medical condition within their competence. As a consequence, changes were made to the regulations from 1 May 2006 to enable suitably trained nurses and pharmacists to qualify as independent prescribers, who are then able to prescribe any licensed medicine (i.e. products with a valid marketing authorisation [licence] in the UK), including some controlled drugs, for any medical condition they are competent to treat. At time of writing (2006), pharmacist independent prescribers cannot prescribe controlled drugs, although this is likely to change. Nurse independent prescribers can prescribe a limited range of controlled drugs for specific medical conditions.

The Medicines and Human Use (Prescribing) (Miscellaneous Amendments) Order of May 2006 and associated medicines regulations enable nurses who have already successfully completed a nurse independent prescribing course (formerly known as an extended formulary nurse prescribing course) to prescribe any licensed medicine (i.e. products with a valid marketing authorisation [licence] in the UK) for any medical condition within their clinical competence. Nurse independent prescribers must only ever prescribe within their own level of experience and competence, acting in accordance with clause 6 of the Nursing and Midwifery Council's Code of Professional Conduct: Standards for Conduct, Performance and Ethics (Nursing and Midwifery Council 2004). A nurse independent prescriber must be a first-level registered nurse, registered midwife or registered specialist community public health nurse whose name in each case is held on the Nursing and Midwifery Council professional register, with an annotation signifying that the nurse has successfully completed an approved programme of preparation and training for nurse independent prescribing.

The Department of Health's working definition of independent prescribing is prescribing by a practitioner (e.g. doctor, dentist, nurse, pharmacist) responsible and accountable for the assessment of patients with undiagnosed or diagnosed conditions and for decisions about the clinical management required, including prescribing. Within medicines legislation, the term used is *appropriate practitioner*. In partnership with the patient, independent prescribing is one element of the clinical management of a patient. It requires an initial patient assessment, an interpretation of that assessment, a decision on safe and appropriate therapy, and a process for ongoing monitoring. The independent prescriber is responsible and accountable for at least this element of a patient's care. Normally, prescribing would be carried out in the context of practice within a multidisciplinary healthcare team, either in a hospital or in a community setting, and within a single, accessible healthcare record.

The selection of nurses who will be trained as independent prescribers is a matter for employing organisations who are best placed to assess local service and patient needs. All individuals selected for prescribing training must have the opportunity to prescribe in the post that they will occupy on completion of training. Increasing numbers of nurses, including practice nurses and hospital nurses in specialist practice, are expected to undertake training in the future. The therapeutic area(s) in which they will prescribe should be identified before they begin training to prescribe. This will almost certainly be in the field in which they already hold considerable expertise. This development is seen as a further opportunity for nurses and midwives to enhance patient care. Its success is dependent on high-quality education provision and multiprofessional support systems. All nurses have a professional responsibility to keep themselves abreast of clinical and professional developments. This is no less true for prescribing. Nurse independent prescribers will be expected to keep up to date with evidence and best practice in the management of the conditions for which they prescribe, and in the use of the relevant medicines.

GOOD PRESCRIBING PRACTICE

Good prescribing is not a fixed aim, and is a process of development towards achieving an outcome whereby the patient receives appropriate medication to ensure maximum benefit. Good prescribing is based on a number of fundamental principles. A seven-step model represented as a prescribing pyramid is advocated (Fig. 5.1; National Prescribing Centre 1999). A thorough, holistic assessment of the patient's needs should always be carried out before any other action is taken. All treatment options should be considered, including not to treat at all. When there is a genuine need to prescribe, care should be taken to select a product that is effective, appropriate for the patient, safe and cost-effective. As far as possible, the patient should be encouraged to participate in the process of deciding on the most suitable product. A regular review of the patient is essential to ensure that the

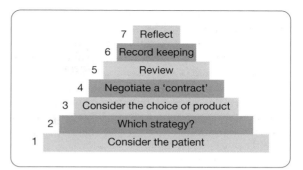

Fig. 5.1 The prescribing pyramid. Each step should be considered carefully before the next is approached. (From National Prescribing Centre 1999 Signposts for prescribing nurses: general principles of good prescribing. Prescribing Nurse Bulletin 1:1–4. With permission of the National Prescribing Centre.)

prescribed treatment is effective, safe and acceptable. Healthcare records are a tool of communication within the team. It is important to ensure that the healthcare record for the patient or client is an accurate account of treatment, care planning and delivery. It should be consecutive, written with the involvement of the patient or client whenever practicable, and completed as soon as possible after an event has occurred. It should provide clear evidence of the care planned, the decisions made, the care delivered and the information shared (Nursing and Midwifery Council 2004). Finally, much can be learned from reviewing prescribing practice. The development of good prescribing is a generic process geared towards achieving an outcome whereby each patient receives appropriate medication to ensure maximum benefit at acceptable cost. The measurement of good prescribing is less to do with comparing one situation against the ideal, but more in measuring an improvement against negotiated targets. An explanation of good prescribing is given in Box 5.1.

When prescribing antibacterials, it is important to consider both the risk:benefits ratio to the individual and the societal effect with the risk of developing resistance. Nurse independent prescribers must ensure that patients are aware that they are being treated by a non-medical practitioner and of the scope and limits of their prescribing. There may be circumstances therefore in which the patient has to be referred on to another healthcare professional to access other aspects of their care. Prescribers are accountable for all aspects of their prescribing decisions. They should therefore prescribe only those medicines that they know are safe and effective for the patient and the condition being treated. They must be able to recognise and

Box 5.1 How good prescribing has been defined

- Recognition by both the clinician and patient of when a medication is appropriate and when a medication is NOT appropriate.
- Prescribing a medication that is appropriate to the illness, at the right dose, quantity and cost, relevant to the patient's, clinician's and community's needs.
- Not prescribing, or stopping medication when it is appropriate and acceptable to the patient.
- Avoiding polypharmacy and interactions where possible, but if unavoidable being aware of the consequences.
- Producing a 'package' of medication which is appropriate and acceptable to the patient.
- Prescribing appropriate medication, which is sensitive to patient need and responsive to demands of colleagues, peers and funding bodies.
- Supplying written and/or verbal information to the patient regarding their illness and their medication.
- Monitoring response to treatment – effectiveness (or lack of benefit), side effects, etc.
- Reviewing at appropriate intervals and recalling, intervening or stopping medication as appropriate.
- Having a robust system and staff, appropriately organised and trained to manage the above.
- Undertaking clinical audits as a means of reviewing and improving practice.
- Communicating in a timely fashion (written and verbally) with other healthcare professionals involved in the patient's medicines management.

(From NHS Grampian 2004, with permission.)

deal with pressures (e.g. from the pharmaceutical industry, patients or colleagues) that might result in inappropriate prescribing.

FUTURE DEVELOPMENTS AND IMPLICATIONS FOR NURSES

The introduction of nurse prescribing brings into even stronger focus the principles of medicine management and associated responsibilities already familiar to the professional nurse. With the advent of full independent nurse prescribing in mid 2006, these responsibilities are even greater. Nurses working both in community practice and in the hospital setting will be able to take advantage of opportunities to extend their roles and practice. Already, we are seeing nurse practitioners providing out-of-hours medical services, and the ability to prescribe independently can only

strengthen this role. Nurses authorised to prescribe are required to utilise to the full their knowledge of the actions and uses of medicines, and their skills in observation, communication and recording. Furthermore, prescribing nurses take a greater part in decision making and thereby have increasing reasons to be accountable for their actions and inactions.

It may be argued that prescribing medicines is simply another medical task that has been devolved to nurses primarily to relieve hard-pressed doctors of a time-consuming chore. Many nurses and other health professionals, however, consider that the development of nurse prescribing is part of a logical progression that recognises the needs of patients and how these can best be met. Nurses have, for many years, exercised considerable influence on the prescribing process. All the indications are that when nurses assume wider professional responsibilities the outcomes are greatly beneficial to patient care. As always, nurses expect to encounter a new set of challenges and opportunities. Prescribing is not a simple mechanistic act. Relationships between patient and prescriber can be subject to tensions and perhaps unreasonable demands on the part of the patient. It is vitally important to ensure that all parties to the prescribing process have a clear understanding of the remit of the nurse and the constraints of a limited formulary within which the nurse is working. Prescribing, whether by doctors or nurses, should never be seen as a substitute for preventive measures or the use of basic household remedies. Patient education, information and counselling must not be neglected. Community nurses are especially well placed to monitor the patient's total use of medicines, both prescribed and non-prescribed. As more potent medicinal products become available without prescription, this aspect of the nurse's responsibilities will become increasingly important. Nurse prescribing must not, and will not, be allowed to become purely a supply service, important though this is. As with all aspects of nursing care, the clinical needs of patients should be uppermost in the minds of nurses when they decide to prescribe for them.

SELF-ASSESSMENT QUESTIONS

1. As a supplementary prescriber, you have to prepare a CMP for a patient to manage her hypertension. What key pieces of information should you include in the CMP?
2. Outline the fundamental principles of good prescribing.

REFERENCES

Blatt B 1997 Nurse prescribing: are you ready? Practice Nursing 8:11–13

Department of Health 1989 Report of the advisory group on nurse prescribing (Crown Report). Department of Health, London

Department of Health 1999 A review of prescribing, supply and administration of medicines: final report (Crown Report 2). Department of Health, London

Department of Health and Social Security 1986 Neighbourhood nursing: a focus for care (Cumberlege Report). HMSO, London

Humphries JL, Green J (eds) 1999 Nurse prescribing. Macmillan, Basingstoke

Jones PGW 2001 How to decide when a patient group direction is needed. Guidelines in Practice 4:78–84

National Prescribing Centre 1999 Signposts for prescribing nurses: general principles of good prescribing. Prescribing Nurse Bulletin 1:1–4

NHS Grampian 2004 Grampian Joint Formulary 2004. NHS Grampian, Aberdeen

Nursing and Midwifery Council 2004 The NMC code of professional conduct: standards for conduct, performance and ethics. NMC, London

Scottish Executive 2001 Extended prescribing of prescription only medicines by independent nurse prescribers. Scottish Executive, Edinburgh

FURTHER READING AND RESOURCES

British National Formulary (http://www.bnf.org)

Courtenay M, Butler M 1999 Nurse prescribing: principles and practice. Greenwich Medical Media, London

Department of Health 2006 Improving patients' access to medicines: a guide to implementing nurse and pharmacist independent prescribing within the NHS in England. Department of Health, London

Medicine and Healthcare products Regulatory Agency (http://www.mhra.gov.uk)

National Prescribing Centre (http://www.npc.co.uk)

Nursing and Midwifery Council (http://www.nmc-uk.org)

Nursing and Midwifery Council 2002 Guidelines for records and record keeping. NMC, London

Nursing and Midwifery Council 2006 Nurse prescribing and the supply and administration of medicines. NMC, London

Patient group directions website (part of the National Electronic Library for Medicines) (http://www.portal.nelm.nhs.uk/PGD/default.aspx)

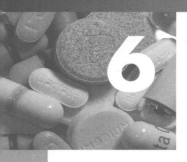

6

Clinical governance and safety in the use of medicines

CHAPTER CONTENTS

KEY OBJECTIVES

After reading this chapter, you should be able to:

- outline the types of errors that can occur with the prescribing and dispensing of medicines
- explain the rationale for a no-blame reporting culture
- detail the role of the nurse in ensuring safe administration of medicines.

INTRODUCTION

Safety is a patient's right and the obligation of all health professionals (Barach and Moss 2001). Systems of healthcare provide a framework within which individual patient care is provided. The concept of clinical governance provides overall guidance to all healthcare staff on the need for high standards in all aspects of patient care. This should be seen as a background to this chapter.

CLINICAL GOVERNANCE/QUALITY STRATEGY

Clinical governance is defined by Scally and Donaldson (1998) as 'a framework through which NHS organisations are accountable for continually improving the quality of their services and safeguarding high standards of care by creating an environment in which excellence in clinical care will flourish'. Health professionals have always worked within their own professional guidelines and relied on their employer to provide facilities, equipment and other resources to enable them to practise safely and effectively. No systematic methods of improving the quality of service were available until the concept of clinical audit was introduced to the NHS in the 1990s. Despite some success within the audit approach, it became clear that sustained progress in improving the quality of care could be achieved only by establishing a quality strategy and by a change in the culture of the NHS (see Box 6.1). Well-publicised failures in the NHS in the late 1990s have given added impetus to the need for change. Attitudes at all levels within the NHS have come under intense public scrutiny. Professional bodies and their members must now revalidate all aspects of the quality of care for which they are responsible. Effective leadership at all levels is essential so that the planning for quality services on the basis of the objective criteria can take place. Implicit in the need to improve the quality of patient care is the need to ensure that safe systems of work are in place throughout the particular organisation. The introduction of clinical governance provides NHS organisations with a powerful imperative to focus on tackling adverse health care events.

A report from the USA shows that 44 000–98 000 unnecessary deaths result each year from a range of preventable errors in hospitals in the USA (Weingart and Wilson 2000). A study from Australia produced even higher error rates. NHS reporting and information systems provide a patchy and incomplete picture of the scale and nature of the problem of serious failures in healthcare. However, every year nearly 10 000 people are reported to have experienced serious adverse reactions to drugs (Department of Health 2000). One study (Ridley et al. 2004) looked at 21 589 systems that can help prevent errors and to make them detectable.

Human error is often a contributory factor in drug errors, but inadequate systems of drug management may also be implicated. Reason (2000) outlines the distinguishing features of a 'high reliability' organisation. In such organisations, human error is expected and systems are put in place to enable the workforce to keep errors to a minimum, to recognise errors when they occur and to cope with the consequences of error. Built into this approach is the need to use each error as a learning experience and to change systems accordingly.

All the key elements are designed to interact with the overall aim of improving the quality of care within the NHS. Clinical governance at local level is supported by the national structures and mechanisms outlined in Box 6.1. Without the supporting framework at national level, clinical governance has only limited potential to improve the overall quality of patient care. Safe and effective systems of medicine management play a very significant role in patient care.

ERRORS IN THE MANAGEMENT OF MEDICINES

With the ever increasing complexity of drug therapy and the need for many patients to receive multiple-drug therapy, the potential for errors in the administration of medicines is great. Indeed, one of the highest risk areas of nursing practice is the administration of medicines (Scholz 1990). A busy, moderately sized hospital might need 5000–10 000 individual doses each day (Ferner 1995). A medical ward with 30 beds may have as many as 60 products in use at any one time and could keep in stock a range of 200 medicinal products, excluding lotions, sterile fluids, etc. Factors other than complexity of therapy also contribute to errors in the administration of medicines.

An error in the administration of medicines may be, at best, inconvenient for the patient or, at worst, catastrophic. In order to gain a balanced perspective, it is necessary first to form a working definition of an error. This is best done by considering how, in practical terms, the overall objective of drug therapy (i.e. therapeutic benefit for the patient with minimal adverse effects) is most likely to be achieved. The assumption is made that the prescriber has taken all relevant factors into account before prescribing and that the choice of drug, dose, route, etc. is appropriate in every respect. To achieve therapeutic benefit for the patient, it is obviously essential to ensure that *the right*

prescriptions (15.3 new prescriptions/patient) written over a 4-week period within 24 critical care units in the UK. Eighty-five per cent (18 448 prescriptions) were error-free, but 3141 (15%) prescriptions had one or more errors. The five most common incorrect prescriptions were for potassium chloride (10.2% errors), heparin (5.3%), magnesium sulphate (5.2%), paracetamol (3.2%) and propofol (3.1%). Most of the errors were minor, having no serious adverse effects, but 618 (19.6%) errors were considered significant, serious or potentially life-threatening.

Unfavourable comparisons have been made between the safe systems used in the aviation industry and those used in the medical professions. Nolan (2000) places great emphasis on the need to design

Table 6.1 Issues linked with drug errors

Stage/source	Aspects to be taken into account
Manufacturer/distributor and faulty product	• Full and prompt recall of affected product undertaken • Investigations of cause and corrective measures taken • May incur significant costs both to supplier and NHS • Purchasers may lose confidence
Prescribing error	• May not be detected by pharmacy • Could result in an administration error
Dispensing error	• Can misinterpret prescriber's intentions • Error can be made in compounding or dispensing product • Dispensing systems may need to be reviewed • Training may be required for pharmacy staff
Administration error	• May result in loss of trust from patient or colleagues • Potential for damage to nurse's confidence and professional future
Patient	• May unwittingly or knowingly take medicines incorrectly • Can misinterpret prescriber's instructions • Many factors influence patient compliance (see Ch. 7)
General	• When errors result in a fatality, manslaughter charges may be made • Can strain/damage professional relationships • Disciplinary action may be taken by professional body or employer • Clear distinction needs to be made between organisational system failure and individual accountability

dose of the right drug is administered at the right time by the right route. Adherence by all healthcare staff to recognised drug procedures is clearly a prerequisite at all times.

Adverse drug reactions and interactions (see Ch. 10) should be avoided if at all possible. However, if an adverse drug reaction is unavoidable, the effect on the patient should be minimised. It therefore follows that monitoring of the patient is essential. All adverse reactions to drugs should be reported to the prescriber.

The National Patient Safety Agency (NPSA) has adopted the US National Coordinating Council definition of a medication error as 'any preventable event that may cause or lead to inappropriate medication use or patient harm while the medication is in the control of a health professional, patient or consumer'.

Such acts may relate to one or more of the practical aspects discussed above. It is obvious that it is not possible to comply to the letter with all aspects of medicine administration throughout all courses of drug therapy for all patients. Clearly, it is essential that, on every occasion, the correct dose of the correct drug is administered by the correct route. However, it must

be recognised that it is often not possible to administer all medicines exactly at the time indicated on the prescription, owing to the time required to complete a medicine round. This is technically an error but will seldom be of clinical significance. There are occasions, however, when the timing of the administration of certain medicines is of vital importance to the patient, such as, for example, with preoperative medication. Whatever the pressures, every effort must be made to eliminate errors by maintaining the highest possible standards of practice.

The definition given above is something of an oversimplification, because it does not reflect all the factors that may contribute to a drug error. Indeed, it is probably impossible to develop a definition that does include all the factors and issues that may contribute to or arise from a drug error. This is because drug administration is a multidisciplinary process that may well involve a chain of events (a cascade) from manufacturer, distributor, prescriber, pharmacist, hospital managers in all disciplines, nurse and possibly patient. Table 6.1 outlines some of the issues for health professionals (and others) who may become involved in a drug error or its consequences.

Box 6.2 Potential sources of drug errors

- Non-adherence to set procedures
- Communications failures
- Failure to comply with drug administration procedures
- Failure to review/cancel prescriptions
- Wrong transcription of information
- Misinterpretation/lack of information on purposes of therapy
- Inadequate training on drug administration procedures
- Use of unofficial abbreviations, non-standard terminology
- Inadequate policies and procedures, poorly designed documents
- Pressure on staff time, interruptions
- Lack of pharmaceutical services, failure to act on pharmaceutical information/advice
- Failure to identify product correctly, misreading labels
- Confusion with drug names; generic and proprietary products
- Poor labelling/packaging
- Calculation of doses
- Drug interactions
- Failure to note a known drug allergy
- Chemical incompatibility: drug additives to parenteral fluids
- Complex drug regimens: variable doses, non-standard intervals
- Improper use of equipment, including infusion pumps
- Failure to identify patient correctly
- Special regimens at extremes of age
- Clinical trials: inadequate information
- Involvement of a third party: possible confusion of roles
- Unauthorised manipulation of dosage form (e.g. crushing slow-release tablet)

SOURCES OF ERRORS

A number of significant potential sources of drug errors are outlined in Box 6.2. It is hoped that by providing this overview, the complex and interactive nature of drug errors will be demonstrated. Seldom will a drug error arise because of the actions or inactions of one individual. A cascade effect is often seen.

THE PRESCRIBER

Full responsibility rests with the prescriber to state clearly and without ambiguity the medicines the patient is to be given. Well-designed prescribing documents undoubtedly contribute to more accurate drug therapy. However, adherence to the prescribing policy is essential if errors are to be avoided, irrespective of the sophistication of the system used. Bad handwriting is probably the commonest potential source of error. Confusion between product names that look alike, especially when badly written, is a well-recognised source of error, e.g. co-codamol, co-codaprin and other approved names with the co- prefix. Even when clearly written, these words have a similar shape. Unofficial abbreviations for medicines are always open to misinterpretation and should not be used. Those who prescribe, dispense and administer medicines should never accept badly written instructions. The omission of essential information (e.g. the strength of the drug) may result in assumptions being made about what is required. When cancellation of a prescription lacks precision, the medicine may continue to be given to the possible detriment of the patient. Errors can arise when the wrong route is prescribed or the patient is not suitable to receive the medicine, i.e. when a patient with existing renal failure is prescribed a non-steroidal anti-inflammatory drug. Electronic prescribing and dispensing systems have the potential to improve the overall quality of prescribing. Such systems are no substitute for effective training and teaching of all staff involved in the use of medicines.

Maxwell and Walley (2002) contrast the training programme available to nurse prescribers with the minimal time currently available for teaching medical students the skills needed to use medicines safely. It is hoped that the General Medical Council will provide clear directions to the UK medical schools about the need for the learning and assessment of the skills needed to use medicines safely, effectively and cost-effectively (Maxwell and Walley 2002). Although the optimum use of medicines can be achieved only by effective team working, the prescribing process is clearly fundamental. If this process is flawed, the patient is highly unlikely to gain benefit from the therapy.

THE PHARMACIST

Errors in the administration of medicines may be due directly or indirectly to failures in the pharmaceutical service. As with clinical departments and wards, standards and procedures in pharmaceutical departments are designed to ensure that, as far as possible, errors are eliminated. Nevertheless, errors can and do occur, which may be due to failures to meet standards and, on some occasions, to lack of effective communication with the prescriber or nurse in charge of a ward or department.

Errors or omissions in the labelling of medicines may cause difficulty, which may lead to an incorrect dose or even a wrong drug being administered. There has been much debate about colour coding of labels and containers, but there can be no substitute for *reading* the label at all times. Coloured rings on ampoule necks may help to identify a 'rogue' ampoule in a box or on a tray.

On occasion, medicines may be required when a full pharmaceutical service is not available. This could result in delay in administering a medicine, which may have serious consequences for the patient.

Regrettably, medicines may be supplied to wards with minimal background information as to the actions, uses or dosage of the product. Ward staff may then have to rely on their own limited information sources, especially if a comprehensive drug information service is not available. On fairly rare occasions, a product or particular batch of a product may have to be withdrawn from use because of a fault or suspected fault. In such circumstances, pharmaceutical staff must ensure the rapid communication of accurate information to wards and departments concerned.

When products are issued to wards for use in connection with a clinical trial, it is very important that sufficient information be made available (without breaking any code) to the medical and nursing staff to enable the product to be used safely. The interest and cooperation of nurses are gained when the background to, and reasons for, a clinical trial are explained. It is also helpful if the results of the work are discussed with those participating.

The role of the pharmacist in drug therapy may be described as that of safety net and overseer. Any failure to discharge this role has serious implications for the safety and well-being of the patient. The community pharmacist has legal liabilities for personal injury caused by medicinal products (Ferguson 1997).

THE NURSE

Nurses are responsible for the safe and accurate administration of medicines to most in-patients and to their patients in the community. In order to discharge this responsibility, the nurse must interpret the prescription, select the correct medicine and make a record of the administration.

The administration of medicines is the culmination of research, development, manufacture, prescribing and dispensing. Although the skills and resources that have gone into producing a medicine are of great benefit to patients, the patient is now dependent on the nurse's skills. The responsibility to ensure safe and accurate administration of a medicine to a patient irrespective of the patient's circumstances should never be underestimated.

IDENTIFICATION OF THE PATIENT

In a study of 79 drug errors, 12.7% were due to the medicine being given to the wrong patient (Gladstone 1995). The NPSA (2005) states that all hospital in-patients in acute settings should wear wristbands (also known as identity bands), with accurate details that correctly identify them and match them to their care. Every precaution may be taken to include accurately the information on the wristband, and to attach the wristband carefully to the right patient, but problems can still arise. Sometimes, a wristband has to be removed – for example when an intravenous infusion is being set up – and it may not be replaced. The patient, unwittingly, may remove the wristband, or may do so while on weekend leave. The writing on the wristband may become indistinct with the passage of time. Even when the wristband remains satisfactorily in position, reference must be made to it. Of course, it was never intended that the wristband should take the place of effective communication between nurse and patient, or that it would obviate the need for regular updating of staff on the patients under their care.

There can be no doubt about the need for identity bands to be used in paediatric units, intensive care units, theatres and in all acute areas where patients are unable to identify themselves. Areas that may pose particular difficulty are care of the elderly units and psychiatric wards. Patients in these wards may understandably have feelings of resentment at being 'labelled'. In addition, staff may feel that this procedure militates against their efforts to reduce any feelings patients may have of being institutionalised, and that they know their patients anyway.

Regularly updated passport size photographs (attached to the prescription sheet) are often used as a more sympathetic aid to patient identification. In any event, health authorities must devise workable policies that are in patients' best interests.

ERRORS IN CALCULATIONS

There is now increasing recognition of the major difficulties young people in the UK from differing backgrounds are having with simple arithmetic (Reid 1996, Clare 1997). With less emphasis placed on the subject in schools and the widespread use of calculators, this is a real cause for concern in nursing. Particular problems relate to the use of quantities less than 1 mg. Efforts to convert 0.125 mg into micrograms have resulted in gross overdosage of digoxin in paediatric practice. It has been suggested that there might be a place for calculators in assisting those who have such difficulty. If the individual's lack of numeracy is so severe as to call for this level of assistance, there must be grave doubts as to whether a calculator could be used safely. Indeed, the improper use of such equipment may be another source of error. Calculators have a place but should probably be used only to make a final check. The Nursing and Midwifery Council (2004) has stated that, when drug administration requires complex calculations to ensure that the correct volume or quantity of medication is administered, it may be necessary for a second practitioner to check the calculation in order to minimise the risk of error. The use of calculators to determine the volume or quantity of medication should not act as a substitute for arithmetical knowledge and skill (Nursing and Midwifery Council 2004).

USE OF INADEQUATE EQUIPMENT/ UNORTHODOX USE OF MEDICINES

Measures for liquid medicines with indistinct markings cannot safely be used. This is especially important in paediatric practice, when potent liquid medicines are often used. Oral syringes must be used.

Using medicines in an unorthodox way may also lead to errors. Some tablets are designed to be broken if a fractional dose is required. Other tablets are not so designed; an attempt to break or divide such a product will almost certainly result in the administration of an incorrect dose. Similarly, the crushing of a modified-release tablet will destroy the essential properties of the formulation, any benefit to the patient being lost. Errors may arise because of the attempted use of an unsuitable presentation such as a very large capsule or tablet that a patient may be unable to swallow.

ERROR REDUCTION/AVOIDANCE

Given that drug errors often arise as a result of a series of failures by the health professionals involved, it follows that programmes designed to improve matters must have the active support of prescriber, pharmacist, nurse and hospital managers. The assumption should not be made that actions by members of one profession acting alone will be all that is required to eliminate or reduce errors. Recognition of the need to improve the safety of healthcare is now apparent at the highest levels of government, in both the UK and the USA. The NPSA has been set up in the UK, and the Agency for Healthcare Research and Quality in the USA

has received additional funding to promote research on the safety of patients (Barach and Moss 2001). Healthcare leaders have embraced patient safety, but it is only within the teams delivering patient care that real advances in patient safety can be made.

THE NURSE MANAGER

The nurse who is in overall charge (nurse manager, ward sister or charge nurse) is accountable for the maintenance of standards of medicine administration in the ward. Insisting on accurate prescribing practice is one of the most demanding aspects of the role. It will be to the benefit of both the nurse manager and the patients to make it known that failure to meet the standard is unacceptable. It is important to ensure that up to date relevant information on drugs is readily available at ward level. All wards and departments should have an up to date copy of the British National Formulary and local formularies. Clear lines of communication must be established with clinical pharmacists and medicine information services.

Whenever possible, the nurse in charge should avoid delegating the administration of medicines to nurses who are unfamiliar with the identity of patients in the ward. Examples include nurses who have recently been appointed to the ward, have just returned from a period of absence or have been sent to assist on a temporary basis from an agency or from another ward. It is important also to assign appropriate members of staff to the administration of medicines. It is irresponsible to ask nurses to participate in the administration of medicines unless they have been taught the theoretical aspects of it. Although in other aspects of care the role of nursing auxiliaries/assistants has developed in recent years, their involvement in relation to the administration of medicines remains as before, i.e. to see that the patient has a drink with which to take the drug, to help the patient into a suitably comfortable position to take the drug, and to report to the person conducting the drug round if for any reason the patient fails to take the drug.

Although care assistants in residential homes may be involved in issuing medicines from previously prepared medicine distribution systems, the responsibility for interpreting the prescription and dispensing the medicines totally rests with the community pharmacist. In some nursing homes, in the absence of a second registered nurse it may be necessary for a care assistant to check controlled drug stock, but a care assistant is not permitted to participate in the administration of the drug.

Efforts should be made to discourage discussion with patients' visitors or visiting members of staff during procedures involving the administration of medicines. It may be useful to display a notice on the medicine trolley – 'DO NOT DISTURB' – with the intention of minimising interruptions during administration of medicines.

In the event of duplications in patients' names in a ward, staff and the patients concerned must be alerted. The nurse in charge must also ensure that identification wristbands/photographs are renewed and replaced as necessary (e.g. if the writing becomes illegible, the band tears or comes apart). Great emphasis is rightly placed on the need for the accurate administration of medicines, but it is also essential to ensure that medicines are discontinued when a course of treatment is complete. Where an instruction to discontinue therapy has been given, and when it is clear that the medicine does not constitute replacement or other long-term therapy, the continuing need for the medicine should be questioned. Prime responsibility for discontinuation of treatment must rest with the prescriber.

All staff are required to keep accurate and legible records (Nursing and Midwifery Council 2004), which include those used in drug administration. Prescribers should be asked to rewrite prescription sheets when they become untidy or when the use of two prescription sheets concurrently could be obviated. The Nursing and Midwifery Council's stance on the transcribing of drugs is discussed on page 34. Kardex or similar holders for prescribing and recording documents should be kept in good repair, and the order of sheets should be rearranged to correspond with the movement of patients within the ward. Nursing staff must adopt a safe and efficient system of storing all medicines and withdraw medicines that are no longer required. Advice from pharmacy staff on appropriate levels of ordering, expiry dates, etc., and on any other aspects of stock management, is readily available. In situations in which drug regimens remain unchanged for long periods of time, every effort must be made to prevent complacency.

It is safer when administering medicines to concentrate fully on the procedure and to leave the discussion of uses, actions, side effects, etc. for a more appropriate time. Because teaching and learning are demanding of time and effort and not without risk for both the clinical supervisor/educator and the person being supervised, it is advisable to limit the experience to a few patients, preferably ones with whose care the learner is already involved.

The administration of medicines should be kept high on the list of priorities in a ward. The nursing staff's awareness of medicines in use in their ward may be increased by referring to patients' prescription sheets in conjunction with the giving of a verbal report on the patients, for example at the changeover of staff. If time permits, a separate reporting session specifically about the medicines in use and any related difficulties that the patient or nurse may be having with them can be valuable to the nurse in charge as well as to more junior nursing staff.

Consideration should also be given to the timing and number of medicine rounds required. Standardised systems of prescribing and administration should allow room for flexibility to meet the needs of individual patients. For example, special account may need to be taken of the timing of administration to patients suffering neurological conditions such as Parkinson's disease. Such flexibility, of course, must reflect the need for effective drug therapy.

Clinical pharmacy services should be fully utilised. Any special needs of the ward will become apparent to the clinical pharmacist, but there is no substitute for active cooperation with the pharmacist. A climate of passive acceptance of any service is not conducive to achieving the highest standard of care for patients.

THE SENIOR NURSE MANAGER

The continuing need to promote safe practice and in so doing reduce drug errors is the responsibility of those involved in policy making, management and education, as well as those in clinical practice. Nurse managers spend time allocating staff to meet service commitments. Along with the many other demands that they try to meet, greater consideration could be given to staff levels needed at the main medicine round times or when pre- and postoperative medications are to be given. The extent to which two nurses should be involved in the administration of medicines continues to exercise the minds of nurse managers and nurses in clinical practice.

Practitioners whose names are on the Nursing and Midwifery Council register (including midwives) are considered competent to administer medicines on their own and are responsible for their actions in so doing. The involvement of a second person in the administration of medicines with a registered practitioner needs to occur when that practitioner is instructing a student nurse. The patient's condition or other circumstances as locally determined may also make it necessary to involve a second person.

Community nurses have, of course, always administered medicines single-handed. Some hospital policies still require that two nurses be involved in the administration of medicines, one of whom is a registered nurse. The possible advantages and

Box 6.3 The advantages and disadvantages of involving two nurses in the administration of medicines in hospital

Advantages
- Presence of second nurse provides an additional check that should improve patient safety by reducing drug errors.
- Presence of second nurse helpful if calculations of drug dosage are required.
- Patient feels reassured that a second person is involved in checking the medicine.
- Provides important learning situation for procedures of medicine administration.
- Impact of interruptions can be minimised, because the medicine round can probably be continued by one nurse.
- Some patients understandably wish to ask questions about their medicines during rounds. This may be difficult for one nurse to cope with, although even if two nurses are present some complex questions may have to be noted for answering later.
- Improved security of medicines during medicine rounds.
- Any emergency arising during the medicine round can be dealt with more promptly.

Disadvantages
- Blurring of responsibility, leading to confusion and perhaps error.
- Student nurse may be reluctant to challenge a trained nurse, assuming that the trained nurse is always right.
- May provide false sense of safety in medicine administration.
- Medicine round may take longer because of double checking.
- Dilution of professional responsibility.
- In some situations (e.g. night duty), staffing levels make it impracticable for two nurses to be routinely involved in medicine administration, leading to delay.

disadvantages of this approach are summarised in Box 6.3. It should be noted that there is little evidence in the literature to confirm or otherwise the views expressed, which is not surprising because a valid comparative study would be very difficult to undertake with so many variables to influence the outcome.

Clearly, the advantages and disadvantages outlined in Box 6.3 do not carry equal weight but will serve as a frame of reference when local policies are being formulated. As with other aspects of nursing care, the procedure to be adopted will always be chosen with the best interests of the patient in mind. The need for two nurses to be involved in the administration of medicines to children is a generally agreed principle.

Equipment and siting of fixtures used in the management of medicines, such as drug trolleys, individual patient medication boxes, medicine cupboards and refrigerators, should be chosen with care so that the particular needs of the ward are satisfied. Nurse managers should always be prepared to take time to consult with practising clinical colleagues as to their requirements. Guidance from the pharmacist should also be sought. Policy makers must ensure that the systems of medicine management, including prescribing and recording documents, reach the required standard, are of suitable design and are relevant to the drug therapy used in all wards. With increased opportunities for healthcare professionals to design and produce documents within their own clinical area, the required standard may not always be reached. Mechanisms are needed to ensure that there is an effective means of updating the design of or introducing new prescription sheets and associated documents in such a way that the needs of all practitioners are fully met.

Continuing education on the subject is essential for all trained nursing staff, along with updating of nurses returning to work after some years' absence. Attendance at regular in-service lectures and seminars on medicine administration should be given a very high priority. There is also considerable scope for operational research into many aspects of medicine management. Nurse managers have a duty to encourage their staff in this direction. Nurse managers must ensure that procedures applicable in the event of errors in medicine administration are not seen as threatening by nurses or a deterrent to the reporting of errors.

Apart from actions taken by individuals or within a particular profession, it is essential to ensure that an active multidisciplinary drug and therapeutics committee or medicines management committee keeps under review all aspects of medicine management and issues guidance when necessary. The establishment of a post of medication safety officer should be considered.

THE PATIENT

The active cooperation of the patient is essential in order to achieve the therapeutic benefit of a course of drug treatment. Nurses and their medical colleagues should, however, never take the patient's cooperation for granted or expect this to be given automatically.

The patient's right to question or even reject treatment must be respected. Nurses must play their part in ensuring that, if a patient does decide to reject a particular treatment, this decision is reached on the basis of a full understanding of the implications for the patient's health and well-being. It would obviously be unfair to attribute the patient's action or lack of action as a source of drug errors, but in some situations the patient will bear some responsibility if the treatment fails. The not uncommon occurrence of finding tablets in the patient's bed or under the cushions of a chair may or may not indicate failure on the part of the patient. This may be the first indication the nurse has that all is not well. Needless to say, great tact and perception may be needed to establish the true cause of this rejection.

Care must be taken when using medicines brought into hospital by patients on admission. Such medicines dispensed for individual patients may have been inappropriately stored in the patient's home. Labels may have been altered or removed, causing difficulty in identifying the contents of a container. It may be appropriate to use patients' own medicines when they are in hospital, but the responsibility for doing so should not be undertaken lightly. All available means, including clinical pharmacy services, must be used to validate the patient's own medicines before using them in hospital. This may involve seeking information from patients and/or their carers. As patient packs are now the norm, the use of patients' own medicines during hospitalisation is often a worthwhile option.

ERROR REDUCTION/AVOIDANCE CHECKLIST

PATIENT

- Pay particular attention to identification of the patient.
- Take extra care at extremes of age. With individual exceptions, the risks to infants and the very old are greater, partly because of the effects of the drugs but also because these patients may be unable to speak for themselves.
- Be especially careful when patients are mobile and when large groups of patients are sitting about at random (e.g. in day rooms).
- Whenever possible, increase involvement of patients in their own drug therapy.

PRESCRIPTION

- Consider benefits of electronic prescribing systems.
- Use correct documentation and report any inadequacies in the documentation design/layout.
- Develop/update documentation in line with changes in practice.
- Follow the policy and do not accept inadequate, unclear instructions.
- Avoid prospective prescribing whenever possible. If this is necessary, ensure that directions are clear.
- Avoid the use of unofficial abbreviations and chemical symbols/nomenclature.
- Take particular care with similar-looking drug names.
- Complex calculations should be checked by a second person.
- Be alert to sudden changes in dosage.
- If it appears that a dose has to be made up of several tablets/ampoules, check carefully that all is in order.
- Pay particular attention to doses expressed in micrograms or units.
- Pay particular attention to doses of drugs that alter key physiological parameters (e.g. insulin injections).
- When two nurses are involved in the administration of medicines, read out the details of the prescription and the label so that each is aware of the other's interpretation of them. Also, when administering a medicine for which a calculation has to be made, make the calculations independently before making comparison.
- Ask, check and ask again if not satisfied. While wishing to trust colleagues, do not passively take the word of a senior member of staff as necessarily correct.
- Report at once any suspicions you may have that all is not in order regarding the prescription.

MEDICINE

- Ensure correct storage of medicines (e.g. do not mix different ampoules in the same container).
- Do not alter any labels on containers of medicines and other pharmaceutical products.
- Do not remove drugs from containers unless for administration to the patient.
- Any medicine removed from its container and not used should be disposed of safely.
- Report any apparent abnormalities to the supplier or senior colleague (e.g. changes in size, shape, colour of a product).
- Use the correct dosage form (e.g. request a supply of 5-mg tablets rather than try to divide a 20-mg tablet).
- When there is no intravenous reconstitution service available and this task has to be undertaken by nursing staff, ensure correct volume of correct diluent is used. (This applies equally to the reconstitution of liquid oral dosage forms.) If in any doubt, always ask advice from the pharmacy department.

- Drugs intended for intrathecal use must be supplied in a presentation that ensures correct administration.
- Use the correct equipment (e.g. measures, syringes).
- Ensure that mechanical equipment is maintained/serviced on a programmed basis.
- Be aware of drug interactions (e.g. drug–drug; drug–food).
- Be aware of any drug that could interfere with laboratory tests.
- Avoid drug incompatibility (e.g. when adding drugs to intravenous fluids). Use pharmacy-based services whenever possible.

ALL STAFF

- Be observant. Here is the distinction between seeing and observing. The ability to take in an overview of a chart or the contents of the medicine trolley/cupboard as well as the details of one prescription or one product has to be developed.
- When a telephoned order for medicines is unavoidable, write the message down and repeat it to the caller.
- Ensure adequate flow of information to other clinical departments. Diagnostic tests may be influenced by patients' current or previous drug therapy.
- Report, discuss and seek views of colleagues, especially if the safety of the patient is involved (e.g. unexplained side effects of a drug).
- When two nurses are involved in administering medicines, the more experienced nurse should check the decisions, calculations and actions of the less experienced nurse.
- Whenever possible, reduce the ward medicine inventory by encouraging the adoption of a ward formulary or prescribing policy.
- Read the literature and keep up to date; ask for more information if it is not provided.
- Make full use of pharmacy services, especially the ward/clinical pharmacy service and drug information services.
- Encourage the development of a questioning, enquiring attitude at all levels.

WARD MANAGERS

- Encourage by all practical means adherence to drug policy.
- Integrate verbal report on current ward drug therapy with nursing report.
- Provide suitable drug information source at ward level (e.g. British National Formulary, Data Sheet Compendium).
- Eliminate borrowing of medicines between wards and departments.

- Reduce interruptions during the administration of medicines.
- Ensure that equipment available for medicine administration is suitable in all respects.
- Improve procedures for checking medicines prior to administration.

SENIOR MANAGERS

- Encourage the development of ward prescribing policies, reduction of ward medicines inventory.
- Make careful choice of new equipment. Establish regular in-service education for nurses on all aspects of drug therapy.
- Develop clinical pharmacy services.
- Improve nurse staffing levels.
- Ensure that nurses have the necessary skills and knowledge relating to the use of medicines.
- Establish educational programmes for junior hospital doctors on procedural aspects of ward medicine management, including prescribing.
- Promote research/clinical audit into all aspects of medicine use.
- Examine and, if necessary, improve procedures for dealing with errors in the administration of medicines.

However accurate and detailed the prescribing, however efficient the pharmaceutical service and however effective the nursing management, there can be no substitute for the greatest care and attention to detail when a medicine is being administered. Understandably, the nurse who undertakes the final act feels in a very vulnerable position. This is because the administration of a medicine is so 'visible' and so final. The medicine has actually been taken by the patient or injected into the patient's tissues. At this stage, any second thoughts are not capable of being translated into action (other than reporting the error or suspected error). Unlike written prescriptions, doses actually given cannot be changed. This situation should be recognised by all those who prescribe and dispense medicines and by those who draw up policy and procedure documents.

In designing safe systems for the management of drugs, it is important to assess the levels of risk involved. It is quite unacceptable to accept different standards, but it must be recognised that the risks involved in administering complex parenteral chemotherapy are greater than the oral administration of a simple analgesic. Managing risk has three main components:

1. the identification of risk
2. the analysis of the risks involved
3. most importantly, the control of risk.

Table 6.2 Risk management (intravenous administration of chemotherapy as an example)

Phase	Questions	Answers
Identification of risk	• What could go wrong? • How could it happen? • What would be the effect?	• Incorrect dose, route; complex regimens • Inadequate information/documentation • Failure of treatment; adverse drug reaction
Analysis of risk	• How often is it likely to happen? • Cost if it does happen? • How severe if it does happen?	• Confining use of chemotherapy to specialist unit helps in this matter • Potentially very high • Outcome potentially catastrophic for patient
Control of risk	• How can risks be eliminated? • How can risks be avoided? • How can they be made less likely? • How can they be made less costly?	• Reduce complexity • Provide drugs in patient-specific presentations • Improve staff training • Use of protocols; use best available technology; use automated processes; manage change effectively

Table 6.2 outlines how these principles could be applied to medicine administration. By applying risk management techniques, it is possible to analyse drug errors in a systematic way. Following such an approach provides the basis for the establishment of safe systems of working.

PREVENTION OF ERRORS

Unfortunately, errors in the administration of medicines can never be completely eliminated (Ferner 1995). In recognition of the risks involved in the administration of medicines, a preventive approach has been used in an effort to help nurses avoid making errors (Downie et al. 1997). The use of up to date documents outlining the requirements and responsibilities at national, health authority and trust levels is essential. Access to written texts, which include the safe and effective use of medicines as well as their pharmacological properties, should be created. The use of an open learning programme on calculating medicine dosages has allowed students to learn in private and at their own pace (Mackenzie, unpublished work, 1996). Links between healthcare professionals and between service and education personnel help to ensure that records used in relation to the management of medicines and the content of policies and procedures are constantly reviewed.

DEALING WITH MEDICATION ERRORS/INCIDENTS

In the past, drug errors were universally viewed in the same way by senior nursing staff, and disciplinary action was often taken against offenders for their mistakes. The belief was that this was necessary to protect the patient. Such action is thought to do the exact opposite (Goodall 1993). Indeed, the fear of being disciplined may actually do the patient harm if the nurse is too frightened to ask for help (Arndt 1994). Punitive measures may also lead to under-reporting of drug errors (Cooper 1995). It is of course right, in healthcare as in any other field, that individuals must sometimes be held to account for their actions – in particular if there is evidence of gross negligence or recklessness or of criminal behaviour. Yet in the great majority of cases, the causes of serious failures stretch far beyond the actions of the individuals immediately involved. Safety is a dynamic, not static, situation. In a socially and technically complex field such as healthcare, a huge number of factors are at work at any one time that influence the likelihood of failure. These factors are a combination of the following.

- Active failures: 'unsafe acts' committed by those working at the sharp end of a system, which are usually short-lived and often unpredictable.
- Latent conditions: factors that can develop over time and lie dormant before combining with other factors or active failures to breach a system's safety defences. They are long-lived and, unlike many active failures, can be identified and removed before they cause an adverse event (Department of Health 2000).

Human error may sometimes be the factor that immediately precipitates a serious failure, but there are usually deeper, systemic factors at work that, if addressed, would have prevented the error or acted as a safety net to mitigate its consequences. It is now considered important to make the distinction between human error caused by, for example, pressure of work and negligence or reckless practice (Nursing and Midwifery Council 2004).

In June 2000, the Government accepted all recommendations made in the report of an expert group, led by the chief medical officer, called *An Organisation with a Memory* (Department of Health 2000). The report acknowledged that there has been little systematic learning from patient safety incidents and service failure in the NHS in the past, and drew attention to the scale of the problem of potentially avoidable events that result in unintended harm to patients.

An Organisation with a Memory proposed solutions based on developing a culture of openness, reporting and safety consciousness within NHS organisations. In summary, it recommended that the NHS needed to develop:

- unified mechanisms for reporting and analysis when things go wrong
- a more open culture, in which errors or service failures can be reported and discussed
- mechanisms for ensuring that, when lessons are identified, the necessary changes are put into practice
- a much wider appreciation of the value of the system approach in preventing, analysing and learning from errors.

National Health Service Quality Improvement Scotland took the lead for patient safety in Scotland when the organisation was established in January 2003. Prior to that, responsibility rested with the chief medical and nursing officers of the Scottish Executive Health Department. England took a slightly different approach when the chief medical officer set up the NPSA in 2001; both Wales and Northern Ireland are now covered by the NPSA. The NPSA was created to coordinate the efforts of all those involved in healthcare and, more importantly, to learn from patient safety incidents occurring in the NHS.

Every effort must be made to develop an open culture in which errors and near misses can be openly discussed and lessons learned. If considered appropriate, an anonymous reporting system may be established, but a system that guarantees confidentiality may be preferred. There is also the view that training should be provided for those involved in an error and support given to restore self-confidence (Williams 1996). One approach being used with student nurses who have been involved in a medication error/incident is based on the application of clinical risk management. The steps of risk management include identification, analysis and

control of the risks involved (Department of Health 1993; Table 6.2). Consideration of any financial implications (and this may be taken to include social costs) is also included. The teaching of subjects such as the management of medicines is, in effect, directed at managing the risks attached to the procedures involved. In the event of an error taking place, the steps of risk management are revisited, but this time in relation to the specific incident. Risk management is thus used in a cyclical way to help identify knowledge deficits or misunderstandings on the part of the student as well as those areas that would benefit from greater emphasis or clarification in future teaching. Both student and teacher thus stand to benefit. Whichever way drug errors are investigated, it is vitally important to have a structured approach to the investigation process. An excellent approach has been described that should ensure that lessons from an incident can be learned, especially about the organisational factors involved (Vincent et al. 2000).

Facing up to drug errors, or any other errors in delivering healthcare, is not easy either for health professionals involved in direct patient care or for those in managerial roles. There are encouraging signs that the problem of drug errors in particular is being addressed in the UK.

Medication safety committees are being established in the UK with a remit to improve patient safety. Reviewing error reporting data in order to determine trends and sharing learning with other healthcare professionals are key to their role.

Patient safety must be approached by all the professions involved on a joint basis. Lessons can be learned from other industries (Helmreich 2000) but, above all, we must learn from our patients and avoid the long-established 'the doctor/nurse/pharmacist knows best' cliché.

SELF-ASSESSMENT QUESTIONS

1. Apart from disciplinary aspects, what could be a significant consequence of not reporting a 'near miss' of a drug error?

2. What are the advantages of BAN for medicines?

3. Do you prefer to use proprietary or official names for medicines? Explain the reasons for your preference. (No answer given.)

4. Suggest one way by which drug errors can be reduced in your practice environment. (No answer given.)

REFERENCES

Arndt M 1994 Nurses' medication errors. Journal of Advanced Nursing 19:519–526

Barach P, Moss F 2001 Delivering safe healthcare. British Medical Journal 323:585–586

Clare J 1997 Survey shows Britons simply can't add up. Daily Telegraph 17 January 1997

Cooper MC 1995 Can a zero defects philosophy be applied to drug errors? Journal of Advanced Nursing 21:487–491

Department of Health 1993 Risk management in the NHS. Department of Health, London

Department of Health 2000 An organisation with a memory. Department of Health, London

Downie G, Mackenzie J, Williams A 1997 Help nurses avoid drug errors. Pharmacy in Practice November:539–543

Ferguson PR 1997 The legal liability of the community pharmacy for personal injury caused by medicinal products: liability for negligence. Pharmaceutical Journal 258:133–135

Ferner RE 1995 Is there a cure for drug errors? [editorial]. British Medical Journal 311:463–464

Gladstone J 1995 Drug administration errors: a study into the factors underlying the occurrence and reporting of drug errors in a district general hospital. Journal of Advanced Nursing 22:628–637

Goodall C 1993 Crimes (and misdemeanours). Nursing Standard 7:46–47

Helmreich RL 2000 On error management: lessons from aviation. British Medical Journal 320:781–784

Maxwell S, Walley T 2002 Using drugs safely. British Medical Journal 324:930–931

National Patient Safety Agency 2005 Wristbands for hospital inpatients improves safety. Safer Practice Notice 11. National Patient Safety Agency, London

Nolan TW 2000 System changes to improve patient safety. British Medical Journal 320:771–773

Nursing and Midwifery Council 2004 Guidelines for the administration of medicines. NMC, London

Reason J 2000 Human error: models and management. British Medical Journal 320:768–770

Reid T 1996 Official: young British workers cannot count. Sunday Telegraph 29 September 1996

Ridley SA, Booth SA, Thompson CM 2004 Prescription errors in UK critical care units. Anaesthesia 59:1193–1200

Scally G, Donaldson LJ 1998 Clinical governance and the drive for quality improvement in the new NHS in England. British Medical Journal 317:61–65

Scholz DA 1990 Establishing and monitoring an endemic medication error rate. Journal of Nursing Quality Assurance 4:71–85

Vincent C, Taylor-Adams S et al. 2000 How to investigate and analyse clinical incidents. Clinical Risk Unit and Association of Litigation and Risk Management protocol. British Medical Journal 320:777–781

Weingart SN, Wilson RM 2000 Epidemiology of medical error. British Medical Journal 320:774–777

Williams A 1996 How to avoid mistakes in medicine administration. Nursing Times 92:40–41

FURTHER READING AND RESOURCES

[Anonymous] 2000 Theme edition. British Medical Journal 320(7237)

[Anonymous] 2001 Compulsory guidelines aim to stop intrathecal chemotherapy disasters [editorial]. Pharmaceutical Journal 267:707

[Anonymous] 2001 Medical errors. British Medical Journal 322:1421–1425

Adcock H 2001 Learning from medication errors. Pharmaceutical Journal 267:287–289

Audit Commission 2001 A spoonful of sugar. Medicines management in NHS hospitals. Audit Commission, London

Drug errors (http://www.medicine-errors.org.uk)

Fradgley S, Pryce A 2002 An investigation into the clinical risks in the use of patients' own drugs on surgical wards. Pharmaceutical Journal 268:63–67

Halligan A, Donaldson L 2001 Implementing clinical governance: turning vision into reality. British Medical Journal 322:1413–1416

Institute of Medicine 1999 To err is human: building a safety health system. National Academy Press, Washington

Kendall MJ 2002 Therapeutics needs to be better taught. British Medical Journal 324:792

Kravitz RL, Melnikow J 2001 Engaging patients in medical decision making. British Medical Journal 323:584–585

Moscrop A 2001 Expert patients will help to manage chronic disease. British Medical Journal 323:653

National Patient Safety Agency (http://www.npsa.nhs.uk)

Nursing and Midwifery Council 2002 Guidelines for records and record keeping. NMC, London

Runciman B, Merry A 2001 Improving patients' safety by gathering information. British Medical Journal 323:298

Scott H 2002 Increasing numbers of patients are being given wrong drugs [editorial]. British Journal of Nursing 11:4

Smith J 2004 Building a safer NHS for patients: improving medication safety. Department of Health, London

The role of patients and carers in medicines management

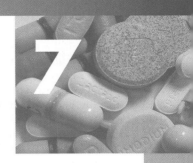

7

CHAPTER CONTENTS

KEY OBJECTIVES

After reading this chapter, you should be able to:

- give reasons why demand for drugs is always rising
- discuss methods used nationally and locally to contain expenditure on drugs
- discuss what is meant by 'postcode prescribing'
- identify sources of drug information available to the public
- discuss the ethical implications of drug testing on humans
- discuss how costs of drug therapy relate to patient outcomes
- define compliance in the context of drug therapy
- identify the factors that contribute to non-compliance
- distinguish between compliance and concordance
- discuss ways in which patient compliance may be improved
- discuss the precautions needed for and benefits to be gained from self-administration of medicines
- outline the role of home carers with regard to medicine administration
- discuss the issues concerning the giving of medicines in schools

- discuss the place of alternative and complementary medicines in society today.

INTRODUCTION

BENEFITS AND COSTS OF MODERN MEDICINES

Today, many patients are enjoying both a longer and better quality of life as a result of drug treatment. Perhaps the most dramatic example of this is the control of certain common infections that, 50 years ago, would almost certainly have had a fatal outcome. Drugs acting on the cardiovascular system, the newer insulins, oncolytics, improved anaesthetics, antiviral agents and psychotropic drugs have prolonged and improved life for many patients. In considering the advances made in drug therapy, the massive progress made in other aspects of health technology should not be overlooked (e.g. diagnostic and scanning equipment).

At a time when the resources available for healthcare are under great pressure, health service managers are required to examine carefully all competing demands.

The drug bill is no exception to this process. There is a need for an informed public debate on this aspect of healthcare, especially when issues of rationing care and inequalities of provision may be involved. Patient pressure groups address such issues as inconsistent availability of anticancer drugs having a significant impact on the provision of care.

The National Institute for Health and Clinical Excellence covers England, and similar bodies have been established in Wales and Scotland. These bodies issue guidance on important new drugs, which is often reproduced in the British National Formulary.

Although most patients derive great benefit from their medicines, the search for the 'magic bullet' goes on, especially in oncology. All medicines have the potential to cause harm to the patient, even when used in standard doses. Many patients, especially older patients, suffer from more than one condition, resulting in multiple-drug therapy (polypharmacy). The risk of drug interactions therefore increases, but the risk of harm to the patient is low in well-managed situations because the professionals involved in the management of medicines take steps to protect the patient from such eventualities. Chapter 3 describes the vital contribution made by the nurse in helping to ensure that the patient derives benefit from the prescribed treatment.

Abuse of substances is of growing concern throughout the world, a particular concern being the use of so-called recreational and lifestyle drugs. Much drug abuse is based on the use of illegal substances, but medicines can be abused, with potentially devastating outcomes for misusers and their families. Dependency on drugs may arise as the result of prescribed medical treatment, but this is rare. Legislation is in place designed to reduce the likelihood of drugs being diverted for abuse (see Ch. 2).

PUBLIC, PERSONAL AND PROFESSIONAL PERCEPTIONS

Health promotion resources are targeted at prevention strategies such as a healthy lifestyle, but the belief that health can be achieved or maintained by the use of medicines is still widely held. All health professionals must seek to ensure that patients (and their carers) have realistic expectations of their drug therapy and know when and why drug therapy is needed. Surveys of public opinion clearly show that people want to be involved in decisions about treatment (Kelham et al. 2005).

Economic and other pressures have led to campaigns designed to encourage people to take more responsibility for their own health. One outcome of this is the increasing sales of proprietary medicines, both traditional and less orthodox. There can be no doubt of the importance of self-medication in healthcare. The NHS would collapse if all the demands for medicines had to be met from NHS resources alone. There are dangers in assuming that proprietary over-the-counter medicines are completely safe and can be treated as placebos. As more medicines are made available for sale without prescription, the possibility of drug interactions must be borne in mind.

The use of complementary and alternative medicine (CAM) appears to be increasing. Issues relating to CAM are discussed on page 118.

One key objective of the NHS is to provide patients with comprehensive information about all aspects of their treatment. Linked with this is the need to ensure that patients and their carers have all the necessary information to enable courses of drug treatment to be completed successfully. A coordinated approach between professionals is called for on the provision of relevant non-conflicting information. The recognition of the need for a wider range of information on treatment is a product of both consumer pressures and changing attitudes within the professions. Care is needed to ensure that the information needs and views of ethnic minorities are recognised and responded to. In all situations, it is important to avoid information overload.

As yet, prescription-only medicines cannot be advertised to the public in the UK. In the USA, such advertisements are allowed and free telephone numbers offer callers a detailed information service. Website addresses are given where detailed information can be accessed. The use of Internet search engines can yield much detailed information on current drug treatments. There can be no doubt that patients and their carers are much better informed today than they were in the early years of the NHS.

PERSONAL FACTORS

The realisation that patients and their families hold, and are entitled to hold, their own beliefs about treatment was recognised by the Patient's Charter (Scottish Office Home and Health Department 1991). Patients (and their families) can formulate views on a proposed treatment only if they are in possession of relevant information about the condition, nature and effects of the treatment, alternatives available and consequences of not accepting treatment. The right of the patient or client follows the principle of informed consent, which is based on the individual having the necessary knowledge to make a decision (Nursing and Midwifery Council 2004). There may be situations, however, when it is in patients' best interests not to provide full information on their drug therapy.

From time to time, it may be necessary to change a patient's drug therapy, the reasons for which must be clearly explained to the patient by the prescriber. A medicine that has proved to be highly successful in treating a particular condition plays an important part in the patient's life. There may be an understandable reluctance on the part of the patient to accept the change. Nurses can play an important part in providing the patient with any necessary reassurance when drug treatment is changed for whatever reason. It should be remembered, too, that the patient has the right to refuse to take the medication. Were this to happen, details of the refusal must be documented. Major problems could arise if insulin or high-dose corticosteroids, for example, were refused.

Ethnic minority groups may have special needs and concerns that must be recognised and met. Cultural barriers may inhibit access to mainstream healthcare. In order to overcome these barriers, novel approaches may be needed. Moberly (2005) describes a service for the review of medicines within a mosque.

SOCIAL FACTORS

The ethical issues relating to medicines with which society is confronted raise many questions. For example, should the pharmaceutical industry be making profits out of illness? Some argue that profits from innovation and high levels of capital investment must be rewarded. Dependence, addiction and over-reliance on drugs raise doubts in the minds of many health professionals. Nurses will enter the debate on the ethical aspects of the use of medicines as part of their professional role. Local ethics committees provide guidance on specific matters, particularly on clinical trials. There may be situations in which, on religious grounds, a nurse cannot be involved in a particular form of treatment. This stance has to be respected and accepted by colleagues without any form of sanction being applied. Nurses in such situations will receive the support they need but, as always, the best interests of the patient must be served.

PROFESSIONAL FACTORS

Nurses want to be able to help their patients get better. There are factors, however, that must be considered before deciding which is the best treatment (or indeed whether or not to treat the patient at all). For example, the decision may be influenced by the likely side effects, the risk of dependence on the drug, the age of the patient and the patient's prognosis.

Downwards pressure on prescribing costs must not be allowed to compromise patient care. Well-researched, evidence-based prescribing policies must take into account cost factors, but all healthcare professionals have a duty to provide the best for their patients in the light of the current state of knowledge. When to withhold treatment may be a more difficult decision than when to initiate treatment.

Medical misadventures may also have a profound and long-term effect on all those unfortunate enough to be involved. Even with more enlightened policies on such matters as drug errors, health professionals may suffer from a lack of confidence that may need expert professionals' help to overcome (see Ch. 6).

THE BRISTOL INQUIRY

The Bristol Inquiry, which examined many failures on the part of cardiac surgeons and others, made numerous recommendations regarding the importance of health professionals treating all patients as partners by regarding them as 'equals with different expertise' (Coulter 2002). Key recommendations in the report of the inquiry are given in Box 7.1.

Although these recommendations were made following major failures in the provision of paediatric cardiac surgery services, the principles involved can be used to encourage greater responsiveness to the needs of patients by all those involved in the provision of drug therapy. Healthcare professionals carry out many functions that help to ensure a good outcome of a patient's drug therapy. However, without the active participation of the patient (and parents or carers), optimal results of the treatment may not be achieved.

Box 7.1 Bristol Inquiry report recommendations

- Involve patients (or their parents) in decisions.
- Keep patients (or their parents) informed.
- Improve communications with patients (or their parents).
- Provide patients (or their parents) with counselling and support.
- Gain informed consent for all procedures and processes.
- Elicit feedback from patients (or their parents) and listen to their views.
- Be open and candid when adverse events occur.

(From Anonymous 2001, with permission.)

The recommendations in Box 7.1 provide the necessary broad guidance for health professionals that, if followed, will help to ensure the achievement of an effective partnership with patients' concordance. Involving patients more in decision making has many benefits, not least in improving patient safety. Prescribing errors could be reduced by actively involving patients in their own care (Coulter 2002). It is recognised that, to achieve this, resource implications will have to be met and cultural and technical barriers overcome (Coulter 2002). Electronic access by patients to a range of relevant information may be the way forward (Coulter 2002). Patients may also become involved in the training of those involved in the provision of healthcare. The concept of the expert patient is being developed. Selected patients suffering from a chronic disease are given short training programmes in anatomy, physiology and the disease process. Drawing on this training and, above all, their own experiences, patients are then able to provide inputs on a range of matters into the training of medical students, doctors and other healthcare professionals.

The key recommendations of the Bristol Inquiry and the implications of these should be kept in mind when reading this chapter.

COMPLIANCE OF THE PATIENT

An essential component for the successful outcome of any treatment plan, drug or otherwise, is the patient's compliance with the prescriber's advice and directions. The compliance of a patient can be defined as the 'extent to which the patient's behaviour coincides with medical or health advice' (Sackett 1976). The term *patient compliance* is often considered to be unsatisfactory, because it has overtones of coercion or compulsion and does not include any reference to treatment outcome. Alternative, less-threatening terms that have been proposed include *therapeutic alliance and treatment adherence* (Blackwell 1976). At no time will the term *compliance* be used here with any implications of coercion of the patient. Increasingly, an approach (concordance) based on a partnership in medicine taking is advocated as a framework for improving patient care.

The key aspects of concordance are:

- there is an understanding of and respect for the patient's view on his or her medicines
- healthcare professional explores/understands the patient's view
- an equal partnership is formed, i.e. patient/healthcare professional

- an agreed plan that incorporates the above is formulated
- in the event of no agreement on the way forwards, the healthcare professional should offer further discussions
- the patient's decision on whether or not to take the medicine/use the therapy is respected
- differences between patient and healthcare professional are recognised
- the whole process depends on consultation – it is a two-way process
- the whole process is patient-centred.

Nurses in both community and hospital practice are well placed to help patients comply with the medical advice and instructions they are given regarding drug treatment. Often, the nurse is the only health professional who has continuing contact with the patient over long periods. As a result, the nurse is able to gain an understanding of the patient's difficulties, offer advice and monitor compliance.

NON-COMPLIANCE OF THE PATIENT

A very crude indication of the extent of non-compliance may be obtained when surveys are undertaken on the vast quantities of prescription medicines returned to pharmacies by patients.

Many studies have been published that demonstrate in detail the extent of non-compliance with directions regarding drug treatment. In long-term therapy, compliance is often inadequate. Patients taking antiepileptics achieved a 76% compliance level, which fell to 39% when the dosage schedule was changed from 8-hourly to 6-hourly (Cramer 1989). With short-term therapy, the position may generally be better. Studies by Donabedian and Rosenfeld (1984) and Mushlin (1972) showed that up to 75% of patients complied with their directions. Few studies relate the extent of non-compliance to the failure to achieve the desired therapeutic outcome. Nevertheless, non-compliance should always be considered as a possible reason for the failure of treatment.

Some patients may need extra help in managing their medicines, because of a disability. The Disability Discrimination Act 1995 applies to many aspects of everyday life, including the supply of medicines. Disabled people have a right to be treated no less favourably than other people. Pharmacists are required to provide the extra help a disabled person may need, for example by providing an aid to the use of medicines (see Table 7.1).

Table 7.1 Factors contributing to non-compliance

Factor	Comment(s)
Personal factors	
Patient's belief as to value of therapy	Patients from all groups of society may have particular views which are influenced by many factors.
Ethnic aspects	May conflict with mainstream western medicine.
Relationship with health personnel involved	Patient's faith in prescriber, especially, often influences outcome.
Ageing process	Loss of recent memory, physical disability, etc. may contribute to non-compliance.
Some psychiatric illnesses	Schizophrenia, for example, may bring particular problems.
Pressures of a busy life	Especially hard to comply when several daily dosage intervals are involved.
Poor understanding of regimen	Increasingly, patients may be receiving multiple therapy and may lack the ability to manage a complex regime.
Limited knowledge of condition	This may arise due to poor explanations by health professionals or denial.
Social factors	
Isolation	May arise from a breakdown in the family structure.
Deprivation	Some patients have to contend with a difficult journey to the surgery or pharmacy. Older people often have to contend with multiple deprivation and are more vulnerable when things do go wrong with their medicine taking.
Poverty	Patients who cannot afford prescription charges will probably need help and guidance not only with use of medicines but with the social security system also.
Factors directly related to medicines	
Tablets	Large tablets may be difficult to swallow; very small tablets may be difficult for a patient with stiff fingers to pick up.
Liquid medicines	Liquid medicines may have an unpleasant taste, colour or 'feel' in the mouth. Many liquid medicines that are used by older patients are formulated for children. Highly coloured, sweet, sickly flavours are generally not very acceptable to older patients, even if children find them acceptable, which often they do not. Measuring liquid medicines will be difficult for many patients, as will handling a 500-mL glass bottle of liquid medicine that may weigh almost 1 kg.
Topical preparations	Stiff ointments may be difficult to use, or there may be difficulty squeezing creams or ointments out of a tube. Products that stain the patient's linen, shower or bath may prove unacceptable.
Packaging	Child-resistant packaging is difficult for many people, although its use has reduced accidental poisoning of children significantly.
Labelling	Labelling systems have been improved with the introduction of machine-printed labels for all dispensed medicines, but the small print on some labels may be impossible for some patients to read.
Prophylactic medicines	Medicines prescribed for prophylaxis may not always be taken as prescribed, because the patient does not feel the benefit directly, e.g. malarial prophylaxis.
Unpleasant side effects	Unpleasant side effects such as headache and nausea may, undoubtedly, be a cause of non-compliance.

MEASUREMENT OF NON-COMPLIANCE

Many difficulties are presented when measuring or assessing patient compliance. The methods available vary from the basic tablet count to the use of electronic monitoring devices (Punchak et al. 1992) and the measurement of the drug (or metabolite) in body fluids. The methods available are listed under two headings: first, methods that are normally available to the nurse, and second, those methods that require considerable technical back-up and are applicable only in structured investigations into patient compliance.

METHODS OF COMPLIANCE ASSESSMENT AVAILABLE TO THE NURSE

- General impressions of the patient's understanding of the drug regimen.
- Tablet counts at suitable intervals.
- Physiological markers (e.g. pulse rate in digoxin therapy).
- Visible presence of drug or metabolites in urine or faeces (e.g. rifampicin produces a reddish discoloration of the urine).

METHODS OF COMPLIANCE DETERMINATION

- Chemical methods of determination of metabolites in body fluids.
- Measurement in body fluids of pharmacologically inert chemical markers added to the medicine.
- Medication monitors that record the withdrawal and time of withdrawal of a dose from the container.
- The presence of some drugs detected by chemical analysis of the patient's hair.
- Electronic devices incorporated into containers that record the date and times that the containers were opened or used (eye drop bottles).

Although these methods of determining compliance may be useful in a research setting, in practice the experienced nurse will rely on a less sophisticated approach.

SIGNIFICANCE OF NON-COMPLIANCE

Does it matter that some patients fail to take their medicines as prescribed? There can be no simple answer to this question. Failure to comply may delay a patient's restoration to full health (failure to complete a course of antibiotic therapy), or it may be life-threatening (inappropriate use of a corticosteroid by an asthmatic patient). Failure to take antirejection therapy following renal transplantation can be catastrophic, for both the patient and the service. Failure to take HIV therapy and antirejection therapy could mean the difference between life and death. Non-compliance with therapy for diabetes could have very serious consequences for the patient. The extent of non-compliance must also be taken into account, because it may well be that for a particular regimen an 80% compliance level by the patient may be adequate to achieve the desired therapeutic outcome. No general rules can be established. The whole situation must be assessed because, in many cases, the patient's condition will vary – and therefore the patient's need for medication will also change. Intelligent non-compliance has been described by Weintraub (1976) as occurring when patients either reduce the dose or stop taking a medicine altogether. The reasons for this behaviour may, when examined, be quite rational, such as the adjustment of a drug dose in response to the occurrence of side effects.

FACTORS IN NON-COMPLIANCE

Many factors have been identified as contributing to patient non-compliance. Haynes (1979) cites more than 200 factors, ranging from doctor–patient relationships to the colour and taste of the prescribed medicine. The factors involved can be classified into three main groups:

- personal factors
- social factors
- factors directly related to the medicines.

Rarely, if ever, will non-compliance be due to a single factor. Often, it will be attributable to a number of interacting factors. Table 7.1 lists the factors that contribute to non-compliance.

Occupational therapists have an important role to play in advising on the use of the various aids to the use of medicines. While the provision of an aid will help many patients, equally, the mere provision of an aid without more supportive action is unlikely to achieve anything.

The practical problems discussed above, although often contributing to non-compliance according to the strict definitions given, may also jeopardise the safe management of medicines by the patient; for example, child-resistant closures, once removed, may be left off, with consequent loss of security. The increasing use of foil-packed tablets etc. is helpful, but difficulties in removing the tablets can arise for patients with stiff fingers. Patients may find more unfamiliar presentations, such as suppositories and pressurised aerosols, difficult to use properly.

PATIENTS' RESPONSES TO PROBLEMS WITH THEIR MEDICINES

Many highly motivated patients, their carers, health personnel and social workers develop their own

DIY compliance aids. A number of approaches have been reported (Williams 1979). The most common is probably the setting out of individual doses, in advance, in household containers such as eggcups, ice trays, egg boxes and the like. Sellotape has been used to stick tablets and capsules to suitable fixtures in the kitchen or living room to act as a reminder that the dose is due. To help the patient select the right medicine, labels on containers and product information leaflets may be supplemented by lay terms such as 'water tablets', 'sleeping tablets', 'heart tablets', etc. Instructions on labels may also be modified, additional labels being added – often using large print or symbols to reinforce the dosage instructions. The timing of a television programme may be used by some patients as a signal that a dose is due. A variety of charts, calendars, etc. have also been used to assist the short-term memory.

It would appear that many of these ingenious aids are of assistance to some patients, and such self-help should not normally be discouraged. Equally, however, there can be no doubt that in some situations the 'homemade' devices may be a further source of problems that may not always be recognised by the patient. By transferring tablets from the original well-closed container, product security and stability may be lost. For example, if glyceryl trinitrate tablets are not stored in a well-sealed glass container, the volatile active ingredient will be lost. Some products (e.g. omeprazole capsules) absorb moisture from the atmosphere and should always be stored in the original foil packaging. Improved packaging such as calendar packs and a more proactive approach by healthcare professionals should remove the need for a DIY approach.

Nurses (and others) can learn from patients' coping strategies, because these may highlight inadequacies in the service provided. Expert patients in particular can provide valuable insights on many aspects of drug therapy (Jardine 2005). Patients are now encouraged to report problems with medicines and medicine equipment directly to the Medicines and Healthcare products Regulatory Agency.

METHODS FOR IMPROVING PATIENT COMPLIANCE

Before embarking on a course of action designed to improve patient compliance, two main questions must be borne in mind. First, does the patient really need drug therapy, or is some other form of therapy more appropriate? Second, will improved compliance assist in the achievement of the therapeutic objective(s)? For instance, it may well be that improved compliance will result in an unacceptable level of side effects. It is also vital to determine the real causes of non-compliance and to ensure that any strategies decided on are within the patient's capabilities, otherwise further problems will be created for the patient.

The available methods can be considered as:
- involving the patient in decision making and, if possible, the prescribing process (see p. 108)
- improving presentation (labelling and packaging) of dispensed medicines (see Table 7.2)
- providing aids to compliance (see Table 7.2)
- providing patient education and counselling (including the provision of patient information leaflets in the form of package inserts [see Fig. 7.1] and/or other suitable specially designed material)
- encouraging predischarge self-administration of medicines
- using financial incentives.

In some situations, a combination of strategies may be required, the patient being given a suitable aid and counselled as to the importance of therapy. While there is no sure way to identify the potential defaulter, it is essential to make every effort to identify the high-risk patient.

EDUCATION AND COUNSELLING

Patient groups are becoming increasingly active on a range of issues relating to drug therapy. Availability of treatments and the need for more information about prescribed medicines are key issues. Along with their professional colleagues, nurses can play a key role in ensuring that patients have sufficient knowledge to enable them to manage their prescribed medicines safely and effectively and thus achieve therapeutic benefit. Herxheimer (1976) has outlined the knowledge needed by patients, or by those responsible for their day-to-day care, in terms of questions to the pre-scriber (see Box 7.2). These questions are still relevant in the new century.

The amount of information given to an individual will vary, depending on particular circumstances.

PATIENT INFORMATION LEAFLETS

Patient information leaflets are made available with all prescribed medicines to supplement and reinforce the counselling of patients (see Fig. 7.1 and Box 7.3). These range from general information on a particular

Table 7.2 Methods for improving patient compliance

Method	Details
Presentation of dispensed medicines	
Appropriate containers and closures	Plastic, lightweight bottles with a cleft for ease of handling by an arthritic patient may be useful. Containers used for tablets should generally be at least the 32-mL size for ease of handling. Plastic containers are generally preferred by patients. Screw caps that can be easily removed have obvious advantages (Le Gallez et al. 1984) for some patients, although there is great need to ensure that containers fitted with such closures are stored out of the reach of children.
Improved labelling	A wide variety of labelling systems is available, each of which is designed to provide the information required for the patient in a clear, unambiguous way. Ideally, the label of a dispensed medicine should bear the following information. • full instructions about the drug and its required frequency • approved name of product and strength • name and address of dispensing pharmacist • date of dispensing • quantity dispensed • expiry date of product • lay term (e.g. 'water tablets') • warning – 'Keep out of reach and sight of children' • any special storage instructions • any special precautions in use • 'For external use only' and/or other appropriate warnings. Illustrations Large print Braille The needs of patients whose command of English is minimal will require attention. Labels written in their mother tongue will be required. The needs of the illiterate must be recognised and dealt with in a sympathetic way. Pictorial labels have been developed, and these may. prove useful in some situations.
Aids to compliance	
Aids in the management of solid dosage forms	The Dosett tray has certain special features, notably the Braille markings and a detailed labelling facility on the reverse. Other compartmentalised trays of the Wiegand type are useful, because each compartment can be labelled with the contents and any special instructions. The Pill Minder has some degree of 'child resistance', unlike the other trays described above. Other products available include the Medidos system, which has the advantage of being highly portable, because each daily tray can be carried separately. Combination products (e.g. diuretic with potassium) may prove useful, because the number of tablets to be taken daily is reduced. Compliance packs (calendar packs) are also made available for some products (e.g. oral contraceptives).
Aids in the management of liquid dosage forms	Measuring liquid medicines with the standard medicine spoon may prove difficult for many patients. Several alternative measuring devices are available. Blind patients may find a special measuring device helpful.
Other aids in the management of medicines	A long-handled ointment applicator has been developed for patients with physical disabilities. A device (Opticare) to aid the instillation of eye drops is available that helps the patient to aim the drop and squeeze the eye drop bottle (Fig. 23.5, p. 469). Other devices for eye drop instillation include Easidrop for aiming and Autodrop for aiming and squeezing. Talking labels allow a voice message to be attached to a standard package of medication.

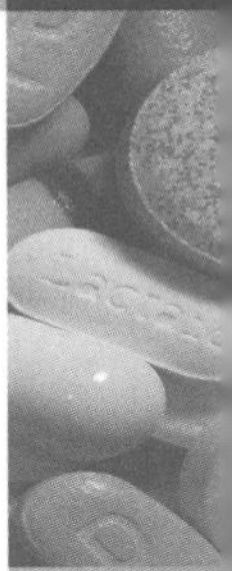

NAME OF MEDICINE

General introduction to medicine

Active ingredients

Information on manufacturer

Main actions of drug

Therapeutic indications

Precautions in use

Basic information on taking/using medicine

Action to be taken if dose exceeded/dose missed

Unwanted effects/need to report to doctor or other health professional

Safe storage

Other useful information, e.g. patient support groups/ sources of other information

Fig. 7.1 Patient information leaflet using lay terms.

Box 7.2 Herxheimer's questions to the prescriber

What for and how?
- What kind of tablets are they, and in what way do you expect them to help?
- How should I take them? How many and how often?
- Will I be able to tell whether they are working?
- How do I keep them?

How important?
- How important is it for me to take these tablets?
- What is likely to happen if I do not take them?

Any side effects?
- Do the tablets have any other effects that I should look out for?
- Do they ever cause any trouble?
- Is it alright to drive when I am taking them?
- Are they alright with other medicines I may need?
- Will alcohol interfere with them?
- What should be done if someone takes too many?

How long for?
- How long will I need to continue with these tablets?
- What should be done with any left over?
- When will I need to see you again?
- What will you want to know at the time?

Box 7.3 Examples of areas explained in a patient information leaflet

- Name of medicine
- What is in your medicine
- What your medicine is for
- What to consider before taking your medicine (e.g. other conditions you may suffer from, allergy)
- How to take your medicine
- What to do if you take too many tablets
- What to do if you miss a tablet
- Undesirable effects you may experience
- How to look after your medicine (including storage)

condition and associated drug therapy to information packages designed to meet the needs of an individual patient. A study by George et al. (1983) found that patients who received a leaflet were more likely to be completely satisfied with the treatment and with the information they had been given. It is vitally important that the information given to patients by different health professionals is complementary and does not give rise to confusion.

EDUCATION PACKAGES

Nurses working in the community can play a wider educational role by presenting talks to organised groups in the community on aspects of the safe use of medicines. The topics covered would naturally be selected in line with the interests and needs of the group (e.g. care of medicines among older people). In both hospital and the community, video recordings of the more common disorders (e.g. diabetes, lymphoma and asthma) sponsored by the bigger drug companies may be used.

SELF-ADMINISTRATION OF MEDICINES

A valuable opportunity to improve patient compliance may be presented during a period of in-patient care by a programme of self-administration of medicines. Such methods of medicine administration have been used over the years, with particular emphasis on the needs of patients in wards providing rehabilitation, care for older people and care for patients with a mental illness. It is recognised that self-administration systems can be used to advantage in acute wards (Bird 1988). The advantages claimed for systems of self-administration include improved patient compliance on discharge from hospital arising from better understanding of the medication(s), and more appropriate timing of medicine administration than can be achieved by the traditional medicine round. Nurses and other professional colleagues may be anxious about the risks that self-administration of medicines may cause, particularly as regards the safety and security of medicines in the ward environment. However, the adoption of a well-structured system will eliminate risk to a very large extent. Well-managed self-administration systems are essential to ensure both patient safety and the achievement of the desired therapeutic outcome. Self-administration systems may be useful when patients use their own prescribed medicines during their hospital stay. The essential components of a system for self-administration of medicines are outlined in Box 7.4.

A number of systems have been used to facilitate self-administration of medicines. In limited circumstances, patients may be given a small supply of certain medicines to keep in their bedside cabinet, or patients can be encouraged to ask for their medicines from the medicine trolley or designated cupboard. A system that gives the patient full involvement and control is based on using an individual, small lockable medicine cabinet. Access to the medicines is given according to the patient's needs and abilities. Patients who have been shown to be capable of managing their medicines well and whose needs are quite specific may be given the key to the medicine cabinet for the period of

---

Box 7.4 Essential components of a system for the self-administration of medicines

- A system that has been fully documented and agreed by all responsible authorities.
- Full patient information made available, and the patient's consent obtained.
- A detailed protocol that includes:
  — assessment of the patient
  — stages of the process once it has been confirmed that the patient is suitable for self-medication and wishes to undertake this detailed documentation, including the prescription sheet, a record of self-administration, a record of checks made on the patient's compliance and any other records of action taken to assist the patient
  — clear guidelines on the role of the healthcare professionals involved, especially nurses and clinical pharmacists.

Box 7.5 Stages in self-administration of medicines

Stage 1: patient assessed
Patient's knowledge of the medication can be assessed, and a general idea of degree of compliance can be established. At this stage, any special needs patient may have can be identified (e.g. need for compliance aid).

Stage 2: patient given access to bedside medicine cabinet under nurse's supervision
Process of assessment can be continued; frequency and nature of any checks on patient's compliance can be determined on a multidisciplinary basis. Value of any aid to compliance can be evaluated.

Stage 3: patient given key to medicine cabinet and allowed to self-administer with only limited supervision/checks
Further information/education on patient's medicines can be given at this stage as patient's confidence develops.

Stage 4: patient allowed to self-administer with reduced level of checks (say, weekly) on compliance
During this stage, patient can be prepared for discharge and any remaining problems resolved.

---

their in-patient treatment. In other situations, the key may be made available to the patient only at specific times.

Opportunities to assess and improve patient compliance are presented at all stages of the self-administration process. The stages are summarised in Box 7.5, together with a brief discussion of patient compliance issues.

If at any stage difficulties are identified, it may be necessary to review the arrangements, which could include discontinuation of the plan or reverting to an earlier stage of the process. This should seldom prove to be necessary if the assessment and checks are made with due care and sensitivity. Patient self-administration of medicines is playing an increasing role in helping patients to achieve good compliance and resulting benefits from their medication.

Patients are encouraged to bring their own supplies of prescribed medicines into hospital on admission. In such situations, it is logical that they should continue to have some control of their medicines during hospitalisation.

FINANCIAL INCENTIVES

In a review of the literature, Giuffrida and Torgerson (1997) found that, in 10 out of 11 studies reviewed, patient compliance was improved with the use of financial incentives. The incentives included cash, vouchers, lottery tickets or gifts. The studies examined were carried out in the USA, and it is not clear whether similar beneficial results could be achieved in other countries. Because patient non-compliance generates additional costs, it may be that provision of financial incentives would be cost-effective in certain situations. Further research is required in different environments, but it would be essential to ensure that any aspect chosen for study was capable of effective monitoring of patient compliance. In the present climate within healthcare in the UK, it does not seem likely that a financial approach to improving patient compliance will be followed, even if the ethical issues involved could be resolved.

THE ROLE OF SOCIAL WORK HOME CARERS IN THE ADMINISTRATION OF MEDICINES

The emphasis on care in the community has resulted in home carers becoming involved in aspects of the administration of medicines on behalf of their clients. The level to which the home carer becomes involved will be a matter for local social services departments to determine. In any event, most home carers will from time to time be required to provide their clients with assistance with their medicines. This assistance could range from helping with the taking of medicines to the disposal of unwanted medicines.

Box 7.6 Contents of a training programme for home carers

- Introduction
- Learning objectives
- Roles and responsibilities
- Taking the medicine – what happens next?
- Risk factors associated with medicines
- Types of medication (formulations)
- Ordering, collection, storage and disposal of medicines
- Dispensing labels – how to take the medicine
- Additional administration instructions – what do they mean?
- Ambiguous labels – or none at all
- Adverse effects of medication
- Over-the-counter medicines – what can be bought in a shop?
- Documentation:
  — medicines chart
  — recording sheet
  — medicines disposal form.
- Medicine administration practice
- Professional help and advice
- Case scenarios
- Good practice points

In order that the role can be discharged safely and effectively, locally recognised training programmes will be beneficial. An outline of what might be included in such a training programme is indicated in Box 7.6.

The training programme defines levels of responsibility in accordance with the needs of clients. Some clients will take full responsibility for their prescribed (and other) medicines. Other clients may need minimal assistance (e.g. ordering, collection and disposal of medicines). In some situations, more assistance will be required; for example, the carer may administer an oral dose or may assist in the use of topical preparations. In all situations, the level of input by the home carer will be clearly defined by supervisors and other social work or health professionals (e.g. community nurse). The home carer may need to be aware of any medicines the client may purchase.

Home carers can play a vital role in helping to ensure that their clients gain the full benefit of their medication and can also alert colleagues to any developing problem.

COMPLEMENTARY AND ALTERNATIVE MEDICINE

The debate about the value of complementary and alternative medicine (CAM) led by HRH Prince Charles has raged for years and no doubt will continue. Equally, there can be no doubt that many people 'vote with their feet' and regularly use one or more of the therapies or other form of treatment (e.g. acupuncture). Moore et al. (1985) found that patients using CAM were not 'cranks' and had not lost confidence in conventional treatments. A high percentage of patients felt benefit from their therapy. A study by Shang et al. (2005) showed that homeopathy effects are no better than placebo. Advocates of holistic medicine support an integrated approach that combines homeopathy and conventional medicine.

Herbal remedies are favoured by many people. Despite the view that herbal remedies being from natural sources are safe and cannot possibly do harm, certain problems may arise. Herbal remedies may interact with conventional medicines (Barnes et al. 2003) and products, especially those of Asian origin, may be contaminated (Ernst 2005).

In the light of the pressure from patients, it may be important for nurses and other health professionals to understand more fully the patient's wishes and whenever possible facilitate the continuation of an orthodox therapy in hospital. It is very important to assess if there are any hazards (interactions, toxicity) in continuing the therapy or otherwise. More research is called for into the benefits or otherwise of CAM. Most herbal remedies available in the UK have been exempt from licensing. A European Union directive came into force in October 2005 designed to ensure product safety of herbal remedies. It is worth remembering that a significant number of highly effective modern drugs were originally derived from natural sources, such as roots, barks and leaves, but these are subject to stringent quality control procedures.

MEDICINES IN SCHOOLS

A significant number of children attending mainstream schools need to take medication during the school day. It is vitally important to ensure that the necessary medication is made available in such a way that the pupil's education is not disrupted. Cooperation between parents/guardians and school authorities is required to ensure this.

Cooperation between the NHS and education authorities is also essential to ensure that systems are put in place to facilitate the safe management of medicines in schools. The overall aim of any system must be to ensure that pupils with medical needs are able to benefit fully from their education. In special schools, it will be necessary to make arrangements that reflect the particular needs of the pupils. Key elements of a safe system of medicine management for specialist and mainstream schools are outlined below.

- An individual care plan or one that is incorporated into a pupil's personal learning plan.
- Cooperation of staff (legal position of staff and school may need clarification).
- Involvement of parents/guardians in provision of information on pupil's medical condition and supply of necessary medicines.
- Involvement of NHS and school health service in such matters as local protocols/procedures and training needs of staff involved in medicine administration.
- Good working relationships with local general practitioners, nurses, pharmacists and other healthcare professionals.
- Guidance of local education authority.
- System of documenting care policy/procedures that can be applied flexibly, with sensitivity, and preserve confidentiality
- Procedures for dealing with mild and severe allergic reactions and other special situations (e.g. asthma). Arrangements for calling emergency service should be made known to all staff.
- Procedures for administration of medicines, including recording of administration of all medicines (consent of pupil or parent/guardian must be secured). Principles of medicine administration are those that apply to administration of a medicine by a health professional, although information available within school may not be as comprehensive as information available to a health professional.
- Arrangements for medicines management during out-of-school activities.
- Safe storage of all medicines at all times. Stocks held should be limited to essential needs only. Disposal of unwanted medicines must be in accordance with local guidance. Inhalers must be readily available on the basis of need.
- Basic hygiene procedures (e.g. in use of topical preparations and inhalers).
- Balance between making medicines available to pupils who need them and safety of all pupils.

Prescribed medicines help many people to live a normal life. The whole aim of medicine management procedures in schools must be to ensure that pupils derive benefit from their medicines, which in turn will enable them to benefit fully from all their educational opportunities.

CASE STUDY

This case history is included to emphasise that, despite all the advances in medical science and treatments based on high technology, relatively trivial (to the health professional) matters can be a cause of concern to patients. Such concerns need to be addressed in a clear and uncompromising way, avoiding information overload (See Q and A paragraph).

The patient suffers from non-Hodgkin's lymphoma and has just been discharged from hospital after $2\frac{1}{2}$ months. The reason for admission was severe diarrhoea and confusion, which led to status epilepticus. After being transferred to the intensive care unit, the diagnosis of thrombotic thrombocytopenic purpura was made. Twenty nine days were spent in the intensive care unit, 18 in the haematology ward and 27 in rehabilitation. In the unit, close monitoring of the patient took place. To control the airway, a tracheotomy was carried out. Numerous plasma exchanges were performed, as well as peritoneal dialysis.

On discharge, the patient was mobile with two sticks, although still very weak and with limited concentration. The medicines on discharge were:

- dispersible aspirin 75-mg tablets × 2 to be dissolved in water daily with or after food
- folic acid 5-mg tablet daily
- sodium valproate enteric-coated tablet 500 mg × 2 twice daily
- phenytoin 100-mg capsule × 2 and 25-mg capsule × 1 at night
- ranitidine 150-mg tablet twice daily
- furosemide 40-mg tablet daily
- dalteparin 2500 units subcutaneous daily, self-administered.

One week later:

- dalteparin was discontinued
- a reducing regimen of phenytoin was begun at a rate of 25 mg per fortnight, having started at 250 mg per day.

Two weeks later:

- neutrophil count 0.2×10^9/L
- commenced G-CSF 263 micrograms subcutaneous daily, self-administered
- full blood count to be done in 1 week's time.

One week later:

- neutrophil count risen dramatically
- G-CSF discontinued.

Four weeks later:

- sodium valproate reduced to 800 mg (i.e. 500-mg tablet, 200-mg tablet and 100-mg tablet) twice daily
- phenytoin to continue as previously described for 2 weeks and then reduced by 25 mg until seen at haematology clinic 1 week later.

PATIENT/NURSE DIALOGUE

Q *I've found this all rather confusing. I wasn't taking in what people were saying all that well at the time I was discharged. I had all these packets, and there was so much to remember. I still felt very fragile and unable to remember what I had just been told. Is there any way things might have been made easier for me?*

A Anyone would have found this a lot to take in. You could have done with more information written down for you. Also, a member of your family could have been present to help in understanding the prescriptions and instructions.

Q *Most of the tablets are in foil packs. The tablets can be awfully difficult to push through sometimes. I find the ferrous sulphate especially difficult. I also once nearly swallowed a fragment of foil.*

A There is a gadget called a pill pusher that can be extremely useful. Because it looks as if you might be on medication for some time, you may find it a good investment to get one. Your local pharmacist will be able to advise you.

Q *Although the 500-mg and 200-mg strength of sodium valproate don't say crushable on the pack, the 100-mg strength does. What does this mean? Will they only work if they're crushed?*

A The tablet will work if not crushed; they are made in this form for ease of use in children. The stronger strength tablets have a special coating to prevent irritation of the stomach. These tablets should not be crushed, so as to keep the benefits of the special coating.

Q *Being on so many medicines, I feel they are taking over my life. Is there any way I could be better organised?*

A A number of aids to medicine taking are available. One such is a compartmentalised system called a Dosette, which might help you. You should speak to your local pharmacist or community nurse.

Q *The tablets and capsules are either very slippery or very sticky when being handled. I am in danger of losing them sometimes. I know of one at least that's under the washing machine! Why are they like this?*

A The tablets are slippery to ease swallowing, and the capsules are sticky because the capsule shell is made of gelatin, which may become sticky in contact with moisture in your hand.

Continued

Q *I sometimes have difficulty pushing in the drug when I've been giving myself an injection from a ready-filled syringe. Can you give me any tips to overcome this?*

A Try slackening the plunger first by pushing the black bung up and down once or twice. Take care, however, that you don't lose any of the drug in the process.

Q *If I'm going on the bus into town in the morning, I find the furosemide has an effect on me and I am in danger of not getting to a toilet in time. Would it be OK if I took it later than prescribed on those days, such as lunchtime?*

A Yes, but you might like to consider your fluid intake and the duration and onset of action of the effect. Decaffeinated tea and coffee may be of some help.

Q *The label says 'BP'. Am I being treated for high blood pressure?*

A BP in this context stands for British Pharmacopoeia.

SELF-ASSESSMENT QUESTIONS

Identify the difficulties the following patients may have in complying with their medication.

1. A 55-year-old female teacher instilling eye drops for glaucoma.
2. An unemployed unskilled worker with type 1 diabetes.
3. A 75-year-old gentleman with three coexisting conditions each being treated with regular daily oral therapy.
4. A 37-year-old middle manager in the oil industry taking fluoxetine for depression and triple therapy for *H. pylori* eradication.
5. A 20-year-old female student nurse taking oral salicylate and prednisolone for Crohn's disease.
6. A socially active widow aged 69 years taking oral therapy for hypertension.
7. A teenager with psoriasis.
8. A retired farmer of 77 years who has been prescribed omeprazole for his gastro-oesophageal reflux disease. He does not take the medication regularly, because he is worried about how much it is costing the NHS.

REFERENCES

[Anonymous] 2001 Learning from Bristol: the report of the public inquiry into children's heart surgery at the Bristol Royal Infirmary 1984–1995. HMSO, London

Barnes J, Anderson LA, Phillipson JD 2003 Pharmaceutical Journal 270:118–121

Bird CA 1988 Taking their own medicine. Nursing Times 84:28–32

Blackwell B 1976 Treatment adherence. British Journal of Psychiatry 129:513–531

Coulter A 2002 After Bristol: putting patients at the centre. British Medical Journal 324:648–651

Cramer JA 1989 How often is medication taken as prescribed?: a novel assessment technique. Journal of the American Medical Association 261:3273–3277

Donabedian A, Rosenfeld LS 1984 Follow-up study of chronically ill patients discharged from hospital. Journal of Chronic Disorders 14:847–862

Ernst E 2005 Contamination of herbal medicines. Pharmaceutical Journal 275:167–168

George CF, Nicholas JA, Waters WE 1983 Prescription information leaflets: a pilot study in general practices. British Medical Journal 287:1193–1196

Giuffrida A, Torgerson DJ 1997 Should we pay the patient?: review of financial incentives to enhance patient compliance. British Medical Journal 315:703–707

Haynes RB 1979 Factors contributing to patient non-compliance. In: Haynes RB, Taylor DW, Sackett DL (eds) Compliance in health care. Johns Hopkins University Press, Baltimore, pp. 1–7

Herxheimer A 1976 Sharing the responsibility for treatment. Lancet ii:1294

Jardine C 2005 Expert patients: not quite what the doctor ordered. Daily Telegraph 9 November 2005

Kelham C, Mynors G, Shaw J 2005 Who decides?: UK public perceptions of decisions about care and medicines. Pharmaceutical Journal 274:215

Le Gallez P, Bird HA, Wright V et al. 1984 Comparison of 12 different containers for dispensing anti-inflammatory drugs. British Medical Journal 288:699–701

Moberly T 2005 Taking medicines review into a mosque. Pharmaceutical Journal 274:585

Moore J, Phipps K, Mareer D et al. 1985 Why do people seek treatment by alternative medicine? British Medical Journal 290:28–29

Mushlin AI 1972 A study of physicians' ability to predict patient compliance. Master's thesis. Johns Hopkins University, Baltimore

Nursing and Midwifery Council 2004 Code of professional conduct. NMC, London

Punchak SS, Goodyer LI, Miskelly FG 1992 Recent developments in electronic monitoring aids in assessing compliance with medication. Hospital Pharmacy Practice 2:167–169

Sackett DL 1976 Introduction. In: Sackett DL, Haynes RB (eds) Compliance with therapeutic regimens. Johns Hopkins University Press, Baltimore, p. 1

Scottish Office Home and Health Department 1991 The patient's charter: a charter for health. SOHDD, Edinburgh

Shang A, Huwiler-Muntener K, Nartey L et al. 2005 Are the clinical effects of homeopathy placebo effects?: comparative study of placebo-controlled trials of homeopathy and allopathy. Lancet 366:726–732

Weintraub M 1976 Intelligent and capricious non-compliance. In: Lasagna A (ed) Compliance. Futura, Mount Kisco, p. 39

Williams A 1979 The role of the pharmacist in improving compliance in the elderly patient. Proceedings of the Guild of Hospital Pharmacists 6:1–22

FURTHER READING AND RESOURCES

[Anonymous] 2004 How does a self-medicating consumer decide what medicine to use? Pharmaceutical Journal 273:440–441

Anadalo D 2006 Medicines management in English care homes: a grim and chaotic picture. Pharmaceutical Journal 275:198–199

Aronson JK, Hardman M 1992 Patient compliance. British Medical Journal 305:1009–1011

Association of the British Pharmaceutical Industry 2005 Code of practice for the pharmaceutical industry. ABPI, London

Bellingham C 2004 Improving medicines management in intermediate care and social services. Pharmaceutical Journal 273:349–350

Bird CA 1990 Patient self-medication. Surgical Nurse 3:22–26

Bloom BS 2001 Daily regimen and compliance with treatment. British Medical Journal 323:647

Bond C (ed.) 2004 Concordance. Pharmaceutical Press, London

Brown ME 2001 What is a drug? Pharmaceutical Journal 267:301–302

Cameron C 1996 Patient compliance: recognition of factors involved and suggestions for promoting compliance with therapeutic regimens. Journal of Advanced Nursing 24:244–250

Davis S 1991 Self-administration of medicines. Nursing Standard 5:29–31

Department of Health 2004 Building a safer NHS for patients: improving medication safety. A report from the Chief Pharmaceutical Officer. Department of Health, London

Department of Health. The expert patient – a new approach to chronic disease management for the 21st century. Online. Available: http://www.doh.gov.uk/whatsnew

Ferguson T 2002 From patients to end users: quality of online patient networks needs more attention than quality of online health information. British Medical Journal 324:555–556

Grills A 1997 An assessment of the pharmaceutical needs of the blind and partially sighted in Dumfries and Galloway. Pharmaceutical Journal 259:381–384

Holloway A 1996 Patient knowledge and information concerning medication on discharge from hospital. Journal of Advanced Nursing 24:1169–1174

Huckerby C, Hesslewood J, Jagpal P 2006 Taking health care into black and minority communities: a pharmacist-led initiative. Pharmaceutical Journal 276:680–682

Ley P 1981 Professional non-compliance: a neglected problem. British Journal of Clinical Psychology 20:151–154

Ley P 1988 Communicating with patients: improving communication, satisfaction and compliance. Croom Helm, London

Mintzes B, Barer ML 2002 Influence of direct to consumer pharmaceutical advertising and patients' requests on prescribing decisions: two site cross sectional survey. British Medical Journal 324:278–279

National Institute for Health and Clinical Excellence (http://www.nice.org.uk)

Nyatanga B 1997 Psychological theories of patient non-compliance. Professional Nurse 12:331–334

Pharmacy Community Care Liaison Group 1997 Medicines in schools. Implementing good practice in mainstream schools: a guide for pharmacists. Pharmaceutical Journal 258:69–71

Raynor DKT, Britten N 2001 Medicine information leaflets fail concordance test. British Medical Journal 322:1541

Rosenbloom K, Wakeman R, Scrimshaw 2005 The Disability Discrimination Act. Pharmaceutical Journal 275:747–750

Runciman B, Merry A 2001 Improving patients' safety by gathering information. British Medical Journal 323:298

Scottish Executive 2001 The administration of medicines in schools. Scottish Executive, Edinburgh

Scottish Executive Health Department (Pharmacy Division) 2000 Guidance on exploring effective strategies to empower patients and the public about their medicines. Scottish Executive Health Department, Edinburgh

Scottish Medicines Consortium (http://www.scottishmedicines.org.uk)

Sculpher M, Drummond M, O'Brien B 2001 Effectiveness, efficiency and NICE. British Medical Journal 322:943–944

Skene L, Smallwood R 2002 Informed consent: lessons from Australia. British Medical Journal 324:39–41

Stockwell Morris L, Schulz RM 1992 Patient compliance: an overview. Journal of Clinical Pharmacology and Therapeutics 17:283–295

Vincent C 2001 The safety of acupuncture. British Medical Journal 323:467–468

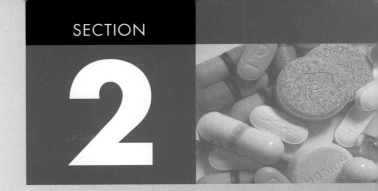

GENERAL PRINCIPLES OF PHARMACOLOGY

Pharmacokinetics and pharmacodynamics

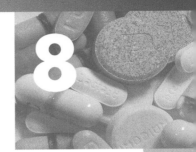

8

CHAPTER CONTENTS

KEY OBJECTIVES

After reading this chapter, you should be able to:

- outline the process that happens to a drug after administration
- explain how the half-life of a drug affects its dosing schedule
- give three examples of drugs that are receptor antagonists
- explain the effects that occur on drug handling due to age.

INTRODUCTION

Patients rely on nursing staff and pharmacists to ensure that medicines are administered appropriately. It is essential that nurses have a sound understanding of what happens to a drug following administration. *Pharmacokinetics* is the term used to describe how the body handles a drug over a period of time, including how the body absorbs, distributes, metabolises and excretes the drug (Fig. 8.1). These processes influence the effectiveness of the drug because, in order for a drug to be effective, it must be available at the site of action in the correct concentration. In the simplest terms, pharmacokinetics can be described as what the body does to the drug, as opposed to pharmacodynamics, which is what drugs do to the body.

PHARMACOKINETICS

ABSORPTION

Except for the intravenous route, a drug must be absorbed across cell membranes before it enters the systemic circulation. The oral route is the one most commonly used for drug administration. Most drugs are absorbed by diffusion through the wall of the intestine into the bloodstream, which is aided by the very large surface of the gut wall. The rate of absorption also depends on the lipid-solubility of the drug. Drugs are normally formulated to make them as lipid-soluble as possible to enable them to cross the cell membranes of the intestinal wall. However, sometimes a drug's low lipid-solubility is used to good effect, because it reaches the colon largely unabsorbed, for example aminosalicylates for use in ulcerative colitis and the antibiotics vancomycin and neomycin. In these examples, the aim is to get the drug into the lumen of the colon for therapeutic purposes while avoiding systemic absorption. A few drugs are absorbed by active transport processes. Iron, levodopa and fluorouracil

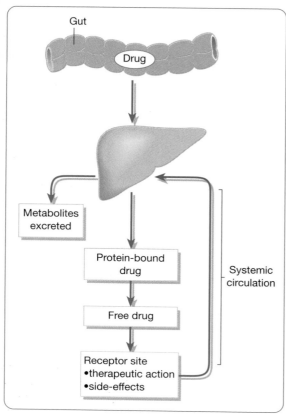

Fig. 8.1 Absorption, distribution, metabolism and excretion of an oral drug.

are examples of drugs actively transported across the intestinal mucosa.

The presence or absence of food in the stomach can affect the rate and amount of drug absorbed. Penicillins, erythromycin and rifampicin are examples of drugs that are better absorbed on an empty stomach and should be given half an hour before meals. Absorption of drugs from the gastrointestinal tract may be complete or incomplete. This can be influenced by the lipid-solubility of the drug and, as a result, the rate it crosses cell membranes, the rate at which the stomach empties and the presence or absence of food in the stomach.

Following absorption from the gastrointestinal tract, drugs are transported via the portal vein to the liver before reaching the general circulation. Many drugs are broken down (metabolised) as they pass through the liver, so that only a proportion of the amount absorbed reaches the general circulation to be carried to the site of action. This is called the first-pass effect. Some drugs show a very significant first-pass effect. Examples include glyceryl trinitrate,

which is often given sublingually, resulting in absorption through the mucosa, and lignocaine (lidocaine), which is given by injection, in both instances bypassing the portal circulation. The manufacturers will, of course, be aware of the first-pass effect and, when drugs are affected by this, they will have tailored the dose accordingly in order to ensure a therapeutic effect.

DISTRIBUTION

When a drug enters the bloodstream, it is rapidly diluted and transported throughout the body. Movement from the blood to tissues is influenced by a number of factors that can greatly affect the resultant drug action. Plasma proteins, particularly albumin, can bind many drugs. Only the *unbound* fraction of the drug is free to move from the bloodstream into tissues to exert a pharmacological effect. The bound drug is pharmacologically inactive, because the drug–protein complex is unable to cross cell membranes. It provides a reserve of drug, because the complex can dissociate and quickly replenish the unbound drug as it is removed from the plasma. The degree of protein binding will thus affect the intensity and duration of a drug's action.

In addition, if a patient suffers from a disease in which plasma proteins are deficient (e.g. liver disease, malnutrition), more of the drug is free to enter the tissues. A normal dose of a drug could then be dangerous, because so little is bound by available protein, thus increasing the availability of unbound drug.

In practice, changes in the protein-bound drug, resulting in increased levels of unbound drug, are important only for highly bound drugs with a narrow therapeutic index, such as warfarin or phenytoin. The term *narrow therapeutic index* is used to describe drugs for which the toxic level is only slightly above the therapeutic range, and a slight increase in unbound drug may therefore result in toxic symptoms. It is important therefore that the nurse has an awareness of these drugs and knowledge of the symptoms that the patient may show should toxic levels be reached.

Drugs diffuse out of the plasma into tissue spaces, and some enter cells and spread through the total water of the body. The total body water represents about 0.55 L/kg. Therefore the more widely a drug diffuses, the lower will be the concentration produced by a given dose. Factors that affect the rate and extent of distribution are cardiac output and regional blood flow. If the patient is nursed in a warm environment,

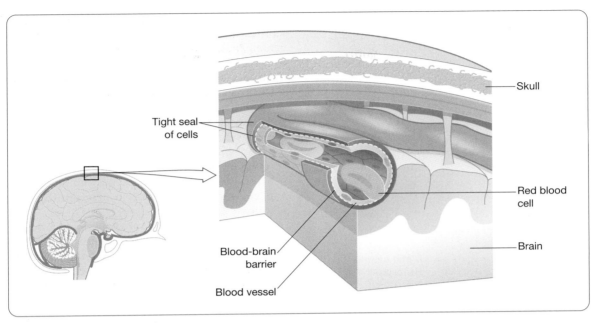

Fig. 8.2 The blood–brain barrier.

this will help to maintain a better blood circulation and improve drug distribution, an important factor in patients receiving antibiotics. Similarly, inflamed tissues have increased vascularity and permeability, which lead to an increased rate of passage of drugs, especially antibiotics.

TRANSFER BARRIERS

The central nervous system is surrounded by a specialised membrane consisting of the blood–brain and blood–cerebrospinal fluid barriers (Fig. 8.2). This membrane is highly selective for lipid-soluble drugs; for example, the penicillins diffuse well into body tissues and fluids but penetration into the cerebrospinal fluid is poor, except when the meninges are inflamed. Chloramphenicol, because of its lipid-solubility, is one of the few antibiotics that reach the cerebrospinal fluid in appreciable concentrations. Dopamine in the treatment of Parkinson's disease cannot be given in this form, because it does not cross the blood–brain barrier. It is administered orally as the precursor, levodopa, which is absorbed, crosses the blood–brain barrier and is broken down to dopamine by the enzyme dopa decarboxylase.

During pregnancy, the placenta provides a barrier between mother and fetus. Some drugs (e.g. chlor-promazine and morphine) cross it relatively easily, while others (e.g. suxamethonium chloride) are not transferred. Because fetal liver and kidney are unable to metabolise or excrete drugs, and the fetus is likely to be more sensitive to them, drugs must be used with caution in pregnancy and, in general, few are used.

METABOLISM AND EXCRETION

The most common route for drug excretion is through the kidneys into the urine. Drugs and their metabolites are filtered out from the plasma through the capillaries within the glomeruli of the kidneys. Drugs and metabolites can also be eliminated by the body in other ways (e.g. salivary glands, sweat glands).

Several factors, including certain characteristics of the drug, affect the kidneys' ability to excrete drugs. To be extensively excreted in urine, a drug or metabolite must be water-soluble and must not be bound too tightly to proteins in the bloodstream. The acidity of urine, which is affected by diet, drugs and kidney disorders, can affect the rate at which the kidneys excrete some drugs. Some drugs, such as atenolol, digoxin and captopril, are water-soluble and are readily eliminated by the kidney without prior metabolism. However, many drugs require to be changed into a form that can be readily eliminated by the body, and this process is called metabolism.

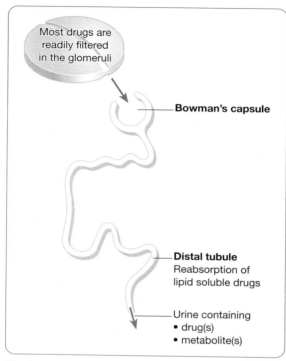

Most drugs are readily filtered in the glomeruli

Bowman's capsule

Distal tubule
Reabsorption of lipid soluble drugs

Urine containing
• drug(s)
• metabolite(s)

Fig. 8.3 Filtration of drugs through the kidney.

Most drugs are very lipid-soluble, and this enables them to cross cell membranes or the blood–brain barrier in order to reach their site of action. If a lipid-soluble drug is filtered by the kidney, it is largely reabsorbed from the distal tubule (Fig. 8.3) and retained in the body. Metabolism increases the water-solubility of the molecule and aids its elimination. Most metabolism takes place in the liver, but it can also be carried out in other organs, including the gut wall, lungs and kidney, and in the plasma.

In the process of metabolism, drugs may be broken down or combined with a chemical. This is brought about by substances called enzymes. The nurse should be aware that the rate at which this occurs in the liver can vary. If the liver cells are damaged or the circulation to the liver is reduced, as in cardiac failure, the inactivation process may be slowed and a lower dose of drug would be indicated.

PHARMACOGENETICS

Pharmacogenetics is the study of the extent to which genetic differences influence the response of individuals to medicines. Its use in drug development research is still at an early stage. The terms *pharmacogenetics* and *pharmacogenomics* are often used synonymously,

but there are subtle differences in their meaning. Pharmacogenetics essentially refers to how a person's genetic make-up influences her or his response to drugs and, in particular, how specific genes affect the responses to specific drugs or drug classes. More recently, since completion of the Human Genome Project, the term pharmacogenomics has come into common use. Pharmacogenomics is a somewhat broader term, referring to the genome-wide search for genes and associated products (such as enzymes or other proteins) that may be suitable targets for new drug discovery or that interact with other genes and environmental factors in determining drug response.

Response to drugs can vary between individuals and between different ethnic populations. The most important aspect is the genetic variability between individuals in their ability to metabolise drugs due to expression of polymorphic enzymes. Polymorphism enables division of individuals within a given population into at least two groups: poor metabolisers and extensive metabolisers of certain drugs. Hydralazine and isoniazid are inactivated by acetylation, a process involving enzyme action. Acetylation proceeds at different rates in different individuals, over half the population being slow acetylators and the remainder fast acetylators. The fast acetylators will require a higher dose than the slow acetylators in order to receive an equivalent therapeutic effect.

RENAL DISEASE

When drugs or their breakdown products are excreted through the kidneys, excretion will be delayed if the kidneys are damaged by disease, and accumulation can occur. Kidney function is also reduced in old age. Because renal impairment results in a decreased capacity of the kidney to eliminate drugs, dosages must be adjusted to achieve therapeutic drug plasma levels.

The severity of renal impairment is expressed in terms of glomerular filtration rate, usually measured by creatinine clearance (Cr Cl). Creatinine is an end product of muscle metabolism and is eliminated from the body by the kidney. Cr Cl is obtained by measuring the plasma creatinine concentration in a 24-h collection of urine. When this is difficult to obtain, the serum Cr Cl is used. Normal Cr Cl is 100–120 mL/min for both men and women. Renal impairment is divided into three grades, as shown in Table 8.1. Renal function declines with age, and many elderly patients have a glomerular filtration rate of less than 50 mL/min.

Table 8.1 The three grades of renal impairment

Grade	Glomerular filtration rate (mL/min)
Mild	20–50
Moderate	10–20
Severe	< 10

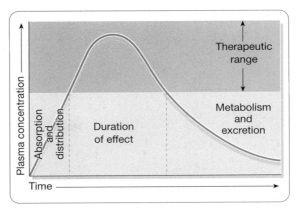

Fig. 8.4 Effects of absorption, distribution, metabolism and excretion on the plasma concentration of an administered drug.

The Cockcroft–Gault equation aims to predict Cr Cl from knowledge of serum creatinine, age and weight (ideal body weight, IBW):

$$\text{Cr Cl (male)} = \frac{[1.23 \times (140 - \text{age}) \times \text{IBW}]}{\text{serum creatinine}}$$

$$\text{Cr Cl (female)} = \frac{[1.04 \times (140 - \text{age}) \times \text{IBW}]}{\text{serum creatinine}}$$

Weight should be lean body mass. Estimate lean body mass for extremes of size.

If the glomerular filtration rate is only 50% of normal, the time for a drug to be eliminated in an unchanged form by the kidney will be doubled. The dose can be adjusted either by being halved or by giving the normal dose at double the time intervals.

The British National Formulary (BNF) provides guidance on the use of an extensive list of drugs when there is mild, moderate or severe renal impairment.

DOSE–EFFECT RELATIONSHIP

Safe and effective therapy can be achieved only with doses that produce optimal concentrations of a drug in the plasma and target tissues. Smaller doses will be ineffective, while larger doses will not increase the benefits and may have toxic effects. Between the minimal dose that gives the required therapeutic response and the dose at which toxic symptoms appear is a dose range called the therapeutic dose range. Some drugs have a narrow range, whereas others have a wide therapeutic range.

After administration of a drug, its plasma level rises; the more rapidly the drug is absorbed, the faster its plasma level rises (Fig. 8.4).

As drug absorption decreases, and distribution, metabolism and excretion rates increase, the curve reaches its peak. It then descends, as elimination

occurs more rapidly than absorption. As previously noted, the route of administration influences the time taken for the drug to reach maximal concentration. This is fastest with an intravenous injection and slower with intramuscular and subcutaneous injections and with oral doses.

As the dose of a drug is increased, its therapeutic effect increases as more receptors are occupied. Eventually, the dose is reached that produces a maximal effect when all the receptors of the target organs are occupied by drug molecules. Increasing the dose further will therefore not increase the therapeutic effect.

HALF-LIFE OF DRUGS

The rate at which drugs are eliminated from plasma is commonly expressed in terms of the drug's half-life ($t_{\frac{1}{2}}$). This is the time required for the concentration of the drug in the plasma to decrease to one-half of its initial value.

The plasma concentration of a drug at one half-life is 50% of its initial value; at two half-lives, 25%; at three half-lives, 12.5%; at four half-lives, 6.25%; and at five half-lives, just over 3%. Thus, most of a drug (almost 97%) is eliminated in five half-lives, regardless of the dose or route of administration. This rule of thumb can be applied in calculating the time required to elapse when discontinuing one drug and starting another that may interact if given in conjunction with the first. It is also useful in estimating how long it will take a toxic plasma concentration (after overdosing) to clear the body.

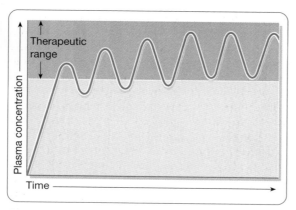

Fig. 8.5 Concentration of drug after repeated dosage.

Half-lives of different drugs vary widely; for example, the half-life of theophylline is 3 h, that of aspirin, 6 h; of metronidazole, 9 h; of digoxin, about 36 h; and of phenobarbital, about 5 days. A short half-life may result from extensive tissue uptake, rapid metabolism or rapid excretion, and a long half-life may be the consequence of extensive plasma protein binding, slow metabolism or poor excretion. The knowledge of half-lives of drugs is essential in determining the intervals between drug doses.

Certain conditions can be treated with a single dose of medication (e.g. analgesics for a headache). Many conditions, however, require continuous drug action (e.g. diabetes mellitus, infections, arthritis). This can be achieved through the administration of repeated doses at regular intervals. In such therapy, the second, third and subsequent doses will add to whatever remains of the previous dose, causing gradual accumulation until stable concentrations are maintained (Fig. 8.5).

The level of drug in the plasma rises after absorption, reaches its peak and then falls to minimal effective concentration. Administration of the next dose raises the drug concentration to a peak. The concentration falls as the drug is metabolised and excreted, then rises again after the next dose. If the interval between doses is too long, or the dose too small, the plasma concentration will have fallen below the therapeutic range before the next dose is given. As a result, the drug concentration is within the therapeutic range only for short intervals.

If a drug is administered too frequently or in too high a dose, the plasma concentration will rise above the therapeutic range and may give rise to toxic effects. In theory, the optimal dosage interval between drug administrations is equal to the half-life of the drug. Initially, the drug accumulates in the body. If 100 mg of drug is given with a half-life of 6 h, when the second dose of 100 mg is given 6 h later, 50 mg of the original dose will still be present in the body – giving a total of 150 mg. After a further 6 h, 75 mg will remain when the third dose of 100 mg is administered – giving a total of 175 mg. At the next dose, 88 mg remains – giving a total of 188 mg. As can be seen, the rate of accumulation becomes less between doses, i.e. 50 mg after the second dose, 25 mg after the third dose and 13 mg after the fourth dose; in practical terms, a steady state maximal concentration is reached after approximately five doses. In the steady state, the plasma level rises and falls between doses but remains within the therapeutic range – the quantity of drug supplied by each dose is equal to the amount eliminated between doses.

The time required to reach a steady concentration depends on the half-life of the drug. The shorter the half-life, the faster the steady state is reached, irrespective of the route of administration. Aspirin, with a half-life of 6 h, will reach equilibrium in five half-lives, i.e. 30 h.

A dosing interval equal to the half-life of a drug may be impractical for drugs with very short half-lives. Penicillin would have to be given every 30 min. This would be inconvenient (if not impossible) for the patient and would lead to poor compliance. Penicillin, however, has a wide therapeutic range, and high doses are relatively non-toxic, so that much higher doses can be given every 6–8 h compared with the dose that would be given every 30 min. This ensures that the therapeutic level in the blood is maintained until the next dose. Short half-life drugs, such as lignocaine (lidocaine), which have a narrow therapeutic range, must be given by intravenous infusion, because larger doses given infrequently would cause toxic effects.

Most drugs obey a simple relationship between steady state concentration and dose. Usually, the dose and steady state concentration are directly proportional: if the dose is doubled, the steady state concentration doubles. For some drugs (e.g. phenytoin, aspirin), however, the rate of clearance decreases with increasing serum concentrations. When dosages of these drugs are increased, steady state concentrations increase more than expected. There are also drugs (e.g. disopyramide, sodium valproate) with the opposite effect, i.e. clearance increases with increasing concentration. In these cases, increased dosages will produce a smaller than expected increase in steady state concentration.

LOADING DOSE

In certain conditions, it is desirable to reach an effective level of drug in the blood without waiting for accumulation to take place (e.g. if a patient has an infection and requires antibiotic treatment). This can be achieved by giving the patient an initial dose that is twice the maintenance dose. The effective blood concentration is reached after the first dose (e.g. 500 mg) and maintained during subsequent dosing intervals by giving appropriate doses (e.g. 250 mg). With a drug that has a long half-life, this regimen is impractical and may be dangerous. It is usually better to allow gradual accumulation following the usual dose and dosage intervals. Patients will then reach their individual steady state concentration in due course.

PROLONGATION OF DRUG ACTION

Because most drugs are absorbed, then cleared from the body fairly quickly, therapeutic effects are maintained for a relatively short time. In order to prolong the therapeutic effect, the drug must be administered either frequently or by constant infusion. It may be desirable to reduce the frequency of dosage, for example when compliance is poor, or to simplify regimens when a number of drugs are being administered. Either or both may be achieved by regulating the release of the active drug from the dosage form in order to maintain therapeutic plasma concentrations (Fig. 8.6).

Absorption can be delayed and the drug's action correspondingly prolonged in a number of different ways. In local anaesthesia with lignocaine (lidocaine),

the addition of adrenaline (epinephrine) causes constriction of local blood vessels, thus delaying absorption of the anaesthetic and prolonging its local effect. Delay can also be achieved by giving the drug as a suspension (e.g. insulin zinc suspension) that is absorbed slowly (depot therapy) (Fig. 8.7).

In certain instances, extremely slow absorption may be desirable. In psychiatric practice, long-acting preparations can be used to avoid frequent drug administration to patients who find it difficult to remember, or who refuse to take their medications by the oral route. The introduction of oily injections of fluphenazine ensures that non-compliant chronic schizophrenic patients can be treated satisfactorily by single intramuscular injections at 2- to 5-weekly intervals. Similarly, long-lasting contraception can be achieved with depot injections of progestogen.

LONGER-ACTING ORAL PREPARATIONS

The sustained release of a drug can be achieved in a number of ways, as discussed below.

COATED GRANULES

The active drug is contained in small granules packed in a gelatin capsule. Some granules have no coating and dissolve immediately. Other granules have coatings of varying thickness of materials such as waxes. The granules with thin coatings will dissolve and release the drug faster than those with thicker

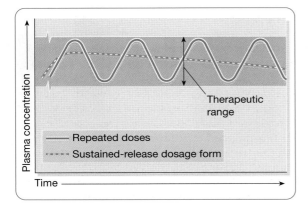

Fig. 8.6   Prolongation of drug action.

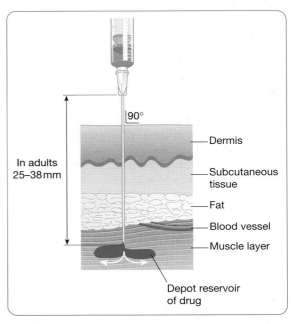

Fig. 8.7   Depot injection.

coatings. It is therefore possible for the active drug to be released over a longer period of time, and for a steady plasma level to be maintained by one dose instead of three or four individual doses of the conventional preparation.

MULTILAYER TABLETS

Sustained action can be achieved by manufacturing tablets that consist of a number of layers or several coats. The drug is dissolved immediately from one layer or the outer coat and more slowly from succeeding layers or coats.

MATRIX PREPARATIONS

The active ingredient is distributed throughout an inert wax or plastic matrix. The drug is slowly leached out of this network, and its action may be sustained for up to 24 h. A variation of this involves the active substance being embedded in a tablet surrounded by a porous coating. The pores are filled with water-soluble crystals that dissolve on contact with aqueous liquids, allowing the active ingredient to be released in a controlled manner by diffusion through the pores. Some preparations of long-acting oral morphine are delivered using matrix formulations.

MINIATURE OSMOTIC PUMP

A novel method of achieving oral controlled release of a drug is the miniature osmotic pump. The traditional tablet structure is replaced by a tablet-sized structure made up of a semipermeable membrane that encloses the active drug and the osmotic driving agent. This system is used to provide controlled release of methylphenidate. As with other controlled-release products, it is important to explain to patients that the tablet must be taken and that the tablet membrane may be passed unchanged.

Controlled-release oral dosage forms may be more convenient than conventional preparations, because they require less frequent administration, therefore improving the patient's compliance. In addition, the gastric mucosa is exposed to a lower concentration of drug than would have been the case with immediate-release products. This may be important when the drug causes irritation or bleeding of the gastrointestinal tract. However, in practice, the results obtained from controlled-release dosage forms may be far from ideal and may vary between patients. The contents of sustained-release preparations may not be released completely and may tail off, giving therapeutic concentrations initially but only subtherapeutic concentrations prior to the next dose.

PHARMACODYNAMICS

MECHANISMS OF DRUG ACTION

In certain cases, the medicine will bring about a normal physiological response when it is a replacement for a deficiency, for example:

- levothyroxine is taken orally in hypothyroidism
- insulin is injected subcutaneously in diabetes mellitus
- hydroxocobalamin is injected intramuscularly in the treatment of pernicious anaemia
- ferrous salts are taken orally to treat anaemia due to iron deficiency
- electrolytes in aqueous solution may be administered orally in cases of severe diarrhoea.

More frequently, however, drugs act by affecting either biochemical or physiological processes in the body or by controlling changes in these processes brought about by disease. One way this is achieved is by affecting receptors.

RECEPTOR AGONISTS AND ANTAGONISTS

The term *receptor* can be used to mean any clearly defined target molecule with which a drug molecule has to combine in order to produce a specific effect. Receptors will interact only with those drugs that are exactly compatible structurally (Fig. 8.8). When

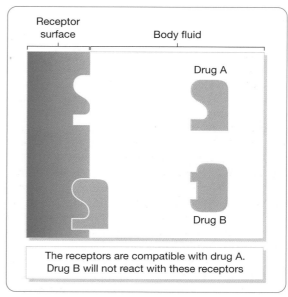

The receptors are compatible with drug A. Drug B will not react with these receptors

Fig. 8.8 Drug–receptor interaction.

the drug binds to the receptor, a complex is formed that may produce two results. First, activation of the receptor may occur, producing a specific result (receptor agonist). The second type of effect is when a drug binds with a receptor, preventing a naturally occurring substance within the body combining with the receptor. In this way, the normal response is blocked (receptor antagonist).

Receptor agonists can be used to alleviate a variety of conditions, examples of which are detailed below.

β_2-adrenoceptor agonists. The main effect is a bronchodilator action directly on the β_2-adrenoceptors of smooth muscle, providing relief in asthma sufferers. Examples include terbutaline, salbutamol and salmeterol.

Sumatriptan. This 5 HT_1 serotonin agonist is used in the treatment of migraine. Headaches, which are a prominent feature of migraine, are believed to result from excessive dilatation of extracerebral cranial arteries, arteriovenous shunts or both. Sumatriptan is a novel selective agonist that blocks these mechanisms.

Bromocriptine. In Parkinson's disease, dopamine production in the brain is greatly reduced. Bromocriptine can be administered to alleviate this condition, because it acts as a direct agonist, stimulating dopamine receptors. It has another action, because it mimics the action of dopamine on the pituitary, which inhibits prolactin release and, as a result, lactation is suppressed.

Receptor antagonists, by preventing a naturally occurring substance combining with the receptor, produce therapeutic outcomes as illustrated by the following examples.

5 HT_3-receptor antagonists. The major sites responsive to emetic stimuli are in the gut and in the brain, areas that are rich in 5 HT_3 receptors. Ondansetron is a potent 5 HT_3 receptor antagonist and, as such, blocks the emetic reflex responses.

β_1-adrenoceptor antagonists. Atenolol blocks the β_1 actions of noradrenaline (norepinephrine) released from cardiac sympathetic stimulation and of circulating adrenaline (epinephrine). It is used to treat angina pectoris and hypertension. In angina pectoris, beta-receptor antagonists reduce the force and contraction of the ventricle, resulting in a reduction in cardiac oxygen consumption, relieving anginal pain.

H_1-histamine receptor antagonists. There are two classes of histamine antagonists: H_1-receptor antagonists and H_2-receptor antagonists. The term *antihistamine* conventionally refers to the H_1-receptor antagonists such as promethazine, cetirizine and loratadine. They are used mainly to block the actions of histamine released during hypersensitivity reactions.

H_2-histamine receptor antagonists. Histamine has numerous actions, including a powerful stimulant effect on gastric secretion. Selective antagonists have been developed that have proved potent in blocking the stimulant action of histamine on the acid-secreting parietal cells of the stomach. H_2-receptor antagonists such as cimetidine and ranitidine are capable of reducing gastric acid secretion by 70% or more.

ENZYME INHIBITORS

An enzyme is a protein that can promote or accelerate a biochemical reaction with a substrate. When the enzyme mistakenly identifies the drug as being the substrate, a drug–enzyme interaction occurs. This interaction could increase or decrease the rate of a biochemical reaction.

Carbidopa and benserazide. In Parkinson's disease, levodopa is given as the precursor to dopamine, because it crosses the blood–brain barrier, which dopamine is unable to do. It is then broken down to dopamine by dopa decarboxylase. However, dopa decarboxylase is present in the gut and liver, resulting in the breakdown of a proportion of the levodopa before it enters the brain. By combining the levodopa with either carbidopa or benserazide, which inhibit the action of dopa decarboxylase, the breakdown of levodopa is reduced and a lower dose can be given.

Vigabatrin. Gamma-aminobutyric acid (GABA) inhibits the spread of seizure activity by blocking synaptic transmission. GABA is metabolised by the enzyme GABA transaminase. The action of vigabatrin in the treatment of epilepsy is to inhibit GABA transaminase irreversibly, thus preventing the breakdown of GABA. The action persists until new enzyme is synthesised.

Neostigmine. This drug is used in the treatment of myasthenia gravis. Acetylcholine is broken down by the enzyme cholinesterase. Neostigmine inhibits the action of cholinesterase, allowing an accumulation of acetylcholine at the muscle motor endplate, thereby alleviating the block in neuromuscular transmission that occurs in this condition.

Omeprazole. Omeprazole reduces secretion of gastric acid by inhibiting an enzyme called H^+K^+-adenosine triphosphatase (the so-called gastric proton pump). This enzyme is responsible for the final stage in the production of acid in the parietal cells of the gastric mucosa. It pumps protons out from the cell into the gastric lumen in exchange for potassium ions. Once in the lumen, the protons (hydrogen ions) meet up with chloride ions to form hydrochloric acid.

DRUGS AFFECTING TRANSPORT PROCESSES

This mechanism of action can apply both to drugs introduced to the body and substances synthesised by the body.

Thiazide diuretics. The thiazide diuretics decrease the reabsorption of sodium in the renal distal tubule. This results in an increased excretion of sodium and water.

Probenecid. In gout, there is an increase in the amount of uric acid in the body. Probenecid inhibits the transport of organic acids across epithelial membranes. The reabsorption of uric acid from the renal tubule is blocked by probenecid, resulting in an increased secretion and relief from the symptoms of gout.

Insulin. Insulin has a number of actions, one of which is to promote the transport of glucose into cells. This action results in a rapid fall in glucose levels in the blood, relieving hyperglycaemic diabetic coma.

CHEMOTHERAPEUTIC AGENTS

In cancer chemotherapy, cytotoxic drugs act by interfering with cell growth and division. Ideally, a drug is required to have a selective action on all abnormal, rapidly dividing cells found in cancerous conditions, with no toxic effect in normal cells. Such a drug is not yet available, because currently used drugs attack normal growing cells as well as malignant cells. All cells that are synthesising DNA go through a cycle that has several different phases. Different cytotoxic drugs act at different phases of the cell cycle:

- methotrexate inhibits the formation of folic acid, which is important in the synthesis of DNA
- bleomycin damages DNA.

In infective disease, an increasing number of drugs affect bacteria and other micro-organisms:

- penicillins and cephalosporins inhibit synthesis of bacterial cell walls
- nystatin and amphotericin act by increasing the permeability of cell membranes of invading organisms
- chloramphenicol and erythromycin inhibit bacterial protein synthesis.

MISCELLANEOUS

There are a significant number of drug actions that can be classed under this heading.

- Antacids such as aluminium hydroxide and magnesium hydroxide have a direct neutralising effect on acid and reduce gastric acidity.

- Ion exchange resins such as calcium polystyrene sulphonate are used to remove excess potassium in mild hyperkalaemia. The sodium in the ion exchange resin exchanges for potassium, which is removed from the body as the resin passes through and is excreted.
- Desferrioxamine chelates ferrous iron in the treatment of iron poisoning.
- Potassium citrate makes the urine alkaline and relieves the discomfort of cystitis in lower urinary tract infections.

DRUGS AFFECTING THE FETUS

DRUGS IN PREGNANCY

During the first 2 weeks of human gestation, the fertilised ovum is already sensitive to drugs and, after this, drugs may produce congenital malformations in the fetus in the first trimester. The time of greatest risk is between the third and eleventh weeks of pregnancy, when differentiation of organs occurs. The development of the embryo is very rapid, with continuous changes resulting from cell division, cell migration and cell differentiation. Each organ and each system undergoes a critical stage of differentiation at a precise period of prenatal development (e.g. the heart from day 20 to day 40, and limbs from day 24 to day 46). It is during this time that specific gross malformations can be produced by particular drugs.

Complete closure of the palate occurs in the fetus at 8 weeks, differentiation of the external genitalia between the fourth and fifth month, and further differentiation of the nervous system from the fourth month until after birth. Drugs administered around these times may interfere with the normal development of the genitalia and nervous system.

As a general principle, drugs should not be administered to a woman during pregnancy unless the potential benefit to the mother outweighs the risk to the fetus. However, serious illness can occur during pregnancy and complications of pregnancy often need to be treated with drugs, so administration cannot always be avoided. The mother may suffer from a chronic condition that requires continuous medication. For example, patients with hypothyroidism require regular doses of levothyroxine. Although the placenta is relatively impermeable to levothyroxine, adequate replacement in hypothyroid patients is extremely important, as it has been shown that children of women who had inadequate replacement therapy scored lower in tests of mental and fine motor development when compared with the offspring of women with adequate replacement therapy.

The transfer of drugs across the placenta is accomplished in a similar manner to the distribution of drugs in body organs and tissues. Most drugs cross the placenta by simple diffusion from an area of high concentration to an area of low concentration. Biochemical and physiological changes occur in women during pregnancy, and therefore drug distribution, metabolism and excretion may be altered. Metabolism of drugs in the maternal liver is reduced during pregnancy, and an increase in plasma volume in conjunction with a reduction in albumin content may increase the amount of free drug in the plasma. Because the fetus is in equilibrium with the maternal circulation, drugs and metabolites that readily cross the placenta and enter the fetal circulation will also be in equilibrium and will then pass back into the mother's circulation when cleared by the fetus.

Care must be taken when drugs are administered shortly before term or during labour, because these may not have been cleared from the fetus before birth. A drug can no longer pass from the fetal to the maternal circulation after the umbilical cord has been clamped, and this may cause adverse effects on the neonate after delivery, owing to problems of metabolism and excretion. If treatment is required, drugs preferred are those that have been used extensively. New or untried drugs should be avoided when an alternative with a known 'safe' history is available.

Antibacterial drugs may be used in pregnancy for the treatment of maternal infection. The penicillins are probably the safest antibiotics for use in pregnancy. Tetracyclines are irreversibly incorporated into fetal teeth, resulting in discoloration and a tendency to develop dental caries. Although the benefits of antiepileptics to the mother may outweigh the risk to the fetus, there is an increased incidence of congenital malformation in infants born to mothers receiving antiepileptic drugs. There is no evidence that general anaesthetics are harmful to the fetus, provided that maternal hypotension and respiratory depression are avoided.

Although a great deal of work is now being done on the adverse effects of drugs administered during pregnancy, the effects of many drugs on the fetus have yet to be determined. Much of the work has been done on laboratory animals, which may react differently to humans. In addition, studies conducted in humans are usually retrospective, and it is difficult to attribute adverse effects on the fetus to a particular drug.

Drug treatment should be avoided whenever possible during pregnancy, especially during the first trimester and prior to delivery. Care should also be taken in administering drugs to women of childbearing age, as major harmful effects of drugs on the fetus will be produced very early in pregnancy, possibly before the woman realises she is pregnant.

DRUG THERAPY IN THE YOUNG

All children, and particularly neonates, differ from adults in their response to drugs. The immaturity of organs involved in drug metabolism and excretion may alter not only the pharmacokinetics but also the toxicity of many drugs. Great variability exists in absorption, protein binding, distribution, metabolism and excretion according to age and weight, and important differences have been observed in premature neonates, full-term babies and older children. These differences become more complex when congenital anomalies or disease states exist. The BNF for children provides information on the use of medicines in children ranging from neonates to adolescents.

ABSORPTION OF DRUGS

Gastrointestinal tract. The absorption of drugs from the gastrointestinal tract is influenced by the pH of the stomach contents and also by gastric emptying time. The pH of the stomach at birth is 6–8 but falls to 1–3 in the first 24 h. (In premature neonates, this fall does not occur, because the acid-secreting mechanism has not fully developed.) The pH then returns to between 6 and 8 for 10–15 days, because no more acid is secreted during this period. This relatively neutral pH of the stomach contents may result in higher blood levels of drugs such as penicillin, because of reduced chemical decomposition resulting in increased availability for absorption. The adult value of gastric pH (approximately 3) is gradually reached between 2 and 3 years of age.

The gastric emptying time may be as long as 6–8 h in neonates, reaching adult values at 6–8 months. This prolonged emptying time may have an important influence on the absorption rate of orally administered drugs.

Intramuscular injection. The absorption rate of drugs following intramuscular injection is influenced by the changes in muscle blood flow that occur in the first days of life and by vasoconstriction resulting from temperature change or circulatory insufficiency.

Skin. Percutaneous absorption is greatly increased in neonates and young infants, who have thin, well-hydrated skin. This increased permeability has led to toxic effects associated with the use of hexachlorophene soaps and powders and preparations containing salicylic acid. The dangers of absorption of corticosteroids from topical preparations are also widely recognised.

THE BINDING OF DRUGS BY PROTEINS

Neonates have reduced plasma protein binding of various drugs. This is because of a reduced plasma protein concentration and because neonatal albumin has a lower binding capacity for drugs than that of adults. These factors may vary in their effects and may lead to drug toxicity. On the other hand, the dose of digoxin required in infants is high compared with that for adults. An average daily maintenance dose for adults is 3–5 micrograms/kg of body weight, whereas in infants it is 10–25 micrograms/kg. This higher dose is required because the digoxin has a lower binding affinity for digoxin receptors in the myocardium of neonates. In addition to reduced plasma protein binding, another factor affecting drug distribution is the total body water in neonates, which is 70%, compared to the adult value of 55%.

HEPATIC METABOLISM OF DRUGS

Drug metabolism by the liver can occur in a number of ways, for example by acetylation or by conjugation. In the newborn, the necessary enzyme systems are developed to varying extents. Conjugation involving glucuronidation is deficient in some newborn infants. A number of drugs, including chloramphenicol, are metabolised in this way. Grey syndrome (abdominal distension, pallid cyanosis, circulatory collapse) may follow excessive doses of chloramphenicol in neonates with immature hepatic metabolism. This deficiency in metabolism disappears in the first or second week of life.

EXCRETION OF DRUGS

At birth, all aspects of renal function are diminished, but they become comparable with those in adults between 6 months and a year. Full-term babies have a reduced glomerular filtration rate compared with adults. Compounds that are not extensively metabolised and depend on renal function for excretion are eliminated more slowly in neonates. The maintenance dose must be adjusted depending on the child's kidney function, increasing as the kidney function develops. On the other hand, drugs such as diuretics, which depend on the glomerular filtration to produce a therapeutic effect, will require a higher dose at birth when the Cr Cl is approximately 20 mL/min, but at age 1 month, when the clearance rate is 60 mL/min, the dose would be reduced accordingly.

DRUGS IN BREAST MILK

Breast milk is the only food the infant needs for the first 4–6 months of life. There are many benefits to be gained from breast-feeding. The composition of human milk is tailored to organ development and growth, and some protection against infection is obtained; compared with cow's milk, there is less likelihood of food allergy and it is more digestible. The advantages for the nursing mother, in addition to maternal bonding, are convenience and a lower cost compared with substitute products.

The contact of the baby's sucking serves to keep prolactin levels high and may delay subsequent pregnancy. Prolactin secretion can be altered by drugs. It is decreased by levodopa and bromocriptine and increased by phenothiazines, methyldopa and theophylline. The production of milk can be affected by diuretics. Bendroflumethiazide (bendrofluazide) has been shown to stop lactation. Spironolactone, however, can be used safely.

Although most drugs are excreted to some extent in breast milk, the significance of their effects depends on the amount excreted in the milk. The newborn metabolise and excrete drugs very inefficiently. Preterm infants are at greater risk than others, but the risk decreases as renal and hepatic functions mature. Because infants have poorly developed renal and hepatic functions, they may be particularly sensitive to the accumulation of drugs. When possible, drugs should be avoided during breast-feeding and mothers should be warned of the possible dangers of self-medication.

Because of their potential toxicity, a number of drugs are absolutely contraindicated while the mother is breast-feeding. These include antithyroid drugs, radioactive isotopes, lithium, chloramphenicol, ergot alkaloids and most anticancer drugs. If some form of drug treatment is essential, then alternatives to these must be used or breast-feeding must be stopped. A number of other drugs are to be avoided or used with caution. For example, atropine may cause intoxication in sensitive infants and calciferol, in high doses, may cause hypercalcaemia in the infant.

If drugs (e.g. penicillins) are secreted in milk in relatively low concentrations, the advantages of breast-feeding probably outweigh the marginal risks involved. Many drugs (e.g. cephalosporins) known to be excreted in breast milk do not appear to produce adverse effects in the infant.

Generally, the mother should breast-feed prior to taking medication. When a nursing mother takes a drug that is potentially hazardous to the infant, breast-feeding may be temporarily discontinued when a single dose or short course is involved. Attention should be paid to the half-life of the drug. In this situation, breast milk should be expressed regularly to maintain lactation, and then discarded.

When drugs are prescribed for a nursing mother, a number of principles are adhered to by the doctor, and the nurse should be aware of these principles:

- never prescribe a drug unless it is essential
- use the safest drug when alternatives are available
- use the lowest effective dose for the shortest possible time.

If there is no alternative to drug therapy and the principles above are adhered to, adverse effects on the baby should not occur. The mother may need reassurance and general guidance so that she is alert for any recognisable effects on the baby.

Appendix 4 of the BNF gives specific guidance on drugs to be avoided or to be used with caution in pregnancy. As with all prescribing, risk–benefit issues must be taken into account. For example, the benefits of treatment of severe asthma with corticosteroids outweigh the risk. Risks of teratogenicity must always be considered, as must the possibility of drug interactions.

As more medicines become deregulated, care must be taken to ensure that a pregnant woman receives good advice on the use of medicines that can be purchased without prescription (over-the-counter medicines). Community pharmacists are well placed to advise women; indeed, there is a professional responsibility to ensure, as far as is practicable, that sales of medicines are made within agreed protocols that are designed to protect the purchaser.

DRUGS IN OLDER PEOPLE

It is wrong to view older people as a homogeneous group, all of whom are suffering from several coexisting disease processes. However, there is no doubt that, as the ageing process continues, there is an increasing likelihood that drug treatment will be required. The physiological changes that occur with ageing have an impact on the distribution and metabolism of drugs. One of the fundamental characteristics of ageing is a progressive reduction in homeostatic mechanisms. A typical example for the consequences of the decrease in homeostatic mechanisms is the increased susceptibility of elderly patients to postural hypotension in response to drugs that lower arterial blood pressure.

The central nervous system is a particularly vulnerable drug target in the elderly. Between the age of 20 and 80 years, brain weight is reduced by 20%, and neuronal loss has been reported for several brain regions. The number of synapses decreases, and the age-related reduction in dopamine content and receptor abundance predisposes to an increased frequency and severity of extrapyramidal symptoms in response to dopaminergic blockade by neuroleptics and metoclopramide.

The need for pharmacotherapy has to be evaluated very carefully in geriatric patients. The number of drugs administered simultaneously should be reduced as much as possible. The list of medications should be reviewed critically and periodically, i.e. drugs no longer needed should be discontinued.

DISTRIBUTION OF DRUGS IN THE BODY

In most older people, total body mass, lean body mass and total body water decrease; total body fat increases. These changes in body composition can affect a drug's concentration in the body. A water-soluble drug is distributed primarily in the aqueous parts of the body and lean body tissue. Because an older person has relatively less water and lean tissue, more of the water-soluble drug stays in the blood, which leads to increased blood concentration levels. As a result, dosage reduction may be required. Body water content falls by 10–15% until the age of 80. The volume of distribution of hydrophilic drugs therefore decreases. The equivalent doses given to younger individuals will result in higher plasma concentrations. This, for instance, is the case for aspirin, tubocurarine, edrophonium, famotidine and lithium.

The older patient has a higher proportion of body fat, and more of a fat-soluble drug is distributed to the fatty tissue. This produces misleadingly low blood levels and may cause dosage to be incorrectly increased. The fatty tissue slowly releases stored drug into the bloodstream, and this explains why a fat-soluble sedative may produce a hangover effect.

A decrease in albumin results in a reduction in the plasma protein binding of some drugs (e.g. phenytoin, warfarin). More non-bound drug is available to act at receptor sites and may result in toxicity. In these cases, a dose reduction should be considered.

METABOLISM OF DRUGS IN OLDER PEOPLE

Hepatic metabolism of some drugs would appear to be altered as a consequence of the ageing process, which results in a reduction of liver blood flow and a reduction in liver mass. General rules cannot be formulated, but for some drugs it appears that decreased hepatic metabolism does result in longer half-life of the drug. The nutritional status of a patient has a marked influence on the rate of drug metabolism. In frail elderly, drug metabolism is diminished to a greater extent than in elderly persons with normal body weight.

RENAL EXCRETION OF DRUGS IN OLDER PEOPLE

The most important pharmacokinetic change in the elderly is the reduction in renal drug elimination, as glomerular filtration rate, tubular secretion and renal blood flow are reduced. If doses are not adjusted for the reduction in drug elimination by the kidneys in the elderly, this will result in increased drug serum levels. The decline in renal function in the elderly is closely related to the incidence of adverse drug reactions. Whereas the effect on drug action of reduced hepatic metabolism is difficult to predict, the effect of reduced renal excretion is more readily determined. Glomerular filtration rate by the age of 80 may have fallen to less than 50 mL/min. Drugs or active metabolites of those that are excreted mainly in the urine will require to be administered in lower dose, particularly those with a narrow therapeutic index (e.g. warfarin, digoxin, lithium, phenytoin and carbamazepine). Tetracyclines are best avoided in older people because, in the presence of poor renal function, they accumulate, causing nausea and vomiting, resulting in dehydration and further deterioration in renal function.

SELF-ASSESSMENT QUESTION

Describe the changes in absorption that can affect pharmacokinetic drug response in the elderly patient.

FURTHER READING AND RESOURCES

Bradley JR 1997 Renal disorders. Hospital Pharmacist 4:137–139

Brice P 2006 Genetics, health and medicine. Pharmaceutical Journal 277:53–56

Kanneh A 2002 Paediatric nursing. Paediatric pharmacological principles: an update part 2. Pharmacokinetics: absorption and distribution. Paediatric Nursing 14:39–43

Kelly J 1995 Pharmacodynamics and drug therapy. Professional Nurse 10:792–796

Thomson A 2004 Back to basics: pharmacokinetics. Pharmaceutical Journal 272:769–771

Thomson A 2004 Variability in drug dosage requirements. Pharmaceutical Journal 272:806–808

Walker D 1999 How relevant is drug metabolism to prescribing? Prescriber 10:139–142

Autonomic nervous system

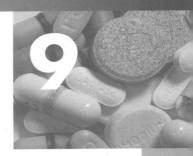

9

CHAPTER CONTENTS

KEY OBJECTIVES

After studying this chapter, you should be able to:

- describe the main effects of muscarinic agonists (parasympathomimetics)
- name two muscarinic agonists (parasympathomimetics)
- name two antimuscarinics
- describe the main effects of adrenoceptor agonists (α_1 and β_2) (sympathomimetics)
- name two adrenoceptor agonists (α and β) (sympathomimetics)
- name two beta-adrenoceptor antagonists (beta-blockers)
- explain the central importance of the autonomic nervous system and health and illness states.

INTRODUCTION

A full appreciation of the autonomic nervous system (ANS) is central to the understanding of the actions and uses of drugs in a wide range of conditions, in particular conditions affecting the cardiovascular, respiratory, genitourinary and gastrointestinal systems. The actions of key drugs used in the treatment of eye diseases also depend on their ability to modify (mimic or block) the action of chemical mediators produced by the ANS. Drugs acting on the ANS are capable of bringing great benefits to patients but, like many other drugs, the dangers of inappropriate use (and side effects) should not be underestimated, especially in vulnerable patients at extremes of age.

Careful study of this chapter, and further reading (before a study of section 3), will be amply rewarded both in the theoretical context and in a very practical sense.

PERIPHERAL NERVOUS SYSTEM

The peripheral nervous system comprises the ANS and other systems that innervate skeletal (striated) muscle. The anatomy and physiology of the ANS will be described in some detail. The ANS has three anatomical divisions: the sympathetic and parasympathetic systems, which convey the outputs from the central nervous system to the main organ systems of the body, and the enteric nervous system. The enteric nervous system is made up of nerve plexuses of the gastrointestinal tract.

The ANS is responsible for the involuntary activity of the body, for example heartbeat and the contraction and relaxation of smooth muscle in the cardiovascular, respiratory and gastrointestinal systems. Other important actions include the regulation of secretions (endocrine and exocrine) and the production of energy in the liver and skeletal muscle.

The basic anatomical plan of the ANS is illustrated in Figure 9.1. In a more detailed and highly simplified form, Figure 9.2 illustrates the similarities and differences between the sympathetic and parasympathetic systems. It will be seen that in the sympathetic system the ganglia are situated close to the central nervous system, whereas in the parasympathetic system the ganglia are mainly close to or within the organ supplied.

The neurones of the enteric nervous system are located in the plexuses of the gastrointestinal tract and are supplied by the sympathetic and parasympathetic systems, but they can also act independently to control functions of the gastrointestinal system. The enteric nervous system is more complex than the other elements of the ANS, because it involves other chemical transmitters. The sympathetic and parasympathetic

139

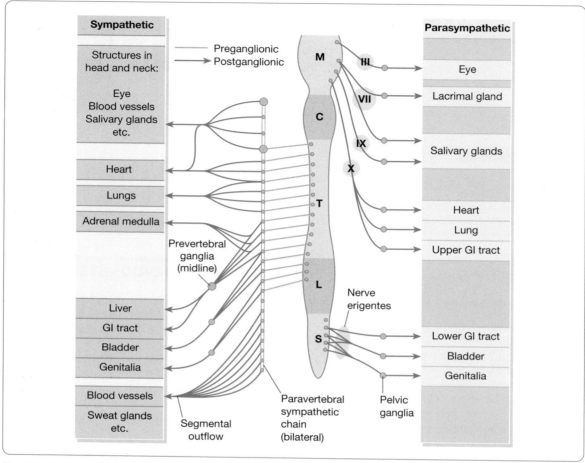

Fig. 9.1 Basic anatomical plan of the autonomic nervous system. C, cervical; GI, gastrointestinal; L, lumbar; M, medullary; S, sacral; T, thoracic. (From Rang HP, Dale MM, Ritter JM et al. 2003 Pharmacology. Churchill Livingstone, Edinburgh. With permission of Elsevier Ltd.) Please see Fig. 9.1, p.124 in Rang and Dale.

systems have opposing actions on some organs of the body, for example the heart (see Tables 9.1 and 9.2). In very general terms, sympathetic activity is associated with stress and activity; parasympathetic activity is associated with inactivity. Under normal conditions, the ANS exerts control on organs of the body on a continuous basis.

CHEMICAL TRANSMITTERS AND THEIR TARGETS (RECEPTORS)

Chemical transmitters are of fundamental importance in the working of the ANS. To be physiologically effective, transmitters (and drugs) must have targets with which they can interact. There are a number of different targets in the organs of the body. These are receptors, ion channels, enzymes and transporters,

all of which are specialised proteins. Receptors play a key role in the functioning of the ANS. In the ANS, the chemical transmitters are noradrenaline (norepinephrine) (sympathetic) and acetylcholine (in both the sympathetic and the parasympathetic systems). The chemical transmitters are produced by complex processes that will not be discussed here. Figure 9.3 illustrates the sites where the transmitters are released. The released transmitters act on different types of receptors, as outlined in Table 9.3. If the chemical transmitter was allowed to accumulate at the sites of action, physiological processes would break down. Table 9.4 outlines the processes (based on enzyme action) that destroy the chemical transmitters or render them inactive in other ways.

The nicotinic and muscarinic actions of acetylcholine were first described by Dale in 1914, before the understanding of receptors was developed. It is not

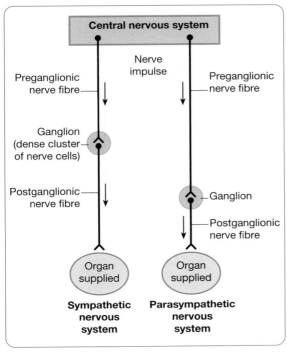

Fig. 9.2 Simplified structures within the autonomic nervous system.

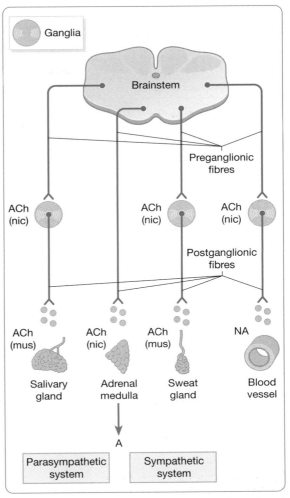

Fig. 9.3 Sites of release of chemical transmitter in the autonomic nervous system.

Table 9.1 Main actions of noradrenaline (norepinephrine) on adrenergic receptors

Organ/body system	Receptors		
	α	β$_1$	β$_2$
Blood vessels (arterioles)	Constriction	–	Dilatation (arterioles in skeletal muscle and veins)
Bronchi	No sympathetic innervation	–	Dilatation by circulating adrenaline (epinephrine)
Gastrointestinal tract	Relax	–	Relax
Gastrointestinal sphincter	Contract	–	Contract
Salivary glands	Secretions increased	–	Secretions increased
Uterus	Contract (pregnant)	–	Relax (non-pregnant)
Heart rate	–	Increase	–

Continued

Table 9.1 Main actions of noradrenaline (norepinephrine) on adrenergic receptors *'cont ...'*

Organ/body system	Receptors		
	α	β$_1$	β$_2$
Heart force of contraction	–	Increase	–
Sweat glands	Secretions are mainly increased by *cholinergic* fibres of sympathetic nervous system	–	–
Eye	See Chapter 23	–	–
Kidney	–	–	Renin secretion increased
Liver	Glycogenolysis, gluconeogenesis	–	Glycogenolysis, gluconeogenesis

Table 9.2 Main actions of acetylcholine on muscarinic receptors

Organ/body system	Receptors	
	Muscarinic	Nicotinic
Blood vessels (arterioles)	Dilatation (erectile tissue and salivary glands)	Nicotinic receptors are found in sympathetic and parasympathetic ganglia; stimulation of these receptors produces complex effects including tachycardia, elevation of blood pressure and increased gastrointestinal activity
Bronchi	Smooth muscle constricted	
Gastrointestinal tract	Peristaltic activity increased	
Gastrointestinal sphincter	Dilatation, gastric secretions increased	
Salivary glands	Secretions increased	
Uterus	Variable effect	
Heart rate	Decreased	
Heart, force of contraction	Decreased	
Sweat glands	No effect	
Eye	See Chapter 23	
Kidney	No effect	
Liver	No effect	

Table 9.3 Chemical transmitters and receptors in the autonomic nervous system[a]

	Sympathetic nervous system		Parasympathetic nervous system
	Acetylcholine	Noradrenaline (norepinephrine)	Acetylcholine
Motor nerve fibres leaving central nervous system (preganglionic fibres)	Nicotinic receptors	–	Nicotinic receptors
Postganglionic fibres	Muscarinic receptors in sweat glands	alpha and beta receptors	Muscarinic[b] receptors[c]

[a]Other chemical transmitters are involved in the autonomic nervous system. These include nitric oxide, various peptides, γ-aminobutyric acid and dopamine. These will not be discussed here.
[b]This term is derived from the name of a substance (muscarine) found in the poisonous toadstool *Amanita muscaria*.
[c]Five types of muscarinic receptors have been identified: the most important are neural, cardiac and glandular.

essential for the nurse to study fully the fine detail of the functioning of receptors, but the nicotinic and muscarinic actions of acetylcholine are fundamental to both the physiology of the ANS and the actions of important drugs. The work of Dale may seem to be ancient history, but the current British National Formulary uses many of the terms originated by him.

Tables 9.1 and 9.2 describe in detail the effects of the transmitters (via the receptors) on organs of the body.

DRUGS ACTING ON THE AUTONOMIC NERVOUS SYSTEM

Many key drugs act by influencing adrenergic or cholinergic transmissions. Some important terms are used to describe the action of these (and other) drugs. An agonist is a chemical substance (or drug) that binds with a receptor to produce a response (the receptor is activated). An antagonist binds with a receptor but produces no activation. Different mechanisms are involved, but the most important is receptor block (see p. 133). Some drugs acting on the ANS depend for their actions on their ability to block the action of cholinesterase, thus enhancing the effects of endogenous acetylcholine. This class of drugs is the anticholinesterases.

Tables 9.5–9.10 summarise some of the main drugs that act on the ANS. These drugs will be fully discussed in the appropriate chapters.

CHANGES IN AUTONOMIC FUNCTION IN AGE AND DISEASE

With increasing age, there is an increase of cardiovascular sympathetic activity and a reduction of cardiac parasympathetic nervous system activity. Both parasympathetic and sympathetic nervous system inputs to the iris are diminished in older persons. Although sympathetic outflows generally increase with advancing age, whether this contributes to the development of hypertension or other cardiovascular disorders as opposed to reflecting adaptive responses to changes in the internal environment (e.g. decreased end organ responsiveness) remains unclear.

Poorly controlled diabetes mellitus can lead to damage to the ANS resulting in disorders of the structures involved.

SELF-ASSESSMENT QUESTION

Discuss the actions and side-effect profiles of non-selective beta-blockers (e.g. propranolol, sotalol) in relation to their action on beta receptors.

Table 9.4 Enzymes that destroy chemical transmitters in the autonomic nervous system

Sympathetic nervous system		Parasympathetic nervous system
Acetylcholine	Noradrenaline (norepinephrine)	Acetylcholine
Cholinesterase (hydrolyses acetylcholine very rapidly)	Monoamine oxidase and catechol-*O*-methyl transferase; these enzymes act more slowly than cholinesterase.[a] Noradrenaline is mainly removed by uptake into the nerve terminals.	Cholinesterase (hydrolyses acetylcholine very rapidly)

[a]These enzymes also destroy circulating adrenaline (epinephrine) and noradrenaline.

Table 9.5 Noradrenergic agonists (sympathomimetics)

Drug	Classification	Main uses
Epinephrine[a] Norepinephrine[a]	Non-selective adrenoceptor agonists	Cardiac arrest, anaphylaxis, emergencies in asthma
Dobutamine	Selective β_1 agonist	Cardiac stimulant – increases cardiac contractility
Isoprenaline	Non-selective adrenoceptor agonist	Originally used as a bronchodilator; now seldom used because of non-selectivity
Phenylephrine	α_1 agonist	Vasoconstriction in nasal congestion
Salbutamol, terbutaline, salmeterol	Selective β_2 agonists	Bronchodilators

[a]Adrenaline and noradrenaline are the names used for the naturally occurring substances.

Table 9.6 Noradrenergic antagonists

Drug	Classification	Main uses
Nadolol Propranolol	Beta antagonists, non-selective (beta-adrenoceptor-blocking drugs – beta-blockers)	Hypertension Antiarrhythmia
Phentolamine	Alpha antagonist, non-selective	To reduce hypertension in phaeochromocytoma
Prazosin	Alpha antagonist	Hypertension
Tamsulosin	Alpha antagonist	Uroselective; used in benign prostatic hyperplasia

Table 9.7   Cholinergic transmission: agonists (parasympathomimetics)

Drug	Classification	Main uses
Bethanechol, carbachol, methacholine	Muscarinic receptor agonist	Urinary retention Side-effects limit use
Pilocarpine	Muscarinic receptor agonist	Orally for dry mouth (increases secretions) (see also Ch. 23 for use in ophthalmology)

Table 9.8   Anticholinesterases

Drug	Classification	Main uses
Neostigmine, physostigmine	Anticholinesterase	Reversal of neuromuscular block (see Ch. 14)
Pyridostigmine	Anticholinesterase	Myasthenia gravis

Table 9.9   Cholinergic transmission: antagonists (antimuscarinics, formerly anticholinergics)

Drug	Classification	Main uses
Atropine (also similar hyoscine, homatropine, cyclopentolate)	Muscarinic receptor antagonist	Reduction of secretions, antispasmodic (gastrointestinal tract); see Chapter 23 for ophthalmic use
Ipratropium	Muscarinic receptor agonist	A bronchodilator by inhalation

Table 9.10   Other drugs acting on the autonomic nervous system

Drug	Classification	Main uses
Pancuronium[a]	Neuromuscular blocking agent (blocks acetylcholine receptors)	Muscle relaxant in surgery for long procedures

[a]Other drugs are available that have different lengths of action, for example vecuronium (intermediate action) and mivacurium (short action).

FURTHER READING AND RESOURCES

Goldstein DS 2001 The autonomic nervous system in health and disease. Marcel Dekker, New York

Rang HP, Dale MM, Ritter JM et al. 2003 Pharmacology, 5th edn. Churchill Livingstone, Edinburgh

Seal DR, Monahan KD, Bell C et al. 2001 The aging cardiovascular system: changes in autonomic function at rest and in response to exercise. International Journal of Sport, Nutrition, Exercise and Metabolism 11(suppl):189–195

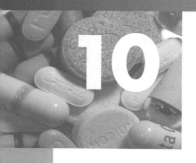

10 Adverse drug reactions and drug interactions

CHAPTER CONTENTS

KEY OBJECTIVES

After reading this chapter, you should be able to:

- explain the two different types of adverse reactions and give examples
- describe the presentation and treatment of anaphylactic reactions
- outline the role of the nurse in the management of adverse drug reactions
- outline the different mechanisms of drug interactions.

INTRODUCTION

An adverse drug reaction (ADR) has been defined by the World Health Organization as 'any response to a drug which is noxious, unintended and occurs at doses used for prophylaxis, diagnosis and therapy'. All pharmaceutical preparations are potentially harmful, and this is a key reason why many medicines are strictly controlled and available only on prescription.

The safe use of medicines is an important issue for nurses, pharmacists, doctors, regulatory authorities, the pharmaceutical industry and the public. Health professionals have a responsibility to their patients, who themselves are increasingly aware of problems associated with drug therapy. It is essential that the practising nurse has a knowledge of the adverse effects of drugs and how to recognise and prevent them. The special roles performed by nurses give them a unique opportunity to help reduce the incidence of ADRs and to minimise their impact on patients.

A tragic event occurred in the early 1960s that involved a hypnotic called thalidomide. This drug proved to be teratogenic, and many babies with congenital limb defects were born to mothers who had taken this preparation in early pregnancy. This major disaster led to the establishment of regulatory agencies that enforce rigorous testing and evaluation of drugs prior to the granting of a product licence and subsequent marketing. In addition to these processes, detection and recording of ADRs that occur when the drug is in use are of vital importance. A well-established reporting system enables ADRs to be reported to the Committee on Safety of Medicines. Both prescribed and non-prescribed medicines are included in this system. Yellow reporting forms for ADRs are included in the British National Formulary (BNF).

CLASSIFICATION

The simplest classification of ADRs is into types A and B.

TYPE A REACTIONS

Type A reactions to drugs include augmented responses that are undesirable. Examples include hypoglycaemia with a sulphonylurea and postural hypotension with an antihypertensive drug. Many type A reactions arise from secondary pharmacological effects of a drug, such as anticholinergic effects with antihistamines and tricyclic antidepressants. Type A reactions are usually dose-dependent and predictable and are often recognised before a drug is marketed.

TYPE B REACTIONS

Type B reactions are unrelated to the drug's pharmacology and are generally unrelated to dosage. Although comparatively rare, they often cause serious illness and may result in death. These reactions are often caused by pharmacogenetic and immunological mechanisms. Genetic differences in the population can result in altered drug metabolism (e.g. fast and slow acetylators).

Allergic reactions are immunologically mediated effects. They vary from rash and angioedema to life-threatening bronchospasm and hypotension associated with anaphylaxis. Features of these reactions are that there is often a delay between the first exposure to the drug and the occurrence of the subsequent adverse reaction, very small doses of the drug may trigger the reaction once allergy is established and the reaction disappears on withdrawal. Documenting of allergic reactions for individual patients is important in order to avoid future exposures to the allergen.

OTHER PREDISPOSING FACTORS

Age may be a factor, and the very old and the very young are more susceptible to ADRs. In older people, the incidence of multiple and chronic diseases is increased, resulting in increased reliance on medication. This results in a higher incidence of ADRs, because of increased drug exposure and also age-related pharmacokinetic changes. Drugs that commonly cause problems in older people include hypnotics, diuretics, non-steroidal anti-inflammatory drugs (NSAIDs), antihypertensives, psychotropics

and digoxin. All children, and particularly neonates, differ from adults in the way they handle and respond to drugs. Hazardous drugs in neonates include chloramphenicol and morphine. A specific example of concern in children is Reye's syndrome with aspirin. Children under 16 years of age should not take aspirin.

PHARMACOVIGILANCE

As part of the stringent conditions for granting a product licence to a newly developed drug, clinical trials with patients must be carried out to assess the efficacy and adverse effects of the product. On average, around 1500 people will have taken the product, and only the common adverse effects will have been experienced. Type B reactions, which occur to a lesser extent, may not be identified. Exclusion criteria for those taking part in the trial may mean that patients with multiple disease states, children, older people and pregnant women are excluded or are not well studied. In addition, the effect of long-term use will be unknown. Postmarketing surveillance or pharmacovigilance is therefore essential in detecting uncommon reactions. Suspicions that an adverse reaction may be related to a drug or combination of drugs should be notified to the Medicines and Healthcare products Regulatory Agency. All reactions should be reported for black triangle drugs, and only serious adverse reactions for established drugs. Yellow reporting cards are available in the back of the BNF. Nurses may report using the yellow card system.

DRUG-INDUCED GASTROINTESTINAL DISORDERS

Adverse drug reactions frequently affect the gastrointestinal tract. This is understandable when one considers that this is the most common route for medication administration and the vast range of oral medicines now available. Nausea and vomiting are one of the commonest adverse effects experienced by patients. However, in many cases symptoms soon resolve with continued use. When this is not the case, a lower dose or an alternative preparation may need to be considered, otherwise a concurrent antiemetic may be required. If nausea and vomiting are severe, treatment may have to be stopped.

Non-steroidal anti-inflammatory drugs including aspirin are very widely used but have a potential to damage the gastrointestinal tract. NSAIDs are administered to reduce pain and inflammation, particularly in arthritis. This is achieved by inhibition of synthesis of certain prostaglandins. However, they also inhibit prostaglandins, which are protective to tissues, resulting in irritant effects on the gastric epithelium.

Adverse drug reactions including abdominal pain, nausea, diarrhoea and dyspepsia are experienced. NSAID-induced erosions can result in bleeding and perforation of the stomach and duodenum. The following guidance can help minimise the risk from NSAIDs.

- When an NSAID is indicated, one with a lower incidence of side effects should be the first choice (e.g. ibuprofen).
- The lowest effective dose should be used. The maximum recommended dose should not be exceeded.
- No more than one NSAID should be used at any one time.
- The patient's medication should be regularly reviewed and NSAIDs stopped or changed to a safer product when possible.
- Should be taken after food.
- Patients should be counselled on how the drug works, the dose to be taken and the side effects to expect. They should be advised to consult their doctor without delay when signs of internal bleeding occur (e.g. blood-stained vomit or black tarry stools).

Table 10.1 provides details of several of the more commonly experienced gastrointestinal adverse effects (dry mouth, taste disturbance, oesophageal reflux, nausea and vomiting, diarrhoea and constipation) and examples of drugs causing these.

Table 10.1 Examples of drugs causing gastrointestinal adverse drug reactions

Adverse drug reaction	Examples of drugs
Dry mouth	Anticholinergics, antihistamines, central nervous system stimulants, ribavirin, tricyclic antidepressants, phenothiazines
Metallic taste	Metformin, metronidazole, zopiclone
Taste disturbance	Angiotensin-converting enzyme inhibitors, penicillamine, terbinafine
Oesophageal reflux	Anticholinergics, calcium-channel blockers, opioids
Nausea and vomiting	Cytotoxics, levodopa, opioids, quinolones, ribavirin
Diarrhoea	Antibiotics, colchicine, gold compounds, misoprostol, proton pump inhibitors
Constipation	Anticholinergics, antihistamines, diuretics, iron preparations, opioid analgesics, tricyclic antidepressants, verapamil

DRUG-INDUCED MENTAL HEALTH DISORDERS

Drug-induced mental health disorders are relatively common. Most adverse psychiatric effects of drugs are classified as type A reactions, as they are dose-related or predictable, although a few are idiosyncratic type B reactions. Psychiatric symptoms are also a common feature of withdrawal reactions, which can occur after certain drug therapy is stopped, particularly when it is stopped abruptly. For example, rapid withdrawal of benzodiazepines may cause rebound insomnia and anxiety.

The risk of an individual experiencing a psychiatric reaction to a drug is greater if mental illness is present or has been experienced in the past. Other associated factors include alcohol or drug abuse. Drugs implicated in psychiatric reactions can cause more than one effect. For example, phenytoin can cause delirium, hallucinations and psychosis.

PSYCHIATRIC CONDITIONS

Psychiatric conditions arising as a result of ADRs include depression, psychosis, mania, confusion and delirium. Depressive reactions to drugs may vary from mild mood changes to more severe adverse effects such as sleep disturbances, loss of appetite and suicidal ideation. When a drug is suspected of causing depression, resolution of symptoms on withdrawal will confirm diagnosis. Psychosis is characterised by delusions, hallucinations and distorted personality. As adverse effects of drugs, these are more common in older people. The effects are usually dose-related and resolve on discontinuation.

Mania is characterised by an elevated mood and also rapid speech, overactivity, insomnia and disinhibition. Drug-induced mania is uncommon, and affected patients usually have a history of mood disorder. Drugs linked to this include levodopa and corticosteroids. The suspected drugs should be discontinued and manic symptoms treated with an antipsychotic.

Table 10.2 Drugs associated with drug-induced mental disorders

Condition	Examples of drugs associated with the condition
Depression	Ciprofloxacin, beta-blockers, calcium-channel blockers, benzodiazepines, levodopa, carbamazepine, phenothiazines, rivastigmine, corticosteroids, disulfiram, levetiracetam, isotretinoin, mefloquine
Psychosis	Quinolones, anticholinergics, antiepileptics, disulfiram, ganciclovir, levodopa, mefloquine, zolpidem
Mania	Baclofen, bromocriptine, corticosteroids, levodopa
Delirium	Anticholinergics, antiepileptics, antipsychotics, corticosteroids, disulfiram, lithium, opioids
Confusion	Diazepam, carbamazepine, mexiletine, omeprazole, spironolactone

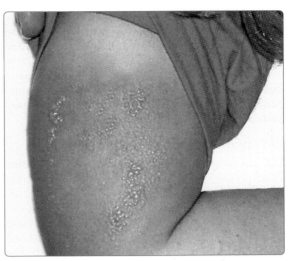

Fig. 10.1 Adverse effect following immunisation.

Patients suffering from acute confusional states have a short attention span, appear bewildered and have difficulty following commands. Delirium is characterised by disorientation and reduced attention, and the patient may be frightened, restless and hostile. Most drug-induced confusional states resolve on withdrawal of the drug. Antimuscarinics are recognised as causing delirium, disorientation, confusion and visual hallucinations. Table 10.2 lists drugs associated with drug-induced mental disorders.

DRUG-INDUCED SKIN DISORDERS

Drug-induced skin eruptions are likely to be the most frequent adverse reaction seen by a nurse, because approximately 30% of reported drug reactions involve the skin. Reactions are frequently seen after immunisations and can range from mild to more severe (Fig. 10.1).

ERYTHEMATOUS ERUPTION

This is a skin rash characterised by erythema (abnormal flushing of the skin) and is the most common type of drug-induced skin reaction. Erythematous rashes may be morbilliform (resembling measles) or maculopapular, i.e. consisting of macules (distinct flat areas, mostly discoloured) and papules (raised lesions). Early reactions start within 2 or 3 days of the administration of the drug and occur in previously sensitised patients, i.e. patients who have built up antibodies after receiving the drug on a previous occasion. In the late-type reaction, the hypersensitivity develops during administration. The peak incidence is around the ninth day, but rashes can occur as late as 3 weeks after starting treatment. A high incidence of erythematous rashes can be expected during or following treatment with penicillins, gold salts and NSAIDs.

PRURITUS

Pruritus (itching) may be the first sign of drug hypersensitivity and should act as an early warning for more severe skin reactions, such as those seen with gold therapy. Anal pruritus can be produced as a contact allergy following the local administration of ointments and suppositories.

URTICARIA

Urticaria is referred to as hives or nettle rash and is an acute or a chronic allergic reaction in which red weals develop. The weals itch intensely and may last for hours or days. Sometimes, urticaria affects areas other than the skin, causing swelling of the tongue, lips and eyelids. This serious variety is called angioedema and requires urgent medical attention. Only acute urticaria is likely to be drug-induced, occurring straight away or shortly after the administration of a drug to a sensitised patient, and it can be regarded as the cutaneous manifestation of anaphylaxis. Urticaria may arise following treatment with, for example, penicillins, vaccines, indometacin, imipramine, aspirin, dextrans and X-ray contrast media.

ERYTHEMA MULTIFORME

The lesions are erythematous maculopapules affecting the hands and feet more than the trunk. They appear over a few days and fade within 1 or 2 weeks. Lesions, which may be 1–2 cm after 48 h, can reach a size of up to 10 cm, with the centre becoming cyanotic – a characteristic iris or target-shaped lesion. Involvement of the mucosa is common. The drugs most likely to cause erythema multiforme are penicillins, phenytoin, carbamazepine, NSAIDs and gold salts.

TOXIC EPIDERMAL NECROLYSIS

This condition usually starts a few weeks after the start of treatment with the drug concerned. It is characterised by a redness of the whole skin with widespread exfoliation. Causes include captopril, carbamazepine, gold salts and thiazide diuretics.

LICHENOID ERUPTIONS

In lichenoid drug eruptions, the characteristic wide, flat, mauve pimples of lichen planus skin disease are present but can be associated with papular, scaling and eczematous lesions. The lesions are found mainly on the forearms, neck and between the thighs. Drugs that can cause this condition include phenothiazines, carbamazepine, gold salts, NSAIDs, penicillamine and thiazide diuretics.

ERYTHEMA NODOSUM

The lesions are painful subcutaneous nodules usually limited to extremities and may be preceded by transient erythema. Although not commonly drug-induced, erythema nodosum has been observed in women taking oral contraceptives. Other suspect drugs are drugs with a sulphonamide component, salicylates, penicillins and gold salts.

PHOTOSENSITIVITY

Increased sensitivity to light may be produced by thiazide diuretics, tetracyclines, chlorpromazine, promazine, carbamazepine, naproxen and amiodarone. Patients should be warned to avoid exposure to strong sunlight.

DRUG-INDUCED BLOOD DISORDERS

Like other ADRs, those affecting the blood can be divided into type A and type B reactions. Type A reactions can be predicted from the therapeutic action of the drug. Bone marrow suppression by cytotoxic drugs is a common type A effect.

The nurse has a role in advising patients prescribed high-risk drugs to seek urgent medical attention should they develop signs or symptoms suggestive of haematological ADRs. Patients will often present with a sore throat, mouth ulcers, rash, malaise, fever, bruising or bleeding. For some high-risk drugs, the risk is such that regular monitoring of the blood count is advised. These include amphotericin, clozapine, gold therapy, penicillamine, phenytoin, sulfasalazine and zidovudine.

Drugs can cause blood dyscrasias by acting at different stages of haemopoiesis from the stem cell through to the mature cells – red cells, white cells and platelets. Aplastic anaemia, agranulocytosis and thrombocytopenia are blood dyscrasias that can occur.

APLASTIC ANAEMIA

In aplastic anaemia, there is suppression of red cells (anaemia), white cells (leucopenia) and platelets (thrombocytopenia), resulting from suppression of bone marrow function (hypoplasia). This condition may persist despite drug withdrawal. The presenting features are anaemia, infection and bleeding, giving rise to the main symptoms of weakness, fatigue and pallor.

AGRANULOCYTOSIS

Leucopenia is the term used to describe a reduction in total white cell count, but agranulocytosis is more common. This is a selective reduction in granulocytes, which include neutrophils, eosinophils and basophils. In agranulocytosis, the absence of neutrophils in the blood results in the patient being very susceptible to serious infection. Common symptoms of acute neutropenia include fever, sore throat and painful mucosal ulcers. Any drug that might be implicated should be stopped immediately. In most cases, there is spontaneous recovery within 2 weeks of drug withdrawal.

Drugs strongly associated with agranulocytosis are listed in Table 10.3.

THROMBOCYTOPENIA

Thrombocytopenia is defined as a reduction in platelet count to less than 150×10^9/L. The main presenting

Table 10.3 Examples of drugs associated with aplastic anaemia, agranulocytosis and thrombocytopenia

Drug group	Drug(s)
Antipsychotics	Chlorpromazine, clozapine
Antiepileptics	Carbamazepine
Antibacterials	Chloramphenicol, co-trimoxazole, sulphonamides, cephalosporins, penicillins
Antithyroid drugs	Carbimazole, propylthiouracil
Anti-inflammatory drugs	Indometacin, phenylbutazone
Rheumatic disease suppressants	Gold, penicillamine, sulfasalazine

Table 10.4 Drugs that may cause headache

Drug group	Example(s)
Antidepressants	Lofepramine, trazodone, venlafaxine
Antipsychotics	Clozapine, risperidone
Anticonvulsants	Gabapentin, lamotrigine, phenytoin, vigabatrin
Non-steroidal anti-inflammatory drugs	Indometacin, naproxen, piroxicam
Nitrates	Glyceryl trinitrate, isosorbide mononitrate
Antiarrhythmics	Amiodarone, digoxin, metoprolol, verapamil
Ulcer-healing drugs	Proton pump inhibitors, ranitidine
Antidiabetic drugs	Glipizide
Diuretics	Bumetanide, furosemide, spironolactone
Angiotensin-converting enzyme inhibitors	Enalapril, lisinopril
Calcium-channel blockers	Amlodipine, nimodipine

feature is haemorrhage, which is most commonly seen in the skin, resulting in purpura and petechiae; there may also be nosebleeds (epistaxis) and bleeding from the gums. The mechanism of drug-induced thrombocytopenia is as a result of either reduction in platelet production due to suppression of the bone marrow or an immune reaction. This results in the production of antibodies that reduce the lifespan of platelets in the circulation from 7–10 days to several hours. Table 10.3 lists the drugs most commonly associated with thrombocytopenia.

Cessation of the drug responsible is often sufficient to restore the platelet count within several days. Platelet transfusions may be required if the count is very low. Future exposure to the likely causative drug should be avoided.

DRUG-INDUCED NEUROLOGICAL DISORDERS

Many drugs have the potential to cause adverse effects on the central nervous system. Headache is a common symptom. Vasodilators such as nitrates, calcium channel blockers and hydralazine may precipitate a vascular headache, but tolerance to this effect usually occurs and the nurse should encourage patients to continue with therapy. Table 10.4 lists drugs commonly associated with headache, particularly on initial therapy.

ADVERSE REACTIONS: CENTRAL NERVOUS SYSTEM

NAUSEA AND VOMITING

Chemotherapeutic agents may cause the release of serotonin in the small intestine, initiating a vomiting reflex by activating serotonin receptors. In addition, serotonin may be released in the brain, which promotes emesis centrally. The emetogenic effect of cancer chemotherapy varies according to the dose and combination of drugs used. High-dose cisplatin therapy is highly emetogenic. Carboplatin is also emetogenic but less so than cisplatin. Other drugs cause gastrointestinal side effects by a more direct

Table 10.5 Examples of drugs associated with dizziness

Class of drug	Example(s)
Antidepressants	Amitriptyline, clomipramine, sertraline, venlafaxine
Antipsychotics	Haloperidol, trifluoperazine
Drugs in Parkinson's disease and parkinsonism	Orphenadrine, trihexyphenidyl
Anticonvulsants	Gabapentin, lamotrigine, phenytoin, vigabatrin
Opioids	Buprenorphine, diamorphine
Non-steroidal anti-inflammatory drugs	Indometacin, piroxicam
Antiarrhythmics	Metoprolol, mexiletine, verapamil
Ulcer-healing drugs	Proton pump inhibitors, ranitidine
Diuretics	Bumetanide
Angiotensin-converting enzyme inhibitors	Enalapril, lisinopril
Calcium-channel blockers	Amlodipine, nifedipine

irritant effect on the gut. When cytotoxic chemotherapy regimens are known to be emetogenic, then the patient is usually prescribed serotonin receptor antagonists (e.g. ondansetron) in advance of therapy to prevent expected side effects.

DIZZINESS

Dizziness is a symptom that can arise from most centrally acting drugs, especially on initiation and at higher doses. The nurse's awareness of drugs that cause dizziness (see Table 10.5) will help to prevent falls.

TINNITUS

This refers to any noise, such as ringing, in the ears. The reaction is dose-related, and the dose must be reduced or the drug stopped. Tinnitus caused by salicylates is an indication of a toxic reaction.

DROWSINESS

Some medicines have special labelling requirements because they cause drowsiness, for example: 'This drug may cause drowsiness. If affected, do not drive or operate machinery. Avoid alcoholic drink'. Drowsiness is a common effect of many drugs that act on the central nervous system.

PARKINSONISM

Parkinson's disease, due to a decrease in dopamine production, is characterised by tremor, rigidity and a poverty of spontaneous movements. Drug-induced parkinsonism resembles Parkinson's disease and occurs to varying degrees in patients treated with antipsychotic drugs. The phenothiazines (e.g. trifluoperazine, fluphenazine), the butyrophenones (e.g. haloperidol) and the diphenylbutyl piperidines (e.g. pimozide, fluspirilene) are associated with a higher incidence of extrapyramidal effects. Drug-induced parkinsonism is reversible on dose reduction or drug withdrawal. Other drugs that have been implicated in parkinsonism include prochlorperazine, metoclopramide and tricyclic antidepressants.

ALLERGIC EMERGENCY (ANAPHYLACTIC SHOCK)

This is a life-threatening reaction with abrupt onset caused by exposure of sensitised individuals to specific allergens. The mechanism in susceptible individuals involves the production of immunoglobulin E antibody directed against the antigens. Immunoglobulin E binds to the surface of the mast cells and basophils. Subsequent exposure to antigen triggers the release of various substances, predominant among which is histamine. This causes:

- vasodilatation
- increased capillary permeability
- tissue oedema.

These changes give rise to:

- hypotension
- urticaria
- erythema of face and neck.

The reaction develops rapidly, reaching a maximum within 5–30 min. Individuals who experience an anaphylactic reaction may have a personal or family history of allergy.

In a severe reaction, the signs and symptoms are:
- pallor or cyanosis with weakening pulse
- skin cold and clammy to touch

- swelling of the glottis
- bronchoconstriction
- feeling of faintness
- loss of consciousness.

Other less serious features include:

- nasal congestion
- rhinorrhoea
- hoarseness.

Death from anaphylactic shock is due mostly to respiratory tract obstruction resulting from laryngeal oedema and bronchoconstriction. The incidence of these serious reactions is low, but in their rarity lies danger.

Common causes include:

- drugs, particularly if given by injection
- blood products
- insect stings
- desensitising agents
- certain foods (nuts, fish, shellfish).

The following groups of drugs are most commonly implicated:

- vaccines
- antibiotics, particularly penicillins
- desensitising solutions
- heparin
- anti-inflammatory analgesics
- neuromuscular blocking drugs
- hydroxocobalamin (rarely)
- cytotoxic drugs.

Anaphylaxis is more likely to occur as the result of an injection than from taking an oral preparation.

PREVENTION

Prior to administering a new medicine, particularly an injectable one, the following actions may help to prevent an anaphylactic reaction.

- Ask patients if they have suffered any previous reaction to drugs.
- Ask patients if they are taking drugs currently, including both prescribed and non-prescribed drugs.
- Ask patients if they have suffered from previous allergies such as asthma, hay fever or eczema.
- If in doubt, discuss with the doctor or other colleague before giving the drug.
- Consider giving a small test dose and carefully observe the patient before giving the full dose (e.g. for sodium aurothiomalate).

TREATMENT

This takes the form of drug therapy and is directed towards antagonising the effects of chemical mediators and preventing the further release of mediator substances.

First-line treatment includes laying the patient flat. For adults, a dose of 0.5 mL of adrenaline (epinephrine) 1:1000 solution (500 micrograms) should be administered intramuscularly, and repeated after about 5 min in the absence of clinical improvement or if deterioration occurs after the initial treatment, especially if consciousness becomes, or remains, impaired as a result of hypotension. In some cases, several doses may be needed, particularly if improvement is transient. Reduced doses are recommended for children by the Resuscitation Council (UK) (2005).

Adrenaline (epinephrine) inhibits the release of mediator chemicals from mast cells, limiting the severity of anaphylaxis. It also stimulates the β_2 receptors in bronchial smooth muscle, causing bronchodilatation. An antihistamine (chlorphenamine) should be administered. Caution is needed to avoid drug-induced hypotension. It is administered either by slow intravenous injection or by intramuscular injection. Its use may be helpful and is unlikely to be harmful. The dose for children and adults is determined by age. The effect of this is to block the H_1 receptor-mediated actions of histamine, reducing vascular permeability and bronchospasm.

Corticosteroids such as hydrocortisone or prednisolone are of no value in the immediate treatment of anaphylaxis, as onset of their therapeutic effect takes several hours. They are, however, very useful in preventing further deterioration in severely affected patients by inhibiting the release of inflammatory mediators and suppressing inflammatory reactions.

Some patients with severe allergy to insect stings may be advised to carry an adrenaline (epinephrine) syringe prefilled with adrenaline solution. Devices for home use are available for adults and children. These autoinjectors can inject 300 micrograms or 150 micrograms, respectively. The drug may therefore have been administered by parents before medical help is available. The doses can be regarded as equally suitable as the 250 micrograms and 125 micrograms more generally recommended for children.

PEANUT ALLERGY

Peanut allergy is probably the most common cause of food anaphylaxis. Peanuts are widely used as both ingredients in processed foods and readily identified peanut products such as peanut butter and roasted peanuts. Peanut oil has wide application as an industrial lubricant and as an ingredient in healthcare products (e.g. Naseptin cream, arachis oil enema and cosmetics). Nurses need to be aware and check that the patient is not a known allergy sufferer.

The allergen is contained in the protein but has been identified in cooking oils. Avoidance of exposure to the allergen is very difficult, but people with a known allergy must take every precaution to avoid exposure by checking carefully the foodstuffs they consume and by not experimenting with unknown foods. This is vitally important, because the allergen is very potent and mere traces can cause severe problems. The anaphylaxis caused by peanuts (and other nuts) is characterised by circulatory collapse and hypotension. Loss of consciousness, shock and cardiac disturbances may occur. As with other allergies, oedema of the larynx, epiglottis and pharynx may cause suffocation, leading to death.

Treatment of peanut anaphylaxis follows accepted practice for the treatment of other allergies. Milder reactions are treated with antihistamines, and adrenaline (epinephrine) is used for severe reactions. Prefilled adrenaline syringes should be carried by those with a history of severe reactions.

ROLE OF THE NURSE IN ADVERSE DRUG REACTIONS

The nurse, in liaison with the doctor and pharmacist, can play an important role in identifying ADRs or situations in which these may occur, and as a result may be able to reduce the incidence or severity of these occurrences. Factors involved in this include:

- recognising when a patient has had a previous allergic reaction and ensuring that there is not an exposure to the allergen that caused the reaction
- identifying drugs that are known to produce predictable dose-related adverse effects and avoiding their use when an equally effective and safer alternative is available
- checking that patients are not unnecessarily exposed to risk through use of unrequired drugs, disregard for warnings, special precautions or contraindications
- ensuring that patients receive patient information leaflets and counselling on the correct use of their medicines.

The role of the nurse in relation to ADRs may be summed up as anticipating and avoiding reactions and as recognising and responding to any that arise. A sound knowledge of the principles of pharmacology and ready access to current data on medicines are essential if the nurse is to play a full part in anticipating those situations in which an adverse reaction to a drug is likely. A thorough initial history of medicine taking and any previous experience of side effects should be taken. Nurses are trained to be active listeners. ADRs may be avoided or at least minimised by following the manufacturer's or pharmacist's instructions. For example, gastrointestinal effects may be avoided by the simple action of taking the medicine with food. Midwives can advise women at what stage in their pregnancy medicines, if they must have them, may be safely taken. Warning patients and/or relatives of possible adverse effects should be done in such a way, however, that they receive sufficient information without at the same time being put into a state of alarm.

To fulfil their role in this field, nurses must not only be observant but must also be able to make connections between their observations and the treatment being given. In any unexplained illness, they should always consider the possibility of an adverse reaction to the medicines the patient is receiving. Particular care should be taken in this regard in relation to older people, because the incidence of ADRs tends to increase with age as a result of metabolic and excretory processes becoming impaired. Having noted signs that they suspect may be linked with the medicines being taken, nurses must know how to respond appropriately. At one extreme, they may simply require to advise the patient to wait and watch; at the other, immediate action may be called for, including the instigation of appropriate resuscitative measures. Finally, nurses must be able to report and record accurately their observations, any significant symptoms described by the patient and any decisions made or advice given.

TREATMENT OF POISONING

At the extreme end of the ADR spectrum is poisoning. The treatment of acute poisoning, either intentional or accidental, presents a major challenge to clinical staff. Careless storage of medicines and household products is a common cause of accidental poisoning in children. Natural products, leaves, berries, etc. may also be implicated. Intentional poisoning is a complex subject. Self-poisoning may be undertaken by people determined to end their life. However, in some cases the ingestion of a poisonous substance, often a medicinal product, may be a cry for help or form part of a manipulative personal situation. Many social factors contribute to the tragic situations that can arise, for example poverty, alcoholism, drug abuse and social deprivation.

The management of a patient who has been poisoned, whatever the cause or circumstances, must be directed towards the maintenance of respiration and circulation. Seldom are the symptoms of poisoning highly specific, but many clues are available to the observant doctor or nurse. Tablets may be found in the victim's possession or at the scene of the tragedy. Family members and/or friends may be able to give useful information. The first priority of treatment is to maintain the patient's vital functions. If necessary, laboratory tests to determine the exact nature of the poison are undertaken. National poisons centres provide back-up, advice and guidance on clinical management in special situations Key aspects in the treatment of poisoning are as follow:

- maintenance of respiration: physical methods
- maintenance of circulation: physical methods and drug treatment
- maintenance of body temperature: physical methods
- maintenance of fluid and electrolyte levels in accordance with biochemical tests
- removal of the poisons (gastric lavage, emesis or active elimination)
- inactivation of the poisons: use of activated charcoal to adsorb the poison
- correction of metabolic complications (e.g. metabolic acidosis).

Once the acute situation has been dealt with and the patient assessed, it may be necessary to call in specialised psychiatric help.

Some poisons have specific antidotes, but there can be no substitute for the general supportive measures outlined above. An outline of the agents available for the treatment of poisoning is given in Table 10.6. These agents will be used together with general supportive measures.

In considering the treatment of acute poisoning, it is important to recognise the place of prevention, especially in children. Some useful guidelines for parents are given in Box 10.1.

The BNF gives an overview of the treatment of poisoning, but it is recommended that either a poisons information centre or Toxbase is consulted when there is doubt about the degree of risk or about management.

Box 10.1 Guidelines on the prevention of child poisoning for parents or guardians

- Keep medicines locked away.
- If your medicine is stored in a fridge, fit a safety lock to the door.
- Teach children not to play with medicines.
- Never share medicines.
- Warn children not to swallow anything unfamiliar.
- Never pretend that medicines are sweets.
- Dispose of medicines at the pharmacy.

If you think that your child has swallowed a medicine or poison
- Get the child to the nearest accident and emergency department as soon as possible.
- Take the drug container with you so that the doctor knows what has been taken.
- Do not try to make the child sick.
- If the child is unconscious, lay on one side to ease breathing and stop choking.

DRUG INTERACTIONS

The term *interaction* can be applied to the effects that drugs, food and other substances can have on the action of a drug. When two or more drugs are administered at the same time, they may exert their effect independently or they may interact. This may result in the action of one drug being more potent or being reduced because of an effect by the other drug. Many drug interactions are harmless, and a particular drug combination may cause harm to only a small proportion of individuals who receive it. The drugs most often involved in serious interactions are those with a narrow therapeutic range (e.g. aminoglycosides, phenytoin) and those for which the dose must be closely monitored according to the response (e.g. anticoagulants, antidiabetic drugs). Patients at increased risk from drug interactions include those with impaired renal and liver function and the elderly, because of changes in physiology due to ageing and also because older people are prescribed proportionately more drugs than younger people.

Drug interactions can be considered under three main headings:

- chemical interactions
- pharmacokinetic interactions
- pharmacodynamic interactions.

The BNF (appendix 1) contains a list of drugs and their interactions.

Table 10.6 Treatment of poisoning

Drug	Uses/indications
Acetylcysteine	This drug is given by intravenous infusion in the treatment of paracetamol poisoning. The dose is determined by reference to plasma paracetamol levels. Treatment with acetylcysteine is designed to reduce the often fatal liver damage caused by paracetamol ingestion in high doses. Treatment must be commenced as soon as possible after ingestion. If a period of more than 24 h has passed after ingestion, the liver damage will be irreversible.
Charcoal (activated)	Used to bind poisons, thus reducing absorption. A single dose of up to 50 g reduces absorption, and repeated doses of activated charcoal enhance the elimination of certain drugs after absorption.
Desferrioxamine	This is a specific antidote for iron poisoning. The drug acts by chelating the iron. Administration is by intravenous infusion, depending on the patient's serum iron level.
Dicobalt edetate	This is a specific antidote used in the treatment of cyanide poisoning.
Dimercaprol (BAL)	In poisoning by metals such as gold and mercury. Also in poisoning by arsenic and antimony.
Haemoperfusion and haemodialysis	These techniques may be used in severely poisoned patients, particularly in the treatment of salicylate and barbiturate poisoning.
Methionine	Given orally in paracetamol poisoning. This may be a useful approach when hospital treatment is not readily available.
Naloxone	Naloxone is a specific antidote for opioid overdosage. The intramuscular, intravenous or subcutaneous routes can be used, the dosage being determined in accordance with the patient's needs (see BNF).
Penicillamine	Lead poisoning by oral administration.
Pralidoxime	With atropine in the treatment of organophosphorus poisoning by intramuscular or slow intravenous injection or infusion.
Sodium nitrite and sodium thiosulphate	Used in combination in the treatment of cyanide poisoning.

CHEMICAL INTERACTIONS

These may occur in a number of situations, especially when drugs are reconstituted prior to administration in either large or small volumes. The use of a central intravenous additive service will help to minimise problems, but if reconstitution has to be carried out at ward level, the manufacturer's instructions must always be followed and the correct diluent used. For example, amphotericin must be diluted in glucose 5% injection with a pH greater than 4.2. Care must be taken when calcium salts and phosphate are added to an intravenous infusion, because above certain concentrations a precipitate is formed. Appendix 6 of the BNF gives a list of suitable infusion vehicles to be used in specific circumstances.

Mixing of drugs in a syringe prior to administration can cause a chemical interaction. Such admixtures may facilitate ease of administration (e.g. in a syringe driver), but pharmaceutical advice should always be taken to help to avoid harmful clinical interactions, particularly if the contents of the syringe become cloudy or opaque.

PHARMACOKINETIC INTERACTIONS

These occur when one drug alters the absorption, distribution, protein binding, metabolism or excretion of another, thus increasing or reducing the amount of drug available to produce its pharmacological effects.

ABSORPTION

Antacids and binding agents such as colestyramine may impair absorption of a drug from the gastrointestinal tract by binding the drug (e.g. iron, tetracycline). Other drugs, such as metoclopramide, may influence the gut transit time and hence the absorption of other drugs. In many cases, this influences the rate of absorption rather than the amount absorbed (extent). Most of these interactions have a low level of clinical significance and can be managed by separating the administration of each drug.

PROTEIN BINDING

Many drugs bind to plasma protein, particularly albumin. At any one time, there is an equilibrium between bound drug (attached to protein) and free drug. In general, the bound fraction is unavailable for activity, and the effect of the drug is exerted by the free fraction.

Protein displacement interactions occur when two drugs compete for the same binding site and one or both is displaced. This increases the concentration of free drug, but this is usually compensated for by increased excretion. The effect is usually transient and of minor importance. There may be exceptions, for example if the excretory mechanisms are unable to cope with the increased load (e.g. in renal or hepatic impairment) or if the therapeutic margin of the drug is so narrow that even transient increases can be damaging.

Displacement from protein binding plays a part in the potentiation of warfarin by sulphonamides, resulting in disturbances of anticoagulant control.

Lithium levels that are within the therapeutic range in a patient stabilised on lithium and a diuretic may be upset during illness, which alters fluid and electrolyte balance.

METABOLISM

Many drugs are metabolised in the body, principally in the liver. The result of metabolism may be inactive metabolites that are excreted (usually in bile or urine), or active metabolites that contribute to the effects of the drug. Some drugs (prodrugs) are inactive until metabolised to their active form.

There are a number of enzyme systems that metabolise drugs, and the most important is called the cytochrome P450 system. Interactions involving enzyme systems fall into two main categories, discussed below.

Enzyme induction. Certain drugs may cause enzyme induction, increasing the level of a particular enzyme. Drugs that are metabolised by this enzyme will therefore be broken down more quickly. Griseofulvin potentiates the enzymes that break down warfarin, and rifampicin potentiates those that break down oestrogens and progestogens. The latter interaction is important when the patient is taking oral contraceptives, because these will be broken down more quickly, resulting in an increased risk of pregnancy occurring.

Enzyme inhibition. Enzyme inhibition results in a lower level of enzymes, resulting in an accumulation of the drug that is metabolised by these particular enzymes. Examples of enzyme inhibitors are allopurinol, erythromycin, clarithromycin, fluconazole and ketoconazole.

RENAL EXCRETION

Drugs are eliminated through the kidney by both glomerular filtration and active tubular excretion. Competition can occur when drugs share the active transport mechanisms in the proximal tubule. Probenecid delays the excretion of all penicillins and some cephalosporins, which leads to their increased plasma levels. A combination of aspirin and methotrexate leads to a risk of toxicity from increased levels of methotrexate, because of competition for tubular secretion. NSAIDs can reduce glomerular filtration rate, especially during stress, and can reduce elimination of renally excreted drugs. Figure 10.2 summarises pharmacokinetic influence in drug interactions.

PHARMACODYNAMIC INTERACTIONS

These are interactions between drugs that have similar or antagonistic pharmacological effects or side effects. They may be due to competition at receptor sites, or occur between drugs acting on the same physiological system. They are usually predictable from a knowledge of the pharmacology of the interacting drugs; in general, those demonstrated with one drug are likely to occur with related drugs. They occur to a greater or lesser extent in most patients who receive the interacting drugs.

These interactions occur between drugs that have similar or antagonistic pharmacological effects or side effects.

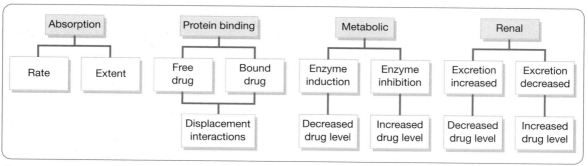

Fig. 10.2 Pharmacokinetic interactions.

INTERACTIONS AT RECEPTOR SITES

These interactions occur when two drugs act on the same site either antagonistically or synergistically.

Antagonism. An example of this, which is therapeutically beneficial, is the reversal of the effects of opiates by naloxone.

Synergism. Aminoglycosides enhance the effect of non-polarising muscle relaxant drugs such as atracurium.

Sedation with anxiolytics and hypnotics is enhanced by many other drugs with sedative properties, including some antihistamines, antidepressants and antipsychotics. Few of these interactions are hazardous, and some may be beneficial in patients for whom a sedative effect is appropriate.

INTERACTIONS BETWEEN DRUGS AFFECTING THE SAME SYSTEM

Acetazolamide, corticosteroids and corticotropin interact with thiazide diuretics, furosemide and bumetanide, causing increased urinary potassium loss resulting in hypokalaemia. Antihypertensive drugs are potentiated by hypnotics, tranquillisers and levodopa, which produce hypo-tension as a side effect.

INTERACTIONS DUE TO ALTERED PHYSIOLOGY

These interactions can occur in a number of ways, for example carbenoxolone and corticosteroids antagonise the effect of antihypertensive drugs because of fluid retention. Potassium-losing diuretics may give rise to digoxin toxicity because of increased potassium loss.

DRUG INTERACTIONS WITH ALCOHOL

Alcohol can interact with many drugs. It has a depressant effect on the nervous system, and when administered concurrently with central nervous system depressants the effect is additive. Alcohol increases the risk of death from an overdose of these drugs. The vasodilator effect of alcohol increases the postural hypotension of antihypertensive drugs. It can cause postural hypotension with peripheral vasodilators (e.g. pentoxifylline [oxpentifylline]) and antianginal drugs (e.g. nitrates, verapamil). This interaction can also occur with metronidazole and procarbazine. Some alcoholic drinks contain tyramine. If this is taken along with monoamine-oxidase inhibitors such as phenelzine or tranylcypromine, there is a risk of a hypertensive crisis. People who abuse drugs may be especially at risk from 'cocktails' of drugs with alcohol.

MINIMISING DRUG INTERACTIONS

AVOID COMBINATIONS OF DRUGS WHEN POSSIBLE

If the potential hazards of adding an interacting drug to existing therapy outweigh any benefit, then the patient may have to be denied the new therapy. However, in most cases an alternative can be found that does not interact in the same manner. If there is no alternative to the 'new' drug, then perhaps the existing therapy can be changed.

The choice of an alternative may depend on whether or not an interaction is a class effect that is likely to apply to any drug with a similar mode of action and/or chemical structure. For example, cimetidine is known to inhibit the metabolism of carbamazepine, phenytoin and valproate, and in this case ranitidine may be considered as an alternative.

ADJUST THE DOSE

If the net effect of an interaction is to increase or reduce the effect of one or more drugs, then modification of the dose of one or both may compensate for this. If a patient on lithium therapy is commenced on an NSAID, the excretion of lithium is reduced, resulting in higher plasma levels. A reduction in dose will compensate for this. Dose modification may be necessary on discontinuation of a drug as well as at introduction.

Dose adjustment can also involve a change to the timing of doses so that plasma concentrations of one drug are relatively low when the second is given. This may or may not be effective depending, for example, on the half-life of each drug.

MONITOR THE PATIENT

Whatever course of action is taken in the face of a potential interaction, it may be prudent to monitor the patient more closely for a realistic period after change of therapy.

SELF-ASSESSMENT QUESTIONS

1. Describe the symptoms of an anaphylactic or anaphylactoid reaction.

2. What is the nurse's role in the prevention/minimisation of adverse drug reactions?

REFERENCES

Resuscitation Council (UK) 2005 Resuscitation guidelines 2005. Resuscitation Council, London

FURTHER READING AND RESOURCES

Barnes J, Anderson LA, Phillipson JD 2003 Herbal interactions. Pharmaceutical Journal 270:118–121

Camm J 2005 Allergic reaction. Community Practitioner 78:234–235

Dawson M, Hodgson SL, Judd A 1997 Poisoning – common exposures and problems. Pharmaceutical Journal 4:111–115

Evans C, Tippins E 2005 Emergency treatment of anaphylaxis. Accident and Emergency Nursing 13:232–237

Freely J, Barry M 2005 Adverse drug interactions. Clinical Medicine 5:19–22

Lucas H 1999 Drug interactions that matter – anti-arrhythmics. Pharmaceutical Journal 262:28–31

Lucas H 1999 Drug interactions that matter – anticonvulsants. Pharmaceutical Journal 262:325–327

Lucas H 1999 Drug interactions that matter – antihypertensives. Pharmaceutical Journal 262:547–551

Mason P 1995 Diet and drug interactions. Pharmaceutical Journal 255:94–97

McGavock H 2002 How to predict and avoid drug reactions. Prescriber 13:107–111

Medicines and Healthcare Products Regulatory Agency 2006 Current problems in pharmacovigulance. Online. Available: http://www.mhra.gov.uk

Royal College of Physicians of London 1997 Medication for older people, 2nd edn. Royal College of Physicians of London, London

Van Dijk KN, De Vries PB, Van Den Berg JRB et al. 2001 Occurrence of potential drug–drug interactions in nursing home residents. International Journal of Pharmacy Practice 9:45–52

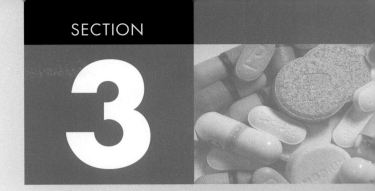
CLINICAL PHARMACOLOGY

Drug treatment of gastrointestinal disorders

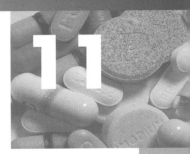

11

KEY OBJECTIVES

After reading this chapter, you should be able to:

- outline the anatomy and normal physiology of the gastrointestinal tract
- discuss the main products used in the management of dyspepsia
- distinguish between gastric and duodenal ulceration
- list the main risk factors for the development of peptic ulcer
- describe what is meant by triple therapy
- list the four main laxative groups and give one example of each
- compare and contrast the features of ulcerative colitis and Crohn's disease
- name the main drug groups used in the treatment of inflammatory bowel disease
- outline the management of haemorrhoids
- describe how to administer rectal medicines
- discuss the care required in prescribing and administering medicines to people with a stoma
- identify lifestyle changes that may help to reduce the incidence of gastrointestinal disease.

INTRODUCTION

A glance at the shelves of your local pharmacy gives a good, if crude, indication of the high prevalence of gastrointestinal disorders in the community. It is perhaps surprising, given the abuse many people subject their digestive systems to, at home and abroad, that problems are not even more widespread. Fortunately, many conditions have no organic cause and resolve with time, simple remedies and possibly a change of lifestyle (smoking cessation and diet). However, given the complex and intricate systems, both hormonal and neuronal, that control the chemical and mechanical functions of the gut, it is perhaps understandable that when physiology becomes disordered very significant illness can result.

Prompt, accurate diagnosis (using modern imaging and endoscopic techniques) and treatment are required in order to prevent more serious longer-term complications developing. An excellent range of drugs is available, designed to act on specific physiological processes and using sophisticated delivery systems. These products have greatly improved treatment outcomes for patients. Side effects are often minimal, and the need for surgery for duodenal ulcer has been reduced, which is good news for patients and NHS budgets.

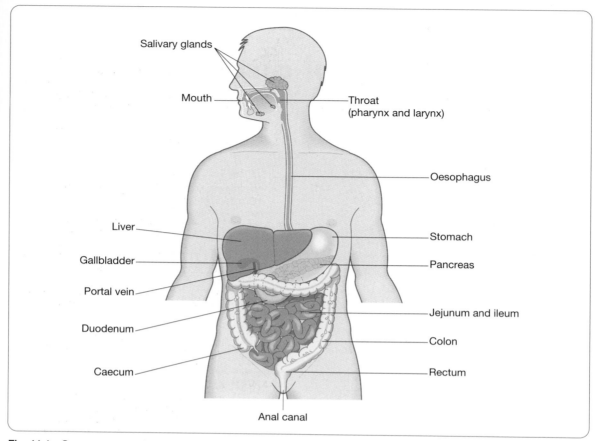

Fig. 11.1 Gross anatomy of the gastrointestinal tract from mouth to anus.

Western lifestyles may be contributory factors in gastrointestinal disorders, especially malignant disease. High intake of alcohol and smoking greatly increase the risk of peptic ulcer disease developing.

DRUG TREATMENT OF DISORDERS OF THE GASTROINTESTINAL TRACT

ANATOMY AND PHYSIOLOGY

The gastrointestinal tract consists of a long, tubular structure extending from the mouth to the anus via the oesophagus, stomach and intestines. Its purpose is to digest, absorb and eliminate substances following the ingestion of food. The process of digestion is assisted by four accessory organs, namely the salivary glands, liver, gall bladder and pancreas (Fig. 11.1).

DIGESTION

Food is digested both mechanically and chemically. Mechanical digestion results from voluntary and involuntary muscle action, i.e. nervous control; chemical digestion is produced by the action of enzymes and hormones. The digestive processes taking place in each section of the gastrointestinal tract are summarised in Table 11.1.

Food allergy is best dealt with by avoidance. Sodium cromoglicate 200 mg four times daily may be useful.

ABSORPTION

The absorption of some nutrients begins in the stomach, and some absorption takes place in the large intestine. By far the most absorption, however, occurs in the small intestine (see Fig. 11.2). Table 11.2 summarises some aspects of the absorption of nutrient materials and drugs from the gastrointestinal tract.

Table 11.1 Stages of digestion

Organ	Mechanical	Chemical
Mouth	Food taken in is masticated (chewed) by the teeth. The muscular action of the tongue and the presence of saliva convert the food into a moist bolus ready for swallowing.	Saliva is produced by the salivary glands under the control of the autonomic nervous system. It consists of water and the enzyme salivary amylase. Salivary amylase converts cooked starches into maltose.
Oesophagus	Bolus is propelled forwards first by voluntary muscle action and then under autonomic nerve control.	No chemical action initiated in the oesophagus.
Stomach	The muscular layers produce a churning action and assist peristalsis. The semisolid mixture produced is known as chyme.	Stimulated by the hormone gastrin, gastric juice is produced by the gastric mucosa. It is composed of: • water, which liquefies food • hydrochloric acid, which acidifies food, kills micro-organisms, and converts the enzyme pepsinogen secreted by the parietal cells into pepsin, an essential factor in the digestion of protein • intrinsic factor, necessary for absorption of vitamin B_{12} • mucus, which, as a lubricant, protects the stomach wall from the harmful effects of hydrochloric acid and protein-digesting pepsin.
Small intestine	Onwards movement of contents by peristalsis and segmental movement.	The hormones secretin and cholecystokinin–pancreozymin stimulate the secretion of pancreatic juice, which consists of: • water • mineral salts • enzymes – pancreatic amylase, which converts starches not affected by salivary amylase to sugars; lipase, which converts fats to fatty acids and glycerol; trypsinogen and chymotrypsinogen, which convert polypeptides into amino acids. Stimulated by cholecystokinin–pancreozymin, bile, secreted by the liver but stored in the gall bladder, passes into the duodenum after a meal has been taken. Bile consists of: • water • mineral salts • mucus • bile salts • bile pigment. Bile is essential for the emulsification of fats and the absorption of vitamin K, and it colours and deodorises the faeces. Intestinal juice is secreted by glands in the small intestine and consists of: • water • mucus • the enzyme enterokinase.
Large intestine	Intermittent waves of peristalsis known as mass movement, often precipitated by the gastrocolic reflex following the entry of food into the stomach.	No secretion of enzymes – the last phase of digestion depends on the presence of bacteria in the colon. Bacteria: • ferment foodstuffs in faecal matter, producing gases that form flatus • break down other nutrients and give faeces their distinctive odour • decompose bilirubin, giving faeces their characteristic colour • synthesise vitamins.

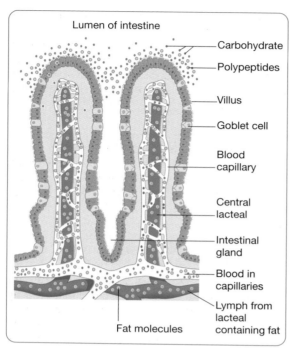

Lumen of intestine

- Carbohydrate
- Polypeptides
- Villus
- Goblet cell
- Blood capillary
- Central lacteal
- Intestinal gland
- Blood in capillaries
- Lymph from lacteal containing fat

Fat molecules

Fig. 11.2 Absorption in the small intestine. (From Waugh A, Grant A 2001 Ross and Wilson anatomy and physiology in health and illness, 9th edn. Churchill Livingstone, Edinburgh. With permission of Elsevier.)

ELIMINATION

Undigested and unabsorbed foodstuffs, along with the bile pigments and bilirubin, are eliminated as waste from the body via the large intestine in the form of faeces. Defecation is the term used to describe the expulsion of faeces from the rectum and anal canal. Prior to the act of defecation, several physiological processes take place; these are shown in Box 11.1.

The act of defecation is voluntarily assisted by contraction of the diaphragm and the muscles of the abdominal wall. Relaxation of the external anal sphincter finally allows the faeces to be expelled.

DISORDERS AND THEIR TREATMENT

DYSPEPSIA

Dyspepsia is characterised by recurrent pain or discomfort in the upper abdomen. Heartburn and acid regurgitation may be accompanied by bloating, nausea or vomiting. Patients may also experience early satiety, feelings of upper abdominal fullness and belching. It is essential to ensure that patients presenting with dyspeptic symptoms are fully investigated so as to eliminate (or treat) serious conditions such as malignancy or ulcer disease.

Duodenal and gastric ulcer disease are significant causes of morbidity and mortality despite the great

Table 11.2 Absorption in the gastrointestinal tract[a]

Organ	Site of absorption and notes	Substances absorbed
Stomach	Walls of the stomach. Systemic absorption influenced by acid environment and gastric emptying time.	Water Alcohol Weak acids (e.g. aspirin, lipid-soluble non-ionised drugs)
Small intestine	The villi and microvilli into the capillaries and lacteals. Largest gastrointestinal surface area for absorption. Alkaline environment may influence absorption of some substances.	Carbohydrates as monosaccharides Proteins as amino acids Fats as fatty acids and glycerol Vitamins Mineral salts Some water (one-tenth only)
Large intestine	Predominantly the caecum and ascending colon.	Water (remaining nine-tenths) Mineral salts, especially sodium Drugs not absorbed in small intestine may be absorbed to some extent

[a]Absorption of drugs from the gastrointestinal tract is very complex and may be affected by a range of factors, including dosage form, pH, gut motility, presence or absence of food, and pathology.

advances made in both their diagnosis and treatment. Well-managed treatment will bring about control of these conditions. Maintenance therapy following healing of an ulcer is frequently required. The key diagnostic features of ulcer disease are localised epigastric pain and nocturnal pain. The pain is often relieved by food and antacids. In some patients, the pain may be relieved by vomiting. Endoscopy is used to confirm the diagnosis. There are significant differences between gastric and duodenal ulcers; these are summarised in Table 11.3.

The importance of accurate diagnosis cannot be overemphasised. Patients with alarm symptoms such as gastrointestinal bleeding, anaemia, jaundice, vomiting, severe pain or the presence of an epigastric mass need referral to a consultant gastroenterologist.

Risk factors in dyspepsia
The risk factors are summarised in Table 11.4.

In healthy people, there is a balance between damaging forces (e.g. acid, smoking, drugs, stress) and protective and repair mechanisms. When these forces become out of balance, ulcers and erosions can occur.

Treatment of uncomplicated dyspepsia
Various aspects of treatment are as follow.

General measures. Many patients who present with peptic ulcer disease are elderly and may have coexisting diseases such as diabetes or cardiovascular problems. Nurses, as well as providing care, can encourage patients to adopt a more healthy lifestyle such as improved dietary habits (avoiding highly spiced foods, fatty foods and heavy meals in the evening), cessation of smoking and avoidance of stress. Weight reduction is also important. Excessive alcohol intake is very harmful.

Box 11.1 Physiological processes prior to defecation

1. Mass movement in pelvic colon
2. Faecal matter enters rectum
3. Rectal wall distended
4. Pressure receptors in wall stimulated
5. Nerve impulses transmitted to sacral cord
6. Motor impulses transmitted back from cord via parasympathetic nerves
7. Rectal muscles contract
8. Pressure in rectum increases
9. Reflex relaxation of internal anal sphincter
10. Desire to defecate

Table 11.3 Peptic ulceration: a comparison

Gastric ulcers	Duodenal ulcers
Rare in patients under 40	Prevalence highest in patients over 60 but occur in all age groups
Pain relief following food intake short-lived	Pain relieved by food intake, pain generally worse before meals
Anorexia and nausea more prominent than in duodenal ulcers	–
Gastric acid secretion may be normal or even below normal	Gastric acid is a major factor
Antisecretory therapy produces healing but more slowly than with duodenal ulcers	Antisecretory therapy often produces healing in 4 weeks; lesions smaller than in gastric ulcers
Healing can occur without active treatment	–
Recurrence rate lower than with duodenal ulcers	Ulcers recur when therapy stopped
Helicobacter pylori infection present in 85% of cases	*H. pylori* infection present in 100% of cases
Very important to exclude gastric cancer in patients who present with symptoms of gastric ulcer	–

Table 11.4 Risk factors in dyspepsia

Risk factor	Notes
Acid	This is especially important in duodenal ulcer patients, who often have twice as many parietal cells as normal subjects.
Mucus	Reduced mucus production may be involved, because the protective effect of mucus may be lost.
Helicobacter pylori	*H. pylori* has the ability to colonise human gastric mucosa, especially the distal antral region of the stomach. The bacteria are found on the mucosal surface and do not penetrate the underlying tissues. The organism stimulates an inflammatory response and produces ammonia (an alkali), which protects the organism from gastric acid. The organism is widely distributed in the population and has a major role in dyspepsia. The mechanisms involved in acquiring *H. pylori* infection are not well understood. The presence of this organism can be confirmed by a breath test. Breath samples are taken before and after ingestion of an oral solution of carbon-13 urea. Laboratory analysis of the samples is required.
Cigarette smoking	The smoking of cigarettes is a major risk factor; peptic ulcers in smokers heal more slowly and are more likely to recur than those in non-smokers.
Drugs	Many NSAIDs (see p. 442) can cause serious gastric damage; the extent to which duodenal ulceration is caused by NSAIDs is still the subject of much debate and research.
Stress	Stress has long been associated with dyspepsia.
Foods	Some foods have been associated with dyspepsia – there is considerable variation between patients; avoidance of foods that cause problems is advocated.
Hereditary factors	There is a proven hereditary component in duodenal ulcers.

NSAID, non-steroidal anti-inflammatory drug.

Simple antacids. Examples include:

- aluminium hydroxide mixture
- magnesium-containing compounds
- combined antacid preparations
- magnesium trisilicate mixture or powder.

Antacids can interact with other drugs (see BNF) and may cause the coating of enteric-coated tablets to break down in the stomach. Antacids do often provide rapid relief of dyspeptic symptoms but have no ulcer-healing properties.

Combination antacid products. Antacids may be combined with anti-foaming agents (dimeticone), which are claimed to be of value in flatulence. Alginates (derived from certain seaweeds) form a gel-like 'raft' that, when combined with sodium bicarbonate, is effective in reflux oesophagitis.

Atropine-like antisecretory agents. Antimuscarinic agents have little antisecretory effect in doses that are practicable because of atropine-like side-effects (see Ch. 9). The more specific antisecretory drugs, the H_2-receptor antagonists, are the basis of the treatment of peptic ulceration.

Peptic ulcer

Dyspepsia may be a symptom of peptic ulcer, which is treated by more sophisticated drugs than simple antacids.

Histamine H_2-receptor antagonists (see p. 133). The introduction of cimetidine and ranitidine (and similar drugs such as famotidine) has played a major part in improving the treatment of peptic ulcer disease. Cimetidine is given orally in a dose of 400 mg twice daily or as a single dose of 800 mg at night. A 4-week course of treatment is given in duodenal ulceration, and a 6-week course in the treatment of gastric ulceration. Once healing has been achieved, a maintenance dose must be given over a long period. Ranitidine is also given orally, 150 mg twice daily or 300 mg at night. The side-effect profile of ranitidine is lower than that of cimetidine. The use of both these drugs has greatly reduced the need for surgical treatment of peptic ulcers. Parenteral forms of the drug are available for use in conditions in which the oral route is inappropriate, for example when there is severe bleeding, for the prevention of stress ulceration in seriously ill patients, and prophylactically

Table 11.5 Similarities of, and differences between, cimetidine and ranitidine

	Cimetidine	Ranitidine
Mode of action	Selective histamine H_2-receptor antagonist	As cimetidine
Indications	Peptic ulcer disease, Zollinger–Ellison syndrome	As cimetidine
Oral dose	400 mg twice daily	150 mg twice daily
Maintenance	400 mg at night	150 mg dose at night
Availability	Tablets, syrup; parenteral	As cimetidine – also granules
Contraindications and warnings	Dose reduced in patients with impaired renal function	As cimetidine
	Prolongs elimination of drugs metabolised by oxidation in the liver	Some changes (transient) have been reported in liver function
	May mask symptoms of gastric carcinoma	As cimetidine
	Some drug interactions, especially with oral anticoagulants and phenytoin (dosage reduction of these drugs may be needed)	Few drug interactions have been reported
	Rare reports of bradycardia and arteriovenous block	As cimetidine
	H_2-receptor antagonism may potentiate falls in blood cell counts caused by other factors (e.g. disease or other drug treatment)	Leucopenia and thrombocytopenia have been rarely reported
	Gynaecomastia has been reported but is reversible on stopping treatment	Few reports with ranitidine

in patients thought to be at risk from acid aspiration syndrome. Although these two drugs have similar properties, there are significant differences (Table 11.5). Ranitidine has been combined with a bismuth compound to form a compound ranitidine bismuth citrate. This drug is used together with antibacterial agents in eradication therapy and to treat duodenal and gastric ulceration associated with *Helicobacter pylori*. A dose of 400 mg twice daily for 8 weeks is used to treat benign gastric ulceration. *H. pylori*

eradication therapy (see p. 170) has replaced low-dose maintenance therapy with H_2-receptor antagonists. It should be noted that a number of H_2 antagonists are available without prescription from pharmacies. The indications for which these products may be sold are defined in the product licence. Dizziness, somnolence and fatigue have been reported.

Although some degree of freedom to adjust dosage (note, *not* in eradication therapy) may be an acceptable part of controlling symptoms, primary carers should be alert for any tendencies the patient may have to increase the dose prior to a planned episode of overindulgence.

Chelates and complexes. Tripotassium dicitratobismuthate is thought to act by an antibacterial action on *H. pylori*. Other actions attributed to this compound include the stimulation of the secretion of prostaglandin (a mucosal protective) and/or the stimulation of bicarbonate secretion. The usual dose is two 120-mg tablets twice daily. Sucralfate (a complex of aluminium hydroxide and sulphated sucrose) has only minimal antacid properties but is an effective treatment for both gastric and duodenal ulcer. The mode of action may be to protect mucosa from acid and pepsin attack. Side-effects include constipation, diarrhoea, dry mouth, aches and pains, and skin rashes. The bismuth compounds may darken the tongue and blacken the faeces, and it is important to warn patients accordingly.

Prostaglandin analogues (see also p. 443). Misoprostol is a synthetic compound similar to prostaglandin E_1. It acts by inhibiting acid secretion, and it promotes the healing of both gastric and duodenal ulcer. It may be given to treat gastric ulceration caused by non-steroidal anti-inflammatory drugs (NSAIDs). Combination products (NSAID and misoprostol) are claimed to be safer than NSAIDs alone for 'at risk' patients (e.g. older people).

Proton pump inhibitors. Esomeprazole, omeprazole, lansoprazole, pantoprazole and rabeprazole are effective drugs used in the treatment of both gastric and duodenal ulcer. These drugs are the treatment of choice in stricturing and erosive oesophagitis. Patients very much welcome rapid relief from the distressing symptoms of this condition.

The mode of action is based on the property of blocking the hydrogen potassium ATP enzyme system (see Fig. 11.3) in the parietal cell. This is also a very effective treatment for Zollinger–Ellison syndrome (see below) and reflux oesophagitis. An oral dose of 20 mg daily for 4 weeks is often effective but can be increased in refractory cases to 40 mg daily. It should be noted that the degree of acid suppression achieved is directly related to the rate of ulcer healing. Omeprazole 20 mg daily can produce healing within 4 weeks. This rate of healing can be achieved with H_2 antagonists given in higher doses (e.g. ranitidine 300 mg twice daily). The dosage range of the other proton pump inhibitors is similar to that of omeprazole.

Triple therapy. Triple therapy, designed to eradicate *H. pylori*, has an important place in the treatment of dyspeptic disease. Eradication of *H. pylori* is achieved in over 90% of cases by the use of triple therapy. The

following regimens, among others, are advocated (see British National Formulary, BNF). Each regimen utilises a proton pump inhibitor (acid suppressant) plus antibiotics. Treatment must be given for 7 days. Eradication therapy should not be given to patients with non-ulcer dyspepsia or oesophagitis. Chest pain caused by *H. pylori* infection may be difficult to distinguish from cardiac pain. If cardiac problems can be eliminated, eradication therapy may be helpful:

- omeprazole 20 mg twice daily (or lansoprazole 30 mg twice daily)
- clarithromycin 500 mg twice daily
- amoxicillin 1 g twice daily

or, if allergic to penicillin,

- lansoprazole 30 mg twice daily
- clarithromycin 500 mg twice daily
- metronidazole 400 mg twice daily.

A 2-week dual therapy regimen using a proton pump inhibitor and a single antibacterial agent is inferior to triple therapy and should not be used. Factors such as acceptance by the patient, bacterial resistance, antibiotic allergy, local policies and cost are taken into account. Successful eradication therapy leads to long-term remission, but reinfection can occur with *H. pylori*.

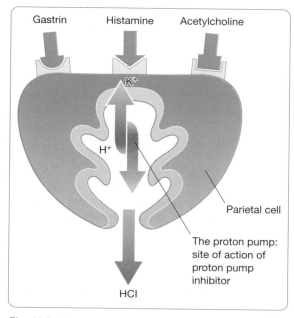

Fig. 11.3 Representation of parietal cell showing site of action of proton pump inhibitors.

If the patient's symptoms persist, this may or may not indicate 'success' of the eradication therapy. If a breath test, carried out 4 weeks after the completion of a course of eradication therapy, indicates the continuing presence of infection, a second but different course of eradication therapy should be given. It is important to check patient compliance before commencing a second course of therapy.

Quadruple therapy may be required for 2 weeks if triple therapy fails. Quadruple therapy comprises a proton pump inhibitor (in standard dosage) twice daily, tripotassium dicitratabismuthate 120 mg four times daily, metronidazole 400–500 mg three times daily and tetracycline 500 mg four times daily.

In view of the nature of the condition, it is essential to ensure that patients comply with treatment regimens, especially in eradication therapy. Concordance by the patient can be improved by explaining to the patient the nature of the condition and the need to take the medication regularly over a period of time. The tendency of some patients to discontinue therapy once the symptoms ease must be recognised and appropriate action taken, otherwise a serious relapse may occur.

Patients receiving eradication therapy must avoid alcohol because of severe interactions.

The availability of H_2 antagonists and a wide variety of antacids over the counter may lead to difficulties if patients receiving prescribed medicines purchase additional medicines. Community nurses (and community pharmacists) will need to be alert to any inappropriate or overuse of non-prescription medicines, especially anti-inflammatory pain-relieving medicines (see pp. 42, 442).

Complications of duodenal and gastric ulceration

Bleeding is a serious complication of ulceration. If uncontrolled, ulceration develops and a blood vessel at the base of the ulcer is penetrated, resulting in serious blood loss. Up to 20% of patients may suffer a bleeding episode and may experience haematemesis and/or melaena. The loss of blood may cause cardiovascular shock, which must be treated urgently. Blood transfusion and resuscitative measures will be needed, together with the combined skills of both gastroenterologist and surgeon.

ZOLLINGER–ELLISON SYNDROME

This condition is characterised by severe and often intractable ulceration caused by very high levels of acid secretion. The high levels of acid result from the continuous stimulation of the parietal cells by the hormone gastrin. Abnormal amounts of gastrin are produced by a gastrinoma (tumour), often situated in the pancreas. In two-thirds of cases, the tumour is malignant.

Treatment is with a proton pump inhibitor such as omeprazole. Doses are higher than those used in the treatment of gastric or duodenal ulcer: omeprazole 60 mg once daily initially, increasing up to 120 mg daily in two divided doses.

Surgery and/or cytotoxic therapy may be valuable if the growth of secondaries is not advanced.

GASTRO-OESOPHAGEAL REFLUX DISEASE (HEARTBURN)

Patients presenting with gastro-oesophageal reflux disease (GORD) complain of a burning sensation, which is often accompanied by severe pains in the chest that may be difficult to distinguish from cardiac pain. Many patients admitted to hospital for suspected myocardial infarction are found to be suffering from GORD. In other patients, the diagnosis creates no difficulty, especially when symptoms occur after a meal. Peptic ulcer disease may coexist with GORD (as may cardiac disease), and it is also important to eliminate gastric neoplasm as a factor. Full diagnostic measures are used to establish the true nature of the patient's condition. Barium meal, endoscopic examination and oesophageal pH monitoring are cornerstones of differential diagnosis, together with a full history of the patient.

Treatment of GORD

The patient's dietary habits must be attended to. Weight loss, smoking cessation and reduction in alcohol intake are also vitally important. The head of the patient's bed should be raised by 20 cm.

Because the pain of GORD is caused by refluxing of gastric contents on to very sensitive oesophageal mucosa, it follows that antacids are the first-line agents (Fig. 11.4). Combinations of antacids with alginates are very useful. If reflux does occur, the stomach contents have been 'neutralised' to some extent and therefore are less likely to cause irritation. If simple antacid therapy does not provide relief, omeprazole or an alternative proton pump inhibitor should be considered. Proton pump inhibitors are more effective than H_2 antagonists and are the treatment of choice.

Metoclopramide may be useful, because this drug improves gastric emptying times, stimulates small intestinal transit and increases the strength of the oesophageal sphincter contraction. Domperidone (a dopamine antagonist) has actions similar to metoclopramide. If medical treatment fails (this

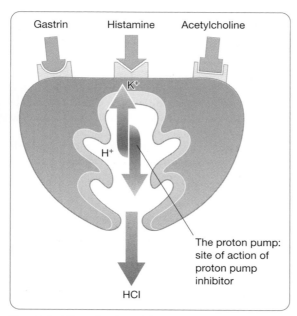

Gastrin   Histamine   Acetylcholine

K^+

H^+

The proton pump: site of action of proton pump inhibitor

HCl

Fig. 11.4 Sites of action of drugs used to treat gastro-oesophageal reflux disease (From Page CP, Hoffman BF, Curtis M et al. 2006 Integrated pharmacology. Mosby, Edinburgh. With permission of Mosby.)

is rare), consideration has to be given to surgical intervention.

DYSPHAGIA

The sensation of food being held up in its passage to the stomach is called dysphagia. It should in all cases be investigated. There are two main types.

In oropharyngeal dysphagia, the patient has difficulty initiating swallowing or in coordinating the swallowing reflex, and presents with pain, choking and regurgitation after swallowing. It can occur in neuromuscular disorders such as stroke (see p. 223) and motor neurone disease.

It is important to elicit whether the difficulty is with solids or liquids or with both, and whether the difficulty is getting progressively worse. Accompanying weight loss may indicate a carcinoma, especially in older people. The reflux symptoms of GORD may lead to a benign peptic stricture, resulting in oesophageal dysphagia.

Diagnosis of these conditions is confirmed by barium swallow and endoscopy. Management includes assessment and supervision of swallowing, modification of diet (especially texture of food) and regular weighing. The specialist inputs of a dietitian and of a speech and language therapist are generally requested.

Nursing staff must minimise the risk of patients choking and be vigilant in observing their ability to swallow, the incidence of coughing, and evidence of any developing chest infection. Feeding may require to be through a percutaneous endoscopic gastrostomy or nasogastric tube. Complete foods, nutritional supplements and thickeners may be prescribed and are listed in the BNF.

DIARRHOEA

The term *diarrhoea* is used to describe an increase in frequency, fluidity and/or volume of stools. It is a leading cause of death in underdeveloped countries. Chronic diarrhoea may occur in conditions such as malabsorption and malnutrition.

In the acute form of diarrhoea, dehydration can quickly develop – especially in infants and older people. Prevention and treatment of dehydration is vital. Fluid and electrolyte replacement takes priority in acute cases requiring the patient's admission to hospital. Abdominal cramp may be relieved by the use of an antispasmodic such as dicycloverine (dicyclomine), alverine and peppermint oil.

Simple gastroenteritis will usually resolve without the need for antibiotic treatment. When there is systemic infection, systemic antibiotic treatment will be needed.

In acute diarrhoea, antimotility drugs such as loperamide, codeine phosphate and co-phenotrope may offer some relief, along with fluid and electrolyte replacement, in adults. The management of chronic diarrhoea that occurs with specific disorders of the bowel appears in the relevant parts of this chapter.

INFLAMMATORY BOWEL DISEASE

The most common presenting symptom of inflammatory bowel disease (IBD) is chronic diarrhoea. However, it is important to recognise that diarrhoea may be due to one of a number of causes. Infection often presents as a sudden episode of diarrhoea, but more sinister causes of diarrhoea are IBD or neoplastic disease. Differential diagnosis is vitally important so as to ensure that the treatment instigated does not mask the underlying condition. The two main conditions are Crohn's disease and ulcerative colitis. These conditions have similar features and yet are distinctly separate diseases (Table 11.6). Both diseases are relatively common; within a general practice of 2000 patients, about four will have some form of IBD.

Table 11.6 A comparison of the main features of Crohn's disease and ulcerative colitis

Crohn's disease	Ulcerative colitis[a]
Can affect any part of the gastrointestinal tract from mouth to anus	Primarily involves large intestine
Most common sites are terminal ileum and ascending colon	–
Rectum affected in approximately 50% of patients	Most patients have rectal involvement
Inflammatory process involves all layers of bowel	Inflammatory process mainly confined to mucosa
Presence of multiple granulomas	Multiple granulomas not seen
Clinical symptoms: bloody diarrhoea, anorexia, pain, fever, weight loss due to malabsorption	Clinical symptoms: similar to Crohn's disease but bloody diarrhoea very common, abdominal pain and fever more prominent, signs of malabsorption not seen
Strictures are common	Strictures very rare
Neoplastic changes may be seen in cases of extensive disease	–

[a]Also known as ulcerative enteritis.

Diagnosis of Crohn's disease and ulcerative colitis

Differential diagnosis relies on clinical examination (including endoscopy) supported by histological examination. Differentiation can be very difficult, as both conditions can be mimicked by enteric infections and pseudomembranous colitis. Figure 11.5 shows the appearance on X-ray of the colon in a patient with Crohn's disease.

Drug treatment. Although the causes of IBD are not yet known, knowledge of the factors involved is increasing. Various theories have been put forward. The fact that corticosteroids and immunosuppressants are beneficial in the treatment of IBD lends support to the theory that these diseases are due to an immunological disorder. An infection and/or sensitising agents may be the trigger for the immunological changes that occur in IBD. The pathogenesis of these conditions may be multifactorial, with infection, genetic influences, diet and environmental agents combining in ways that are not fully understood. Prostaglandins (see p. 443) have been shown in animal studies to act with other agents such as histamine to alter lymphocyte function and increase vascular permeability. The treatments available do ameliorate the symptoms of IBD, which can be very distressing and debilitating. Table 11.7 gives an outline of the main drugs used in

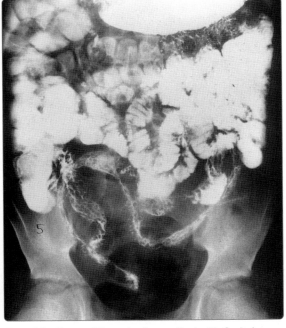

Fig. 11.5 X-ray of the colon in a patient with Crohn's disease. (From Andreoli TE, Carpenter CCJ, Griggs RC et al. (eds) 2004 Cecil essentials of medicine. Grune & Stratton, New York. With permission of Elsevier Inc.)

Table 11.7 Treatment of inflammatory bowel disease

Drug	Dose/formulation	Notes
Antidiarrhoeal agents		
Codeine phosphate Loperamide	15–30 mg three or four times daily. 4 mg initially, then 2 mg after each loose stool, with a maximum of 16 mg daily for 5 days.	Reduce gastrointestinal motility; antidiarrhoeal agents should not be used in patients with acute ulcerative colitis.
Colestyramine	12–24g with water; powder	Used for the treatment of diarrhoea in some patients with ileal Crohn's disease.
Corticosteroids		
Prednisolone	Variable dose depending on the condition; 10 mg three or four times daily is a typical dose given for 2–3 weeks. Above this level, side effects may be troublesome.	Small bowel diarrhoea reduced by oral corticosteroids. Beneficial action thought to be due to anti-inflammatory and immunosuppressive action. Corticosteroids are especially useful in the acute phase of inflammatory bowel disease.
Budesonide	Available as 3-mg capsules in two formulations for the treatment of mild/moderate Crohn's disease affecting the ileum or ascending colon. Two capsule formulations are available; both are controlled-release formulations. Budenofalk is a pH-sensitive formulation that has different release characteristics compared with Entocort CR. Comparative clinical trials are needed to determine the relative advantages of the formulations. In each case, the daily dose is 9 mg for up to 8 weeks. Dosage during the last 2 weeks of treatment should be reduced. The Entocort CR formulation is given as a once-daily dose. A budesonide enema is available (2 mg/100 mL). One enema at bedtime is given for 4 weeks.	This corticosteroid has fewer adverse effects than prednisolone, because it has less systemic bioavailability. Its activity is mainly topical, because it has a high affinity for corticosteroid receptors. In clinical trials, budesonide achieved similar rates of remission to oral prednisolone but with a lower incidence of adverse effects.
Antimicrobial agents		
Metronidazole Tetracycline	Doses given in relation to body weight and carefully monitored by blood level determinations.	Bacterial overgrowth in small bowel due to active Crohn's disease may cause diarrhoea, which is amenable to treatment with antimicrobial agents in normal doses.
Immunosuppressive therapy		
Ciclosporin	–	Potent immunosuppressive drug (see p. 411). Place in treatment of refractory ulcerative colitis remains to be further investigated.
Azathioprine	3 mg/kg of body weight per day, reducing to smaller maintenance dose according to response.	Not first-line therapy but reserved for patients who are intolerant of or who do not respond to corticosteroids. Used to reduce corticosteroid dosage levels in patients with ulcerative colitis. Has been reported to induce remission in patients with Crohn's disease. Adverse effects limit its use (see p. 411).
Infliximab	For severe active Crohn's disease, 5 mg per kg by intravenous infusion over 2 h, repeated	This drug is a monoclonal antibody active against tumour necrosing factor. Very careful

Table 11.7 Treatment of inflammatory bowel disease *'cont …'*

Drug	Dose/formulation	Notes
	at 2 and 6 weeks after the first infusion. Specialist supervision is essential.	monitoring is essential for signs of acute reactions. This treatment is reserved for patients with a disease state that is not treatable by conventional therapy (aminosalicylates and corticosteroids). The treatment is safe to use in combination with standard drugs.
Salicylates		
Sulfasalazine	1–2 g four times daily in acute attack. Maintenance dose of 500 mg four times daily. Corticosteroids may be needed in the acute phase.	Used for the treatment of active Crohn's disease and is the first-line agent of choice for maintenance therapy in ulcerative colitis. Combination of a salicylate and a sulphonamide. Salicylate part of compound has desired therapeutic effect; sulphonamide part associated with side-effects. An enteric-coated tablet may be useful for patients who are intolerant of the uncoated tablet. Topical sulfasalazine also available in the form of suppositories or retention enema. Drug colours the urine yellow, and patients should be warned about this.
Mesalazine (5-ASA)	For acute ulcerative colitis, 800 mg (two tablets) three times daily with corticosteroid therapy when necessary. Maintenance dose should be lowest that will maintain remission. 400 mg three times daily up to 800 mg three times daily may be required. A foam enema containing 1 g per metered dose is used for acute attacks affecting the rectosigmoid region; 2 g daily is administered for 4–6 weeks.	Sulfasalazine is metabolised to sulfapyridine and 5-ASA, and it is thought that the sulfapyridine component is the major cause of side effects. Mesalazine is the active component of sulfasalazine. Presented for use as a tablet coated with special resin designed to release active ingredient in the terminal ileum and colon. Suppositories of 250 and 500 mg also available for use in patients with distal disease. The drug should not be given to patients with renal impairment; large doses have been shown to cause renal damage in experimental animals. Should not be given to patients with salicylate intolerance. Anti-inflammatory effect not achieved if intestinal transit time rapid owing to diarrhoea.
Balsalazide sodium	2.25 g three times daily for up to 12 weeks. 1.5 g daily for maintenance.	This is a prodrug of 5-ASA. It is designed to avoid the side-effects associated with the sulfapyridine portion of mesalazine. Side-effects due to the 5-ASA are not eliminated.
Olsalazine	For acute mild ulcerative colitis, 1 g daily in divided doses up to maximum of 3 g daily over 1 week. 250 mg twice daily will often maintain patient in remission.	Compound that is a combination of two molecules of 5-ASA. Specifically designed to reach the colon, where the compound breaks down to release 5-ASA. Almost no systemic absorption of 5-ASA, therefore available to act topically on colonic mucosa. Side-effects reported similar to other salicylates; gastrointestinal problems such as watery diarrhoea may occur.
Electrolytes and fluid		
	In accordance with the needs of the patient.	The need for the correction of electrolyte imbalance arises from the profuse diarrhoea.
Intravenous nutrition		
	In accordance with the. nutritional status of the patient	Impaired ability to absorb nutrients must be recognised and treated in both the short and long term.

5-ASA, 5-aminosalicylic acid.

the treatment of ulcerative colitis and Crohn's disease. In resistant or relapsing cases of IBD, azathioprine or mercaptopurine may be used under specialist supervision. In addition to drug treatment, attention must be given to diet, although direct links between diet and IBD are not clear. Foods that have a high residue content are best avoided.

Systemic manifestations of IBD are often seen. Joint disease (arthritis), skin problems (erythema nodosum), aphthous ulcers, eye disease (iritis), gallstones (patients with Crohn's disease of the ileum) and inflammation of the veins of the legs occur in ulcerative colitis.

Treatment given to control the gastrointestinal tract symptoms will help to resolve the systemic manifestations, but specific local treatment may be required (e.g. for inflammatory eye conditions). Regular follow-up and review of medication are essential. Attention should be paid to diet.

IRRITABLE BOWEL SYNDROME AND GUT MOTILITY PROBLEMS

Although not all sufferers present for investigation, as many as 20% of adults in the western world, mostly young and female, suffer from the functional disorder of the digestive system known as irritable bowel syndrome (IBS). The condition is characterised by abdominal pain (relieved by defecation), abdominal distension, loose frequent stools after the onset of pain, rectal mucus and a feeling of incomplete evacuation. The major presenting features are diarrhoea and constipation. As well as physical signs and symptoms, many IBS sufferers have high stress levels.

Before establishing that the patient does in fact have IBS, it is essential that more serious conditions of the bowel are excluded by studying the history and carrying out haematological investigations as well as sigmoidoscopy. These would include IBD, infection, malabsorption and carcinoma of the colon.

The contribution that drugs can make to the treatment of IBS is limited. Treatment is directed at whatever is the predominant symptom. Considerable relief can be achieved from bulk laxatives (see Table 11.8) and antispasmodics, many of which can be bought over the counter. Antispasmodics fall into two main categories: antimuscarinics such as atropine, dicycloverine (dicyclomine), hyoscine and propantheline, and smooth muscle relaxants such as alverine, mebeverine and peppermint oil. Antimuscarinics in high doses may cause dry mouth, blurred vision, constipation and urinary retention. In certain individuals, there may be a place for anxiolytics and antidepressants.

Attention to diet is important. Regular meals with a rich fibre content are advocated. Exercise is to be encouraged. Some patients may benefit from alternative therapies such as homeopathy and psychotherapy. There is an extremely important placebo effect in IBS.

CONSTIPATION

Normal bowel habit is influenced by upbringing and culture. As a result, constipation is often interpreted in different ways. It arises from decreased colonic activity. Bowel contents pass slowly through the colon, becoming dehydrated and hard with loss of faecal volume. Decreased colonic activity can arise in old age and with immobility, and is often associated with a low dietary fibre intake and dehydration.

In considering the causes of constipation, a detailed drug history (including the use of over-the-counter medicines) should be taken. Drugs with antimuscarinic activity are especially liable to cause constipation. Constipation is often present in patients suffering from depression and confusional states. Certain metabolic disorders, such as hypercalcaemia and myxoedema, may also cause constipation. Constipation may occur when the call to stool is neglected. This has the effect of decreasing the sensitivity of rectal sensors. If the patient is too ill to respond to the call to stool or for some other reason is unable to respond, such as pressure of duties, the stimulus is gradually lost and the rectum becomes overloaded with faecal material.

All patients complaining of constipation should be carefully investigated so as to eliminate a more serious condition. Pain (arising from a malignant condition) on bowel evacuation may result in constipation. Whenever possible, constipation should be treated by attention to diet and exercise, and the encouragement of a healthy lifestyle. For example, the simple step of adding bran or other dietary products to food may be all that is required.

If drug treatment is required, a wide range of products is available (Table 11.8). Laxatives may be classified into four main groups.

- Bulk-forming laxatives act by drawing water into the colon and thus help to expand and soften the faeces. The increased bulk stimulates receptors in the colonic mucosa that promote peristalsis. It is vital that there is a concurrent increase in fluid intake so as to avoid intestinal obstruction. These laxatives generally take a few days to work. Only when it is not possible to increase fibre in the diet should they be used.

Table 11.8 Main laxative drugs

Drug	Dose	Notes
Bulk-forming agents		
Ispaghula husk	3.5 g twice daily with water.	Important to ensure that patient has good fluid intake to avoid intestinal obstruction. For ease of use can be made into a jelly.
Methylcellulose	Available as 500-mg tablet. Three to six tablets daily with 300 mL of water.	Good fluid intake essential. Bulk-forming agents should be carefully swallowed with water and should not be taken immediately before going to bed. An increase in dietary fibre is preferable to the use of bulking agents, but this may not be possible when dietary intake is compromised (e.g. in older patients).
Stimulants		
Bisacodyl	5–10 mg orally at night. Also available as suppository.	Like other stimulant laxatives, can cause local irritation and griping pain.
Dantron	Available as co-danthramer (i.e. dantron 25 mg with poloxamer 200 mg in 5 mL). Normal dose 5–10 mL.	Because of possible carcinogenic effects, reserved for use in older patients. Especially valuable when essential that bowel movements are not accompanied by straining. Also widely used in patients receiving opioids in palliative care.
Docusate sodium	Orally up to 500 mg daily in divided doses.	–
Glycerol (glycerin)	Given in suppository form.	Mild irritant.
Senna	Two to four tablets, each containing 7.5 mg of sennosides at night.	Also used prior to radiological examination, endoscopy and surgery.
Sodium picosulfate	Available as elixir containing 5 mg/5 mL. Dose: 5–15 mL at night.	Indications similar to those of senna.
Faecal softeners		
Arachis oil	130 mL given as retention enema.	Warmed before use. Used to soften impacted faeces. As with all enemas, should be used with caution in patients with intestinal obstruction and a history of peanut allergy.
Iso-osmotic laxatives		
Macrogol solutions (polyethylene glycol)	Low doses of macrogol solutions help to increase bowel frequency and improve defecation. Stools are also softened.	Contraindicated in a number of conditions (e.g. inflammatory bowel disease).
Osmotic laxatives		
Lactulose (a disaccharide)	Available as an elixir containing 3.35 g in 5 mL. Initial dose 15 mL twice daily, reducing when patient's condition warrants.	Lactulose passes through the small intestine unchanged. It is broken down in the colon by bacteria to substances (acetic and lactic acids) that exert their osmotic effect in the gut lumen. May cause cramps and flatulence.

Continued

Table 11.8 Main laxative drugs 'cont ...'

Drug	Dose	Notes
Magnesium sulphate	5–10 g in water.	Produces rapid bowel clearance (2–4 h). Other magnesium salts also used (e.g. magnesium citrate and magnesium hydroxide).
Phosphates	Sodium acid phosphate 12.8 g and sodium phosphate 10.24 g in the form of an enema (128 mL).	Contraindicated in patients with ulcerative or inflammatory bowel conditions. Local irritation may occur, and sodium absorption can cause problems in patients who have a low sodium requirement.
Sodium citrate	Given in form of a microenema together with a surfactant.	Small volume (5 mL) of these enemas makes for ease of use.
Lubricants		
Liquid paraffin	–	The long-term use of this may interfere with the absorption of fat-soluble vitamins (A, D and K). Lipid aspiration pneumonia has been reported (inhalation of liquid paraffin following vomiting). Leakage of oil from the anus often occurs. There is some evidence that the long-term use of liquid paraffin may cause cancer of the large bowel. Liquid paraffin is no longer prescribed.

- Stimulant laxatives increase intestinal motility by nerve stimulation. There is a risk of causing abdominal cramp, and long-term use may lead to colonic atony and hypokalaemia.
- Faecal softeners lubricate and soften the faeces, thus easing their passage.
- Osmotic laxatives act by retaining fluid in the lumen of the gut by osmosis, leading to a softening of the stools and stimulation of intestinal contractions.

Despite the 'homely' image of laxatives, it must not be forgotten that these are drugs with potentially serious adverse effects. Overuse of laxatives can cause hypokalaemia and an atonic non-functioning colon. Inappropriate use of laxatives in situations in which the diagnosis of the cause of the constipation is inadequate can be very dangerous. Patient group directions may permit the prescription of laxatives by nurses. Nurses have an important role to play in advising patients about their use of laxatives. Laxatives should be used only when other measures have failed. These would include attention to the amount of dietary fibre (wholewheat cereals, wholemeal bread and whole fruit), fluid intake and exercise. Attention to details such as the provision of warmth and privacy when attending to toileting needs and exploiting the gastrocolic reflex after breakfast can greatly assist the constipated patient. When laxatives are indicated, patients should be encouraged to continue with these simple measures and to take only the recommended dose. There are, of course, very important indications for the use of laxatives on a routine basis, especially in patients receiving opiates for palliative care.

The modes of action of laxatives are illustrated in Figure 11.6.

Bowel-cleansing solutions

Prior to colonic surgery, radiological examination and colonoscopy, it is essential to ensure that the bowel is free of solid faecal matter. A range of preparations are available. Most are based on inorganic salts, such as phosphates, magnesium compounds and a combination of electrolytes. Patient counselling on the need for compliance with the regimen and reconstitution of the powder is vitally important in achieving a good clearing of the bowel (see specialist literature for dosage details). There are a number of contraindications to the use of these products, in particular known gastrointestinal disease (e.g. ulceration, obstruction and

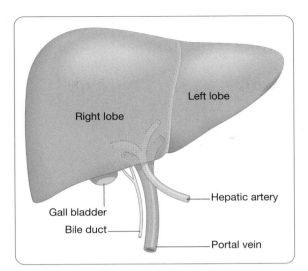

Fig. 11.6 Mode of action of laxatives. (From Page CP, Hoffman BF, Curtis M et al. 2006 Integrated pharmacology. Mosby, Edinburgh. With permission of Mosby.)

gastric retention). Congestive cardiac failure is also a contraindication to the use of these agents.

HAEMORRHOIDS AND OTHER PERIANAL CONDITIONS

Painful, itching and bleeding conditions of the perianal region are common. Usually, the lesions are benign and may often be amenable to treatment by topical application of soothing, emollient, anti-inflammatory and anaesthetic agents, alone or in combination. The most common perianal condition is haemorrhoids. The condition may present in a variety of ways, ranging from superficial bleeding to permanently prolapsed haemorrhoids. The causes of haemorrhoids are not fully understood, but the condition is associated with congestion of the superior haemorrhoidal venous plexus. Surgical treatment or local injection with a sclerosing agent (oily phenol injection) may be required. Considerable relief can be obtained by the use of rectal ointments designed to relieve itching and pain. Application of the ointment is aided by using a rectal nozzle. In some cases, a suppository with active ingredients similar to those of the ointments may be used. Some active ingredients of rectal ointments are listed in Table 11.9. Unprolapsed haemorrhoids may

Table 11.9 Active ingredients, (often used in combination) of rectal ointments, foams and sprays and suppositories.

Ingredient	Normal strength in ointment (%) W/V	Action/notes
Aluminium acetate	3.5	Astringent
Benzoylbenzoate	1.2	Mild antiseptic
Bismuth compounds	Various	Mild astringent
Cinchocaine	0.5	Local anaesthetic
Hydrocortisone[a]	0.5	Anti-inflammatory
Lidocaine (lignocaine)	0.5	Local anaesthetic; as with other anaesthetics, may be absorbed to produce toxic effects
Prednisolone hexanoate[a]	0.19	Anti-inflammatory
Zinc oxide	Range 10–18	Mild astringent

[a]All corticosteroid topical preparations should be used for limited periods to avoid absorption and possible side effects (see p. 499).

be treated by local injection of a sclerosant, usually phenol in an oily base.

Anal fissures require stool softening and increased dietary fibre. Surgical treatment may be required, and glyceryl trinitrate ointment may be helpful.

MALIGNANT DISEASE

See Chapter 19.

DRUG TREATMENT OF HEPATIC DISORDERS

ANATOMY AND PHYSIOLOGY

The liver can be considered as the chemical factory of the body. It is the largest organ in the body, weighing up to 2.3 kg (range 1–2.3 kg). The liver has four lobes and occupies the greater part of the right hypochondriac region (see Fig. 11.7). The most obvious lobes are the right and left lobes. Closely associated with the liver are the organs of the gastrointestinal tract, large blood vessels and the gall bladder (see Fig. 11.8). At the microscopic level, hepatocytes make up the lobules, which are just visible to the naked eye.

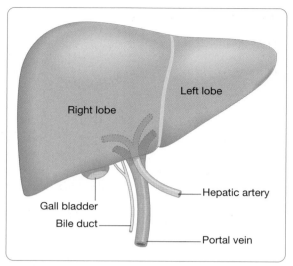

Fig. 11.7 The liver.

The liver carries out a great range of chemical functions that are essential to health. These functions are summarised in Table 11.10.

Liver diseases disrupt the functions of the liver, which may have profound consequences for the patient.

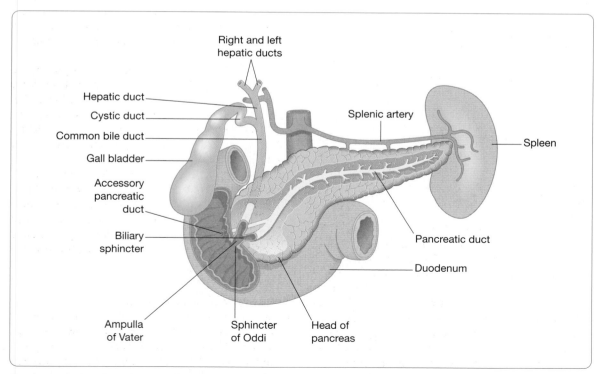

Fig. 11.8 Organs associated with the liver.

Table 11.10 Functions of the liver

Main function	Outline of functions
Amino acid metabolism	Breakdown of certain amino acids to form urea; formation of uric acid from nucleoprotein
Bile production	Bile salts, pigments and cholesterol produced in liver cells
Carbohydrate metabolism	Glucose is converted to glycogen (after a meal), and glycogen is broken down to glucose to meet energy requirements (see also Ch. 21)
Detoxification processes	Drugs and other noxious substances (e.g. toxins produced by micro-organisms); also metabolises ethyl alcohol taken in alcoholic drinks (see p. 182)
Fat metabolism	Fat is converted into a form that can be used by the body as an energy source
Heat production	Because a great number of chemical processes are carried out in the liver, heat is produced, which is the main source of body heat
Inactivation	A wide range of hormones are inactivated (e.g. insulin, thyroid hormones, sex hormones and aldosterone)
Storage functions	Vitamins, both fat- and water-soluble, iron and copper; glucose in the form of glycogen
Synthesis	Vitamin A, non-essential amino acids and blood-clotting factors

HEPATIC DISEASE

The main diseases of the liver are potentially life-threatening, but unfortunately some are not very amenable to drug treatment. Drug treatment in combination with general supportive measures, and alteration to diet, can help to ameliorate symptoms.

HEPATITIS

Hepatitis may be caused by one of a number of viruses or by a toxic chemical, very often a drug. In both virus- and drug-induced hepatitis, there is extensive cell damage throughout the liver, although there may be variation in the extent of the damage in different lobes of the liver.

Hepatitis due to the A virus is associated with anorexia, nausea, malaise, fever and joint pain. The liver is tender, and jaundice occurs as the fever abates. The virus is spread by the faecal–oral route, and contaminated food or drink may be involved. The course of the A infection generally lasts 3–6 weeks. A vaccine is available (see p. 404).

Hepatitis due to the B virus is a much more serious condition. The virus is spread by blood, secretions and sexual intercourse. In view of the seriousness of hepatitis B, special attention must be given to protecting people at particular risk. Health and

other vulnerable workers should be protected by vaccination, and great care must be taken with all procedures involved in taking blood and other invasive techniques. Safe disposal of contaminated equipment is essential (see p. 71).

In both forms of infection, the symptoms are similar, although much more severe in the B form of the disease. Symptoms include chills, headache, general malaise, gastrointestinal disturbances and anorexia. Abdominal pain and dark urine will be followed by jaundice. Liver enlargement occurs, and the liver is often tender.

Hepatitis C may be acquired via infected blood, plasma derivatives, unsafe sex, injecting drug abuse, tattoos and piercings. It has an insidious onset, with vague abdominal discomfort, anorexia, nausea and vomiting, and eventually jaundice. Peginterferon alfa-2a combined with ribavirin is used to treat the chronic form.

Treatment of acute hepatitis

Care must be taken to determine the cause of the condition. It is particularly important to exclude drugs as a cause. If a drug is implicated (see p. 147), the treatment should be stopped and further exposure to the drug avoided. Exposure to toxic chemicals in the workplace must also be considered as a possible cause. Key elements of the treatment of hepatitis are dietary measures and bed rest. It is important to maintain a high-calorie diet, although patients' gastrointestinal problems may restrict the range of foods they are able to tolerate. Bed rest is very important so as to avoid exhaustion, to which the patient may be especially prone. Fluid and electrolyte therapy should be given in the acute phase of the condition. Corticosteroids may be of value for their appetite-stimulating properties, although the side effects of corticosteroids are so hazardous that their use should be minimised. All drugs with a potential to cause liver damage must be avoided, as must alcohol, a well-recognised liver toxin.

Treatment of chronic hepatitis

Corticosteroids are useful in the form of chronic hepatitis that is not due to viral infection.

Hepatitis B and hepatitis C viruses are major causes of chronic hepatitis. Interferon alfa is of limited use in the treatment of chronic hepatitis B and is contraindicated in decompensated liver disease. Lamivudine may be used as an alternative.

The antiviral agent ribavirin in combination with interferon alfa-2b may be of value in the treatment of chronic hepatitis C. Therapy needs to be continued for 6 months. Peginterferon alfa-2b may be used when ribavirin for any reason cannot be given, but therapy with a single agent is less effective than combination therapy.

HEPATIC FAILURE

This is a very serious condition for which no specific treatment is available. Because the liver performs so many vital functions, it follows that liver failure has very serious consequences. The usual cause of fulminant hepatic failure is an acute viral infection, but it may be caused by drugs, pregnancy or Wilson's disease.

The symptoms of hepatic failure include cerebral disturbance. Encephalopathy arises from the accumulation of toxic substances in the blood, which arise because the damaged liver cannot metabolise the range of chemical substances a healthy liver can cope with. A wide range of neurological symptoms are seen, including restlessness, behavioural abnormalities, mania, drowsiness and coma. Jaundice develops and physical signs are abnormal. Mortality is age-related. Profound biochemical disturbances such as electrolyte disturbance, alkalosis and coagulation disorders are common during the course of the illness.

Treatment plans include general supportive measures together with measures designed to sustain the patient in the hope that the hepatic tissue will regenerate. Nutritional needs should be met with glucose orally or parenterally. Bacteria that produce toxic nitrogenous products in the colon should be suppressed with a suitable antibiotic such as neomycin orally. Neomycin is a non-absorbable antibiotic, but small amounts may be absorbed over time to produce potentially dangerous side effects. Infection and electrolyte disturbances must be treated, and if renal failure occurs, haemodialysis and other measures may be required. The physical and biochemical parameters must be monitored and corrective measures taken. Disorders of blood coagulation may lead to bleeding from the gastrointestinal tract. Ranitidine by intravenous injection may be required to control this. Lactulose (orally) is used to acidify the colonic contents so as to reduce the level of nitrogen-producing bacteria.

CIRRHOSIS OF THE LIVER

Cirrhosis is caused by alcohol abuse, chronic hepatitis or biliary cirrhosis. Alcohol has a direct toxic effect on the liver. A daily substantial intake over a number of years will result in cirrhosis. Women are at greater risk than men from a prolonged and regular intake of alcohol. Other causes of cirrhosis include certain metabolic disorders, viral infections and drugs. Obstruction in the biliary network may also cause cirrhosis. Cirrhosis of the liver has a number of clinical features. The presentation of the condition varies but often includes portal hypertension, blood disorders, ascites, circulatory changes and jaundice. Treatment of hepatic cirrhosis is based on attempting to halt the progression of the condition, because there is no treatment that can reverse it.

Substance abuse (alcohol and/or drugs) must be dealt with by complete abstinence. A high-calorie diet is advisable, together with bed rest. Fluid and sodium intake must be restricted. Diuretics should be used with care in conjunction with monitoring of electrolytes and blood urea.

A common complication of hepatic cirrhosis is bleeding from oesophageal varices. These are caused by portal hypertension. Various techniques are used to deal with this condition. Pressure can be applied to the varices by special tubes with inflatable 'cuffs', or surgical treatment can be used. Any treatment designed to arrest bleeding by constriction of the splanchnic arterioles may be useful. Vasopressin is given by intravenous infusion in a dose of 20 units over a period of 15 min.

Blood transfusions may be required to correct losses from recurrent bleeds. The possibility of injecting the varices with a sclerosing agent may be worth considering.

Because the liver plays an important part in the metabolism of drugs, it follows that drug choice/dosage for patients with liver disease must be given special consideration.

DRUG TREATMENT OF BILIARY TRACT DISORDERS

ANATOMY AND PHYSIOLOGY

The gall bladder is attached to the posterior surface of the liver. Its function is to concentrate and store bile. Bile is secreted by the liver, from where it passes into the gall bladder via the hepatic duct and cystic duct. The bile from the liver already contains bile salts, bile pigment and cholesterol. In the gall bladder, mucus and water are added. When fatty foods enter the duodenum, the hormone cholecystokinin is released, which in turn causes the gall bladder to contract, expelling its contents into the bile duct and thence to the duodenum.

DISORDERS AND THEIR TREATMENT

The reasons for the formation of gallstones are not fully understood. They are made up of cholesterol, although some gallstones contain a high proportion of calcium in the form of salts of bilirubin. Gallstones are frequently asymptomatic but can cause a variety of symptoms, including biliary colic or cholecystitis relieved by strong analgesia and treatment with antibiotics. Figure 11.9 shows the presence of a gallstone in the common bile duct.

Treatment is by surgical removal, often by laparoscopic cholecystectomy or, in the case of small stones, by the oral administration of ursodeoxycholic acid. This drug has no effect on large radio-opaque stones. Ultrasound is used as a non-invasive method of breaking up gallstones.

DRUG TREATMENT OF PANCREATIC DISORDERS

ANATOMY AND PHYSIOLOGY

The pancreas is located in the abdomen, with its head in the curve of the duodenum. It is both an exocrine

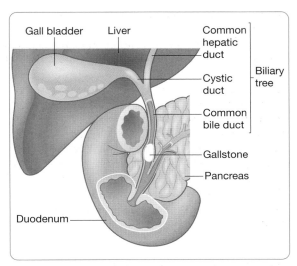

Fig. 11.9   Gallstone in the common bile duct.

and an endocrine gland. Its exocrine function is to produce pancreatic juice, which enters the duodenum. Pancreatic juice contains enzymes involved in the digestion of carbohydrate, protein and fat. The pancreas also contains specialised cells known as the islets of Langerhans, which secrete insulin and glucagon (see p. 338).

DISORDERS AND THEIR TREATMENT

The main conditions affecting the pancreas are pancreatitis (often caused by either gallstones or alcohol abuse), pancreatic tumours and failure of the organ to produce pancreatic (exocrine) secretions.

Pancreatitis may be acute or chronic. A necrotic process is established that often leads to infection and organ dysfunction. A severe attack requires urgent hospitalisation, and even patients with mild pancreatitis require supportive therapy in hospital. In the mild condition, intravenous fluids (crystalloids) are required and suitable analgesics will be needed. Antibiotic therapy may be required for coexisting infections. In severe cases, specialist care in a high-dependency unit is required. Hypovolaemic shock must be dealt with by suitable (often large) volumes of crystalloids and colloids. Prophylactic antibiotics in high doses (cefuroxime and imipenem) may be worthwhile, because these penetrate pancreatic tissue. No specific drug treatment is available and prognosis is poor in patients who exhibit signs of both necrosis and infection. Surgical intervention to remove necrotic tissue will be required. Gallstones are dealt with by laparoscopic cholecystectomy. Chronic pancreatitis is treated using suitable analgesics and the control of metabolic complications (diabetes and fat malabsorption). Alcohol intake must be eliminated completely in all cases of pancreatitis.

PANCREATIC ENZYME DEFICIENCY STATES (EXOCRINE SECRETIONS)

When pancreatic enzyme secretions are absent or reduced, pancreatin is given by mouth. The deficiency state may be caused by cystic fibrosis or chronic pancreatitis, or as a result of certain surgical procedures. Pancreatin (of porcine origin) is inactivated by gastric acid and heat. Drugs that reduce acid secretion (cimetidine or ranitidine) are given 1 h before food, and heat should be minimised if pancreatin is to be added to food. Dosage of pancreatin is adjusted to meet the individual patient's needs. Stool consistency and frequency give a good indication of the need to adjust dosage levels. Preparations of pancreatin include granules and capsules containing protease, lipase and amylase. A range of strengths is available. A Committee on Safety of Medicines warning regarding the high-strength pancreatin preparations is in force, because of the possibility of the development of bowel strictures (see BNF). Pancreatin may cause irritation of the perioral skin and buccal cavity.

PANCREATIC TUMOURS

Pancreatic tumours range from benign to highly malignant. Most tumours develop in the head of the pancreas. Back pain, pruritus due to biliary obstruction, and appetite disturbances are presenting symptoms. Prognosis is poor. Surgery may be beneficial when the tumour is suitable for resection. Radiotherapy and chemotherapy are seldom helpful. The search continues for an effective treatment.

VOMITING

Persistent vomiting is a potentially dangerous condition in both children and adults; untreated, it can lead to severe dehydration. The treatment of vomiting is dealt with in Chapters 14 and 26.

HICCUP

This is a common condition that can occur at any age, even in utero. Minor events may last for a few hours, but prolonged attacks are not uncommon. These are very distressing and potentially highly debilitating

(see also Ch. 26). Mechanism of hiccup is based on an interaction between random contractions of the diaphragm and the inspiratory muscles. Treatment of prolonged hiccup must be based on investigation of any underlying condition. An initial approach to an attack may comprise 'homely' remedies such as granulated sugar, holding one's breath or sipping iced water.

Once a serious underlying cause has been eliminated or to give time for investigations to be completed, various physical manoeuvres may be used in an attempt to disrupt the hiccup reflex (e.g. Valsalva manoeuvre).

Drug treatment includes chlorpromazine 25 mg three times daily or haloperidol 1.5 mg three times daily. Increased doses may be required in some cases. Metoclopramide and other drugs have been recommended but are not licensed for this treatment. Simeticone (an antifoaming agent) may be useful in the relief of hiccup.

ADMINISTRATION OF RECTAL MEDICINES

Drugs can be administered via the rectum (Box 11.2):

- in solid form, as a suppository that melts at body temperature
- as a solution, suspension or foam in the form of an enema.

The rectal route may be utilised for local or systemic action when:

- drugs cannot be swallowed (e.g. because of vomiting, coma, stricture)
- drugs cause severe irritation of the upper gastrointestinal tract (e.g. indometacin)
- a prolonged action is desired (e.g. oxycodone)
- the drug must be delivered close to the site of the lesion(s) (e.g. corticosteroid).

The absorptive surface area of the rectum is small, although the blood supply is extremely efficient and therefore absorption can be rapid. However, the presence of faeces may slow absorption, and irritation may cause early evacuation. Laxatives are administered in order to evacuate the rectum and are retained there for approximately 20 min. All other drugs given rectally are for retention and are normally administered on retiring to bed so that they may be retained overnight. Before administering rectal medicines, the nurse should ensure that the patient

---

Box 11.2 Administration of medications by the rectal route

Documentation
- Prescribing and recording sheet

The medicine
- Suppository or enema as prescribed

The environment
- Patient in bed
- Privacy, warmth, comfort
- Incontinence pad(s) to protect clothes and bedding
- Call bell to hand
- Commode positioned at bedside if appropriate

The nurse and the patient
- Patient identified
- Explanation given of what is involved and consent obtained
- Patient instructed to breathe through the mouth to relax the anal sphincter
- Patient assisted into left lateral position with head on one or two pillows, buttocks in line with edge of bed and knees drawn up towards chin

Technique
- Nurse ensures hands are socially clean before and after procedure
- Disposable gloves are worn for insertion of suppositories

- *Suppositories*:
  - suppository lubricated using, for example, KY Jelly or tip melted in hot water as directed on packet
  - anus carefully located, avoiding external haemorrhoids if present
  - suppository slowly and gently inserted – tapered end first when used to evacuate rectum, blunt end first when suppository to be retained
  - finger withdrawn smoothly.
- *Enemas*:
  - enema warmed then nozzle lubricated after air expelled
  - anus carefully located, avoiding external haemorrhoids if present
  - enema nozzle inserted for 4–6 cm and then pack slowly rolled up to introduce contents
  - nozzle withdrawn gently.
- Anal region wiped and patient left comfortable
- For evacuant medications, patients encouraged to postpone first urges to defecate and to make medication work; for retention medication, elevating foot of bed may help patient to retain medication

Hazards
- Local irritation
- Trauma

---

has no history of allergy. Arachis oil enemas are contraindicated in patients with nut allergy.

Given the option, perhaps more patients on long-term drug therapy would choose this route of administration. When this is the chosen method, patients should be encouraged to insert suppositories themselves (e.g. paracetamol, diclofenac) and may be taught self-administration of a small disposable enema containing a soluble form of prednisolone in the treatment of colitis. In the event of the nurse requiring to administer the medicine, it is important to gain the patient's informed consent, otherwise the procedure could be construed as a form of assault. In the case of a male nurse and a female patient, a female chaperone would be required.

STOMA MANAGEMENT

Modern methods of stapling anastomoses in the rectum have resulted in fewer people requiring the formation of a stoma. Nevertheless, nurses will encounter patients who have had a stoma operation performed recently, as well as those they meet for other reasons who happen to have a stoma. Ostomists are individuals who happen to eliminate in a different way. Each, naturally, will have particular problems and individual methods of overcoming them. Patients and health professionals can benefit from the knowledge and expertise of the specialist stoma nurse.

TYPES OF STOMA

A stoma is usually created when it has been necessary to form a surgical diversion of faeces or urinary flow. There are three main types.

- An operation that necessitates removal of the rectum and sigmoid colon results in the formation of a *colostomy*. At this point in the intestinal tract, the faeces are generally well formed and evacuation is fairly predictable.

- When the large intestine has been entirely removed, or diverted, the stoma is made at the lower end of the small intestine and is known as an *ileostomy*. With this type of stoma, waste is looser because more of the intestine has been removed, or diverted, resulting in loss of reabsorptive capacity.
- In the treatment of certain bladder disorders, the ureters may be transplanted into a short segment taken from the ileum to form an *ileal conduit*, or they may have been brought to the skin surface in the formation of a *urostomy*. Waste in these cases is urine.

In all forms of stoma, because no voluntary muscles are involved, the excretory flow cannot be controlled at will. Management therefore is directed towards modifying waste when this is possible, and applying some form of device for its collection.

DIET

For those who have a colostomy or ileostomy, correct diet comes before anything else. The aim is to produce faeces that are as well formed as possible without causing constipation. Sensible eating can help to achieve this aim and can minimise other problems (e.g. odour, flatus and excoriation of the skin). In time, the ostomist usually finds that most foodstuffs can be taken in moderation, with a few exceptions. Wind-producing foods are soon identified. Highly spiced foods and onions are to be avoided, as they can produce loose and odorous faeces and much flatus. Pulse foods and Brussels sprouts can cause flatus and noise, although not so much odour. The timing of liquid in relation to food is important. It is safer not to drink immediately before, during or until about half an hour after a meal, so as to avoid loosening the faeces. Fizzy drinks are to be avoided, and advice on which alcoholic drinks may be safely taken should be sought.

ODOUR

Odour is caused by either faeces or flatus, and therefore good dietary management helps to keep it to a minimum. Very careful hygiene is essential of course, although deodorants also may be used. Deodorant drops or powders are available for placing in the stoma appliance, although care should be taken not to allow liquid deodorants to touch the stoma or surrounding skin, otherwise they may cause severe irritation. Some ostomy bags have a small vent at the top for inserting deodorant liquid or have a charcoal filter incorporated. A deodorising spray may be used at the time of emptying the appliance and a deodorising air device may be placed as appropriate.

APPLIANCES

All ostomists are entitled to free prescriptions for all their stoma needs, and these may be obtained through a local pharmacy or a dispensing appliance contractor. Many of the items are listed in the Drug Tariff. It is advisable to liaise with the community pharmacist to ensure the availability of the correct product(s). No single appliance is suitable for all those who have a stoma, and this is reflected in the wide range of products currently available. The aim is to find a device that not only serves the purpose of satisfactorily collecting the waste but is discreet, rustle-free and acceptable. A detailed description of all the different appliances is beyond the scope of this book, but there are several aspects that should be understood when considering appliances generally. Stoma bags may or may not be disposable and/or drainable. They are available as either one- or two-piece systems. One-piece appliances consist of a disposable collection bag complete with its own adhesive seal. Two-piece appliances comprise an adhesive flange to which a separate disposable collection bag may be fitted. The flange may be left attached for 3–4 days, while the bag is replaced as often as necessary.

The type and site of the stoma, manual dexterity and skin sensitising all influence the choice of appliance. Many modern appliances involve the use of skin protectives such as hydrocolloid wafers that, because of their malleability, impermeability and skin protection properties, provide a good skin seal. Microporous adhesives may also be used and are mostly well tolerated. A belt may be attached to some appliances for added support. Filler pastes are useful for filling dips and creases peristomally, thus making the surface level prior to putting on an appliance. These pastes must not be used on sensitive skin, as they are spirit-based.

SKIN PROTECTION

In the same way as a person who is paraplegic lives with the threat of pressure sores, the ostomist must constantly take care to prevent irritation and breakdown of the skin that surrounds the stoma. A routine of changing the appliance right to the skin will be followed by each individual. Care must be taken to remove plasters without tearing the skin. The area around the stoma is washed using, for example, cotton wool and warm, soapy water, taking care to remove all traces of faeces, mucus, and skin applications. It is important to rinse off all soap to reduce irritation and to pat the skin dry. Any traces of adhesive should be removed using an adhesive solvent. Additional applications of barrier cream and skin gel may be used for protection of the skin. Creams should be applied sparingly to a radius of about 10 cm from the stoma but not on the stoma itself.

SKIN BREAKDOWN

In the event of the skin becoming red and weepy, adhesives may have to be temporarily replaced with some form of dressing. This may be left in position for several days with the appliance being placed on top of the dressing. Efforts should then be made to identify the cause of the excoriation. It may be that the motions are too loose, calling for a change in diet or a bulking agent. Changing the bag more promptly helps to reduce faecal contact with exposed skin. The size of the aperture may be too big, causing a similar problem, and may have to be reduced. Ideally, there should only be about 0.5 cm of a gap between the stoma and the appliance. Antiseptic solutions tend to be painful when applied to sore skin, causing further irritation, and are best avoided in preference to soap and water, thorough rinsing with cool water, and careful drying.

MEDICINES AND OSTOMISTS

Certain precautions have to be taken by doctors prescribing medicines for patients with an ileostomy or colostomy. Nurses should also be aware of these and other problems relating to medicines that may arise for the ostomist.

PATIENTS WITH A COLOSTOMY

Constipation may be a problem for many colostomy patients and should always be borne in mind in their treatment. For the management of constipation, colostomy patients should increase their fluid intake or make some dietary adjustments in preference to taking medication. If this approach does not help, then bulk-forming laxatives such as ispaghula husk or methylcellulose may be used. These act by increasing faecal mass, which stimulates peristalsis and effects expulsion of faeces provided that sufficient fluid intake is maintained. These medicines are supplied in tablet and granule form. Tablets may be broken up and should be chewed with a little water half an hour before a meal. Liquids are then withheld until about half an hour after the meal. Because these preparations have a hygroscopic action, the timing of fluid is important, otherwise the medication absorbs fluid recently taken instead of the fluid content of the faeces. The granular form of agents such as methylcellulose is found by patients to be less manageable, because there is a tendency for the granules to swell in the mouth and thus be difficult to swallow. Ispaghula husk is available

in granule form in different flavours and when added to water makes an acceptable drink. Lactulose, which is an osmotic laxative, is another useful preparation in this situation, as is the stimulant laxative senna.

Antacids. Those containing aluminium salts may cause the colostomy patient to become constipated.

Antidepressants. The antimuscarinic effects of some antidepressants can lead to a number of troublesome side effects, including constipation.

Opioid analgesics. Analgesics such as dihydrocodeine are especially constipating. Other opioid analgesics such as codeine and morphine may also be troublesome.

PATIENTS WITH AN ILEOSTOMY

Diarrhoea with subsequent loss of water and potassium is a very real threat to the ileostomist at any time, and may be exacerbated by taking medicines.

Digoxin. The improvement in renal perfusion that results from digoxin therapy may cause additional potassium depletion. Potassium supplements (preferably in liquid form) may be needed when digoxin therapy is indicated.

Diuretics. These should be avoided whenever possible, owing to the risk of dehydration and potassium loss. If diuretic therapy is essential, a potassium-sparing diuretic should be used.

Antacids. Magnesium-containing antacids tend to be laxative.

Iron preparations. The intramuscular route should be used instead of by mouth if it is vital that iron is given. Modified-release preparations should not be given.

Laxatives, enemas and bowel washouts. Any form of laxative or washout is contraindicated because of the severe risk of dehydration rapidly occurring.

Tablets. Those with slow-release properties are unsuitable. Such preparations are designed to release the drug from the tablet during its passage through the digestive tract over a period of 3–6 h. In ileostomy patients, this period is shortened, with the result that drug release may be incomplete, leading to underdosage. For this reason, if potassium replacement therapy is required, a liquid form is used to ensure full absorption of potassium.

PATIENTS WITH AN ILEOSTOMY OR COLOSTOMY

For any patient with an ileostomy or a colostomy, oral antibiotics, oral iron preparations and antacids containing magnesium salts should be avoided whenever possible because of the likelihood of diarrhoea. If necessary, concurrent intestinal sedatives such as codeine phosphate, loperamide or co-phenotrope may be given. Salt may have to be replaced in the form of oral rehydration salts, a glucose and electrolyte powder that requires to be reconstituted.

DIETARY SUPPLEMENTS

In certain conditions, some foods have characteristics of drugs. Some of these foods are prescribable within the NHS. The Advisory Committee on Borderline Substances issues advice on which foods may be regarded as drugs within the NHS. The BNF contains details of these foods in a special appendix. Examples of products include gluten-free foods, protein-free foods, protein and carbohydrate combinations for use in malnutritional states and foods for lactose/glucose/galactose intolerance.

Television viewers and readers of glossy magazines will be well aware of foods claimed to help reduce cholesterol, control blood pressure and help improve cardiac health. It will be for the individual to decide if it is preferable to adopt a healthy lifestyle rather than pay premium prices for what some may consider to be basic foodstuffs.

SELF-ASSESSMENT QUESTIONS

1. What investigations are likely to be carried out in a patient with a suspected gastrointestinal disorder?
2. Match the following drugs to their mode of action.

Ranitidine	Neutralises gastric acid
Omeprazole	Inhibits gastric acid by blocking the hydrogen potassium ATP enzyme system of the gastric parietal cell
Misoprostol	Inhibits acid secretion and protects gastric mucosa
Magnesium trisilicate	Suppresses gastric acid production by blocking the action of histamine of receptors in the stomach

3. Gastric and duodenal ulcers are commonly associated with *H. pylori*.
   a. *H. pylori* is a:
      i. virus
      ii. bacterium
      iii. fungus.
   b. Which part of the stomach does it colonise?
      i. The fundus
      ii. The pyloric sphincter
      iii. The pyloric antrum.
   c. How is its presence confirmed?
   d. Which of the following may be the best treatment?
      i. An antacid
      ii. An H$_2$ blocker
      iii. A proton pump inhibitor
      iv. An antibacterial agent
      v. More than one antibacterial agent
      vi. A combination of iii and v.
4. A patient confides in you that he has been taking ranitidine regularly for the past 4 months, which he has purchased from various pharmacies without prescription. What action would you take and why?
5. Which of the following drugs used in the treatment of gastrointestinal disorders should be avoided in patients with glaucoma?
   a. cimetidine
   b. atropine
   c. omeprazole.
6. Which of the following has a constipating effect and which a laxative effect?
   a. codeine phosphate
   b. sodium picosulfate
   c. magnesium trisilicate
   d. magnesium sulphate
   e. atropine
   f. morphine
   g. aluminium hydroxide
   h. loperamide
   i. lactulose
   j. colestyramine.
7. A patient says he needs a purgative. What does he mean?
8. What are the potential side effects of prolonged laxative use?
9. In what circumstances would regular laxative use be justified?
10. Detail a nurse's professional responsibility when administering rectal medicines.
11. Why are H$_2$ receptor antagonists preferred to antimuscarinic drugs for the treatment of peptic ulcer?
12. Explain why ostomists may experience constipation if taking some antidepressants.

FURTHER READING AND RESOURCES

Anderson S, Wilkinson M 2005 Today's optimum management of dyspepsia and ulcers. Prescriber 19 January:41–45

Beckingham IJ, Bornman PC 2001 ABC of diseases of liver, pancreas and biliary system: acute pancreatitis. British Medical Journal 322:595–598

Bennett J 2001 Oesophagus: atypical chest pain and motility disorders. British Medical Journal 323:791–794

Bornman PC, Beckingham IJ 2001 ABC of diseases of liver, pancreas and biliary system: pancreatic tumours. British Medical Journal 322:721–723

Bryan J 2006 Possible treatments for hepatitis C: what's currently in the pipeline? Pharmaceutical Journal 276:43–44

Caestecker JD 2001 Oesophagus: heartburn. British Medical Journal 323:736–739

Calam J, Baron JH 2001 Pathophysiology of duodenal and gastric ulcer and gastric cancer. British Medical Journal 323:980–982

Fuchs GJ 2001 A better oral rehydration solution? British Medical Journal 323:59–60

Gow PJ, Mutimer D 2001 Treatment of chronic hepatitis. British Medical Journal 323:1164–1167

Harris HE, Ramsay ME 2002 Clinical course of hepatitis C virus during the first decade of infection: cohort study. British Medical Journal 324:450–453

Johnson CD 2001 ABC of the upper gastrointestinal tract: upper abdominal pain: gall bladder. British Medical Journal 323:1170–1173

Mayberry J 2001 Explaining inflammatory bowel disease to patients. Prescriber 12:30–38

Meenan J 2000 IBD: a guide to successful drug management. Prescriber 11:93–104

Mpofu C, Ireland A 2006 Inflammatory bowel disease: the disease and its diagnosis. Hospital Pharmacist 13:153–158

Parsonnet J 2005 Clinician-discoverers: Marshall, Warren and *H. pylori*. New England Journal of Medicine 353:2421–2423

Spiller RC 2001 ABC of the upper gastrointestinal tract: anorexia, nausea, vomiting and pain. British Medical Journal 323:1354–1357

St Clair Jones A 2006 Inflammatory bowel disease: drug treatment and its implications. Hospital Pharmacist 13:161–166

Wilcock M 2005 The role of *Helicobacter pylori* in gastrointestinal disease. Pharmacy in Practice January: 36–39

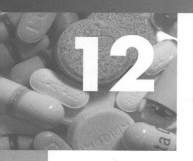

12 Drug treatment of cardiovascular disorders

CHAPTER CONTENTS

KEY OBJECTIVES

After reading this chapter, you should be able to:

- describe the mode of action of the different diuretics and list their indications
- explain the use of the different drugs in the management of arrhythmias
- outline the treatment strategy in the management of hypertension
- describe the mode of action of angiotensin-converting enzyme inhibitors
- discuss the factors contributing to an increased risk of cardiovascular disease
- list the different types of nitrates used in the prophylaxis and treatment of angina pectoris
- list the therapeutic indications for calcium-channel blockers
- discuss the risk and benefits of the use of anticoagulants
- outline the primary treatment for a myocardial infarction
- name four drugs, with different modes of action, used to treat high cholesterol
- outline the aims of drug therapy in the management of heart failure
- discuss the drug treatment of the stroke patient.

INTRODUCTION

Diseases of the heart and circulatory system are the main cause of death in the UK and accounted for just over 216 000 deaths in 2004 (British Heart Foundation 2006). More than one in three people (37%) die from cardiovascular disease (CVD). The main forms of CVD are coronary heart disease (CHD) and stroke. About half (49%) of all deaths from CVD are from CHD, and more than a quarter (28%) are from stroke. Around one in five men and one in six women die from CHD. Death rates from CVD have been falling in the UK since the early 1970s. For people under 75 years, they have fallen by 38% in the past 10 years. Just under one in three of all deaths under 65 years resulting from social class inequalities is due to CHD. Death rates from CHD are highest in Scotland and the North of England, lowest in the South of England, and intermediate in Wales and Northern Ireland. The premature death rate for men living in Scotland is 57% higher than in the South West of England, and 103% higher for women.

The incidence of myocardial infarction (MI) varies around the UK, but on average the incidence rate for men aged between 30 and 69 is about 600 per 100 000 and for women is about 200 per 100 000. Using data from Morbidity Statistics from General Practice, the British Heart Foundation estimates that there are about 183 000 new cases of angina in all men living in the UK and about 161 000 in women. Studies of the incidence of heart failure are scarce, and different studies use different methods, particularly for diagnosing the condition. The Hillingdon Heart Failure Study found a crude incidence rate of 140 per 100 000 for men and 120 per 100 000 for women. Data from the 2003 Health Survey for England suggest that the prevalence of CHD in England is 7.4% in men and 4.5% in women. Prevalence rates increase with age, with around one in four men and one in five women aged 75 years and above living with CHD. It is estimated that there are just over 1.5 million men living in the UK who have had CVD (either angina or heart attack) and about 1.1 million women, giving a total of around 2.6 million.

ANATOMY AND PHYSIOLOGY

THE HEART

The heart lies between the lungs, behind the lower sternum, in front of the oesophagus and above the diaphragm, on which it rests. It is roughly conical in shape, with a base and an apex. It consists of four chambers: the right and left atria above, and the right and left ventricles below. The atria and ventricles are separated by, on the right side, the tricuspid valve and, on the left side, the mitral valve. The walls of the heart have three layers: outermost, a fibrous envelope called the pericardium; in the middle, a thick muscle known as the myocardium; and the innermost layer, a smooth lining called the endocardium (Fig. 12.1).

Venous blood returns from various parts of the body to the heart. It enters the right atrium via the superior and inferior venae cavae and passes through the tricuspid valve to the right ventricle. The right ventricle pumps the blood to the lungs via the pulmonary artery. In the lungs, the blood is oxygenated and carbon dioxide is removed. The blood then returns via the four pulmonary veins into the left atrium, from where it passes through the mitral valve into the left ventricle. The left ventricle pumps the oxygenated blood through the aortic valve into the aorta and out into the body.

The heart derives its own blood supply from the two main coronary arteries that originate from the aorta just above the aortic valve.

The activity of the heart is rhythmical, consisting of contraction (*systole*) and relaxation (*diastole*). The impulse to contract is generated by a microscopic area of specialised cardiac muscle known as the sinoatrial (SA) node, situated at the junction of the superior vena cava and the right atrium. The wave of excitation spreads throughout the muscle layer of both atria, causing them to contract, forcing blood into the ventricles. The impulse is picked up by another small mass of specialised cardiac muscle called the atrioventricular (AV) node, situated in the septal walls of the right atrium. It is relayed by the fibres of Purkinje down the bundle of His and along the right and left branches, causing the ventricles to contract and drive blood into the pulmonary artery and the aorta. The heart then relaxes, refills with venous blood, and awaits the next stimulus for contraction. Although the heart initiates its own impulse to contract, the fine adjustments to its activity required to meet the body's constantly changing needs derive from the autonomic nervous system (see Ch. 9). Sympathetic innervation increases the heart rate, and parasympathetic innervation slows the heart rate.

The SA node is normally the pacemaker for the heart, because of its rapid firing rate of 60–100 electrical discharges per min. Although the specialised cells at the AV node and at the bundle of His are also capable of spontaneously producing an electrical discharge and taking over control of the rhythm, they are normally required to do so only if the SA node fails or becomes unduly slow. The cells of the AV node emit discharges at 50 per min, and those of the ventricles at 40 or fewer per min.

Every time the heart beats, approximately 70 mL of blood is pumped out of each ventricle. The heart rate is normally around 70 beats/min. These two figures multiplied together are termed the *cardiac output*.

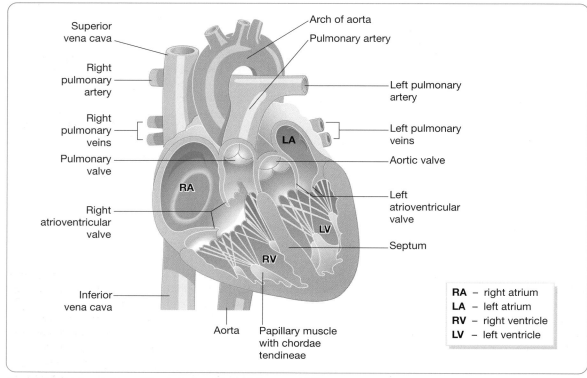

Fig. 12.1   The heart. (From Waugh A, Grant A 2001 Ross and Wilson anatomy and physiology in health and illness, 9th edn. Churchill Livingstone, Edinburgh. With permission of Elsevier.)

THE BLOOD VESSELS

The blood is transported round the body via the blood vessels, which comprise arteries and arterioles, veins and venules, and capillaries. As a rule, arteries convey oxygenated blood and veins convey deoxygenated blood, which has a high percentage of carbon dioxide. Arteries convey blood away from the heart; veins transport blood back to the heart. Capillaries are tiny blood vessels in the periphery of the arteriovenous system. It is through the capillary walls that oxygen and nutrients pass to the tissues and cells and that waste products return from the cells into the circulation.

Like the heart, the walls of the blood vessels consist of three layers: the fibrous outer *tunica adventitia*; the middle muscular layer, the *tunica media*; and the smooth lining, the *tunica intima*. The outer coat of an artery allows it to stand open, whereas a vein collapses when it is cut. The proportion of muscle tissue depends on the size of the vessel, with much more in arteries than in veins. Some veins have valves that allow the blood to flow back to the heart but prevent flow in the opposite direction. The walls of the capillaries are only one cell thick; this readily facilitates gaseous and nutrient exchange (Fig. 12.2).

POSITIVE INOTROPIC DRUGS

CARDIAC GLYCOSIDES

These drugs are used almost exclusively in two conditions:

- cardiac failure
- cardiac arrhythmias.

DIGOXIN

Digoxin is used in the management of atrial flutter and fibrillation, as it reduces conduction through the AV node and the bundle of His, allowing fewer of the excitatory transmissions from the atria to pass and hence slowing ventricular rate and restoring rhythm. In chronic congestive cardiac failure, digoxin is given to increase the force of myocardial contraction, hence increasing cardiac output for any given filling pressure.

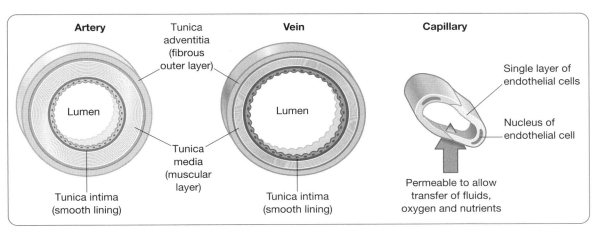

Fig. 12.2 Cross-section through blood vessels.

Mode of action. The actions of digoxin are complex and revolve around its ability to inhibit sodium transport out of cells through inhibition of the enzyme Na$^+$, K$^+$-ATPase, which allows increased intracellular myocardial calcium concentrations. This, in turn, improves contractility.

Pharmacokinetics. Digoxin may be given orally as either tablets or a liquid preparation. It may also be given intravenously, but this is relatively rare. Intravenous digoxin should always be given very slowly to minimise the risks of exposing the myocardium to localised high concentrations that may induce arrhythmias. Digoxin should be added to an intravenous infusion of sodium chloride 0.9% and administered using an intravenous infusion pump over 2 h. Because digoxin is 80% renally eliminated, the dose must be adjusted according to renal function in order to minimise the risks of toxicity. In the elderly, the renal clearance is lower than that in young healthy adults, so a lower maintenance dose is required. The elimination half-life of digoxin in a patient with normal renal function is 36 h, which means that up to 7 days may be required after any dosage alteration to ensure that a steady state has been reached.

Dose. Digoxin is now rarely used for the rapid control of heart rate, as even with intravenous administration it may take many hours to reduce the heart rate. In patients who have mild heart failure, a loading dose is not required and a satisfactory plasma concentration can be achieved over a period of about a week using a dose of 125–250 micrograms orally twice a day, which may then be reduced having special regard to renal function. Because of its long half-life, maintenance doses need be given only once daily. The maintenance dose in atrial fibrillation can usually

be governed by ventricular response, which should not normally be allowed to fall below 60 beats/min. Digoxin plasma concentrations during maintenance treatment are not necessary unless problems are suspected. They relate only partially to the therapeutic effect, because so many other factors can contribute to myocardial excitability (e.g. electrolyte concentrations, catecholamines and hypoxia). The likelihood of toxicity increases progressively through the range 1.5–3 micrograms/L.

Complications of digoxin therapy. Digoxin treatment is particularly hazardous because the toxicity of digoxin is difficult to recognise and it has the potential to cause fatal arrhythmias. The drug's toxicity is more pronounced in the presence of metabolic and electrolyte disturbances (especially hypokalaemia but also hypomagnesaemia, hypercalcaemia, alkalosis, hypothyroidism and hypoxia). The patient's renal function should be taken into account when deciding the digoxin dose in order to minimise the risk of toxicity. Excessive digoxin dose should be considered in any patient who is unwell or who has suddenly deteriorated. Important signs of toxicity are abdominal pain, nausea/anorexia, tiredness/weakness, diarrhoea, confusion and any change in vision, mobility or mood. Toxicity can often be managed by discontinuing therapy and correcting hypokalaemia if appropriate. Serious occurrences require urgent specialist management. Digibind, digoxin-specific antibody fragments in injectable form, is available for reversal of life-threatening overdosage.

Interactions. Hypokalaemia predisposes to toxicity, so that diuretics used with digoxin should be either potassium-sparing or given with potassium supplements. Drugs such as amiodarone, verapamil

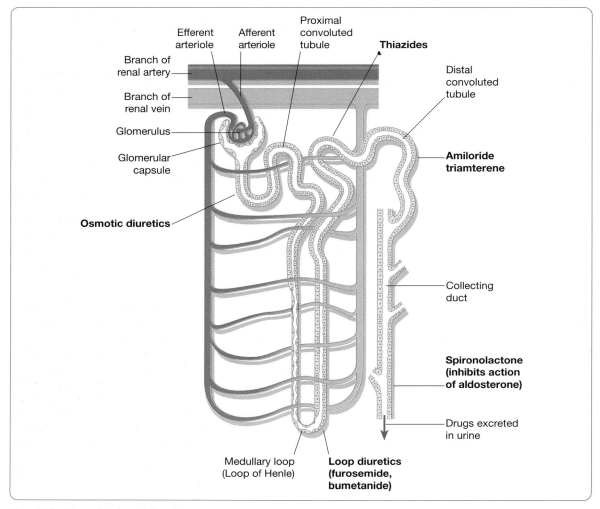

Fig. 12.3 Sites of action of diuretics.

or nifedipine may cause an increase in plasma digoxin concentrations and increase the risk of toxicity.

PHOSPHODIESTERASE INHIBITORS

Enoximone and milrinone are also used in the management of cardiac failure. They are both selective phosphodiesterase inhibitors exerting their effect on the myocardium. This increases cellular calcium ion concentration, enabling the muscle fibres to contract with greater force. The heart pumps out blood more efficiently, thus reducing the strain of congestion in a failing heart. Haemodynamic benefit has been noted after administration, but there is no evidence to date to show benefit on survival rates. They are both given intravenously for short-term use only.

DIURETICS

There are a number of different diuretics that produce the same end result but through a different mode of action (Fig. 12.3). In order to understand their differing modes of action, it is necessary to have a basic understanding of the physiology of the kidney.

PHYSIOLOGY OF THE KIDNEY

Each kidney is made up of approximately 1 million nephrons, each nephron comprising a glomerulus and a proximal and distal tubule that are connected by the loop of Henle (see Ch. 18). The glomerulus consists of a group of capillaries, and as the blood passes through these it is filtered. A large amount of water and dissolved salts is filtered from the blood and passes on to the tubules. In the tubules, a selective reabsorption takes place. Glucose is normally completely reabsorbed. Water and electrolytes, including sodium, potassium, chloride and bicarbonate, are selectively reabsorbed and pass back into the circulation. Urea, excess water, salts and other unwanted substances are excreted as urine. The exact amount of each substance excreted in the urine is controlled in order to maintain the composition of the body fluids at normal levels. The urine is further concentrated and, depending on the electrolyte balance, more sodium is absorbed in exchange for potassium. In the distal tubule, antidiuretic hormone (ADH, vasopressin) excreted by the posterior pituitary gland is an important controlling factor. Increased ingestion of water results in an increased urine flow. When water is absorbed from the gastrointestinal tract, it causes the plasma to become more dilute, and this in turn decreases the release of ADH by the posterior lobe of the pituitary gland. Less ADH reaches the kidney, and this causes the tubules to reabsorb less water so that more is excreted as urine (see Ch. 8 for renal drug excretion).

DISEASE STATES RESULTING IN OEDEMA

In health, the kidney maintains the composition of the blood within narrow limits. Disease can upset this delicate balance. When the blood supply to the glomerulus is reduced because of impaired blood circulation, filtration slows. However, tubular reabsorption continues at the normal rate, and excess water and salts accumulate in the body tissues, resulting in oedema. This can arise in cardiac failure. Oedema can also arise in renal disease (nephrotic syndrome) and cirrhosis of the liver.

Diuretics are used in the treatment of these conditions and also in the treatment of hypertension. They cause a net loss of sodium and water from the body by decreasing the reabsorption of sodium and chloride. Because a large proportion of the salt and water that passes into the tubule is reabsorbed, a small decrease in reabsorption can result in a marked increase in excretion.

THIAZIDE AND RELATED DIURETICS

Mode of action. Thiazide diuretics act by inhibiting the reabsorption of sodium and chloride in the distal tubule of the nephron, resulting in increased sodium, chloride and water secretion. There is also an increased secretion of potassium. The mode of action in relieving hypertension is unclear.

Pharmacokinetics. These diuretics are well absorbed orally and are excreted unchanged by the kidney. Compared with loop diuretics (see later), the potency is lower, with a slow onset and longer duration of action. Because the duration of action is about 12 h, a thiazide diuretic should be given in the morning.

Indications. Thiazide diuretics such as bendroflumethiazide (bendrofluazide), cyclopenthiazide, indapamide, metolazone and xipamide are used to treat hypertension and oedema resulting from cardiac failure, liver disease and nephrotic syndrome. In the management of hypertension, a low dose of a thiazide (e.g. bendroflumethiazide 2.5 mg daily) produces a near-maximal blood pressure–reducing effect with very little biochemical disturbance. Higher doses may cause more marked changes in plasma potassium, uric acid, glucose and lipids, with no advantage in blood pressure control, and should not be used. Optimal doses for the control of heart failure may be larger, and long-term effects are of less importance. Metolazone is particularly effective when combined with a loop diuretic. Profound diuresis may occur, and therefore the patient should be monitored carefully.

Adverse effects. The most important adverse effects are hypokalaemia, hyponatraemia and dehydration. Hypomagnesaemia may also occur. Impotence is reversible on withdrawal of treatment. Competition with uric acid for secretion into the proximal tubule may cause hyperuricaemia, and this may result in gout. Impaired glucose tolerance can occur. Hypotension, headache and dizziness may be experienced.

Hypokalaemia is a common side-effect of thiazide diuretics, particularly at higher doses. Combination products are available containing diuretic plus potassium, but the quantity of potassium is insufficient to correct hypokalaemia. When potassium supplements are necessary, these should be given routinely in tablet or liquid form. Alternatively, the addition of a potassium-sparing diuretic can alleviate the need for supplementation.

Interactions. Lithium excretion is reduced by thiazide diuretics. Dosages should be halved initially and adjusted with careful monitoring of plasma concentration. Hypokalaemia potentiates the effects of digoxin, and toxicity may result.

LOOP DIURETICS

Mode of action. This group of diuretics gets its name because sodium and chloride reabsorption in the ascending limb of the loop of Henle is inhibited. In addition, potassium secretion in the distal tubule is increased (greater with furosemide (frusemide) than with bumetanide).

Pharmacokinetics. Bumetanide is almost completely absorbed after oral administration, while furosemide is 60–70% absorbed. Bumetanide is partially metabolised in the liver, and about 80% of a dose is excreted in the urine – 50% as unchanged drug. Furosemide is excreted primarily unchanged in the urine. Onset of action occurs in 30 min after an oral dose and within a few minutes of intravenous administration. The duration of action lasts between 3 and 6 h after an oral dose.

Indications. The loop diuretics are the most potent diuretics available. They are used in:

- pulmonary oedema (may arise due to left ventricular failure)
- congestive heart failure no longer responding to thiazide diuretics
- hepatic disease
- acute and chronic renal failure.

Adverse effects. The most important adverse effects are hypokalaemia, hyponatraemia and dehydration. Hypokalaemia may be treated with potassium supplements or potassium-sparing diuretics. Other side-effects include hypotension, nausea, gastrointestinal disturbances, hyperuricaemia and gout. Tinnitus and deafness may occur with large parenteral doses and rapid administration, particularly with furosemide.

Interactions. Hypokalaemia potentiates the effects of cardiac glycosides. Lithium excretion is diminished by furosemide, and the dose should be halved. Furosemide also potentiates the nephrotoxic and ototoxic effect of the aminoglycosides.

POTASSIUM-SPARING DIURETICS

Mode of action. Amiloride and triamterene cause increased sodium and chloride excretion in the distal tubule, resulting in an increase in water excretion. The secretion of potassium in the distal tubule is inhibited (unlike thiazide and loop diuretics). The potassium-sparing diuretics have weaker diuretic and antihypertensive effects than other diuretics, but they have the advantage of conserving potassium. For this reason, they are often prescribed with thiazide or loop diuretics.

Pharmacokinetics. Following oral administration, approximately 50% of triamterene and 20% of amiloride is absorbed. Triamterene is extensively metabolised by the liver, but amiloride is excreted unchanged in the urine.

Indications. Amiloride and triamterene are used on their own or, more usually, in combination with thiazide or loop diuretics in the treatment of oedema,

as they are weak diuretics. Dose will be dependent on indication and whether they are used in combination with other diuretics.

Adverse effects. The more common adverse effects are hyperkalaemia, dehydration and hyponatraemia. Other adverse effects include gastrointestinal disturbances, dry mouth, rashes, confusion and hypotension.

ALDOSTERONE ANTAGONIST: POTASSIUM-SPARING DIURETIC

Spironolactone and eplerenone are both aldosterone antagonists. Spironolactone is also used as a potassium-sparing diuretic.

Mode of action. Spironolactone is metabolised to canrenone, which is an antagonist of the action of aldosterone on the distal tubule of the nephron. Aldosterone promotes the retention of sodium and the excretion of potassium by the kidneys. Canrenone reverses this effect, causing increased excretion of sodium and water and retention of potassium. Eplerenone prevents the binding of aldosterone. Eplerenone has relative selectivity in binding to mineralocorticoid receptors compared with its binding to glucocorticoid, progesterone and androgen receptors. As a consequence, the Scottish Medicines Consortium has recommended that eplerenone should be restricted to patients who cannot tolerate the hormonal side effects of spironolactone.

Pharmacokinetics. Spironolactone is well absorbed (approximately 70%). It is metabolised to its active form, canrenone, in the liver. The onset of action occurs in 2–4 h. It has a long duration of action (up to 96 h), and its maximum effect takes several days to occur. The absolute bioavailability of eplerenone is unknown. Maximum plasma concentrations are reached after about 2 h, and a steady state is reached within 2 days. Absorption is not affected by food.

Indications. Spironolactone is used to treat fluid retention due to cardiac failure, the nephrotic syndrome and hepatic disease. In the first two conditions, it is usually used in combination with a thiazide or loop diuretic. In oedema caused by excessive aldosterone activity (e.g. cirrhosis of the liver, primary aldosteronism), it counteracts these effects by competing with aldosterone for receptor sites. Eplerenone is used, in addition to standard therapy, to reduce the risk of cardiovascular mortality and morbidity in stable patients with left ventricular dysfunction and clinical evidence of heart failure after recent MI.

Adverse effects. Hyperkalaemia is the major risk, and potassium supplements must not be given with either spironolactone or eplerenone, as the body potassium could rise to a dangerous level. Gastrointestinal disturbances may occur, and gynaecomastia can sometimes be seen with spironolactone.

GENERAL PRECAUTIONS TO BE OBSERVED IN THE USE OF DIURETICS

Caution must be exercised when administering diuretics to patients with impaired liver or kidney function and also to patients suffering from diabetes. The patient should always be observed for signs of fluid and electrolyte imbalance.

Diuretics can cause acute toxic reactions in patients to whom digitalis glycosides or non-depolarising muscle relaxants have already been administered, by depleting serum potassium. They also enhance the effects of antihypertensive drugs (e.g. methyldopa, hydralazine), and this enables the dose of these drugs to be reduced when treating hypertension.

The thiazides and loop diuretics can lead to potassium depletion. In these cases, potassium supplements may have to be given.

POTASSIUM SUPPLEMENTS

The potassium loss produced by certain diuretics may lead to a severe degree of hypokalaemia, with its associated muscle weakness, mental disturbances, cardiac effects and increased risks of digitalis toxicity. Potassium supplements may be given with the thiazide and loop diuretics, but combination therapy with a potassium-sparing diuretic is usually preferred. Potassium chloride in solution is poorly tolerated because of its nauseous effects and it is not often used. Apart from the use of diuretics, deficiency of potassium may occur for various reasons (e.g. ulcerative colitis, diarrhoea, vomiting), but the most common cause is diuretic therapy.

ANTIARRHYTHMIC DRUGS

DISORDERS OF CONDUCTION

Under certain circumstances, the cycle of contraction and relaxation of the heart may be disturbed. These disturbances are known as cardiac arrhythmias. There are several types of arrhythmia for which antiarrhythmic drugs are used. An antiarrhythmic drug is a drug that is used to control or correct abnormal rhythms of cardiac action. These drugs may be used for several different types of cardiac arrhythmia, and it is essential that the specific type of arrhythmia is diagnosed by electrocardiogram prior to commencement of treatment.

SUPRAVENTRICULAR ARRHYTHMIAS

As their name implies, these involve arrhythmias arising from above the ventricles and are normally tachyarrhythmias (i.e. faster than normal). The most common of these are atrial flutter and atrial fibrillation, which are often a result of ischaemic heart disease.

Atrial flutter and atrial fibrillation. Atrial flutter is very rapid, but regular, contractions of the atria of the heart that the ventricles may follow exactly, producing a very fast, regular pulse. Atrial fibrillation is an arrhythmia that may develop following atrial flutter and involves very rapid (400–600 per min) disordered contractions of the atria. This results in irregular stimulation of the AV node and, coupled again with AV block, a fast irregular pulse. Either of these conditions may lead (sometimes rapidly) to exhaustion of the myocardium, other arrhythmias and cardiac failure. In both atrial flutter and atrial fibrillation, AV block develops because of, and its degree is determined by, the refractoriness of the bundle of His and the AV node. After each stimulation, there is a period during which the fibres cannot be restimulated, and this is known as the refractory period.

In atrial fibrillation and flutter, messages from the atria will reach the AV node during this refractory period and hence be missed. The length of the refractory period will determine how many atrial beats are blocked for each that is passed, and hence the ventricles may contract only for every second, third, fourth or more atrial beats.

Ectopic beats. Ectopic beats, also called premature beats or extrasystoles, arise from a focus other than the pacemaker. They rarely require drug treatment, but it should be remembered that they may precipitate other types of arrhythmia. In certain cases, they do become troublesome and may be treated with beta-adrenoceptor blocking drugs.

Supraventricular tachycardias. These tachycardias may arise for a number of reasons, for example following MI, in patients with thyrotoxicosis or in patients suffering from Wolff–Parkinson–White syndrome. (This is a condition whereby impulses are conducted not only through the AV node but also through an anomalous pathway connecting the atria to the ventricles.) Paroxysmal supraventricular tachycardia (coming on in sudden bursts) does not usually require drug treatment, and normal rhythm can often be achieved by, for example, respiratory manoeuvres, prompt squatting or pressure over one carotid sinus.

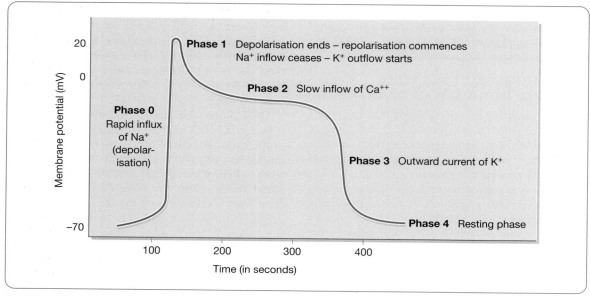

Fig. 12.4   Phases of an action potential in the Purkinje fibre cell and the cationic changes that take place.

VENTRICULAR ARRHYTHMIAS

Ventricular tachycardia is potentially more dangerous than supraventricular tachycardias. These arrhythmias are common following acute MI or can be precipitated by supraventricular tachycardias. A ventricular ectopic beat may initiate ventricular tachycardia, followed by ventricular fibrillation with loss of cardiac output and death.

BRADYCARDIA

Bradycardia is a slowing of the heart, is supraventricular in origin, and may occur, for example, following MI or can be a side effect of beta-adrenoceptor blocking drugs.

THE CARDIAC ACTION POTENTIAL

Antiarrhythmic drugs are used to treat abnormal electrical activity of the heart. To understand the actions of these drugs, it is necessary first to examine the cardiac action potential (Fig. 12.4).

Phase 4. This is the resting phase in cells normally capable of spontaneous depolarisation (cells in SA node, AV node and His–Purkinje system). There is a voltage difference across the surface membrane of all myocardial cells that is called the resting trans-membrane voltage or potential. During the resting phase, there is a slow drift from the maximum negative potential (around 290 mV) to a potential of about 270 mV. This is due to a small influx of sodium ions

into the cell and a small efflux of potassium ions. This depolarisation is spontaneous and continues until it reaches the threshold at which an action potential is initiated automatically (phase 0). Atrial and ventricular cells do not normally exhibit spontaneous depolarisation but remain at rest (diastole) until stimulated by a propagatory impulse.

Phase 0. When the threshold potential is reached and the cell is stimulated, there is a very rapid influx of sodium ions into the cell, causing a rapid rise in transmembrane potential (depolarisation) until it reaches a given value (above 120 mV in Purkinje fibres). This inward current of sodium is very intense and very brief.

Phase 1. The potential starts to fall rapidly as repolarisation takes place, until it plateaus.

Phase 2. This phase is known as the plateau phase. There is a slow current of calcium ions into the cell, which is balanced by a small outward current of potassium ions. These calcium ions are important to the strength of cardiac contraction, which is discussed under calcium antagonists (p. 211).

Phase 3. Repolarisation continues, marked by an outward flux of potassium ions. As the transmembrane potential falls to its maximum negative value, the outward flux is terminated and phase 4 commences with sodium ions entering the cell and potassium ions leaving the cell.

REFRACTORY PERIOD

During phases 1–3 (repolarisation), depolarisation cannot normally occur. This period is called the refractory period, although when about 50% of repolarisation has occurred a larger than normal stimulus can cause depolarisation.

ANTIARRHYTHMIC DRUGS

These drugs limit cardiac electrical activity to normal conduction pathways and decrease abnormally fast heart rates. They may be classified in a number of ways:

- those that act on supraventricular arrhythmias (e.g. verapamil)
- those that act on both supraventricular arrhythmias and ventricular arrhythmias (e.g. disopyramide)
- those that act on ventricular arrhythmias (e.g. lignocaine [lidocaine])
- by the Vaughan Williams classification, which classifies drugs into four distinct classes according to their effects on the electrical behaviour of myocardial cells during activity (termed the *action potential*).

A drug may show more than one of the classes of antiarrhythmic action. The main function of this classification is to define drugs with similar modes of action and to identify possible antiarrhythmic compounds by their effects on cardiac conduction. The clinical value of this classification is limited, and it excludes some antiarrhythmic agents such as the cardiac glycosides.

TREATMENT OF SUPRAVENTRICULAR ARRHYTHMIAS

Adenosine causes rapid reversion of sinus rhythm of paroxysmal supraventricular tachycardias. It is given by rapid intravenous injection into a large peripheral vein. The dose is 3 mg over 2 s, with cardiac monitoring. If required, this is followed by 6 mg after 1–2 min, then by 12 mg after a further 1–2 min. Adverse effects include transient facial flush, dyspnoea, lightheadedness, choking sensation and nausea.

Cardiac glycosides are the treatment of choice in slowing ventricular response in atrial flutter or atrial fibrillation.

Verapamil is usually effective for supraventricular tachycardias. An initial intravenous dose may be followed by oral treatment. It should not be injected into patients recently treated with beta-blockers, because of the risk of hypotension and asystole.

TREATMENT OF SUPRAVENTRICULAR AND VENTRICULAR ARRHYTHMIAS

Amiodarone should be initiated only under hospital or specialist supervision. It is used for treatment of other arrhythmias when previous treatments have failed (e.g. paroxysmal supraventricular, nodal and ventricular tachycardias; atrial fibrillation and flutter; and ventricular fibrillation). It may also be used to treat tachycardia associated with the Wolff–Parkinson–White syndrome (this is a congenital abnormality occurring in about 0.2% of the population and results from an additional conducting system between the atria and the ventricles). Amiodarone can be given orally or by intravenous infusion. It has a long half-life (30–45 days). Its onset of action may take 1–2 weeks, and effects can be seen months after the drug is withdrawn. Most patients on amiodarone develop corneal microdeposits, usually reversible on withdrawal of the drug. This may lead to drivers being dazzled by headlights at night. As it contains 37% iodine, it can affect thyroid hormone metabolism. Pulmonary toxicity may also be a problem and can result in pneumonitis and fibrosis.

The antiarrhythmic properties of beta-blockers are conferred mainly through their β_1-blocking actions, which oppose the electrophysical effects of catecholamines and raise the threshold for ventricular fibrillation. The different beta-blockers have different selectivity for the two receptors β_1 and β_2. For example, atenolol, acebutolol and bisoprolol are relatively β_1-selective when compared with propranolol, oxprenolol and sotalol, which have equal activity for β_1 and β_2. Beta-blockers are useful in preventing arrhythmias induced by exercise, emotion or anaesthesia, and for controlling the ventricular rate in atrial fibrillation. Intravenous esmolol gives rapid beta blockade of short duration (a few minutes) and is particularly useful for the rapid control, for instance, of perioperative tachyarrhythmias. Sotalol has specific antiarrhythmic properties. It may reverse or prevent recurrence of atrial fibrillation and paroxysmal junction tachycardia associated with the Wolff–Parkinson–White syndrome (see below) and may prevent recurrent life-threatening ventricular arrhythmias. However, sotalol may itself cause serious ventricular arrhythmia, including torsades de pointes, especially in patients with depressed left ventricular function, hypokalaemia, or if given with other drugs that prolong the QT interval. Sotalol should be reserved for patients with serious arrhythmias likely to benefit specifically from its antiarrhythmic actions.

Disopyramide is very effective against ventricular extrasystoles and is also used for ventricular arrhythmias, especially where MI is suspected or has been proven. It suppresses the frequency of ectopic ventricular beats as well as the frequency and duration of self-limiting bursts of ventricular tachycardia. It can be given orally or by intravenous infusion. Too rapid an infusion rate can lead to hypotension and cardiac failure. It has anticholinergic side effects, including dry mouth and blurred vision.

Flecainide is of value for serious symptomatic ventricular arrhythmias and paroxysmal atrial fibrillation. It delays intracardiac conduction, but it may precipitate serious arrhythmias in certain patients. It should be initiated in hospital under specialist supervision.

Procainamide is used to control ventricular arrhythmias. The rate of metabolism will depend if the patient is a fast or slow acetylator. (Variation in the *N*-acetyltransferase gene divides people into slow acetylators and fast acetylators [see Ch. 8], with very different half-lives and blood concentrations of such important drugs as isoniazid as well as procainamide.)

Propafenone is used for the prophylaxis and treatment of ventricular arrhythmias and also for some supraventricular arrhythmias. It is rapidly absorbed after oral administration but can cause antimuscarinc side effects, including constipation, blurred vision and dry mouth.

Quinidine may be effective in suppressing supraventricular and ventricular arrhythmias and is rarely used now. It is best used under specialist advice.

TREATMENT OF VENTRICULAR ARRHYTHMIAS

Lidocaine is the first choice in an emergency. In patients without gross circulatory impairment, 100 mg is given as a bolus over a few minutes (50 mg in lighter patients or those whose circulation is severely impaired); this is followed immediately by infusion of 4 mg/min for 30 min, 2 mg/min for 2 h, then 1 mg/min. The infusion concentration is reduced further if continued beyond 24 h. It is effective in suppressing ventricular tachycardia and reducing the risk of ventricular fibrillation following MI. It can be given only by slow intravenous injection, as it is not available in an oral formulation due to a high first-pass metabolism effect. Although effective when used in an emergency, it has not been shown to reduce mortality when used prophylactically. In patients with cardiac or hepatic failure, doses may need to be reduced to avoid convulsions, depression of the central nervous system, or depression of the cardiovascular system. It can cause central nervous system disturbances, including convulsions, drowsiness and paraesthesia.

Mexiletine may be given as a slow intravenous injection if lidocaine is ineffective, and it has a similar action. Unlike lidocaine, it is well absorbed from the gastrointestinal tract. Adverse cardiovascular and central nervous system effects may limit the dose tolerated; nausea and vomiting may prevent an effective dose being given by mouth. Its effect is antagonised by hypokalaemia.

MANAGEMENT OF ARRHYTHMIAS

Management of an arrhythmia, apart from treatment of the associated heart failure, requires precise diagnosis of the type of arrhythmia, and an electrocardiograph is essential. In atrial fibrillation, the ventricular rate can usually be controlled with digoxin. A beta-blocker or verapamil may be added if control is inadequate. In valvular or myocardial disease, anticoagulants may be indicated. In atrial flutter, the ventricular rate can similarly be controlled by digoxin. Synchronised direct current shock can be utilised when reversion to sinus rhythm is indicated.

Paroxysmal supraventricular tachycardia usually remits spontaneously or can be returned to sinus rhythm by reflex vagal stimulation, by prompt squatting or respiratory control. If drug treatment is required, intravenous adenosine is usually the first choice. Digitalisation, an intravenous beta-blocker, intravenous verapamil or direct current shock may be tried.

When arrhythmias occur after MI, lidocaine should be given intravenously. Bradycardia, especially if complicated with hypotension, should be treated with intravenous atropine sulphate (0.3–1 mg).

β-ADRENOCEPTOR BLOCKING DRUGS

Adrenaline (epinephrine) and noradrenaline (norepinephrine), which are produced by the adrenal glands and at sympathetic nerve endings, exercise their physiological actions via α and beta adrenoceptors (see Ch. 9).

Beta adrenoceptors are widely distributed in the body, being present in the heart, bronchi, blood vessels, eyes, pancreas, liver and gastrointestinal tract. The β receptors can be divided into two groups:

- β_1 receptors, which predominate in the heart
- β_2 receptors, which are found mainly in the airways and blood vessels.

Stimulation of β_1 adrenoceptors in the heart and coronary arteries will lead to an increase in heart rate, increase in conduction velocity and force of contraction in the heart, and vasodilatation of coronary arteries. Excitation of β_2 adrenoceptors will lead to dilatation of peripheral arteries.

Beta adrenergic blocking agents interfere with catecholamine binding at beta adrenoceptors. Several beta-blockers (acebutolol, atenolol, bisoprolol and metoprolol) are said to be cardioselective. These agents have the ability to antagonise the action of catecholamines at β_1 receptors at doses smaller than those required to block β_2 receptors. They are not, however, cardiospecific. They have a smaller effect on airways' resistance but are not free of this side-effect. Others block both β_1 and β_2 receptors (i.e. cardiac plus bronchial plus peripheral blood vessel receptors) and are called non-selective beta-blockers. Blocking β_2 receptors causes bronchospasm, which may be of little consequence in normal subjects but in asthmatic patients may make bronchospasm worse and increase dyspnoea. Beta-blockers should be used only in patients with asthma or in those with a history of obstructive airways disease when no alternative treatment is available.

Some beta-blockers (pindolol, oxprenolol, acebutolol and celiprolol) demonstrate various degrees of intrinsic sympathomimetic activity, which represents the capacity of beta-blockers to stimulate as well as block adrenergic receptors. These drugs cause a slight agonist response at the beta receptor while blocking the effect of endogenous catecholamine. Patients given a drug with intrinsic sympathomimetic activity experience a smaller reduction in resting heart rate than those receiving a beta-blocker without intrinsic sympathomimetic activity. They tend to cause less bradycardia and less coldness of the extremities than the other beta-blockers, which is a problem particularly in patients with peripheral vascular disease.

Some beta-blockers are water-soluble and some are lipid-soluble. Lipophilic beta-blockers are able to cross the blood–brain barrier and exert effects on the central nervous system. Nightmares and hallucinations are more of a problem with the lipophilic agents. The most water-soluble are atenolol, celiprolol, nadolol and sotalol. They are less likely to enter the brain and may therefore cause fewer sleep disturbances and nightmares. Water-soluble beta-blockers are excreted by the kidneys, and dose reduction may be required in renal impairment.

All beta-blockers slow the heart; the output of blood is reduced and the work done by the heart is thus decreased. They should not therefore be given to patients with heart block.

Labetalol is a mixed alpha-and non-selective beta-adrenergic antagonist that reduces peripheral resistance but has little effect on heart rate or cardiac output. Positive hypotension occurs. Labetalol may be useful in hypertension of pregnancy and in patients with renal failure.

Beta-blockers are contraindicated in asthma or obstructive airways disease, second- or third-degree heart block, sinus bradycardia, sick sinus syndrome, severe peripheral arterial disease and uncompensated cardiac failure.

The side effects of beta-blockers include fatigue, cold extremities, bronchoconstriction, interference with autonomic and metabolic responses to hypoglycaemia, bradycardia, heart block, negative inotropic effect and impotence.

USES OF BETA-BLOCKERS

HYPERTENSION

Beta-blockers are effective in the treatment of many medical conditions but are most widely used for the treatment of patients with hypertension, in whom they may reduce the long-term morbidity and mortality, and for the prevention of angina. Beta-blockers lower the diastolic blood pressure to less than 95 mmHg in about 40–50% of patients with mild to moderate hypertension. The mechanism of hypotensive action of the beta-blockers is not fully understood. Reduction of cardiac output, resetting of baroreceptors, suppression of renin (which is directly responsible for the production of angiotensin, a circulating vasoconstrictor hormone), release of vasodilator prostaglandins, prejunctional beta-receptor blockade and a direct action on the central nervous system have all been proposed. It may be due to a combination of several of these factors. Blood pressure can usually be controlled with few side-effects. Although atenolol lowers blood pressure, there is some doubt whether it is as effective as other antihypertensive drugs for reducing the incidence of stroke, MI, or cardiovascular mortality.

The 2006 Joint British Societies' guidelines on prevention of CVD in clinical practice amended the algorithm with regard to beta-blockers. This is because several trials, including a large randomised comparison of beta-blocker/thiazide against calcium channel blockers/angiotension-converting enzyme (ACE) inhibitors in primary prevention of CVD, have all revealed an increased risk of developing diabetes in people treated with beta-blockers, especially when combined with thiazide/thiazide-like diuretics. As diabetes further increases the risk of CVD, it is advisable to limit the dose of beta-blockers and not to combine them with a diuretic, particularly in people at high risk of developing diabetes, i.e. those:

- with a strong family history of diabetes
- with obesity
- with impaired glucose regulation and/or features of the metabolic syndrome
- in specific ethnic groups at higher risk of developing diabetes (e.g. Asians and those of African origin).

Beta-blockers are no longer preferred as a routine initial therapy for hypertension. They can be considered for younger people, particularly women of childbearing potential, patients with evidence of increased sympathetic drive, and patients with intolerance of or contraindications to ACE inhibitors and angiotensin-II receptor antagonists.

ANGINA

Beta-blockers, competitive inhibitors of catecholamines, decrease the heart rate, thereby reducing the cardiac workload and increasing the diastolic interval, allowing better coronary perfusion during exercise and reducing the myocardial oxygen demand.

In patients with stable angina, beta-blockers have been shown to be important therapeutic agents as monotherapy or as adjuncts to nitrates. They are particularly useful in the treatment of exertional angina, because of their negative inotropic and chronotropic actions. The most commonly prescribed beta-blockers are atenolol, bisoprolol and metoprolol, which are all cardioselective. A sudden withdrawal of a beta-blocker in patients with angina may cause an exacerbation of the symptoms because of an increase in the number of beta receptors available for stimulation when the antagonist is no longer being given. Stopping a beta-blocker should therefore be by gradual withdrawal.

MYOCARDIAL INFARCTION

Beta-blockade in the first 12 h after MI, when myocardial damage (e.g. rupture) and risk of serious arrhythmias are greatest, is reliably achieved only by intravenous administration (e.g. metoprolol and atenolol may reduce early mortality after intravenous and subsequent oral administration in the acute phase).

Intravenous treatment reduces mortality, reinfarction rate and incidence of cardiac arrest. Follow-on oral treatment with a beta-blocker reduces the risk of reinfarction and death by about 20–25% over 3 years. When there is pre-existing heart failure, hypotension, bradyarrhythmias or obstructive airways disease, this group of drugs is unsuitable.

HEART FAILURE

Beta-blockers may produce benefit in heart failure by blocking sympathetic activity. Bisoprolol and carvedilol reduce mortality in any grade of stable heart failure. Treatment should be initiated by those experienced in the management of heart failure.

OTHER USES OF BETA BLOCKERS

Beta-blockers are used in preoperative preparation for thyroidectomy 4 days before surgery. Propranolol reverses clinical symptoms of thyrotoxicosis. The thyroid is rendered less vascular, making surgery easier. Beta-blockers are also used:

- to relieve anxiety – patients with palpitations, tremor and tachycardia respond better
- in prophylaxis of migraine
- topically in glaucoma (see Ch. 23).

PHARMACOKINETICS

Beta-blockers are usually well absorbed from the gastrointestinal tract (atenolol is an exception – about 50%). Acebutolol, labetalol, metoprolol, propranolol and timolol undergo extensive first-pass metabolism in the liver. The duration of action ranges from 4 h for oral timolol to 24 h for oral atenolol.

ANTIHYPERTENSIVE DRUGS

BLOOD PRESSURE

Blood pressure may be defined as the force exerted on the walls of the blood vessels. Arterial blood pressure is the pressure exerted when the heart pumps blood into the already full aorta. The factors determining the blood pressure are:

- cardiac output
- blood volume
- peripheral resistance
- viscosity of the blood
- venous return.

Blood pressure is maintained by sensory receptors found in several of the arteries close to the heart. These baroreceptors convey information to the vasomotor centre in the medulla of the brain in response to changes in the blood pressure. The vasomotor centre in turn transmits impulses via the sympathetic nervous system to the smooth muscle in the walls of the arterioles, which are stimulated to contract. The chemical transmitter between neurone and muscle is noradrenaline (norepinephrine). The arterioles are kept in a state of partial vasoconstriction by the vasomotor centre. If the vasomotor activity increases, the blood vessels will constrict and the blood pressure will rise and vice versa.

HYPERTENSION

Blood pressure changes with emotion, posture, exercise, etc. In such circumstances, the changes are brought about by reflex adjustments, the aim of which is to keep the pressure at the most appropriate level for the body's needs. Physicians have difficulty agreeing what constitutes hypertension. An elevation of the resting blood pressure above the 'normal' for the patient's age, weight and height is a broadly acceptable definition. This would be the result of taking several readings under resting conditions. The British Hypertension Society guidelines (2006) defined optimal blood pressure as < 80 mmHg diastolic and < 120 mmHg systolic, normal blood pressure as < 85 mmHg diastolic and < 130 mmHg systolic, and high normal as 85–89 mmHg diastolic and 130–139 mmHg systolic. Some 95% of all cases are described as essential hypertension for which there is no known cause. The remainder of cases are associated with renal disorder, adrenal disorder, coarctation of the aorta or toxaemia of pregnancy. In many instances, there are no symptoms. Some cases are picked up on routine examination or when the patient presents with one of the complications of hypertension, such as stroke, ischaemic heart disease or renal failure. Malignant hypertension is a rare condition that affects fairly young males. It has a rapid onset and causes severe headache, dizziness, left ventricular failure and papilloedema. The diastolic blood pressure may be as high as 140 mmHg.

In patients with hypertension, controls are not able to maintain the blood pressure at the normal level. This may be due to a number of factors:

- rigidity of blood vessels due to atheroma that inevitably occurs with age
- hormonal changes that alter peripheral resistance or blood volume
- other factors that may set the baroreceptors at the wrong level.

If there is an identified cause for hypertension (e.g. phaeochromocytoma), this must be treated, but this is rare. In the relatively few cases in which a cause can be found, the hypertension is designated as secondary hypertension.

Hypertension requires to be treated because serious cardiovascular complications may result, such as stroke, heart failure, renal failure or MI. When the cause cannot be removed, high blood pressure is treated with antihypertensive agents. The methods by which these are effective are based on the fact that blood pressure depends on:

- the peripheral vascular resistance
- the output of blood from the heart
- the volume of blood within the circulation.

By decreasing one or more of these, it is possible to lower the blood pressure.

Ambulatory blood pressure monitoring (24-h blood pressure monitoring) provides more information than either home or clinic measurements, for example 24-h profile with mean daytime (generally 7 a.m. to 10 p.m.), night time values and blood pressure variability. However, routine use of automated ambulatory blood pressure monitoring or home monitoring devices in primary care is not currently recommended. Possible indications for ambulatory blood pressure monitoring include:

- if there is unusual variability of clinic blood pressure measurements
- if there are symptoms suggestive of hypotension
- to aid the diagnosis of 'white coat hypertension'
- informing equivocal treatment decisions
- evaluation of nocturnal hypertension
- evaluation of drug-resistant hypertension
- determining the efficacy of drug treatment over 24 h
- diagnosis and treatment of hypertension in pregnancy.

AETIOLOGICAL FACTORS IN HYPERTENSION

A family history of hypertension is common in patients who present with raised blood pressure. There is also a positive correlation between obesity and blood pressure. It is accepted that a reduction in body weight will reduce blood pressure in hypertensive patients. A high salt and high alcohol intake may elevate blood pressure and these should be corrected.

ANTIHYPERTENSIVE THERAPY

Initiation of antihypertensive therapy is recommended by the British Hypertension Society for the following thresholds.

- Accelerated (malignant) hypertension (with papilloedema or fundal haemorrhages and exudates) *or* acute cardiovascular complications, admit for immediate treatment.
- When the initial blood pressure is systolic ≥ 220 mmHg *or* diastolic ≥ 120 mmHg, treat immediately.
- When the initial blood pressure is systolic 180–219 mmHg *or* diastolic 110–119 mmHg,

confirm over 1–2 weeks then treat if these values are sustained.

- When the initial blood pressure is systolic 160–179 mmHg *or* diastolic 100–109 mmHg, *and* the patient has cardiovascular complications, target organ damage (e.g. left ventricular hypertrophy, renal impairment) or diabetes mellitus (type 1 or 2), confirm over 3–4 weeks then treat if these values are sustained.
- When the initial blood pressure is systolic 160–179 mmHg *or* diastolic 100–109 mmHg, but the patient has *no* cardiovascular complications, no target organ damage or no diabetes, advise lifestyle changes, reassess weekly initially and treat if these values are sustained on repeat measurements over 4–12 weeks.
- When the initial blood pressure is systolic 140–159 mmHg *or* diastolic 90–99 mmHg, *and* the patient has cardiovascular complications, target organ damage or diabetes, confirm within 12 weeks and treat if these values are sustained.
- When the initial blood pressure is systolic 140–159 mmHg *or* diastolic 90–99 mmHg, *and* there are *no* cardiovascular complications, target organ damage or diabetes, advise lifestyle changes and reassess monthly; treat persistent mild hypertension if the 10-year CVD risk is ≥ 20%.

The aim of antihypertensive treatment is to reduce the blood pressure to within normal limits, thereby reducing the number of subsequent cardiovascular events. Optimum blood pressure treatment targets are given below.

- Elevated blood pressure 140/90 mmHg with a CVD risk 20% over 10 years and/or target organ damage: target ≤ 140/85 mmHg.
- Elevated blood pressure 140/90 mmHg with diabetes or chronic renal failure or established atherosclerotic disease: target ≤ 130/80 mmHg.

This will be difficult to achieve for some people, especially the target for systolic blood pressure, and combinations of drugs are invariably required.

The British Hypertension Society and National Institute for Health and Clinical Excellence (NICE) clinical guideline 18, issued in August 2004, gave recommendations on the management of hypertension. The section on drug treatment for hypertension was updated in June 2006 in line with new evidence in relation to beta-blockers (Fig. 12.5). The partial update was developed by the National Collaborating Centre for Chronic Conditions and the British Hypertension Society in conjunction with NICE. The new recommendations state that in hypertensive patients aged 55 or older or black patients of any age, the first choice for initial therapy should be either a calcium-channel blocker or a thiazide-type diuretic. For this recommendation, black patients are considered to be those of African or Caribbean descent, not mixed race, Asian or Chinese. In hypertensive patients younger than 55, the first choice for initial therapy should be an ACE inhibitor (or an angiotensin-II receptor antagonist if an ACE inhibitor is not tolerated). Beta-blockers are no longer recommended as a first-line choice.

In head-to-head trials, beta-blockers were found to be usually less effective than a comparator drug at reducing major cardiovascular events, particularly stroke. Beta-blockers were also less effective than an ACE inhibitor or a calcium-channel blocker at reducing the risk of diabetes, particularly in patients taking a beta-blocker and a thiazide-type diuretic. Calcium-channel blockers or thiazide-type diuretics are the most likely drugs to confer benefit as first-line treatment for most patients aged 55 or older. In people younger than 55 years, the evidence suggests that initial therapy with an ACE inhibitor may be better than initial therapy with a calcium-channel blocker or a thiazide-type diuretic. Adding an ACE inhibitor to a calcium-channel blocker or a diuretic (or vice versa) is a logical combination and has been commonly done in trials. There is little evidence on using three drugs, so the NICE recommendation is based on the most straightforward option.

DIURETIC THERAPY

Thiazide diuretics are regarded as first- or second-choice drugs for hypertension. The hypotensive effect of thiazides is not related solely to their promotion of salt and water loss, but they also dilate arterioles, leading to reduced resistance. Only low doses are needed for maximal hypotensive effect, and increasing the dose merely increases the incidence of adverse effects. A thiazide such as bendroflumethiazide (bendrofluazide) 2.5 mg is inexpensive and allows once-daily dosing. Larger doses can cause more metabolic disturbances without any improvement in blood pressure control. Routine use of low doses minimises adverse effects such as hypokalaemia, hyperuricaemia, glucose intolerance, insulin resistance and elevation of serum cholesterol and calcium. Indapamide is a thiazide-like diuretic. While the incidence of hypokalaemia and hyperuricaemia is the same as with thiazides, indapamide produces no adverse effects on the lipid profile, blood glucose

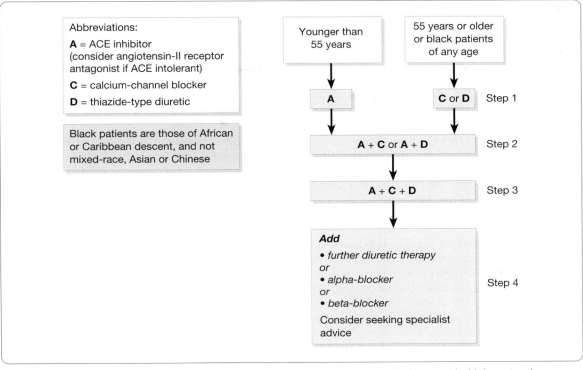

Fig. 12.5 Recommendations for combining blood pressure drugs for patients newly diagnosed with hypertension.

or insulin levels. Indapamide is thought to inhibit progression of left ventricular hypertrophy.

Thiazides are contraindicated in gout, diabetes and hypercalcaemia. Important interactions occur with lithium (lithium toxicity), digoxin (risk of arrhythmia) and non-steroidal anti-inflammatory drugs (hypotensive action reduced).

Loop diuretics have less antihypertensive action than thiazides in uncomplicated patients and are not routinely used for hypertension. They have a valuable role in patients with resistant hypertension, renal impairment and coexistent heart failure, and in patients taking the potent vasodilator minoxidil (for further information on diuretics see pp. 194–197).

BETA-ADRENOCEPTOR BLOCKING DRUGS
See page 200.

CALCIUM-CHANNEL BLOCKERS
Calcium-channel blockers have efficacy similar to that of beta-blockers and thiazide diuretics and are normally used as add-on second-line therapy. Within the calcium-channel blocking group of drugs, which includes diltiazem, verapamil, nifedipine, nicardipine, felodipine and amlodipine, there are important differences (see p. 211).

ANGIOTENSIN-CONVERTING ENZYME INHIBITORS
These drugs are commenced at low doses, because they may cause a profound fall in blood pressure after the first dose, particularly in patients with renal impairment or receiving diuretic therapy (for further details see pp. 207–209).

OTHER DRUGS
Vasodilators (diazoxide, hydralazine, minoxidil), alpha-adrenoceptor blocking drugs (prazosin, terazosin, doxazosin) and centrally acting drugs (methyldopa) are generally reserved for patients whose blood pressure is not controlled by, or who have contraindications to, the drugs already mentioned.

HYPERTENSION IN PREGNANCY

This can be safely treated with methyldopa. Beta blockers may cause intrauterine growth retardation early in pregnancy but are safe from the third trimester onwards.

MALIGNANT HYPERTENSION (ACCELERATED HYPERTENSION)

Malignant hypertension (diastolic blood pressure in excess of 140 mmHg) requires urgent hospital treatment. Although it is desirable to reduce diastolic blood pressure below 120 mmHg within 24 h, this can normally be achieved by oral therapy. If it is lowered too rapidly, cerebral blood flow may fall and brain damage and death can occur from cerebral anoxia, cerebral oedema and cerebral infarction. Normal treatment should be with a beta-blocker (atenolol or labetalol) or a calcium-channel blocker (amlodipine or modified-release nifedipine). Only rarely is parenteral treatment necessary (e.g. in patients with acute dissection of aortic aneurysm or hypertensive encephalopathy). Sodium nitroprusside by infusion is the drug of choice.

VASODILATOR ANTIHYPERTENSIVE DRUGS

Diazoxide, hydralazine, sodium nitroprusside and minoxidil cause peripheral arteriolar dilatation by a direct relaxing effect on vascular smooth muscle. The peripheral dilatation causes a fall in blood pressure. This in turn may cause a resultant reflex tachycardia, negating the fall in blood pressure. This reflex tachycardia can be prevented by administering along with hydralazine or minoxidil a beta-blocker that potentiates their action. For this reason, combination therapy is common when these vasodilators are used.

Diazoxide, hydralazine, minoxidil and sodium nitroprusside are potent drugs, especially when used in combination with a beta-blocker or a thiazide. However, they are generally reserved for patients whose blood pressure is not controlled by, or who have contraindications to, the drugs previously described – thiazides, beta-blockers, calcium-channel blockers and ACE inhibitors.

Diazoxide is available only as an injection and is used only in hypertensive emergencies. It acts within a few minutes and its actions can last from 3 to 12 h.

Hydralazine is rapidly absorbed from the gastro-intestinal tract and has an onset of action of 20–30 min when given orally. When given by intravenous injection, this is much faster. When used alone, it can cause tachycardia and fluid retention. At higher dose, it can induce a systemic lupus erythematosus–like syndrome.

Minoxidil is well absorbed from the gastrointestinal tract, its onset of action is approximately 30 min and its therapeutic effect may last several days. It is usually reserved for the treatment of hypertension resistant to other therapies. It causes vasodilatation accompanied by increased cardiac output, tachycardia, and sodium and water retention. For this reason, a beta-blocker and a diuretic (usually furosemide in high dosage) are required. Other side-effects include weight gain and hypertrichosis.

Sodium nitroprusside is given by intravenous infusion to control severe hypertension when parenteral therapy is indicated. The half-life of sodium nitroprusside is only a few minutes. Its effects can therefore be accurately controlled when administered by infusion.

Bosentan and iloprost are reserved for the specialised treatment of some types of pulmonary hypertension.

CENTRALLY-ACTING ANTIHYPERTENSIVE DRUGS

METHYLDOPA

Methyldopa is converted in the body to methylnoradrenaline (methylnorepinephrine). In the central nervous system, this compound stimulates the α-adrenergic receptors, which results in decreased activity of the sympathetic system. Vascular peripheral tone and arteriolar vasoconstriction are decreased, which lowers standing and supine blood pressures. There is little effect on cardiac output, and there is less orthostatic hypotension compared with peripherally-acting agents.

Although methyldopa is effective in the treatment of hypertension and is easy to use because the fall in blood pressure is not precipitous, it is no longer widely used, because of a high incidence of adverse effects. However, it still has a role in treatment of hypertension during pregnancy.

Central nervous system adverse effects include depression and drowsiness. It may also cause dry mouth, diarrhoea, fluid retention, failure of ejaculation, liver damage, and, rarely, haemolytic anaemia. When fluid retention is a problem, this can be controlled by a diuretic. Side-effects can be minimised if the dose is kept below 1 g/day.

MOXONIDINE

A second class of binding sites termed *imidazoline receptors* has also been shown to influence central sympathetic activity. Moxonidine is the first of a new generation of centrally-acting agents that binds selectively and with high affinity to imidazoline-1 receptors. Occupation of the imidazoline-binding site by moxonidine leads to reduced peripheral sympathetic activity and a consequent reduction in peripheral resistance of the arterioles, while cardiac output and pulmonary haemodynamics remain generally unaffected.

Moxonidine is well absorbed from the gastrointestinal tract and is used in the treatment of mild to moderate hypertension when other antihypertensive agents such as beta-blockers and ACE inhibitors are not appropriate or are ineffective. It can cause dry mouth, headache, fatigue, sedation, dizziness, nausea, sleep disturbances and vasodilatation. Moxonidine is contraindicated in patients with history of angio-edema, cardiac conduction disorders, bradycardia, life-threatening arrhythmia, severe heart failure, severe coronary artery disease, unstable angina, severe liver disease or renal impairment.

ALPHA-ADRENOCEPTOR BLOCKING DRUGS

α_1-adrenoceptor antagonists are effective and well-tolerated drugs that can be used alone or in combination with other groups of drugs in a wide range of hypertensive patients (see Ch. 9). Alpha-blockers reduce left ventricular hypertrophy. They may be considered in patients who fail to respond to, or have toxicity associated with, diuretics and/or beta blockers, including hypertensive patients with lipid disorders or diabetes. Doxazosin, indoramin, prazosin and terazosin selectively block α_1 receptors, interfering with sympathetic stimulation and directly relaxing arteriolar smooth muscle. This interference reduces peripheral vascular resistance and produces vasodilatation without causing tachycardia or reducing cardiac output. They are usually used in combination with other drugs in the treatment of mild to moderate hypertension, They are also used in the treatment of benign prostatic hyperplasia.

Phentolamine and phenoxybenzamine act directly on both α_1 and α_2 adrenoceptors, blocking the pharmacological action of noradrenaline (nor-epinephrine), thereby producing vasodilatation by reducing peripheral resistance. Their action is not selective on α_1 receptors, and reflex tachycardia occurs. They are used in the treatment of hypertensive crisis due to phaeochromocytoma.

All these drugs can cause postural hypotension and dizziness, most evident after the first dose. Other side effects include fatigue, oedema, urinary frequency or incontinence and failure or impairment of ejaculation.

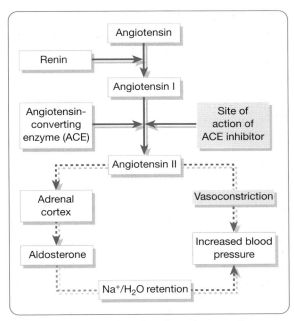

Fig. 12.6 Sites of action of angiotensin-converting enzyme inhibitors.

ANGIOTENSIN-CONVERTING ENZYME INHIBITORS

Angiotensin-converting enzyme inhibitors act on the renin–angiotensin–aldosterone system (see Fig. 12.6) by inhibiting ACE. This system plays an important role in regulating blood pressure, blood volume and electrolyte concentrations. Renin is released from the kidney in response to reduced renal perfusion. It converts angiotensinogen to form angiotensin I. Angiotensin I is then converted in both plasma and tissue to angiotensin II by ACE. Angiotensin II is a potent vasoconstrictor and, in addition, stimulates the release of aldosterone, which promotes water and sodium retention. Both these actions serve to raise blood pressure. ACE inhibitors, by inhibiting the production of angiotensin II, thus effectively lower blood pressure.

Angiotensin-converting enzyme also inactivates certain neuropeptides, including bradykinin. ACE inhibitors therefore increase levels of bradykinin, which may play an important role in preventing left ventricular hypertrophy. Bradykinin is also a vasodilator and may have a key role in the cardio-protective actions of ACE inhibitors. In the kidney, they reduce proteinuria by local inhibition on the postglomerular efferent arteriole. This causes greater dilatation of the efferent than the afferent arteriole, reducing the intraglomerular pressure and thereby reducing proteinuria. This forms the basis of ACE inhibitors as the antihypertensives of choice in diabetics, thus protecting the kidney from further damage. These drugs are now being increasingly used to protect the kidney in non-diabetic kidney disease, except in polycystic disease.

Indications. Angiotensin-converting enzyme inhibitors are used to control hypertension, particularly when thiazides and beta-blockers are contraindicated or ineffective. They are particularly indicated for hypertension in insulin-dependent diabetic patients with nephropathy and possibly for hypertension in all diabetics. In some patients, they may cause a very rapid fall in blood pressure. This is termed *first-dose hypotension*, and treatment should be commenced at low dose, being taken at bedtime. In patients receiving concomitant diuretic therapy at a dose greater than 80 mg of furosemide, or equivalent, then ACE inhibitors should be initiated under close supervision. In some patients, the dose of the diuretic may need to be reduced or discontinued at least 24 h beforehand.

Angiotensin-converting enzyme inhibitors are also used in the treatment of heart failure, either as an adjunct to diuretics or in cases in which there is no response to diuretics. They may also be used, when appropriate, with digoxin. Dilatation of the arterioles reduces the load on the heart and improves its function. Potassium-sparing diuretics or potassium supplements should not be given concomitantly with ACE inhibitors, as dangerous hyperkalaemia may result.

Profound first-dose hypertension can occur in patients with heart failure when an ACE inhibitor is introduced. In those patients receiving high doses of a loop diuretic, withdrawal of the diuretic can result in rebound pulmonary oedema. Therefore in these cases introduction of an ACE inhibitor may need to be initiated under specialist supervision.

Angiotensin-converting enzyme inhibitors are also used in early and long-term management after an MI. Following MI, compensatory changes occur in the heart that lead to ventricular hypertrophy and ultimately heart failure. ACE inhibitors given after MI can reduce these compensatory changes.

Angiotensin-converting enzyme inhibitors range from relatively short-acting ones such as captopril, which is taken two or three times daily, to longer-acting ones such as lisinopril and ramipril, which are taken only once daily. Not all ACE inhibitors are licensed for all indications. Other ACE inhibitors include cilazapril, enalapril, fosinopril, imidapril, moexipril, perindopril, quinapril and trandolapril.

In certain circumstances in risk groups, therapy should be commenced under close medical supervision, usually in hospital, with facilities to treat profound hypotension. These include patients on high-dose loop diuretics (> 80 mg of furosemide); with hypovolaemia or hyponatraemia; with renal failure, unstable heart failure or hypotension; and aged over 70 years.

Side-effects. Angiotensin-converting enzyme inhibitors are generally well tolerated. Dry cough caused by the inhibition of bradykinin breakdown is a feature of ACE inhibitor therapy in up to 15% of patients. This is unresponsive to antitussives and can be severe enough to cause patients to discontinue therapy.

Hypotension, which may be profound, can occur after the first dose of an ACE inhibitor. Patients most at risk include those with congestive cardiac failure, volume depletion and high-renin hypertension. The risk may be minimised by stopping or reducing existing diuretic therapy and administering a low test dose of an ACE inhibitor with a short half-life. ACE inhibitors have produced acute renal failure in patients with bilateral renal artery stenosis and atherosis of the artery supplying a single functioning kidney, because of loss of perfusion pressure. ACE inhibitors are contraindicated in such patients. Hyponatraemia, high-dose diuretic therapy and severe congestive cardiac failure are other predisposing factors to worsening renal function. Haematological side effects may occur, in particular when ACE inhibitors are administered with other drugs causing blood dyscrasias; these side-effects are generally reversible. ACE inhibitors may have a lesser antihypertensive response in Afro-Caribbean patients.

A maculopapular or pruritic rash occurring early on in therapy may be a feature, although this is often self-limiting. Rarely, photosensitivity may occur. Similarly, taste disturbance (characterised by a metallic taste) or taste suppression may arise within the first 1–3 months but is also self-limiting. Hyperkalaemia may occur due to renal potassium retention and may become clinically significant in patients with renal impairment or those taking potassium-sparing diuretics or potassium supplements. Angioedema involving the face and lips, and more dangerously the larynx, may rarely occur.

Contraindications. Angiotensin-converting enzyme inhibitors are best avoided in patients with known or suspected renovascular disease, including patients with symptomatic peripheral vascular disease or severe generalised atherosclerosis. Bilateral renal artery stenosis or arterial stenosis to a single kidney is a contraindication. ACE inhibitors should not be used in aortic stenosis or outflow tract obstruction.

All ACE inhibitors are contraindicated in any trimester of pregnancy, as they may adversely affect fetal growth, neonatal blood pressure control and renal function.

ANGIOTENSIN-II RECEPTOR ANTAGONISTS

Mode of action. There are two classes of angiotensin-II receptors, termed AT_1 and AT_2. The AT_1 receptor appears to be responsible for the known effects of angiotensin II. AT_1 receptors are found mainly in the heart and blood vessels, kidney, adrenal cortex, lung and brain. The exact role of AT_2 receptors is unclear. Among the functions of these receptors are vasoconstriction, promotion of aldosterone release and sodium retention. Antagonism, or blockade, of these receptors therefore leads to an effective blood pressure-lowering response.

Angiotensin-II antagonists are licensed for use in hypertension, and some may also be used as an alternative to an ACE inhibitor in the management of heart failure or diabetic nephropathy. Candesartan, irbesartan, losartan and valsartan were some of the first angiotensin-II antagonists to be licensed. Eprosartan, olmesartan and telmisartan have been introduced latterly.

Side-effects. Unlike ACE inhibitors, the angiotensin-II receptor antagonists do not inhibit the breakdown of bradykinin and other kinins. As a result, they do not appear to cause the persistent dry cough commonly occurring in ACE inhibitor therapy. They are therefore a useful alternative for patients who have to discontinue an ACE inhibitor because of persistent cough. Side-effects are usually mild and transient in nature. Hypotension, hyperkalaemia, gastrointestinal disturbances, dizziness and myalgia have been reported.

Cautions. Angiotensin-II receptor antagonists should be used with caution in renal artery stenosis. Plasma potassium monitoring is advised, particularly in the elderly and in patients with renal impairment. These drugs should be avoided in pregnancy.

ISCHAEMIC HEART DISEASE

Ischaemia arises when the normally smooth endo-thelial surface of one or more of the coronary arteries becomes roughened. Narrowing occurs as a result of deposits (atheroma) that partly occlude the artery. Atheroma starts at an early age and consists of abnormal plaques of fatty compounds that develop in the muscular layer of an artery. As they grow, they project into the lumen of the artery, thus reducing blood flow. The resulting reduction in blood flow leads to a reduction of oxygenated blood supply to the myocardium (see p. 217 for MI).

ANGINA PECTORIS

Angina pectoris is the clinical sign of transient myocardial ischaemia. It occurs when the metabolic demands of the heart for oxygen exceed the ability of diseased coronary arteries to supply adequate blood flow to the myocardium (physical exercise, anaemia). Angina is one of the principal symptoms of CHD. It is characterised by tightness of the chest that may or may not radiate to the jaw, down one or both arms or through into the back. The pain tends to occur during exertion and is of an alarming nature.

Chronic stable angina is by far the commonest form and is characterised by brief (10 min) episodes of pain closely related to precipitants that increase cardiac output, such as exertion, emotion and, less commonly, heavy meals. The treatments used have little or no effect on the obstructed coronary artery itself but prevent angina by reducing or limiting the work of the heart. As its name suggests, this form of angina often follows a stable pattern for many years but may be complicated by MI, unstable angina or sudden death.

Unstable angina presents as a worsening pattern of pre-existing angina, or with episodes of pain that are prolonged (30 min or longer) or that occur spontaneously. It is caused by a non-occlusive thrombus forming on an atherosclerotic plaque that has developed a fissure or had a haemorrhage into its substance. Unstable angina is a threatening condition, because it confers a high risk of MI or sudden death within weeks or months.

MANAGEMENT OF STABLE ANGINA

All patients with angina who smoke should be advised to stop. Cigarette smoking approximately doubles the risk of morbidity and mortality from ischaemic heart disease compared with a lifetime of not smoking, and the risk is related to the duration and amount of smoking. Diet should be modified in line with healthy eating advice:

- increase fruit and vegetable consumption to five portions per day
- increase consumption of oil-rich fish to three portions per week
- decrease total fat consumption

- increase starchy food intake and reduce sugary food intake.

All patients with angina should have their cholesterol level measured. Appropriate dietary measures should be recommended. If required, drug therapy should be initiated to reduce total cholesterol to < 5 mmol/L.

Patients should be encouraged to increase exercise levels within limits set by their disease state. Alcohol consumption should be limited to three units per day for men and two for women.

Patients with stable angina should be treated with aspirin 75 mg per day. In the event of true aspirin intolerance or allergy, clopidogrel 75 mg daily should be considered.

All patients with symptomatic CHD should be prescribed sublingual glyceryl trinitrate and should be educated as to its use for short-term symptom control.

Patients who require regular symptomatic treatment should be treated initially with a beta-blocker and warned not to stop the treatment suddenly.

Patients intolerant of beta-blockers and who show no left-sided ventricular systolic dysfunction should be treated with one of the following:

- a rate-limiting calcium-channel blocker
- a long-acting dihydropyridine (e.g. amlodipine, felodipine)
- a nitrate
- a potassium-channel opening agent.

If symptoms are not controlled in patients taking beta-blockers, isosorbide mononitrate, a long-acting dihydropyridine (e.g. felodipine) or diltiazem can be added.

NITRATES

The nitrates are used in the prophylaxis and treatment of angina pectoris and also to treat left ventricular failure. Beta-blockers and calcium-channel blockers are widely used to treat angina; however, short-acting nitrates retain an important role both for prophylactic use before exertion and for chest pain occurring during exercise.

Mode of action. Nitrates have several effects:
- dilatation of vessels in the venous system decreases venous return and thus the preload to the heart; the reduced preload prevents the left ventricle from overfilling and reduces the symptoms of cardiac failure

- dilatation of arterioles lowers peripheral resistance and left ventricular pressure, reducing myocardial work and oxygen demand
- dilatation of coronary arteries increases blood supply (and therefore oxygen supply) to the myocardium.

The mode of action of nitrates to produce these effects is as follows. Mononitrates enter the walls of veins and arteries, combine with sulphydryl groups and form the vasodilating substance nitric oxide. (The nitric oxide activates guanylate cyclase to produce cyclic guanosine monophosphate, which causes relaxation of vascular smooth muscle with dilatation of veins and arterioles.)

SUBLINGUAL GLYCERYL TRINITRATE

Glyceryl trinitrate is used as soon as an attack of angina occurs or may also be used prophylactically before physical activity. It undergoes extensive first-pass metabolism when taken orally, but the sublingual administration bypasses the hepatic circulation. The tablets are placed under the tongue and allowed to dissolve. Rapid symptomatic relief of angina is normally obtained within a minute, but the effect lasts for only 20–30 min. Initially, one tablet should be used, but if no relief is obtained a second and then a third may be taken at 5-min intervals. If no relief is obtained after three tablets, the patient should seek medical attention.

Patients should be advised that when they get chest pain and need to take a glyceryl trinitrate tablet, they should sit down. The purpose of this is twofold: first, sitting down may in itself relieve the angina symptoms, and second, by sitting, any dizziness caused by the glyceryl trinitrate will be minimised. Patients should be warned of the possible side-effects to expect, such as headache, facial flushing, dizziness, nausea and lightheadedness. These effects can be minimised by spitting out or swallowing any tablet remaining when the pain has subsided. The side-effects usually subside after a few weeks of regular glyceryl trinitrate use.

Patients should be advised to store the tablets in a cool dry place in the original container with the original cap. Any tablets left 8 weeks after first opening the bottle should be discarded and replaced with a fresh supply. If the bottle has not been opened, the contents can be kept until the expiry date on the bottle. Some patients prefer using glyceryl trinitrate spray, as it offers more convenience in terms of longer expiry and easier storage. It is more expensive, but for those patients who do not use tablets frequently it may be a better option. The tablets are available in 300-, 500- and 600-microgram strengths. An aerosol spray provides an effective alternative to tablets.

BUCCAL NITRATE

Buccal nitrate tablets consist of glyceryl trinitrate impregnated in an inert polymer matrix, allowing slow diffusion across the buccal mucosa. The tablet is placed under the top lip without chewing, where a gel-like coating forms around the tablet. This allows adherence to the buccal mucosa, with the release of drug over 3–5 h.

TRANSDERMAL PREPARATIONS

Several transdermal preparations, as either patches or ointment, have been developed for prophylaxis of angina. They bypass first-pass metabolism. Using the patches, therapeutic blood levels are achieved within an hour and last up to 24 h. The patches should be applied to a clean, dry, non-hairy part of the skin (extremities should be avoided). Absorption depends on site of application and blood flow. Skin irritation and variable absorption may limit their use. If tolerance is suspected during the use of transdermal patches, they should be left off for several consecutive hours in 24 h (during a period of time when the patient is least likely to develop chest pain) in order to have a nitrate-free interval.

INTRAVENOUS NITRATES

Glyceryl trinitrate or isosorbide mononitrate may be tried by intravenous injection when the sublingual form is ineffective in patients with chest pain due to MI or severe ischaemia. Intravenous injections are also useful in the treatment of acute left ventricular failure. It may not always be possible to proceed to doses that are high enough to relieve symptoms, because of adverse effects such as headache or hypotension. In the longer term, the infusion rate may need increasing owing to the development of tolerance, because a continuous infusion of glyceryl trinitrate does not permit a nitrate-free period and tolerance may develop within 24–48 h of commencing the infusion.

ISOSORBIDE MONONITRATE AND ISOSORBIDE DINITRATE

Isosorbide mononitrate and isosorbide dinitrate are effective when taken orally, and the mononitrate is less readily metabolised than glyceryl trinitrate in the liver. Isosorbide dinitrate is active sublingually and orally but has a short half-life (0.5–1 h). It undergoes extensive first-pass metabolism, with the main active metabolite being isosorbide mononitrate. No matter which long-acting nitrate preparation is used, the dose has to be titrated to attain the desired response or until the dose is limited by side effects such as headache. The dose varies greatly between patients (see Table 12.1 for further information).

NITRATE TOLERANCE

The release of the vasodilating substance nitric oxide depends on the presence of sulphydryl groups. Continuous 24-h nitrate therapy leads to the depletion of sulphydryl groups, preventing further release of nitric oxide and the development of tolerance. Development of tolerance can be avoided by allowing the plasma nitrate concentration to fall at some period during the 24 h. A nitrate-free gap of several consecutive hours in each 24-h period is necessary for the regeneration of sulphydryl groups. This can be achieved by removing glyceryl trinitrate patches for a period of 6 h. A dosage schedule in which an oral nitrate is taken three times daily, but with the last dose at the time of the evening meal, allows an appropriate interval to counter the development of tolerance. Sustained-release nitrate preparations provide a nitrate-free interval if given once daily.

CALCIUM-CHANNEL BLOCKERS

Mode of action. Calcium ions play an important role in the maintenance of vascular smooth muscle tone. Calcium-channel blockers inhibit the influx of calcium ions into the muscle cells in the arterial walls, resulting in relaxation of the muscle and dilatation of the artery. As a result, coronary or systemic vascular tone may be diminished and calcium-channel blockers are used to

Table 12.1   Onset and duration of action of nitrates

Drug	Onset of action (min)	Duration of action
Sublingual glyceryl trinitrate	2–5	10–30 min
Buccal glyceryl trinitrate	2–5	30–300 min
Glyceryl trinitrate ointment	15–60	3–8 h
Glyceryl trinitrate patch	30–60	18–24 h
Oral isosorbide dinitrate	15–45	2–6 h
Oral isosorbide mononitrate	60	5 h

Table 12.2 Calcium-channel blockers

Drug	Hypertension	Angina	Dose
Amlodipine	√	√	5–10 mg once daily
Diltiazem	√	√	Angina, 60 mg three times daily- to 360 mg daily; longer-acting formulations used in hypertension
Felodipine	√	√	Angina, 5–10 mg once daily hypertension, 2.5–20 mg once daily
Isradipine	√	–	1.25–10 mg twice daily
Lacidipine	√	–	2–6 mg daily
Lercanidipine	√	–	10–20 mg daily
Nicardipine	√	√	20–30 mg three times daily
Nifedipine	√	√	Varies according to which of the many available preparations are used; also used in Raynaud's phenomenon
Nisoldipine	√	√	10–40 mg daily
Verapamil	√	√	Angina, 80–120 mg three times daily; hypertension, 240–480 mg daily in two to three divided doses; also used to treat supraventricular arrhythmias 40–120 mg three times daily

lower blood pressure in hypertension and to dilate coronary arteries in angina. (In addition, verapamil slows conduction in the AV node and is used to treat cardiac arrhythmias.)

Although their actions are similar, the balance of their effects on the myocardium, on conducting tissue and on blood vessels varies, and so there is variation between the drugs in this class. There are important differences between verapamil, diltiazem and the dihydropyridine calcium-channel blockers such as amlodipine, felodipine and nifedipine. They are all given orally and broken down by the liver. Table 12.2 gives an overview of their indications.

The smooth muscle relaxant effect of nimodipine acts preferentially on cerebral arteries. Its use is confined to the prevention of vascular spasm following subarachnoid haemorrhage.

Side-effects. Headache, flushing and ankle oedema can occur because of vasodilatation, but they become less of a problem after a few days. Constipation may be a problem with verapamil. Great care is necessary in patients who have heart failure, as several calcium-channel blockers may further depress cardiac function and cause clinically significant deterioration.

POTASSIUM-CHANNEL ACTIVATORS

NICORANDIL

Nicorandil combines the properties of an organic nitrate with those of a potassium-channel opener, thereby causing dilatation of coronary arteries and arterioles, and also large veins (see Fig. 12.7).

Nicorandil is a nitrate derivative of nicotinamide. Similar to other organic nitrates, it relaxes vascular smooth muscle, particularly on the venous side, reducing the preload (ventricular filling and myocardial work). In addition to dilatation of coronary arteries, nicorandil activates ATP-dependent potassium channels and increases the efflux of potassium ions. This hyperpolarises the cell membrane, inhibits calcium entry and causes arterial vasodilatation (similar to calcium-blockers). The commonest side-effect of nicorandil is headache (especially in initiation, usually transitory).

Pharmacokinetically, nicorandil is rapidly and almost completely absorbed into the circulation with little or no first-pass metabolism in the liver. Nicorandil has a half-life of 1 h and is mainly

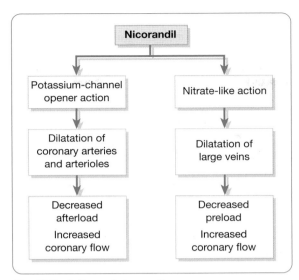

Fig. 12.7   Actions of nicorandil.

metabolised through the liver and excreted via the kidneys.

The commonest side effect of nicorandil is headache (especially on initiation, usually transitory). Other adverse effects may include nausea, vomiting, malaise, dizziness, palpitations and fatigue. Continuous treatment may lead to the development of tolerance to the organic nitrate component of nicorandil, but the drug's efficacy tends to be maintained owing to the potassium-channel-opening effect.

PERIPHERAL VASODILATORS

The blood supply to the limb may be diminished by disease or spasm of the peripheral arteries. This leads to an inadequate oxygen supply to the muscle and thus pain in the muscle on walking (intermittent claudication). The cause of this is occlusion of the vessels either by spasm or by sclerotic plaques. Vasodilators may increase blood flow at rest but have not been shown to be of benefit during exercise.

Because most vasodilators dilate the blood vessels to the skin rather than those to the muscle, they are more useful in the treatment of Raynaud's syndrome, in which spasm is a major factor in poor circulation. It is important that non-drug measures be carried out (e.g. stopping smoking, reducing weight and fat intake, increasing exercise to improve muscle efficiency and prevent build-up of metabolites, avoidance of exposure to the cold).

Many of these drugs have unpleasant side effects, such as gastrointestinal disturbances, headache and dizziness. They may adversely affect patients suffering from angina, those who have had recent MI (by diverting blood from ischaemic areas), those taking antihypertensives (by potentiating their effects) and diabetics (may potentiate insulin and oral hypoglycaemics). Examples of drugs in this class include cilostazol, cinnarizine, nicotinic acid derivatives, pentoxifylline (oxpentifylline), moxisylyte (thymoxamine) and naftidrofuryl oxalate (also a cerebral vasodilator). Most of these are deemed less suitable for prescribing by the British National Formulary.

SYMPATHOMIMETICS

Inotropic and vasoconstrictor sympathomimetics are discussed in this section (see Ch. 9).

INOTROPIC SYMPATHOMIMETICS

The properties of the sympathomimetics vary according to whether they act on alpha or on beta adrenergic receptors (see Ch. 9). Adrenaline (epinephrine) acts on both α and β receptors:

- α effect – vasoconstriction
- β_1 effect – increase in heart rate and contractility
- β_2 effect – peripheral vasodilatation.

Although a powerful sympathomimetic agent, adrenaline is used less frequently, as more selective drugs are available. It is of value in anaphylaxis and bronchospasm and is the first drug given in cardiac arrest. In the latter indication, it has a direct myocardial stimulatory effect, improving the quality of ventricular contraction and improving cardiac output. Adrenaline 1 in 10000 (1 mg per 10 mL) is recommended in a dose of 10 mL by central intravenous injection.

Dopamine is a naturally occurring substance that is changed to noradrenaline (norepinephrine) in the body. However, dopamine has pharmacological actions of its own:

- β_1 effect – potent inotropic action (i.e. it increases the force of contraction more than the rate of the heart)
- stimulates α receptors in the peripheral vascular system, causing vasoconstriction at higher doses
- stimulates dopamine receptors in the mesenteric, coronary, intracerebral and renal vascular systems; this causes dilatation, and in the renal system, blood flow and urinary output are increased, which

is useful in shock when there is a decline in renal function – this effect occurring at low dosage
- causes release of noradrenaline from sympathetic nerves.

Dopamine is used in cardiogenic shock in infarction or cardiac surgery. It is administered by intravenous infusion (2–5 micrograms/kg per min), the dose being adjusted according to response.

Its use requires considerable care, as higher doses lead to vasoconstriction and may exacerbate heart failure. Once the condition is under control, the drug should be withdrawn slowly.

Dobutamine has a more selective action than dopamine, acting mainly on the beta adrenoceptors, and it does not cause release of noradrenaline (nor-epinephrine). It produces an increase in the force of contraction of the heart and at high doses causes peripheral vasodilatation. For the latter reason, it is not appropriate in the treatment of shock when there is marked hypotension. However, it is preferable to dopamine if blood pressure is normal.

Dopexamine is indicated as inotropic support and vasodilator in exacerbations of chronic heart failure and in heart failure associated with cardiac surgery. It is a synthetic catecholamine, structurally related to dopamine, with marked intrinsic agonist activity at β_2 adrenoceptors and lesser activity at β_1 adrenoceptors. Its use in critically ill patients is often aimed at improving vital organ perfusion, specifically gastrointestinal tract, renal, hepatic and splanchnic blood flow, thus preventing the translocation of endotoxins and micro-organisms.

Isoprenaline is less selective and increases both heart rate and contractility. It is now used only as emergency treatment of heart block or severe bradycardia. It is now only available on special order.

VASOCONSTRICTOR SYMPATHOMIMETICS

Although some people have a naturally low blood pressure and come to no harm, when the blood pressure is unusually low there is an inadequate blood supply to the brain, which causes the person to faint. When this is caused by shock of haemorrhage, the patient may lose consciousness and die. In older people, postural hypotension can result from rising from bed or chair too quickly and may provide the reason for some falls. Delay in baroreceptor response may account for this. The danger of vasoconstrictors is that they may raise blood pressure at the expense of the kidneys by reducing kidney perfusion.

Vasoconstrictor sympathomimetics raise blood pressure by acting on α-adrenergic receptors to constrict peripheral vessels. They are used in emergencies to raise blood pressure. They are also used in general and spinal anaesthesia to control blood pressure, because spinal and epidural anaesthesia may result in sympathetic block with resultant hypotension.

Ephedrine is given by slow intravenous injection to reverse hypotension associated with bradycardia following spinal or epidural anaesthesia. It can cause tachycardia, anxiety, restlessness, insomnia and arrhythmias. Noradrenaline (norepinephrine) is used in the treatment of acute hypotension following cardiac arrest. Given by intravenous infusion, it can cause bradycardia, headache and arrhythmias. Metaraminol and phenylephrine are given parenterally for acute hypotension and also for priapism.

ANTICOAGULANTS

BLOOD COAGULATION

Platelets, disc-shaped cells 1–2 micrometres in diameter, are formed in the bone marrow under the control of a regulator called thrombopoietin. Aggregation of platelets occurs in response to blood vessel injury and the platelets plug the disrupted vessel wall. Platelet aggregates are reinforced by precipitation of the insoluble protein called fibrin from soluble precursors in the plasma. Erythrocytes then become enmeshed within this fibrin framework. The formation of fibrin depends on the activation of the clotting cascade along extrinsic and intrinsic pathways (Fig. 12.8).

Exposure of collagen in damaged blood vessels initiates the action of factor XII, and this leads to activation of the intrinsic pathway. The extrinsic part of the cascade is stimulated by tissue thromboplastin released from damaged tissue, which activates factor VII. Once triggered, the coagulation process accelerates. Platelet aggregation leads to release of various mediators, including phospholipid factor III, which is a major accelerating influence on blood coagulation. Thrombin generation also acts as a further stimulus to platelet aggregation. Thrombin (IIa) stimulates the conversion of fibrinogen to fibrin in the presence of calcium ions. The initial fibrin clot is soluble and is converted to an insoluble polymer when factor XIII is activated by thrombin and calcium. The initial conversion of fibrinogen to fibrin is rapid; the conversion to the polymer is slow and complete cross-linking takes several hours.

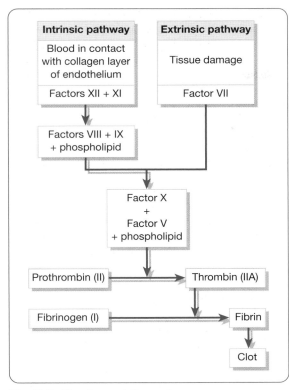

Fig. 12.8   Blood coagulation system.

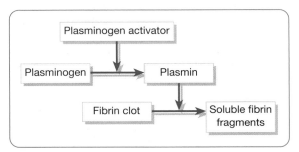

Fig. 12.9   Action of plasmin in fibrinolysis.

Eventually, the process terminates because of the action of physiological inhibitors of coagulation factors (e.g. antithrombin), as well as through the inactivation of factors V and VII by high concentrations of thrombin. Phagocytosis facilitates the removal of precipitated fibrin complexes. Fibrin thrombus undergoes enzymatic digestion to soluble polypeptides by the process of fibrinolysis. The proteolytic enzyme involved is called plasmin.

Plasminogen is incorporated in the clot and is converted to plasmin when the activators diffuse into the clot (Fig. 12.9). In addition to converting fibrin clot to soluble fragments, plasmin acts on fibrinogen, prothrombin and factors V and VIII, rendering them ineffective in the coagulation system, thus preventing excessive coagulation.

TYPES OF ANTICOAGULANT

PARENTERAL ANTICOAGULANTS

Mode of action. Heparin promotes the action of antithrombin III, which in turn inhibits factor X at low (prophylactic) doses and factors IX and XI in anticoagulant doses. The outcome is inhibition of the conversion of prothrombin to thrombin, and this prevents the conversion of fibrinogen to fibrin. This results in the prolongation of clotting time.

Indications. Heparin is used as an anticoagulant in the treatment of deep vein thrombosis (DVT) and pulmonary embolism or in the prevention of DVT.

Pharmacokinetics. Heparin is not well absorbed from the gastrointestinal tract, so it must be administered parenterally. The intravenous route is preferred for high-dose treatment of acute thrombotic episodes, while the subcutaneous route is preferred for low-dose prophylactic therapy. The intramuscular route should be avoided because of the danger of local bleeding. With intravenous administration, the onset of action of heparin is almost immediate, and peak concentration levels occur within minutes. The patient's clotting time will return to normal within 2–6 h after administration of an intravenous bolus. With subcutaneous administration, onset is delayed for about 2 h. The serum half-life of heparin is dose-related, the duration of action being extended with higher doses.

The enzyme heparinase metabolises heparin in the liver. Half-life, approximately 1–1.5 h, is dose-related. The anticoagulant effect is measured by the activated partial thromboplastin time (APTT) test and the partial thromboplastin time. Dosage is adjusted daily, with laboratory monitoring and adjustment according to the APTT.

Dose. Treatment of DVT and pulmonary embolism by intravenous injection: loading dose of 5000 units (10 000 units in severe pulmonary embolism) followed by continuous infusion of 15–25 units/kg per h or by subcutaneous injection of 15 000 units every 12 h (laboratory monitoring essential, preferably on a daily basis). Given by subcutaneous injection, the prophylaxis of DVT is given at a dose of 5000 units 2 h before surgery, then every 8–12 h for 7 days or until the patient is ambulant. Heparin flushes are used to maintain the patency of cannulae intended to be in place for longer than 48 h. They are available as solutions of 10 units/mL and 100 units/mL. For under 48 h, sodium chloride injection 0.9% is effective.

Side-effects. Haemorrhage, thrombocytopenia, hypersensitivity reactions and osteoporosis can occur after prolonged use. Its use is contraindicated in haemophilia and other haemorrhagic disorders, thrombocytopenia, peptic ulcer, cerebral aneurysm, severe hypertension and severe liver disease.

Bleeding due to overdosage may occur with heparin. As with all anticoagulants, this often first appears as haematuria but may develop from any site. Protamine sulphate is a strong base that neutralises acidic heparin by binding with it to form a stable compound with no anticoagulant effect. One milligram of protamine sulphate will neutralise approximately 100 units of heparin. The dose to be given should be carefully calculated bearing in mind the short half-life of heparin. The maximum dose is 50 mg. Protamine sulphate is given slowly by intravenous injection. Rapid injection can cause complications such as dyspnoea, flushing, bradycardia and hypotension. If used in excess, protamine has an anticoagulant effect. It is derived from fish sperm, and hypersensitivity reactions may occur in patients with allergies to fish.

LOW MOLECULAR WEIGHT HEPARIN

Low molecular weight heparins are used for prophylaxis of DVT by subcutaneous injection, particularly in high-risk orthopaedic surgery. A number of similar drugs are available (bemiparin, dalteparin, enoxaparin, reviparin and tinzaparin), the timing of the first dose varying from 12 h before surgery to 1–2 h before surgery. The regimen is continued daily for 7–10 days or until the patient is ambulant. Some low molecular weight heparins are also used in the treatment of DVT, for unstable coronary artery disease and for the prevention of clotting in extracorporeal circuits. Low molecular weight heparin has a longer half-life than heparin, which facilitates once-daily dosing. The standard prophylactic regimen does not require monitoring.

HEPARINOIDS AND HIRUDINS

Danaparoid is a heparinoid used for prophylaxis of DVT in patients undergoing general or orthopaedic surgery and with a history of heparin-induced thrombocytopenia. Lepirudin, a recombinant hirudin, is licensed for anticoagulation in patients with type 2 (immune) heparin-induced thrombocytopenia who require parenteral antithrombotic treatment. The dose is adjusted according to APTT. Bivalirudin, a hirudin analogue, is a thrombin inhibitor that is used for patients undergoing percutaneous coronary intervention who would have been considered for treatment with unfractionated heparin combined with a glycoprotein IIb/IIIa inhibitor; it should not be used alone.

FONDAPARINUX AND EPOPROSTENOL

Fondaparinux sodium is a synthetic pentasaccharide that inhibits activated factor X. It is licensed for prophylaxis of venous thromboembolism in medical patients and in patients undergoing major orthopaedic surgery of the legs or abdominal surgery, and for the treatment of DVT and of pulmonary embolism. Epoprostenol (prostacyclin) can be given to inhibit platelet aggregation during renal dialysis, either alone or with heparin. It can also be used for the treatment of primary pulmonary hypertension resistant to other treatment, usually with oral anticoagulation. It has a half-life of about 3 min, so must be given by continuous intravenous infusion. As it is a potent vasodilator, it causes flushing, headache and hypotension.

ORAL ANTICOAGULANTS

There are three substances in the coumarin group: warfarin, acenocoumarol (nicoumalone) and phenindione. The drug of choice is warfarin, the others being seldom used.

Mode of action. Warfarin is effective by mouth. It antagonises the synthesis of vitamin K-dependent clotting factors in the liver, including prothrombin and factors VII, IX and X. The resulting therapeutic anticoagulant effect does not occur until the already circulating clotting factors are depleted. This takes from several hours for factor VII to 2–3 days for prothrombin. It therefore takes several days before the anticoagulant effect develops, and heparin is used until warfarin is effective. Liver disease, in which synthesis of clotting factors is defective, potentiates warfarin.

Indications. Warfarin is indicated for:

- prophylaxis and treatment of venous thrombosis and pulmonary embolism
- prophylaxis of embolisation in rheumatic heart disease and atrial fibrillation
- prophylaxis after insertion of a prosthetic heart valve to prevent emboli developing on the valves.

Pharmacokinetics. Warfarin is absorbed rapidly and almost completely after oral administration; it is highly protein-bound, although binding and half-life may vary considerably between patients. Dosage must therefore be individualised. The anticoagulant effect must be carefully monitored when other drugs that alter protein binding or metabolism are introduced or withdrawn.

Dose. Whenever possible, the baseline prothrombin should be determined before the initial dose is given. An initial adult dose of 10 mg is given once daily for 2 days with daily measurements of international normalised ratio (INR) for prothrombin time and adjustments as required. The daily maintenance dose of warfarin is usually 3–9 mg (taken at the same time each day). The indications and target INRs currently recommended by the British Society for Haematology are:

- INR 2.5 for treatment of DVT and pulmonary embolism (or for recurrence in patients no longer receiving warfarin), atrial fibrillation, cardioversion, dilated cardiomyopathy, mural thrombus following MI, and rheumatic mitral valve disease
- INR 3.5 for recurrent DVT and pulmonary embolism (in patients currently receiving warfarin with INR above 2) and mechanical prosthetic heart valves.

Adverse reactions. The main adverse reaction of all oral anticoagulants is haemorrhage. The level of INR at which bleeding occurs varies from patient to patient. However, an INR of 8 or over is considered dangerously high and usually necessitates the administration of plasma and possibly blood if haemorrhage has already occurred. Phytomenadione (vitamin K) 5 mg by slow intravenous injection will counteract the effects of warfarin, but it is not ideal because it takes up to 6 h to act and will render the patient resistant to anticoagulants for several weeks. When the INR is raised but to a lesser extent (4.5–7 without haemorrhage), it may be sufficient to withdraw warfarin for 1 or 2 days and then review. Anticoagulant treatment cards are supplied by the pharmacist and must be carried by the patient.

Warfarin is contraindicated in pregnancy, because it is teratogenic. It is also contraindicated in peptic ulcer, severe hypertension and bacterial endocarditis.

Interactions. Drug interactions occur commonly with warfarin for a number of reasons, for example:

- protein-binding displacement – warfarin is highly bound and is displaced (e.g. by salicylates and sulphonamides), which enhances its action
- inhibition of metabolism increases its effect (e.g. metronidazole, cimetidine)
- induction of metabolism by drugs that induce microsomal enzymes (including phenytoin, rifampicin, carbamazepine) reduces the effect of warfarin.

MYOCARDIAL INFARCTION

In western countries, heart attacks are responsible for 30–50% of all deaths. The incidence increases with age and is greater in men. Factors that may contribute to the development of MI include:

- family history of CHD
- stress
- cigarette smoking
- lack of exercise
- hypertension
- raised serum cholesterol
- obesity
- oral contraceptives
- diet rich in saturated fats and cholesterol.

Myocardial infarction occurs when there is a prolonged reduction in the oxygen supply to a region of myocardium (heart muscle). Tissue death follows, and the area is said to be infarcted. This occurs primarily in patients with coronary artery disease when there is significant narrowing of one or more of the three major coronary arteries (Fig. 12.10). As a result of turbulent blood flow at the site of the atheroma, platelets aggregate to form thrombi and blockage of the coronary artery occurs.

Typically, the symptom of MI is severe chest pain that is sudden in onset and prolonged. The pain is characteristically tight or 'band-like' and may radiate to the jaw, shoulders, neck, back or arms. It is often associated with breathlessness, anxiety, weakness, sweating, nausea and vomiting.

The diagnosis is made primarily on the individual's history supported by evidence from an electrocardiogram (Fig. 12.11) and biochemical tests. As infarcted myocardium breaks down, enzymes are liberated into the bloodstream and these can be measured. The three enzymes most frequently assayed are creatine kinase, lactate dehydrogenase and aspartate aminotransferase. Each enzyme has a particular time course for release from damaged myocardial cells during MI.

The most common causes of sudden death following an MI are ventricular fibrillation, heart block (blockage of electrical conduction in the heart) or asystole (total absence of heartbeat).

DRUG INTERVENTION FOLLOWING MYOCARDIAL INFARCTION

Patients with suspected MI are best transferred to hospital, particularly because the risk of early cardiac arrest makes it crucial to ensure rapid access to a

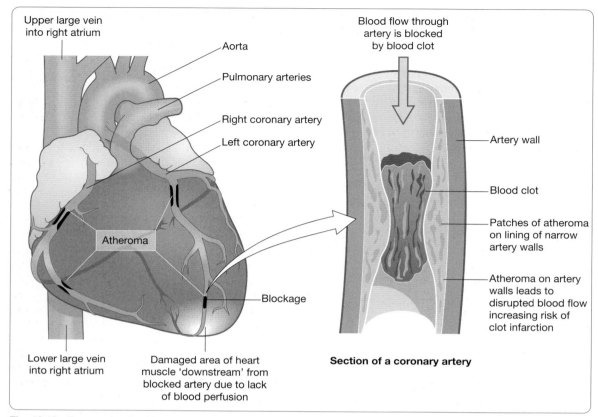

Fig. 12.10 Process involved in a myocardial infarction.

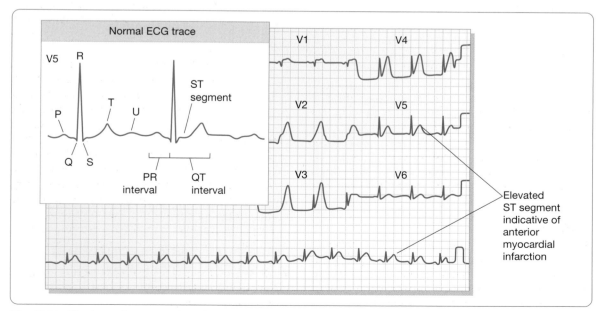

Fig. 12.11 Electrocardiogram tracing of anterior myocardial infarction.

defibrillator. Also, patients should be in a position to receive reperfusion therapy as soon as infarction is confirmed by prompt clinical and electrocardiographic assessment.

The patient should have an intravenous cannula inserted and, to relieve pain and distress, should be given intravenous injections of diamorphine (2.5–5 mg) and an antiemetic (e.g. metoclopramide 10 mg), with further doses if pain persists. Injections should not be given intramuscularly, because this delays pain relief, can increase serum creatine kinase levels and could lead to intramuscular bleeding with thrombolytic therapy. The patient should be given aspirin unless there is a clear contraindication. A single dose of 300 mg of aspirin should be given at the onset of MI. This reduces the risk of death by about 25%. Aspirin irreversibly inhibits cyclo-oxygenase, the main enzyme involved in the synthesis of prostaglandins and ultimately thomboxane, thereby blocking this pathway of platelet aggregation. Aspirin should be continued indefinitely at a dose of 75 mg daily. Clopidogrel should be considered for patients in whom aspirin is contraindicated.

Thrombolysis (see p. 220), in addition to aspirin, can further reduce the risk of death by 20–25%, with the largest benefit seen when given early. Ideally, thrombolytic therapy should be started within 1 h of onset of symptoms.

Beta-blocker therapy should be considered for patients following MI unless there are contraindications. Beta-blockers reduce myocardial ischaemia by lowering blood pressure and heart rate. They could also block arrhythmogenic effects of catecholamines released in acute MI. Beta-blockers have been shown to prolong life following MI by reducing the risk of reinfarction and both supraventricular and ventricular arrhythmias.

Beta-blockade added to ACE inhibitor therapy (see p. 205, 207–209) can also reduce mortality and progression to severe heart failure. Serum cholesterol and low-density lipoprotein (LDL) cholesterol are major risk factors for recurrent cardiac events in patients following MI. Statins (see p. 220) are the drugs of choice for lipid lowering for secondary prevention of CHD following MI.

ANTIPLATELET DRUGS

Arterial thrombosis, such as occurs in coronary thrombosis and strokes, is partly due to an aggregation of platelets that ultimately form plugs in blood vessels. By decreasing platelet aggregation, thrombus formation on the arterial side of the circulation is inhibited (anticoagulants have little effect on arterial

thrombis, and antiplatelet drugs have little effect in venous thromboembolism).

Dipyridamole is used orally as an adjunct to warfarin for prophylaxis of thromboembolism associated with prosthetic heart valves. The dose is 300–600 mg daily in three to four divided doses before food. The most common adverse effects are headache and diarrhoea. Peripheral vasodilatation may result in facial flushing and hypotension.

Aspirin is used in the prophylaxis of cerebrovascular disease or MI; 75–150 mg is given daily. Low-dose aspirin (75 mg daily) is given following bypass surgery. Adverse reactions include gastrointestinal bleeding and bronchospasm. It is contraindicated in children under 16 and in breast-feeding because of the risk of Reye's syndrome.

Clopidogrel is licensed for the prevention of ischaemic events in patients with a history of sympto-matic ischaemic disease. Clopidogrel, in combination with low-dose aspirin, is also licensed for acute coronary syndrome without ST segment elevation; in these circumstances, the combination is given for at least 1 month but usually no longer than 9–12 months. Use of clopidogrel with aspirin increases the risk of bleeding, and there is no evidence of benefit beyond 12 months of the last event of acute coronary syndrome without ST segment elevation.

Glycoprotein IIb/IIIa inhibitors prevent platelet aggregation by blocking the binding of fibrinogen to receptors on platelets. Abciximab is a monoclonal antibody that binds to glycoprotein IIb/IIIa receptors and to other related sites and should be used once only (to avoid additional risk of thrombocytopenia). Eptifibatide and tirofiban also inhibit glycoprotein IIb/IIIa receptors.

The National Institute for Health and Clinical Excellence has recommended (September 2002) that a glycoprotein IIb/IIIa inhibitor (abciximab, eptifibatide, and tirofiban) should be considered in the management of unstable angina or non–ST segment elevation MI. In adddition, a glycoprotein IIb/IIIa inhibitor is recommended for patients at high risk of MI or death when early percutaneous coronary inter-vention is desirable but does not occur immediately; either eptifibatide or tirofiban is recommended in addition to other appropriate drug treatment.

A glycoprotein IIb/IIIa inhibitor is recommended as an adjunct to percutaneous coronary intervention:

- when early percutaneous coronary intervention is indicated but it is delayed
- in patients with diabetes
- if the procedure is complex.

FIBRINOLYTIC DRUGS

Fibrinolytic drugs act as thrombolytics by activating plasminogen to form plasmin, which degrades fibrin and breaks up thrombi. Streptokinase, alteplase (recombinant human tissue-type plasminogen activator), reteplase and tenecteplase are used for the treatment of MI. Alteplase, reteplase and streptokinase need to be given within 12 h of an MI, ideally within 1 h; use after 12 h requires specialist advice. Tenecteplase should be given within 6 h of an MI. Heparin or low molecular weight heparin is used as adjunctive therapy with alteplase, reteplase and tenecteplase to prevent rethrombosis; heparin treatment should be continued for at least 24 h. Antibodies to streptokinase appear after 4 days, and streptokinase should not therefore be used again after this time. Streptokinase is, in addition, indicated for DVT, pulmonary embolism, acute arterial thromboembolism and thrombosed arteriovenous shunts.

The potential for benefit in MI lessens as the delay from onset of major symptoms increases, the value of treatment within the first 12 h being well established. An alternative to streptokinase should be used in patients who have received therapy in the previous 12 months or when an allergic action has occurred.

Streptokinase is an enzyme made by haemolytic streptococci. The initial dose is 250 000 units by intravenous infusion over 30 min in sodium chloride 0.9% solution. The maintenance dose is 100 000 units every hour for 24–72 h. Administration by bolus injections of fibrinolytic drugs such as alteplase, tenecteplase or reteplase by first responders in the community (e.g. GPs and paramedics) can reduce the event to needle time (i.e. the time taken from the onset of an MI to the administration of a fibrinolytic drug), especially in rural locations.

The most common adverse effects are nausea, vomiting and bleeding.

ANTIFIBRINOLYTIC DRUGS AND HAEMOSTATICS

Tranexamic acid has the opposite effect to streptokinase by inhibition of plasminogen activation and fibrinolysis. It is useful in stemming haemorrhage in dental extraction or prostatectomy and in streptokinase overdose.

Aprotinin inhibits the action of plasmin. It is indicated for blood conservation in open heart surgery. A loading dose is given after induction of anaesthesia, and maintained by intravenous infusion until the end of the operation.

LIPID-LOWERING DRUGS

Cardiovascular disease is the most common cause of mortality in the UK. One in four men and one in five women die from CHD. Lowering the concentration of LDL cholesterol and raising high-density lipoprotein cholesterol reduces the progression of coronary atherosclerosis. Lowering total cholesterol by 20–25% (or lowering LDL cholesterol by about 30%) is effective in lowering the risk of atheroma and coronary thrombosis.

Lipoproteins are substances that are composed of fats and proteins and are produced by the liver. The concentration of blood lipoproteins is determined partly by the dietary intake of fats and partly by metabolic processes within the body. There are several ways of lowering lipoprotein levels. These are by decreasing the intake of fats or by reducing absorption or reducing the synthesis of these.

A decrease in the total fat intake and the proportion of saturated (animal) fat to unsaturated (fish and vegetable) fat will reduce plasma cholesterol but requires adherence to a strict diet. Oxidised LDL is highly atherogenic, but naturally occurring anti-oxidants are present in fruit and vegetables and may be protective against CHD. At least five portions of fruit and vegetables daily are recommended.

Statins (e.g. atorvastatin, fluvastatin, pravastatin, rosuvastatin and simvastatin) are the drugs of first choice for treating hypercholesterolaemia. The relative potency per dose varies between these drugs. They block the synthesis of cholesterol in the liver, resulting in a lower blood level. Statin therapy is recommended by NICE (2006) for adults with clinical evidence of CVD. In addition, statin therapy is recommended by NICE as part of the management strategy for the primary prevention of CVD for adults who have a 20% or greater 10-year risk of developing CVD. This level of CVD risk should be estimated using an appropriate risk calculator, or by clinical assessment for people for whom an appropriate risk calculator is not available (e.g. older people, people with diabetes or people in high-risk ethnic groups).

For primary and secondary prevention of CVD, statin treatment should be adjusted to achieve a target total cholesterol concentration of less than 5 mmol/L (or a reduction of 25% if that produces a lower concentration); in terms of LDL cholesterol, the target should be below 3 mmol/L (or a reduction of about 30% if that produces a lower concentration). Increasingly, there is evidence that a cholesterol target even lower than 5 mmol/L may be recommended in future. Liver function tests should be carried out before and within 1–3 months of starting treatment and thereafter at intervals of 6 months for 1 year. Treatment with statins reduces MI, coronary deaths, the risk of stroke and overall mortality rate, and they are the drugs of choice in patients with a high risk of CVD. The statins are well tolerated, and side effects are generally mild and transient. They include headache and gastrointestinal effects. They are taken at night, because cholesterol synthesis is greatest at this time.

Fibrates such as bezafibrate, ciprofibrate, fenofibrate and gemfibrozil lower blood cholesterol and triglycerides, and have been shown to reduce the risk of CHD. Their side effects include nausea, gastric pain, headache, fatigue and rashes.

Anion exchange resins are used in the management of hypercholesterolaemia. Colestyramine and colestipol are examples. They bind to bile acids in the gut, preventing their absorption. This promotes the conversion of cholesterol in the liver to bile acids, effectively reducing LDL cholesterol. However, they may cause abdominal discomfort and diarrhoea.

Ezetimibe inhibits the intestinal absorption of cholesterol. It is used as adjunctive therapy to dietary manipulation in patients with primary hypercholesterolaemia either in combination with a statin or alone (if a statin is inappropriate). It can also be used in patients with familial hypercholesterolaemia or sitosterolaemia. It can cause gastrointestinal disturbances, headache, fatigue and myalgia.

CARDIAC FAILURE

The volume of blood passing through the heart per minute is known as the cardiac output. This output varies considerably depending on the needs of the body, being low at rest and rising with exercise. The healthy heart has a great functional reserve and can cope with the demands for increased output that occur from time to time. In cardiac failure, the cardiac output is reduced (Fig. 12.12). At first, this may be apparent only on exercise, but as the condition progresses it may be insufficient for the needs of the body even at rest. As a result, the tissues and organs receive an inadequate blood supply and therefore insufficient oxygen and nutrients.

Drug therapy can control the symptoms of cardiac failure, but the natural course of the condition is often one of progressive deterioration. Cardiac failure is common, affecting 1–2% of the population, and is becoming more prevalent as older people form a larger part of the population.

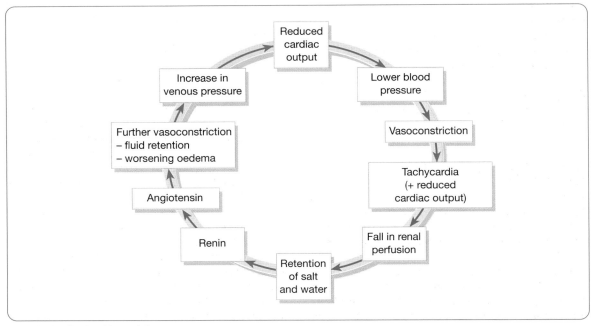

Fig. 12.12   Cycle of heart failure.

Table 12.3   Types of heart failure

Causes	Clinical features
Left heart failure Hypertension Aortic valve disease Coronary artery disease	Those associated with increased venous pressure: • dyspnoea (in acute pulmonary oedema, the patient will also be acutely anxious sweating, pale and very ill-looking) • cough (this may or may not be accompanied by sputum; sputum is generally copious, frothy and tinged with blood) • cyanosis. Those associated with low cardiac output and poor peripheral perfusion: • tiredness • weakness.
Right heart failure Chronic lung disease (e.g. chronic bronchitis) Pulmonary valve disease Congenital defects	These are predominantly the result of increased venous pressure: • raised jugular venous pressure • hepatomegaly, jaundice • anorexia, nausea, vomiting • constipation • peripheral oedema.
Biventricular failure (congestive cardiac failure) Left heart failure	Those associated with left heart failure: • dyspnoea • cough • cyanosis. Those associated with increased venous pressure: • raised jugular venous pressure • hepatomegaly, jaundice • constipation • peripheral oedema. Those associated with insufficient cardiac output: • mental confusion, Cheyne–Stokes respirations • oliguria, proteinuria • fatigue.

TYPES AND CAUSES OF HEART FAILURE

Heart failure is not a diagnosis in itself, rather a 'state' that patients can move into and out of. For example, in otherwise healthy people, a profound anaemia, hyperthyroidism or an overwhelming infection may precipitate heart failure. As these conditions are treated, so the failure will improve. For many patients, however, heart failure exists to a greater or lesser extent as the result of a specific condition, and this will dictate which part of the heart's pumping mechanism is failing and therefore which features present. Table 12.3 summarises the types of heart failure, what causes them to develop and the resulting clinical features. This is based on the kidneys helping to regulate blood pressure through the renin–angiotensin system (see p. 207).

MANAGEMENT OF HEART FAILURE

The aims of management in heart failure are to decrease symptoms, limit progression and prolong survival. Related aims include improving the potential for activity and quality of life.

NON-PHARMACEUTICAL MEASURES

Non-pharmaceutical measures include dietary advice. Because sodium and fluid retention are hallmarks of heart failure, sodium restriction is indicated: salt-rich foods and the addition of salt in cooking or at table should be avoided.

Reducing obesity will reduce the work of the heart, help lower blood pressure and improve the lipid profile. However, stepped changes towards a modest target will have greater success than aiming for large weight loss. In addition, heart failure patients may suffer from malnutrition and muscle wasting. Therefore dietary interventions may require the contribution of a dietician.

Alcohol is absolutely contraindicated in those with alcohol-induced cardiomyopathy. In other patients with heart failure, it should be restricted to small quantities (e.g. one or two units a day). Smoking is harmful and should be stopped if the patient will cooperate.

Rest is an essential element of the management of acute heart failure; however, there is a large body of evidence to suggest that appropriate exercise is beneficial for patients with chronic heart failure.

DRUG MANAGEMENT

The use of ACE inhibitors (see p. 207) is central to the management of heart failure. ACE inhibitors reduce symptoms, mortality rates, hospital admissions and the risk of developing MI in patients with mild to severe heart failure.

All patients with signs of sodium and water retention should be considered for treatment with diuretics to reduce breathlessness and oedema and to improve exercise tolerance. Thiazide diuretics are effective in patients with normal renal function and mild heart failure. Loop diuretics are more effective in older people, in patients with impaired mental function and when heart failure is severe. Digoxin (see p. 192) has long been used to relieve symptoms, increase exercise tolerance and reduce the need for hospital admission due to acute exacerbations in patients with heart failure. It tends to be reserved for patients with atrial fibrillation or those with moderate to severe heart failure who remain symptomatic despite treatment with a diuretic, an ACE inhibitor and a beta-blocker.

In general, because of their negative inotropic effects, beta-blockers can cause worsening of heart failure. However, beta-blockers can reduce mortality when small, carefully titrated doses are added to conventional therapy in patients with stable, mild-to-moderate heart failure. Carvedilol and bisoprolol are both licensed for use in selected patients with heart failure.

While aldosterone is indirectly suppressed by ACE inhibitors, this may be incomplete and transient in some patients. Spironolactone (see p. 196) is a potassium-sparing diuretic but unlike triamterene and amiloride is a direct antagonist of aldosterone. Spironolactone is associated with improved survival and morbidity when added to ACE inhibitor and diuretic therapy.

The use of hydralazine and isosorbide dinitrate combination in heart failure is now reserved for those patients in whom ACE inhibitors or beta-blockers are contraindicated.

STROKE

Stroke is a common condition and, for those who survive, a source of functional disability to varying degrees. The two types of stroke are haemorrhagic stroke and ischaemic stroke.

Some patients experience a minor episode known as a transient ischaemic attack, which lasts for a few minutes or hours; for others, the event is catastrophic, resulting in death or severe disability.

Stroke usually occurs without warning. Occasionally, there may be preceding headache, especially with intracerebral or subarachnoid haemorrhage. Neurological symptoms most often develop within a few minutes, although they can develop in an irregular manner over several hours. Classically, haemorrhage develops rapidly and is associated with headache, vomiting and sometimes clouding of consciousness.

The symptoms that a patient presents with will depend on which part of the brain has been damaged. No one patient is likely to be the same as any other, making predictions as to the likely outcome of the stroke almost impossible to make with any degree of certainty. The basic organisation of the brain differs from one person to the next, and there are differences in the degree to which certain functions are represented in both cerebral hemispheres. This means that if one hemisphere is affected by the stroke, some people will carry on regardless because the other side of the brain can compensate, although others will be severely affected. There are also differences in the ability of individual brains to compensate for localised damage.

The major risk factor for stroke is hypertension. Smoking increases the risk of stroke by around 50%. Cholesterol-lowering using statins reduces the stroke risk by around 25%.

DRUG MANAGEMENT OF STROKE

- All patients should have their blood pressure checked, and hypertension persisting for over 1 month should be treated.
- All patients with ischaemic stroke, not on anticoagulation, should be taking aspirin (75–150 mg) daily or low-dose aspirin and dipyridamole modified release. When patients are aspirin-intolerant, clopidogrel 75 mg daily or

dipyridamole modified release 200 mg twice daily should be used.

- Anticoagulation should be started in every patient with ischaemic stroke who also has atrial fibrillation, unless contraindicated.
- Anticoagulation should not be started until brain imaging has excluded haemorrhage and 12 days have passed from the onset of an acute ischaemic stroke.
- Anticoagulation should not be used after transient ischaemic attacks or minor strokes unless cardiac embolism is suspected.
- Therapy with a statin should be considered for patients following an ischaemic stroke.

SELF-ASSESSMENT QUESTIONS

1. What general health and lifestyle guidance should be given to patients to reduce their risk of coronary artery disease?
2. Describe the main physiological outcome of stimulating β_1 adrenoceptors.
3. How can the outcome (to Qu.2) be modified?
4. How may acute hypotension be treated?
5. What type of drug is ephedrine?

REFERENCES

British Heart Foundation 2006 Statistics database. Online. Available: http://www.heartstats.org June 2006

National Institute for Health and Clinical Excellence 2006 Hypertension: management of hypertension in adults in primary care. NICE, London

FURTHER READING AND RESOURCES

[Anonymous] 2000 Tackling myocardial infarction. Drug and Therapeutics Bulletin 38:17–22

British Cardiac Society, British Hypertension Society, Diabetes UK, Heart UK, Primary Care Cardiovascular Society, Stroke Association 2005 Joint British Societies' guidelines on prevention of cardiovascular disease. Heart 91:v1–v52

Lip GYH, Kamath S 2000 Antiarrhythmic agents. Pharmaceutical Journal 264:659–663

Livingston S 2003 Stroke. Pharmaceutical Journal 271:19–21

National Institute for Clinical Excellence 2003 Management of chronic heart failure in adults in primary and secondary care. NICE, London

National Institute for Health and Clinical Excellence 2006 Statins for the prevention of cardiovascular events. NICE, London

Sani M 2004 Chronic heart failure: diagnosis of the disease. Hospital Pharmacist 11:87–91

Sani M 2004 Chronic heart failure: management of the disease. Hospital Pharmacist 11:92–100

Sani M, Lacey J, Rudd A 2002 The management of stroke. Hospital Pharmacist 9:37–41

Scottish Intercollegiate Guidelines Network 2001 Management of stable angina: a national clinical guideline. SIGN, Edinburgh

Scottish Intercollegiate Guidelines Network 2005 Management of patients with stroke. SIGN, Edinburgh

Smith AJ, Wehner JS, Manley HJ et al. 2001 Current role of beta-adrenergic blockers in the treatment of chronic congestive heart failure. American Journal of Health-System Pharmacists 58:140–145

Stevens M, Williams H 2002 Secondary prevention of heart disease. Pharmaceutical Journal 269:784–786

Topol A, Bijarboneh A, Bakhai A et al. 2001 Myocardial infarction and angina: current drug therapy. Hospital Pharmacist 8:125–132

Williams H 2002 Acute coronary syndromes. Pharmaceutical Journal 269:747–749

Williams H 2003 Arrhythmias: part 1. Pharmaceutical Journal 271:368–370

Williams H, Greenwood E, Paisey J 2003 Arrhythmias: part 2. Pharmaceutical Journal 271:547–549

Williams H, Keaney M 2002 Chronic heart failure. Pharmaceutical Journal 269:25–327

Williams H, McRobbie D, Davies R 2003 Primary prevention of heart disease. Pharmaceutical Journal 270:86–88

Williams H, Stevens M 2002 Stable angina. Pharmaceutical Journal 269:363–365

Williams H, Stevens M 2003 Cholesterol control. Pharmaceutical Journal 270:688–690

Drug treatment of respiratory disorders

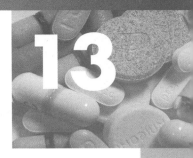

13

CHAPTER CONTENTS

KEY OBJECTIVES

After reading this chapter, you should be able to:

- outline the anatomy and physiology of the respiratory system
- explain the clinical features of asthma
- outline the management of asthma
- explain how the main groups of drugs used to treat asthma work
- explain the clinical features of chronic obstructive pulmonary disease (COPD)
- outline the management of COPD
- explain how the main drugs used in the treatment of COPD work
- explain how to instruct a patient in the use of an inhaler
- explain the indications and function of spacer devices
- describe the care of nebulisers
- describe how to minimise the risks associated with the administration of oxygen.

ANATOMY AND PHYSIOLOGY

The organs of the respiratory system comprise the nose, pharynx, larynx, trachea, bronchi, bronchioles, alveoli and lungs (Fig. 13.1).

The main functions of respiration are to take in oxygen and to give off carbon dioxide. In health, the respiratory epithelium is protected by a mucous blanket of secretions, and ciliary activity ensures that the airways remain clear to allow the transport of gases between the alveoli and the atmosphere. The commonest disorders of the respiratory system are the result of:

- upper respiratory tract infection
- inhaled irritants
- allergens
- intrinsic causes.

Changes to mucus production and cilia lead to cough, while narrowing of the airways produces dyspnoea and, in some cases, wheezing. Depending on the body's capacity to compensate for diminished oxygen intake, the patient may or may not become

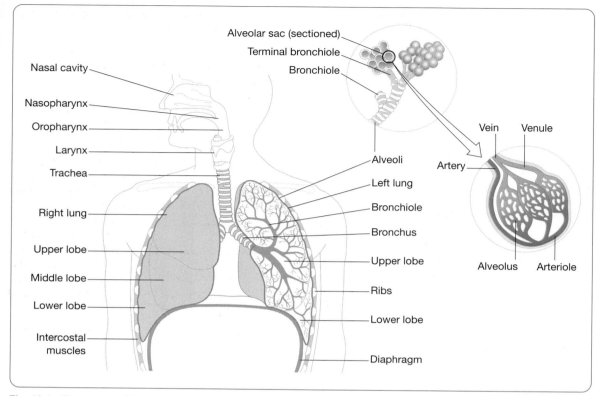

Fig. 13.1 The organs of the respiratory system: the lungs and an alveolus.

cyanosed. Drug treatment is directed primarily towards getting the airways to function normally. A variety of pulmonary function tests assists the doctor in both making a diagnosis and selecting the appropriate drug therapy.

ASTHMA

OVERVIEW

Asthma is a common condition placing a heavy burden on healthcare resources. It has been estimated that 5.1 million people in the UK (1.4 million children and 3.7 million adults) currently receive treatment for asthma (National Asthma Campaign 2001). Most asthma care is provided in primary care. Estimates place the current annual cost of treating asthma within the NHS at £850 million.

People with asthma may suffer from a variety of symptoms, none of which is specific for asthma (British Thoracic Society and Scottish Intercollegiate Guidelines Network 2005). The hallmark of asthma is that these symptoms tend to be:

- wheeze
- shortness of breath
- chest tightness
- cough
- variable
- intermittent
- worse at night
- provoked by triggers, including exercise.

Asthma can be divided into two broad types.

- Early onset, which occurs in childhood or adolescence, is allergy-related and occurs in patients who develop allergic disorders such as eczema or hay fever; there is a strong familial tendency.
- Late onset, which affects older people, has no allergic cause and is often referred to as intrinsic asthma.

Various factors can aggravate both types, and these include dust, tobacco smoke, environmental pollution, rapid changes in humidity or temperature, respiratory tract infection, exercise and stress.

While allergic asthma often resolves after a few years, intrinsic asthma rarely does. Severe acute asthma is a medical emergency clinically recognised by severe wheeze, inability to speak sentences without pausing for breath and a pulse rate over 110 per minute in the adult.

ALLERGIC CONDITIONS

Allergic conditions vary from mild forms of hay fever, skin rashes and eczema to more severe forms such as asthma and anaphylactic shock. Allergens that provoke this response in certain individuals include pollen, animal hair, dust, components of various foods (such as fish and eggs), some food dyes (notably tartrazine), drugs and feathers.

Initial exposure to an allergen inhaled or ingested into the body stimulates the production and release of immunoglobulin E from lymph nodes in atopic individuals. The immunoglobulin E becomes fixed to mast cells (sensitised mast cells), which, on a second exposure to the allergen, causes release of inflammatory mediators including histamine, the cysteinylleukotrienes and prostaglandin D_2.

In allergic asthma, the initial response to allergen provocation occurs abruptly and is due to spasm of the bronchial smooth muscle and results in inflammation with oedema of the bronchial mucosa.

NON-PHARMACOLOGICAL MANAGEMENT

ALLERGEN AVOIDANCE

Allergen avoidance measures may be helpful in reducing the severity of existing disease.

SMOKING CESSATION

Smoking cessation for patients, relatives and carers should be encouraged, as it is good for general health and may decrease asthma severity.

WEIGHT REDUCTION

Weight reduction is recommended in obese patients with asthma to improve asthma control.

PHARMACOLOGICAL MANAGEMENT

The aims of pharmacological management of asthma are the control of symptoms, including nocturnal symptoms and exercise-induced asthma, prevention of exacerbations and the achievement of best pulmonary function with minimal side-effects. Individual patients will have different goals and may also wish to balance these against the potential side-effects or inconvenience of taking the medication necessary to achieve ideal control. In general, control of asthma is assessed against the following:

- minimal symptoms during day and night
- minimal need for reliever medication
- no exacerbation
- no limitation of physical activity
- normal lung function, in practical terms forced expiratory volume in 1 s (FEV_1) and/or peak expiratory flow > 80% predicted or best.

A stepwise approach aims to abolish symptoms as soon as possible and to optimise peak flow by starting treatment at the level most likely to achieve this. Patients should start treatment at the step most appropriate to the initial severity of their asthma. The aim is to achieve early control and to maintain control by stepping up treatment as necessary and stepping down when control is good. Before initiating a new drug therapy, practitioners should check compliance with existing therapies and inhaler technique, and eliminate trigger factors.

Drugs used in the management of asthma include:
- β_2 agonists
- antimuscarinic bronchodilators
- theophylline
- corticosteroids
- cromones
- leukotriene receptor antagonists.

ADMINISTRATION OF DRUGS FOR ASTHMA

Inhalation delivers the drug directly to the airways, requiring a smaller dose than with the oral route, resulting in reduced side effects. Various devices are available for delivering a measured dose (see p. 235). The use of a spacer device may improve drug delivery. Solutions for nebulisation are available for use in acute severe asthma. They are administered over a period of 5–10 min from a nebuliser (see p. 237).

Oral preparations are taken when administration by inhalation is not possible. Systemic side effects occur more frequently when a drug is given orally rather than by inhalation, because of the higher dose required orally. Drugs given by mouth for the treatment of asthma include β_2 agonists, corticosteroids, theophylline and leukotriene receptor antagonists.

In acute severe asthma, drugs such as β_2 agonists, corticosteroids and aminophylline may be given by injection when administration by nebulisation is inadequate or inappropriate.

SELECTIVE β_2 AGONISTS

Mild to moderate symptoms of asthma respond rapidly to the inhalation of a selective short-acting β_2 agonist such as salbutamol. These drugs have a rapid onset of action – about 15 min – and their effects last between 4 and 6 h. They are indicated in step 1 of the advice on the management of acute asthma based on the recommendations of British Thoracic Society and Scottish Intercollegiate Guidelines Network (2005; see p. 232). If β_2-agonist inhalation is required three or more times a week, there should be a move to step 2.

Salmeterol and formoterol are longer-acting β_2 agonists that are administered by inhalation. They are not suitable for relief of an acute asthma attack and are administered as a preventive. β_2 agonists are highly effective at preventing bronchoconstriction when used shortly before exercise or exposure to known allergens. The longer-acting β_2 agonists are included in step 3 (see p. 232) for regular, twice-daily use as second-line controlling treatment in conjunction with a standard dose of inhaled corticosteroid. Dosages of β_2 agonists are shown in Table 13.1.

Table 13.1 β_2 agonists

Drug	Dose
Formoterol	Dry powder for inhalation: 12–24 micrograms twice daily By turbohaler: 6–24 micrograms twice daily
Salbutamol	Aerosol inhalation for persistent symptoms: 100–200 micrograms three or four times daily; for prophylaxis in exercise-induced bronchospasm, 200 micrograms (one or two puffs) Inhalation of powder: 200–400 micrograms for persistent attacks three to four times daily; for prophylaxis of exercise-induced bronchospasm 400 micrograms Inhalation of nebulised solutions: 2.5–5 mg up to four times daily Oral: 2–8 mg three to four times daily
Salmeterol	By inhalation: 50–100 micrograms twice daily
Terbutaline	Inhalation of powder: 500 micrograms up to four times daily Inhalation of nebulised solution: 5–10 mg two to four times daily Oral: 2.5–5 mg three times daily

Mode of action. β_2 agonists act by directly stimulating β_2 receptors in the smooth muscle of the airways, producing bronchodilation. They also stabilise mast cells, preventing release of inflammatory mediators and histamine on exposure to allergens.

Side-effects. Only small doses of β_2 agonists are required by the inhalation route. In this way, side-effects are minimised. Side-effects may occur with the much higher doses required by the oral route and include fine tremor in the hands or headaches.

CORTICOSTEROIDS
Inhaled corticosteroids

Inhaled corticosteroids are the mainstay of preventive therapy in asthma. Inhaled steroids are best started at high dose and reduced as control is achieved. High-dose steroids via metered dose inhalers should be taken through spacers (see p. 236).

Mode of action. Inhaled corticosteroids act by inhibiting a variety of inflammatory agents, reducing inflammatory aspects of asthma and decreasing bronchospasm.

Inhaled corticosteroids are also recommended for prophylactic treatment of asthma when patients are using a β_2 agonist more than once daily. Corticosteroid inhalers must be used regularly to obtain maximum benefit; alleviation of symptoms usually occurs 3–7 days after initiation. Beclometasone dipropionate, budesonide and fluticasone propionate appear to be equally effective. If a patient is using a β_2 agonist inhaler and a corticosteroid inhaler concurrently, the β_2 agonist should be inhaled first, as the resulting bronchorelaxation will result in a more effective dose of corticosteroid.

Patients who have been taking long-term oral corticosteroids can often be transferred to an inhaled corticosteroid, but the transfer must be slow, with gradual reduction in the dose of oral corticosteroid and at a time when the asthma is well controlled. High-dose inhalers are available for patients who respond only partially to standard dose inhalers.

Systemic therapy may be necessary during episodes of infection or if asthma is worsening, when higher doses are needed and access of inhaled drug to small airways may be reduced.

Side-effects of corticosteroids. Because of the much smaller dose administered, inhaled corticosteroids have considerably fewer systemic effects than oral corticosteroids, but adverse effects have been reported, including a small increased risk of glaucoma with prolonged high doses of inhaled corticosteroids; cataracts have also been reported with inhaled corticosteroids. Higher doses of inhaled corticosteroids may induce adrenal suppression, and patients on high doses should be given a steroid card (see Ch. 16).

Bone mineral density is reduced following long-term inhalation of higher doses of corticosteroids, and this may predispose patients to osteoporosis (see Ch. 16).

Patients on inhaled steroids should wash out the mouth and teeth after treatment to reduce the occurrence of fungal infection. Use of a large-volume spacer device may be helpful for those experiencing side effects.

Oral corticosteroids

Acute attacks of asthma should be treated with short courses of oral corticosteroids starting with a high dose, for example prednisolone 40–50 mg daily for at least 5 days. Patients whose asthma has deteriorated rapidly usually respond quickly to corticosteroids. The dose can usually be stopped abruptly in a mild exacerbation of asthma. When patients take long-term steroids (greater than 7.5 mg daily for more than 3 months), side effects may be experienced: indigestion, water retention, muscle weakness, signs of diabetes, hypertension, depression and cataracts.

ANTIMUSCARINIC BRONCHODILATORS

Ipratropium can provide short-term relief in chronic asthma, but short-acting β_2 agonists act more quickly and are preferred. Ipratropium by nebulisation may be added to other standard treatment in life-threatening asthma or when acute asthma fails to improve with standard therapy.

Antimuscarinic bronchodilators are regarded as being more effective in relieving bronchoconstriction associated with chronic obstructive pulmonary disease (COPD, see pp. 231–234) than in relieving asthma.

THEOPHYLLINE

Theophylline is a bronchodilator used for reversible airways obstruction. It may have an additive effect when used in conjunction with small doses of β_2 agonists. The bronchodilatory effect of theophylline has been used for many years in the treatment of patients with persistent symptoms. Theophylline is indicated in step 3 of the British Thoracic Society and Scottish Intercollegiate Guidelines Network (2005) guideline as an addition in patients taking high-dose (800 micrograms daily) inhaled corticosteroids whose asthma is still uncontrolled following a trial of a long-acting β_2 agonist. Patients who suffer from nocturnal asthma may benefit from slow-release preparations of theophylline, as these can provide therapeutic plasma concentrations overnight.

Theophylline acts by inhibiting the enzyme phosphodiesterase in bronchial muscle, causing it to relax and thus relieve bronchospasm. Theophylline may also have an anti-inflammatory effect and may therefore be of benefit when used in combination with inhaled corticosteroids, providing an alternative to increasing the dosage of corticosteroids in suitable patients.

Theophylline has a narrow margin between the therapeutic and the toxic dose. In most patients, a plasma theophylline concentration of 10–20 mg/L is usually required for satisfactory bronchodilation. A dose of theophylline of 125–250 mg three or four times daily is given after food. However, theophylline modified-release preparations are usually able to produce adequate plasma concentrations for up to 12 h. When given as a single dose at night, they have a useful role in controlling nocturnal asthma and early morning wheezing.

Theophylline is given by injection as aminophylline: a mixture of theophylline with ethylenediamine, which is 20 times more soluble than theophylline alone. Aminophylline must be given by *very slow* intravenous injection (over at least 20 min); it is too irritant for intramuscular use.

Intravenous aminophylline has a role in the treatment of severe attacks of asthma that do not respond rapidly to a nebulised β_2 agonist. Measurement of plasma theophylline concentration may be helpful and is essential if aminophylline is to be given to patients who have been taking oral theophylline preparations, because serious side effects such as convulsions and arrhythmias can occasionally precede other symptoms of toxicity.

Side-effects. Side-effects can occur within the 10–20 mg/L plasma theophylline concentration, but their frequency and severity increase at concentrations above 20 mg/L. These include nausea, insomnia and palpitations. These may be the initial signs of toxicity, and the patient should be referred to the doctor as soon as possible.

Metabolism/drug interactions. Theophylline is metabolised in the liver; there is considerable variation in its half-life, particularly in smokers, in patients with hepatic impairment or heart failure, or if certain drugs are taken concurrently. The half-life is *increased* in heart failure, cirrhosis, viral infections and in the elderly, and by drugs such as cimetidine, ciprofloxacin, furosemide, calcium-channel blockers, erythromycin, fluvoxamine and oral contraceptives. The half-life is *decreased* in smokers and in chronic alcoholism, and by drugs such as phenytoin, carbamazepine, rifampicin and barbiturates.

These differences in half-life are important because theophylline has a narrow margin between the therapeutic and toxic dose, and will necessitate a reduction or an increase in dosage in order to maintain the plasma level between 10 and 20 mg/L. Conversely, if a smoker decides to quit, the effect of the theophylline dose may be increased.

LEUKOTRIENE RECEPTOR ANTAGONISTS

Cysteinyl leukotrienes cause potent stimulation of bronchial smooth muscle, release of eosinophils and production of secretions in the airways. Leukotriene receptor antagonists block these effects, relieving smooth muscle bronchoconstriction and preventing inflammation.

Montelukast and zafirlukast are indicated for the prophylaxis of asthma. They are also useful in preventing exercise-induced asthma and aspirin-sensitive asthma.

The dose for montelukast is 10 mg daily at bedtime and for zafirlukast is 20 mg twice daily.

Side-effects appear to be mild but include gastrointestinal disturbances.

CROMONES

The cromones consist of sodium cromoglicate and nedocromil sodium. The cromones improve symptom control in mild to moderate asthma but are less effective than corticosteroids and have therefore been superseded by inhaled steroids, and their use in practice has declined.

Cromones inhibit the release of substances from mast cells responsible for bronchospasm by causing mast cell stabilisation, and are therefore referred to as mast cell stabilisers. Both cromoglicate and nedocromil reduce allergen-induced early- and late-phase responses to immunological stimuli, and they inhibit bronchospasm during and after exercise and exposure to cold or dry air. They tend to be more effective in patients with mild atopic asthma, in particular children with exercise- or allergen-induced asthma.

Because of their short duration of action and four times daily dosing, compliance with therapy can be a problem. However, cromones are well tolerated and rarely cause adverse effects.

STEPWISE MANAGEMENT

The steps involved in the management of asthma in adults are illustrated in Figure 13.2.

STEPPING DOWN

Stepping down treatment once asthma is controlled is recommended but often not implemented, leaving some patients overtreated. Regular review of patients as treatment is stepped down is important. When deciding which drug to step down first and at what rate the severity of asthma, the side-effects of the treatment, the beneficial effect achieved and the patient's preference should all be taken into account.

Patients should be maintained at the lowest possible dose of inhaled steroid. Reduction in inhaled steroid dose should be slow, as patients deteriorate at different rates. Reductions should be considered every 3 months, decreasing the dose by approximately 25–50% each time.

CHRONIC OBSTRUCTIVE PULMONARY DISEASE

INTRODUCTION

Chronic obstructive pulmonary disease is a major cause of morbidity and is the fifth major cause of death in the UK (Calverly and Bellamy 2000). The long-term and progressive nature of COPD means that it imposes a devastating burden on the patient's health status and emotional well-being, as well as on the NHS as a whole, because patients with COPD may be seen frequently in both primary and secondary care. The estimated annual cost of COPD to the NHS is just short of £1 billion, up to half of which may arise from hospitalisations alone (National Institute for Clinical Excellence 2004).

Chronic obstructive pulmonary disease is a chronic disease of the lungs, characterised by airflow obstruction. Most commonly, although not exclusively affecting smokers, there is a progressive decline in lung function leading to increasing breathlessness, particularly on exertion. Significant airflow obstruction may be present before the individual is aware of it. COPD is now the preferred term for the conditions in patients with airflow obstruction who were previously diagnosed as having chronic bronchitis or emphysema.

Chronic bronchitis refers to chronic mucus hypersecretion caused by inflammation in the large airways (usually due to cigarette smoke), leading to proliferation of mucus-producing cells in the respiratory epithelium. The result is a chronic productive cough and frequent respiratory infections. Emphysema is a pathological process in which there is destruction of the terminal bronchioles and distal airspaces. This

Step 5: continuous or frequent use of oral steroids
- Use daily steroid tablet in lowest dose providing adequate control.
- Maintain high-dose inhaled steroid at 2000 micrograms/day.
- Consider other treatments to minimise the use of steroid tablets.
- Refer patient to specialist care.

Step 4: poor control on moderate dose of inhaled steroid and add-on therapy: addition of 4th drug

Consider trials of:
- Increasing inhaled steroid up to 2000 micrograms/day (beclometasone or equivalent).
- Addition of a 4th drug, e.g. leukotriene receptor antagonist, slow release theophylline, β_2 agonist tablet.

Step 3: add-on therapy
- Add inhaled long-acting β_2 agonist (LABA).
- Assess control of asthma:
  - Good response to LABA – continue LABA.
  - Benefit from LABA but control still inadequate – continue LABA and increase inhaled steroid to 800 micrograms/day (if not already on this dose).
  - No response to LABA – stop LABA and increase inhaled steroid to 800 micrograms/day. If control still inadequate, institute a trial of other therapies, e.g. leukotriene receptor antagonist or slow-release theophylline.

Step 2: introduction of regular preventer therapy

Add inhaled corticosteroid, 200 to 800 micrograms/day (beclometasone or equivalent).

Inhaled steroids should be prescribed for patients with recent exacerbations, nocturnal asthma, impaired lung function or inhaled β_2 agonist 3 times a week or more.

Start at dose of inhaled steroid appropriate to severity of disease.

400 micrograms/day is an appropriate dose for many patients.

Initially give dose twice daily. Titrate the dose of inhaled steroid to the lowest dose at which effective control of asthma is maintained.

Beclometasone 200 micrograms $\equiv$ budesonide 200 micrograms fluticasone $\equiv$ 100 micrograms.

Step 1: mild intermittent asthma

Inhaled short-acting β_2 agonist as required.

Fig. 13.2 Stepwise management of asthma in adults.

leads to a loss of alveolar surface area and therefore the impairment of gas exchange (see Fig. 13.3).

DIAGNOSIS

A diagnosis of COPD should be considered in patients over the age of 35 who have a risk factor (generally smoking) and who present with exertional breathlessness, chronic cough, regular sputum production, frequent winter 'bronchitis' or wheeze. The presence of airflow obstruction should be confirmed by performing spirometry. Increasingly, nurses are trained in the use of a spirometer, which measures airflow obstruction. The patient blows into the spirometer until the lungs are completely empty. Two measurements are taken: the FEV_1 and the FVC (forced vital capacity). Airflow obstruction is confirmed if FEV_1 is < 80% predicted and the FEV_1:forced vital capacity ratio < 80% (Fig. 13.4). As well as confirming the diagnosis of COPD, spirometry gives a measure of the severity of airflow obstruction (see Table 13.2).

NON-PHARMACOLOGICAL MANAGEMENT

Normally, FEV_1 declines with age. In smokers who are susceptible to COPD, this decline is accelerated. In those who stop smoking, this rate of decline slows to that expected in a non-smoker. Stopping smoking is therefore the single most important way of affecting outcome in patients at all stages of COPD, whether severe or at earlier stages of the disease. Although the lost function cannot be restored, those who stop smoking will deteriorate more slowly.

If the basal metabolic index is low, patients should be given nutritional supplements to increase their total calorific intake and be encouraged to take exercise to augment the effects of nutritional supplementation. Pulmonary rehabilitation should be offered to all patients who consider themselves functionally disabled by COPD (not suitable for patients, for example, who are unable to walk or have unstable angina).

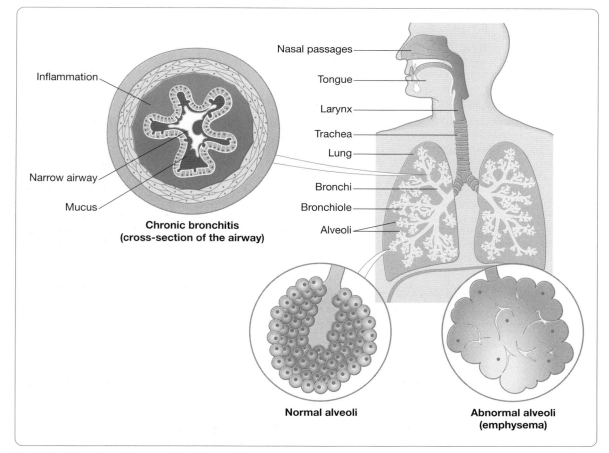

Inflammation
Narrow airway
Mucus
**Chronic bronchitis
(cross-section of the airway)**

Nasal passages
Tongue
Larynx
Trachea
Lung
Bronchi
Bronchiole
Alveoli

Normal alveoli

Abnormal alveoli
(emphysema)

Fig. 13.3   Normal and abnormal physiology of the lungs.

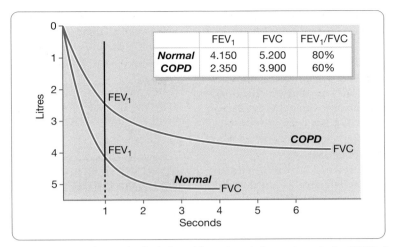

Fig. 13.4 Example of spirometric tracing and calculation of forced expiratory volume in 1 s (FEV$_1$), forced vital capacity (FVC) and FEV$_1$/FVC ratio.

Table 13.2 Signs and symptoms of chronic obstructive pulmonary disease relating to severity

Category of chronic obstructive pulmonary disease	Forced expiratory volume in 1 s	Symptoms and signs
Mild	60–80	No abnormal signs Smoker's cough Little or no breathlessness
Moderate	40–59	Breathlessness (± wheeze) on moderate exertion Cough (± sputum) Variable abnormal signs (general reduction in breath sounds, presence of wheeze)
Severe	< 40	Wheeze and cough often prominent Lung overinflation usual; cyanosis, peripheral oedema and polycythaemia in advanced disease, especially during exacerbation

Pulmonary rehabilitation is a programme of exercise reconditioning, a multidisciplinary intervention aimed at maximising physical and social functioning for patients with chronic lung disease. Exercise training is the core component, but education on the disease and its treatment is often provided. Pulmonary rehabilitation has been shown to improve exercise capacity and quality of life and to reduce breathlessness (Lacasse et al. 2002).

Pneumococcal vaccination (once only) and an annual influenza vaccination should be offered to all patients with COPD.

PHARMACOLOGICAL MANAGEMENT

As with the initial diagnosis of COPD, spirometry plays a key role in individualising treatment to a patient's response.

BRONCHODILATORS

Bronchodilator drugs reduce airway smooth muscle tone and increase airway calibre.

Short-acting β$_2$ agonists

Short-acting inhaled β$_2$ agonists (e.g. salbutamol, terbutaline) are the most commonly used bronchodilators. They are best used as required for symptom relief (see p. 228).

Long-acting β₂ agonists

The advantage of long-acting β₂ agonists (formoterol and salmeterol) is that they produce a sustained relaxation of the airway for approximately 12 h. Long-acting formoterol lasting 24 h has been introduced.

Antimuscarinic bronchodilators

The inhaled antimuscarinic bronchodilator ipratropium is at least as effective as short-acting inhaled β₂ agonists in the short term at relieving symptoms and improving lung function. It differs, however, in having a slower onset of action (approximately 30 min) and a more sustained bronchodilatory effect (up to 8 h).

Tiotropium is a longer-acting antimuscarinic with a duration of action of approximately 24 h. As a result, it requires only once-a-day administration (hard capsules of powder for inhalation using the HandiHaler device). It has been shown to significantly reduce dyspnoea, improve exercise capacity and reduce exacerbation frequency in COPD patients (Casaburi et al. 2002, Celli et al. 2003, O'Donnell et al. 2004).

Antimuscarinics are specific antagonists to muscarinic receptors. They inhibit muscarinic-induced bronchoconstriction.

The dosages of antimuscarinics are given in Table 13.3.

Side effects. Dry mouth can be experienced.

Table 13.3 Dosages of antimuscarinics

Drug	Dose
Ipratropium	Aerosol inhalation: 20–80 micrograms three to four times daily Inhalation of powder: 40 micrograms three to four times daily Inhalation of nebulised solution: 100–500 micrograms up to four times daily
Tiotropium	Inhalation of powder 18 micrograms once daily

CORTICOSTEROIDS

There is no evidence of benefit on lung function from corticosteroids. However, they may reduce the occurrence of exacerbations.

LONG-TERM OXYGEN THERAPY

Oxygen is given to patients with more advanced disease who are chronically hypoxaemic.

ADMINISTRATION OF INHALED DRUGS

The fact that drugs can be introduced directly into the pulmonary system is highly advantageous. Not only is their absorption through the lungs rapid, but also high concentrations of drugs can be obtained in the bronchial mucosa and smooth muscle with minimal systemic side-effects. Inhaled drugs are available in the form of a spray (wet), a powder (dry) or a gas. Some drugs are inhaled via the mouth, some via the nose and some through both mouth and nose. The appliances used include:

- handheld inhaler, with or without any additional device
- nebuliser
- face mask
- nasal cannulae.

INHALER DEVICES

PRESSURISED METERED DOSE INHALERS

HOW THEY WORK

Most commonly, drugs are delivered to the lungs as sprays from pressurised metered dose inhalers. The drug and an inert propellant, such as freon, are maintained under pressure in a small canister. When the valve is activated, a measured quantity of propellant carrying the drug is released through the mouthpiece.

ADMINISTRATION

Maximum benefit is obtained by the patient only when the proper technique of inhalation is used. It has been estimated that 30% of adults and 80% of children have difficulties with aerosol inhalers. The problems include coordinating activation and inhalation, too rapid inspiration and too short breath holding after inspiration (Price 1997). Difficulties arise because:

- patients are not always adequately taught to use the devices prescribed
- the technique is difficult for some patients to master
- patients who are competent often develop poor technique, and need reassessment and education.

INHALER TECHNIQUE

Counselling the patient on proper technique is vitally important, with periodic checks to ensure that efficiency is being maintained (Howard 2005). Instruction in inhaler technique takes time. Oral instruction should be backed up by demonstration using a placebo inhaler and by written guidelines. Although technique will have some bearing, it does not necessarily relate to clinical effectiveness. In one study, of 2467 patients, teaching improved the correct usage score from a mean of 60% to 79% (Scottish Intercollegiate Guidelines Network 2005).

First, the cover should be removed from the mouthpiece and the inhaler shaken vigorously. With the inhaler held upright, the patient breathes out gently and then places the mouthpiece in the mouth and closes the lips around it. The patient should breathe in through the mouth, press the canister to release the medication and continue to breathe in steadily and deeply. The breath is held while the inhaler is removed from the mouth and should continue to be held for as long as is comfortable. The patient should breathe out slowly. If a second puff is to be taken, the inhaler should be kept upright and, after a pause of 0.5–1 min, the procedure repeated. On completion, the cover is replaced. People lacking the necessary power to depress the canister may find it easier to use both hands.

The dose delivered from the inhaler can be seen as a fine mist. If any can be seen escaping from the mouth or nose, the inhaler is not being used correctly. In patients with an ideal technique, only about 12% of the dose enters the lungs (Fig. 13.5). Although this is only a tiny fraction of the oral dose, it is enough to be effective. The remainder of the dose lands on the tongue or the back of the throat and is swallowed, but in such a small quantity that it has no systemic effect.

SPACER DEVICES

In certain situations, spacer devices are particularly useful, for example in:

- patients with poor inhalation technique
- patients requiring higher doses
- children
- patients susceptible to candidiasis with inhaled corticosteroids.

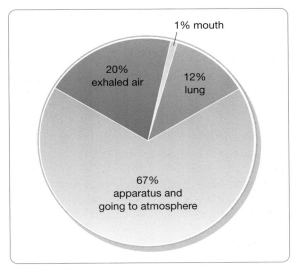

Fig. 13.5   Destinations of an inhaled 'dose'.

A spacer device attached to a metered dose inhaler improves dose delivery to 15%. The device must be compatible with the metered dose inhaler. Spacer devices provide a space between the inhaler and the mouth, so allowing for a reduction in the velocity of the aerosol. There is thus less impaction of particles on the oropharynx and this, together with the greater time for evaporation of the propellant, results in a larger proportion of particles reaching the lungs. The drug should be administered by repeated single actuations of the metered dose inhaler into the spacer, each followed by inhalation. In utilising a spacer device, coordination of inspiration and actuation of the aerosol is less important. It is important, however, that the patient inhales as soon as possible after actuation, because the aerosolised drug is short-lived. The pressurised aerosol is activated at one end of the spacer device, and the patient breathes in through a one-way valve at the other. On expiration, the valve returns to the closed position and a hole in the mouthpiece allows the escape of gas that prevents rebreathing and build-up of carbon dioxide. Spacer devices range in size from the Aerochamber Plus, a medium-volume device, to the Volumatic (Fig. 13.6) and the Nebuhaler, much larger devices.

Patients who are prescribed a spacer for the first time should be treated in the usual way and monitored for worsening symptoms or adverse effects.

Spacer device care

Large-volume spacer devices should be washed in soapy water, rinsed and allowed to dry naturally on a

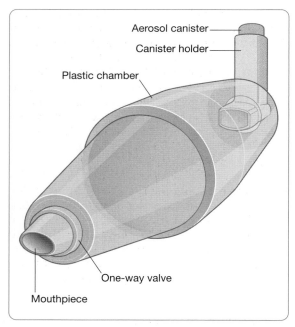

Fig. 13.6 The Volumatic device.

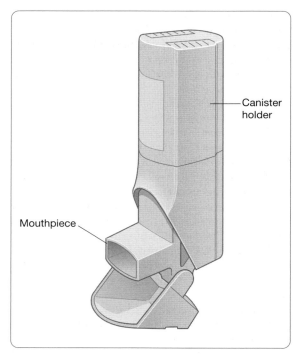

Fig. 13.7 The breath-actuated Easi-Breathe.

monthly basis. The mouthpiece should be wiped with an alcohol wipe. An electrostatic charge may be set up by wiping with a cloth or paper, which could interfere with delivery of the drug. The spacer device should be replaced after 12 months, but some may need to be changed at 6 months.

BREATH-ACTUATED INHALER

For those who cannot coordinate aerosol inhalation, several alternative methods of administration are available. The breath-actuated inhaler, when used correctly, is automatically activated by breathing in. An example is the Easi-Breathe (Fig. 13.7).

DRY POWDER INHALERS

Examples of dry powder inhalers include the Turbohaler (e.g. terbutaline and budesonide) and the Accuhaler (salbutamol and fluticasone).

PATIENT EDUCATION

Compliance is more likely to be achieved if the patient is well informed. The patient should know:

- how to use and care for the inhaler
- the dose to be taken
- the time interval
- the maximum number of inhalations that should be taken in 24 h.

Aerosol inhalers are easily carried in the pocket or handbag, helping the patient to be independent. Nurses supervising patients using this type of device should discreetly observe patients' inhaling techniques but avoid giving any impression of hurrying them in the process. The patient needs to concentrate on what he is doing at this time and so cannot engage in conversation.

More cooperation can be achieved if the patient is informed about the disease, the purpose of the therapy, how to recognise deterioration in his condition and what to do if deterioration is suspected.

It is the responsibility of doctors, nurses, pharmacists and physiotherapists to promote understanding of the technique involved by teaching, demonstrating and checking the patient's performance at intervals. On this basis, alterations in the choice of device may be made so that the patient derives maximum benefit.

NEBULISERS

For the treatment of acute breathlessness and wheeze in patients with airflow obstruction, for example COPD and asthma, the method of choice for administering bronchodilator drugs is by inhalation via a nebuliser. This route is particularly useful for patients in respiratory distress (e.g. emergency treatment of asthma) or who are unable to inhale properly. The aim of nebuliser therapy is to deliver a therapeutic dose of the desired drug as an aerosol in the form of respirable particles within a fairly short period of time, usually 5–10 min. Nebuliser solutions contain the same type of active ingredients as those used in an aerosol inhaler. However, the doses used are up to 25 times greater than those in inhalers, which is why the nebuliser is used in states of acute bronchoconstriction.

HOW THEY WORK

A nebuliser is an apparatus for converting a liquid into a fine spray. A high-pressure gas source is used to suck up the bronchodilator solution from a reservoir. The particles of drug produced impinge on a baffle. Particles of the correct size, i.e. small enough to reach the bronchioles and, in some cases, the alveoli, pass on and are breathed in by the patient via a face mask, while larger particles fall back to be nebulised again (Fig. 13.8).

Because a nebuliser has a 'dead space', a quantity of respirator solution has to be nebulised to fill this space before the particles start to leave the nebuliser and achieve a therapeutic effect. Depending on the design of the nebuliser, this volume of solution should be at least 2 mL and, for the nebuliser to

function efficiently (i.e. 80% of the drug to reach the patient), it must have a starting volume of fluid of not less than 4 mL. In order to achieve this volume, sufficient diluent must be added to the bronchodilator solution(s). Sterile sodium chloride 0.9% w/v is chosen, because it is isotonic, non-irritant and compatible with commercially available bronchodilator solutions; 25-mL sachets of sodium chloride 0.9% solution are available for this purpose. Water would result in hypotonic solutions, which may cause bronchoconstriction.

An increasing number of drugs are given by this route, with the result that more than one agent may be required for the treatment of any patient at one time. The question of stability of drug admixtures in this situation may therefore arise. Drugs can be mixed when there is evidence of compatibility as stated in the relevant data sheet (Harriman and Purcell 1996) otherwise, as a general principle, drugs should not be mixed.

TYPICAL DRUG REGIMENS

Solutions required for administration via a wet nebuliser are:

- β_2-adrenoceptor stimulant respirator solution made up to 4 mL with sodium chloride 0.9% solution *or*
- antimuscarinic bronchodilator solution made up to 4 mL with sodium chloride 0.9% solution *or*
- a combination of β_2-adrenoceptor stimulant and antimuscarinic bronchodilator solutions.

It is common practice in patients receiving a combination of β_2-adrenoceptor stimulant and antimuscarinic bronchodilator solutions for the drugs to be mixed in the same nebuliser and administered concurrently. Other combinations of drugs should not be mixed without consulting the pharmacy.

Nebulised drugs are normally administered 4-hourly. In severe cases of airways obstruction, however, provided that pulmonary function tests show reversibility of the obstruction to be possible, the frequency may be increased to 2-hourly or even hourly. When the obstruction is irreversible, artificial ventilation must be begun.

THE CARRIER GAS

The carrier gas used may be either compressed air or oxygen. The choice of air or oxygen, however, depends on each individual patient's clinical status.

Oxygen. Oxygen must not be used for patients with COPD and carbon dioxide retention. In such cases, air must be used. Oxygen may be used for asthmatics and some patients with COPD but must

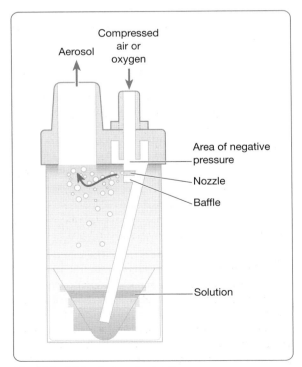

Fig. 13.8 Wet nebuliser (in detail).

Aerosol

Compressed air or oxygen

Area of negative pressure

Nozzle

Baffle

Solution

be prescribed indicating the flow rate in L/min as well as the percentage of oxygen to be used. When the prescribed driving gas is oxygen, a piped supply should be used wherever possible. Patients receiving controlled oxygen should have the prescribed flow rate re-established following nebulisation.

Air. Air is supplied via a portable air compressor or a medical air cylinder. It should be used for patients with chronic bronchitis and evidence of carbon dioxide retention. The use of air in patients with respiratory failure without carbon dioxide retention will aggravate their hypoxia.

ADMINISTRATION

Patients who are to receive nebulised drugs should preferably be in the sitting position, either in bed or in a chair. By a gentle approach, the nurse can encourage the patient to relax. The patient should be advised to breathe through the mouth.

Face masks should be close-fitting. Mouthpieces rather than face masks should be considered in elderly patients susceptible to glaucoma and those using high doses of antimuscarinic drugs. They should also be used for nebulised steroids to prevent deposition on the face.

As with the administration of any medicine, the patient is identified, the prescription carefully read and the expiry date on the respiratory solution checked. When a multidose bottle is being used, it must be discarded 1 month after opening. The nurse should therefore record the date opened on any container used.

Sachets of sodium chloride 0.9% solution used to give the necessary volume to the bronchodilator solution may be used for more than one patient during a medicine round but must be discarded immediately thereafter.

The required amount of each solution used is drawn up using a sterile syringe and needle to avoid bacterial contamination. However, as there is no patient contact there is no need to change the syringe and needle when drawing up the same drug for use in a number of patients.

To produce particles of the correct size, a minimum flow rate of 6 L/min is required. This flow rate will deliver at least 65% of the droplets in a size that enables drug penetration into the distal airways. During nebulisation, it is helpful to tap the nebuliser periodically so that large droplets may be shaken down and to ensure maximum delivery of the drug. Optimal nebulisation of 4 mL takes 5–10 min. A proportion of respirator solution (approximately 0.5 mL) will remain in the nebuliser chamber.

NEBULISER CARE

After each use, the nebuliser chamber and mask should be washed in hot, soapy water, rinsed thoroughly and dried using a paper towel to reduce the risk of bacterial contamination and prevent a build-up of crystallised drug in the nebuliser. The inner tubing should be washed once a week in hot soapy water and dried by attaching it to the gas supply for about 3–4 min. If the patient has a chest infection, then nebuliser, tubing and mask should be changed every week.

PORTABLE NEBULISERS

A portable nebuliser unit is designed to allow greater mobility and independence, and is therefore suitable for use by patients at home. The unit consists of an electrically driven compressor that provides clean breathable air, nebuliser, mask, mouthpiece, supply tube and filters. In addition, a 12-V connection cable and adapter are available for operating the unit from a car, boat or caravan.

PEAK FLOW METERS

Peak flow meters are used in helping to diagnose airflow obstruction, as in COPD and asthma, and in measuring the effectiveness of treatment prescribed for the individual patient.

Peak flow or the peak expiratory flow rate is the maximum flow of air achievable while breathing out as hard as possible. It is an indication of how wide the airways are at the time the measurement is taken. The speed of air passing through the meter is measured in L/min and will vary according to sex, age and height (see Table 13.4). Peak flow readings are usually higher in men than in women. Peak flow varies throughout the day, and the morning reading is often lower than that of the evening. It is the difference between these two readings that is important. When asthma is out of control, great swings occur, with the morning readings being much lower and the evening readings much higher than normal.

TYPES OF PEAK FLOW METER

Mini-Wright and Vitalograph peak flow meters are available on prescription. The use of peak flow meters is the same whichever type is used. The marker is first set to zero. Those able to stand to use the meter are advised to do so. Patients may be taught how to make an accurate recording of peak flow. Some patients may be instructed as to what action to take in the event of a low reading. Readings should be taken at the same time every morning and evening, and a careful record kept to show to their doctor at the outpatient clinic.

Table 13.4 Table of predicted peak flow (litres/min)*

Height	Age									
	25	30	35	40	45	50	55	60	65	70
Males										
5'3" (160 cm)	572	560	548	536	524	512	500	488	476	464
5'6" (167 cm)	597	584	572	559	547	534	522	509	496	484
5'9" (175 cm)	625	612	599	586	573	560	547	533	520	507
6'0" (183 cm)	654	640	626	613	599	585	572	558	544	530
6'3" (191 cm)	679	665	650	636	622	608	593	579	565	551
Female										
4'9" (144 cm)	377	366	356	345	335	324	314	303	293	282
5'0" (152 cm)	403	392	382	371	361	350	340	329	319	308
5'3" (160 cm)	433	422	412	401	391	380	370	359	349	338
5'6" (167 cm)	459	448	438	427	417	406	396	385	375	364
5'9" (175 cm)	489	478	468	457	447	436	426	415	405	394

Standard deviation: 60 min. Negligible ethnic variation
*A severe asthmatic attack is recognised when the peak expiratory flow is less than 40% of the predicted peak flow.
(Figures produced by the National Asthma Campaign.)

ANTIHISTAMINES

Antihistamines compete with histamine and block its action at histamine receptor sites. They do not reverse histamine effects once established. Some antihistamines have antiemetic properties.

USAGE

Antihistamines are used in the treatment of allergic skin rashes, nasal allergy (particularly the seasonal type, e.g. hay fever), pruritus, insect bites and stings, drug allergies and anaphylactic shock (see pp. 152–153), and for the prevention of urticaria and motion sickness.

DRUGS USED IN THIS GROUP

Non-sedating antihistamines such as acrivastine, cetirizine, desloratidine, fexofenadine, levocetirizine, loratadine and mizolastine cause less sedation than the older antihistamines, because they penetrate the blood–brain barrier only to a slight extent. All older antihistamines cause sedation. These include alimemazine, clemastine, chlorphenamine, hydroxyzine and promethazine.

Formulation and dosage. Most antihistamines are available only in the oral form. Following oral administration, symptomatic relief of allergic reactions and side effects may begin within 15–30 min, lasting for 3–6 h.

Chlorphenamine and promethazine are also available as injections to treat severe conditions. Chlorphenamine can be administered by subcutaneous or intramuscular injection (10–20 mg) or by slow intravenous injection (10–20 mg) over 1 min.

Side-effects include influence on the central nervous system, namely drowsiness (may affect the ability to drive or operate machinery), headaches and dulling of mental alertness. With newer antihistamines, there are greatly reduced sedative and psychomotor impairment effects. Antimuscarinic effects such as urinary retention, dry mouth, blurred vision and gastrointestinal disturbances can occur.

Interactions. Antihistamines may enhance sedative effects of central nervous system depressants such as

239

alcohol, analgesics, sedatives and antipsychotics. The newer antihistamines do not seem to potentiate the effect of alcohol.

Caution. Sedating antihistamines have significant antimuscarinic activity and should be used with caution in prostatic hyperplasia, urinary retention and glaucoma. Caution may be required in epilepsy and hepatic disease.

Important point. Patients should be advised to take antihistamines with or after food to avoid gastric disturbances.

OXYGEN

Oxygen, which comprises approximately 21% of air, is essential to all forms of animal life.

Tissue hypoxia results from failure of any one or a combination of the following:

- adequate ventilation
- gas exchange
- circulatory distribution.

Arterial blood gas analysis provides accurate information on pH, partial pressure of oxygen, oxygen saturation and partial pressure of carbon dioxide.

Medical uses of oxygen include maintaining tissue oxygenation during anaesthesia; treatment of diseases including chronic lung disease, myocardial infarction and pulmonary embolism; treatment of cardiopulmonary arrest; and the treatment of newborn babies with respiratory distress.

ADMINISTRATION OF OXYGEN

Medical grade oxygen is regarded as a drug. It should therefore normally be prescribed by a doctor on the patient's prescription sheet, stating:

- the word OXYGEN
- the type of appliance to be used (i.e. mask, nasal cannulae)
- in the case of a mask, the appropriate percentage of oxygen
- the flow rate in L/min
- the duration of administration.

Oxygen may be delivered to the patient using either a *variable oxygen delivery system* or a *fixed oxygen delivery system*. These terms refer to the rates of oxygen delivered by the equipment.

Variable oxygen delivery systems that include nasal cannulae and face masks deliver oxygen at flow rates that supplement the oxygen concentration in room air.

The range can vary from as low as 21% to as high as 90%. The exact concentration, however, depends on the flow rate of oxygen and the patient's rate and depth of breathing. Variable delivery systems are commonly used postoperatively and in pulmonary oedema and pulmonary embolus.

Fixed oxygen delivery systems, which include masks and nebulisers incorporating the Venturi principle, provide the person's total inspiratory needs and can deliver a precise and accurate concentration of oxygen that is not significantly affected by the rate and depth of the patient's breathing and is largely independent of the oxygen flow rate. It is essential that patients with COPD who require oxygen receive a fixed concentration, such as 24 or 28%.

In health, there are two drives for breathing. The predominant drive is the presence of carbon dioxide; the less important one is lack of oxygen. In COPD, the sensitivity to carbon dioxide may be lost, in which case the hypoxic drive predominates. If the patient then receives high concentrations of oxygen, the hypoxic drive will also disappear, leaving the patient respiratorily depressed and likely to develop carbon dioxide narcosis, resulting in loss of consciousness.

As well as ensuring that the patient receives the correct percentage of oxygen at the correct flow rate, it is important to note how long the oxygen should be given. The administration of high concentrations of oxygen (60%) for more than 48 h may damage the alveolar membrane of the lungs.

Oxygen may be administered on a nurse's own initiative only in a life-threatening situation, because in an inappropriate concentration it has potentially harmful effects in some patients.

DEVICES FOR THE ADMINISTRATION OF OXYGEN

Face mask. This is the commonest method for administering oxygen. Face masks are designed to deliver different concentrations of oxygen according to the flow system involved. The main ones are:

- *high-flow* masks that accurately deliver *low concentrations* of oxygen (24–35%) used in COPD
- *low-flow* masks achieving *high concentrations* of oxygen (up to 60%) used in pulmonary oedema and pulmonary embolus.

A variety of masks is available that are lightweight, efficient, and, for most patients, comfortable, and that allow for observation of lip colour. Care must be taken to ensure that the mask fits snugly and that its position is maintained for effective delivery. Redness and sores can result from pressure and chafing from the mask over the bridge of the nose and from the elastic strap over the temporal region and above the ears. When discomfort persists after adjusting the tension of the elastic, this may be relieved by inserting a neat layer of cotton wool between the appliance and the skin. In the course of time, the mask can become moist and sticky, and patients appreciate having it removed for a few moments to allow the face and the mask to be wiped clean and dry. Unless it is delivered at a flow rate of more than 4 L/min, oxygen taken through a mask or nasal cannulae does not require to be humidified, as the air with which it mixes on inspiration contains sufficient water vapour.

Nasal cannulae. These have an advantage over face masks in that they do not interfere to the same extent with feeding and communication. In addition, those patients who experience feelings of claustrophobia with a mask may find nasal cannulae acceptable. Before inserting nasal cannulae, the patient is asked to blow the nose, or else the nostrils are cleaned with moist cotton-tipped applicators.

SAFETY

Oxygen administration is a potentially dangerous procedure, and every precaution must be taken to ensure that standards of safety are maintained.

Although in most hospitals oxygen is piped to the bedside or operating theatre, portable cylinders still have to be used, for example on patient trolleys and during emergencies outside the ward. All nurses must therefore be able to identify a cylinder of oxygen correctly, i.e. black with a white shoulder and marked with the word OXYGEN. Because the oxygen in cylinders is in compressed form, removal of valves or flow meters should be carried out only by those trained to do so and in accordance with local policy. This noisy procedure should take place outside patient areas. At all times, cylinders should be supported in a stand so that they cannot be knocked over, and they should be stored away from direct heat to prevent explosion. Nurses require to anticipate when a replacement cylinder will be needed, taking into account that there will be a rapid decrease in pressure as the gauge reaches the empty mark. Sufficient time also needs to be allowed for a new supply to be delivered to the ward.

Emergency equipment should be checked daily!

PRECAUTIONS

Because oxygen supports combustion and can convert a spark into a flame, precautions must be taken in the immediate area of its use. The patient involved, the surrounding patients and any visitors should have these precautions explained to them. Printed warnings should be in evidence. Items likely to be a danger should be removed, for example matches and cigarette lighters, electric shavers and battery-operated gadgets. Care should be exercised when bed making and combing hair to reduce risk of sparks created by static electricity.

OBSERVATIONS

Periodic observations must be made by the nurse as long as the patient is receiving oxygen. A check should be made of the patient's condition, generally, and respirations, specifically. It is important to recognise whether the oxygen is benefiting the patient. Acute hypoxaemia produces alterations to rate and depth of respiration, bounding pulse, high blood pressure, cyanosis, restlessness and confusion. Pulse oximetry provides non-invasive continuous monitoring of the state of oxygenation.

Other observations include the flow of oxygen, the volume of oxygen remaining in the cylinder and the general environment to ensure that safety is being maintained. When working with the patient receiving oxygen, care should be taken to prevent obstruction of the oxygen tubing by, for example, a bed rail, backrest or the patient herself.

EFFECTS OF OXYGEN THERAPY

To counteract the drying effect of oxygen, patients should be assisted and encouraged to increase their fluid intake. For the same reason, the frequency of oral and nasal hygiene should be increased. Because flammable materials such as paraffin-based lubricants are unsafe to use in the presence of oxygen, water-soluble lubricants such as glycerin should be used for soothing the lips or nasal mucosa. Soft paraffin should not be used.

OXYGEN THERAPY AT HOME

Patients with COPD may require to have oxygen therapy continued on their discharge from hospital. Time must be spent with the patient and, if possible, a member of her family, giving clear instructions on the safe and effective use of oxygen. The community nursing service should be informed so that a domiciliary visit may be arranged.

Cylinders for home use in the UK contain 1360 L of oxygen, providing 11 h of treatment at a flow rate of 2 L/min. Portable cylinders containing 300 L are also available but last for only 2 h at a flow rate of 2 L/min.

An oxygen concentrator for domiciliary use may be supplied for those patients who would otherwise require many cylinders. This device, which is powered by electricity, draws in air from the atmosphere and then filters out unwanted gases to produce oxygen in a concentrated form. The concentrator is an economical method of supplying oxygen. A back-up cylinder should also be available, however, for use in the event of a power cut.

In England and Wales, oxygen and concentrators may be ordered on the home oxygen order form and be contracted out to a supplier. In Scotland, oxygen and its accessories may be dispensed from a prescription by pharmacies contracted to provide domiciliary oxygen; the provision of a concentrator may be made only by a respiratory consultant through the Common Services Agency (British National Formulary 2006).

Clearly, education of the patient and family in the safe use of oxygen in the home is an important aspect of the work of community nurse, doctor and pharmacist. In some districts, supervision of patients at home is undertaken by a respiratory nurse.

MUCOLYTICS

Mucolytics such as carbocisteine are used to ease expectoration by reducing sputum viscosity in chronic asthma and bronchitis. Their therapeutic value, however, is doubtful. Steam inhalation is beneficial in some cases.

INHALATIONS

Decongestants such as steam and menthol may be helpful when breathed in from a Nelson-type inhaler.

COUGH PREPARATIONS

COUGH SUPPRESSANTS

The cough reflex is important in maintaining an open airway. A productive cough expels secretions and foreign material and should not be suppressed.

Cough suppressants act directly on the medullary mechanism in the brain, suppressing the cough reflex.

Usage. The effectiveness of cough suppressants is dubious. Therefore they are only occasionally useful in the treatment of:

- a dry, hacking, non-productive cough that disturbs sleep (codeine, dextromethorphan and pholcodine)
- an extremely distressing cough associated with lung cancer; in this case, the most powerful narcotics are used.

Side-effects and contraindications. All cough suppressants tend to cause constipation. Large doses cause respiratory depression and are contraindicated in patients suffering from asthma.

Important point. Cough suppressants are not recommended for children under the age of 1 year, and only occasionally in older children.

EXPECTORANTS

Theoretically, expectorants liquefy mucus and facilitate its removal from the lungs through coughing, but there is no scientific basis for this.

DEMULCENTS

Demulcent cough preparations contain soothing, moistening substances such as syrup or glycerol. Some patients find this useful in relieving a dry irritating cough. A demulcent such as simple linctus may be helpful.

NASAL DECONGESTANTS

Local nasal decongestants cause vasoconstriction and reduce congestion and oedema of the nasal mucosa.

Systemic decongestants also cause broncho-dilatation.

Preparations. Local preparations such as nasal drops and sprays contain, for example, ephedrine and xylometazoline.

Systemic preparations contain mixtures of para-cetamol, antihistamines and nasal decongestants such as pseudoephedrine. These preparations are of doubtful therapeutic value.

Side-effects. Local decongestants are subject to tolerance and rebound vasodilatation, and cause damage to the nasal mucosa and cilia. They are not generally effective for more than a few days and therefore have limited usefulness.

The sympathomimetic (e.g. pseudoephedrine) component in systemic preparations may cause tachycardia and a rise in blood pressure.

The antihistamine component may cause drowsiness and affect the ability to drive or operate machinery.

Caution. Systemic nasal decongestants should be avoided in patients with hypertension, hyperthyroidism, coronary heart disease, diabetes (they interfere with blood sugar control) and in patients taking monoamine oxidase inhibitors.

SELF-ASSESSMENT QUESTIONS

A.

Mr W has just arrived as an emergency to your ward with severe dyspnoea. His colour is poor, and he has difficulty speaking to you. His wife is with him.

1. What is the immediate nursing care?

He is receiving oxygen.

2. What precautions should be taken?

You are assigned the task of admitting him.

3. What observations and recordings would you carry out?

Several medical investigations are ordered.

4. What are these likely to include?

Mr W's medical notes state that he has COPD. He has smoked for 55 years.

5. What changes may there be to his respiratory tract?

The doctor prescribes medication for Mr W, including oxygen.

6. By what route(s) are medicines likely to be prescribed for this patient?
7. Why is it essential that a precise percentage of oxygen is prescribed?
8. What type of drug(s) may be used to treat COPD?
9. Can you give an example of each?

Some of the drugs are to be given via a nebuliser.

10. How would you minimise infection in a patient using a nebuliser?
11. For what reasons is oral hygiene especially important in patients having nebuliser therapy?

The overall aim is to help Mr W reach his full potential.

12. Which allied health professionals are likely to be involved in the management of his condition?

Mr W's condition improves, and he is fit enough to be discharged.

13. What could Mrs W do to help her husband's condition during the winter months?

B.

1. Name a short-acting β_2 agonist.
2. Name an antimuscarinic bronchodilator.
3. What are the advantages of continuing a β_2 agonist with a corticosteroid in the treatment of asthma?
4. Why should drugs with a muscarinic action (side-effect) be avoided in patients with respiratory disease?

REFERENCES

British Medical Association and Royal Pharmaceutical Society of Great Britain 2006 British National Formulary, no. 51. BMA and RPSGB, London

British Thoracic Society and Scottish Intercollegiate Guidelines Network 2005 Management of Asthma: chronic and acute. In: British Medical Association and Royal Pharmaceutical Society of Great Britain. British National Formulary, no. 51. BMA and RPSGB, London, pp. 141–142

Calverly P, Bellamy D 2000 The challenge of providing better care for patients with chronic obstructive airways disease: the poor relation of airways obstruction? Thorax 55:78–82

Casaburi R, Mahler DA, Jones PW et al. 2002 A long-term evaluation of once-daily inhaled tiotropium in chronic obstructive pulmonary disease. European Respiratory Journal 19(2):271–224

Celli B, Zu Wallack R, Wang S et al. 2003 Improvement in resting inspiratory capacity and hyperinflation with tiotropium in COPD patients with increased static lung volumes. Chest 124:1743–1748

Harriman A-M, Purcell N 1996 Can we mix nebuliser solutions? Pharmacy in Practice 6(9):347–348

Howard R 2005 Asthma medication: methods of improving patient adherence. Prescriber 16(17):13–20

Lacasse Y, Brosseau L, Milne S et al. 2002 Pulmonary rehabilitation for chronic obstructive pulmonary disease. Cochrane Library 3

National Asthma Campaign 2001 Out in the open: a true picture of asthma in the United Kingdom today. Asthma Audit 2001. Asthma Journal 6(3)

National Institute of Clinical Excellence 2004 Chronic obstructive pulmonary disease: national clinical guidelines for management of chronic obstructive pulmonary disease in adults in primary and secondary care. Thorax 59(suppl 1):1–232

O'Donnell DE, Fluge T, Gerhen F et al. 2004 Effects of tiotropium on lung hyperinflation, dyspnoea and exercise tolerance in COPD. European Respiratory Journal 23:832–840

Price D 1997 Improving compliance with asthma therapy. Update 7 May:619–624

Scottish Intercollegiate Guidelines Network 2005 Improvement in MDI usage. SIGN, Edinburgh

FURTHER READING AND RESOURCES

[Anonymous] 2005 Common questions about hay fever. MeReC Bulletin 14(5):17–20

Chandra MO, Steiner MC 2004 COPD: the disease and non-drug treatment. Hospital Pharmacist 11:359–364

Chung F 2006 COPD management. Prescriber 17(11):23–24

Corrigan C 2005 Today's stepwise management of asthma in primary care. Prescriber 16(3):53–70

Corrigan C 2006 Asthma management. Prescriber 17(5):66–69

Currie GP, Douglas JG 2006 Oxygen and inhalers. British Medical Journal 333:34–36

Currie GP, Douglas JG 2006 Pharmacological management: oral treatment. British Medical Journal 332:1497–1499

Dyer C 2006 Asthma: diagnosis and management in the older person. Prescriber 17(14):38–41

Farooque S, Fitzharris P 2004 Allergic rhinitis: current approaches to management. Prescriber 16(8):19–38

Faulding S 2004 New treatments may provide benefit for chronic obstructive pulmonary disease. Pharmacy in Practice 15(12):144–146

Hind C 2005 Smoking cessation: advice and NRT in community pharmacies. Prescriber 16(9):12–20

Meisner S 2006 Current management of lower respiratory tract infections. Prescriber 17(6):48–58

Murphy AC, Steiner MC 2004 COPD: pharmacological management. Hospital Pharmacist 11:367–376

Ohri CM, Steiner MC 2004 COPD: the disease and non-drug treatment. Hospital Pharmacist 11:359–364

Wedzicha J 2005 Oxygen therapy in the home for chronic respiratory conditions. Prescriber 16(22):50–53

Drugs acting on the central nervous system

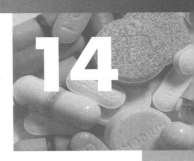

14

CHAPTER CONTENTS

KEY OBJECTIVES

After reading this chapter, you should be able to:

- distinguish between neurosis and psychosis
- be able to identify both non-pharmaceutical and drug therapy used in the treatment of anxiety
- describe the clinical features associated with extrapyramidal side effects of drug treatment for schizophrenia
- discuss manic–depressive disorders
- discuss the effects of lithium
- state how tricyclic antidepressants, monoamine oxidase inhibitors and selective serotonin reuptake inhibitors work
- give the causes of nausea and vomiting
- name the factors that can trigger a migraine attack
- distinguish between a generalised and a partial seizure

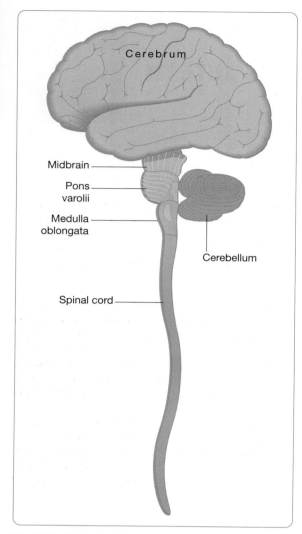

Fig. 14.1 The brain. (From Waugh A, Grant A 2001. Ross and Wilson anatomy and physiology in health and illness, 9th edn. Churchill Livingstone, Edinburgh. With permission of Elsevier.)

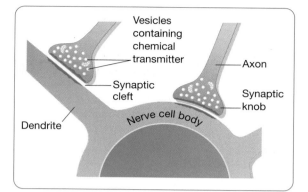

Fig. 14.2 Synaptic cleft. (From Waugh A, Grant A 2001. Ross and Wilson anatomy and physiology in health and illness, 9th edn. Churchill Livingstone, Edinburgh. With permission of Elsevier.)

otherwise termed a *neurone* and its processes, axons and dendrites. The neurones conduct nerve impulses that are akin to tiny electrical charges. Axons, which are usually longer than dendrites, carry nerve impulses away from the cell. Large axons are surrounded by a myelin sheath. Dendrites are nerve fibres that carry impulses towards nerve cells. They form synapses with dendrites of other neurones or terminate in specialised sensory receptors such as those in the skin.

SYNAPSE AND CHEMICAL TRANSMITTERS

A synapse is where nerve impulses are transmitted from one neurone, called the presynaptic neurone, to another neurone, called the postsynaptic neurone. The space between them is the synaptic cleft. Chemical transmitters carry nerve impulses across the synaptic cleft (Fig. 14.2). Noradrenaline (norepinephrine), gamma-aminobutyric acid (GABA), acetylcholine, dopamine and serotonin (5-hydroxytryptamine) are examples of chemicals that act as transmitters. The endings of autonomic nerves supplying smooth muscle and glands release a transmitter substance that stimulates or depresses the activity of the structure.

THE BRAIN

The parts comprising the brain are the:

- cerebrum
- midbrain
- pons varolii   } brain stem
- medulla oblongata
- cerebellum.

- describe the features of Parkinson's disease
- state the key principles of caring for a person with Alzheimer's disease.

ANATOMY AND PHYSIOLOGY

The central nervous system comprises the brain, spinal cord and peripheral nerves (Fig. 14.1). There is a vast number of nerves, each consisting of a nerve cell

Table 14.1 The vital centres of the brain

Centre	Effect of stimulation
Cardiac centre	Sympathetic stimulation increases the rate and force of the heartbeat; parasympathetic stimulation has the opposite effect
Respiratory centre	Controls rate and depth of respiration
Vasomotor centre	Controls diameter of blood vessels; the vasomotor centre may be stimulated by baroreceptors, body temperature, emotion
Reflex centre	Irritating substances in the stomach or respiratory tract cause nerve impulses to pass to the medulla oblongata, which initiate reflex actions such as vomiting, coughing or sneezing

The peripheral part of the cerebrum is composed of nerve cells or grey matter forming the cerebral cortex, and the deeper layers consist of nerve fibres or white matter. The types of activity associated with the cerebral cortex are:

- mental activities – memory, reasoning, learning
- sensory perception – pain, temperature, touch, sight, hearing, taste, smell
- control of voluntary muscle contraction.

The midbrain consists of nerve cells and fibres connecting the cerebrum with lower parts of the brain and with the spinal cord. The medulla oblongata extends from the pons varolii and is continuous with the spinal cord. The vital centres, comprising groups of cells associated with the autonomic reflex activity, lie within the medulla oblongata; they are listed in Table 14.1.

The cerebellum coordinates voluntary muscle movement, posture and balance. The sensory input is derived from the muscles, joints, eyes and ears. Damage to the cerebellum results in uncoordinated muscular movement such as staggering gait.

COMMON DISORDERS

INSOMNIA

Normal sleep is of two kinds.

- Slow wave sleep (SWS):
  — heart rate, blood pressure, respiration are steady or in decline
  — muscles are relaxed
  — growth hormone secretion is maximal.
- Rapid eye movement (REM):
  — heart rate, blood pressure, respiration fluctuate
  — cerebral blood flow increases above that during wakefulness
  — skeletal muscles are profoundly relaxed, although body movements are more pronounced (dreaming sleep).

A 'normal' night consists of a sleep latency period that varies from person to person (the 'dropping off' stage), followed by SWS sleep for about 1 h, REM sleep for about 20 min, SWS for approximately 90 min and REM sleep for about 20 min, and the rest of the night alternates between SWS and REM sleep until wakefulness. Both kinds of sleep appear necessary for normal health.

Insomnia affects most of us at some time in our lives. For the majority it is transient, but for some people insomnia becomes a chronic problem. Many people who sleep badly complain of tiredness during the day and mood disturbance. Insomnia may be characterised by:

- difficulty in falling asleep
- difficulty in staying asleep
- short unrefreshing sleep.

However, individual requirements differ, some people finding that only 4–6 h is adequate, whereas others require 8 or 9 h to feel refreshed the following day. In general, the elderly require less sleep than the young.

Hypnotics are often prescribed without adequate clinical evaluation to recognise underlying emotional or physical causes that may respond to specific psychotherapy or pharmacotherapy.

When insomnia is caused by the following symptoms, treatment of these primary symptoms may relieve the problem: pain, dyspnoea, cough, frequency of micturition, excitatory drugs (e.g. caffeine), pruritus.

Insomnia is a common feature of psychiatric illness, particularly in anxiety states and depressive illness. Difficulty in getting to sleep is found in both depression and anxiety, and early morning awakening is common in depression. Choosing a medication to treat the illness with a secondary hypnotic activity can assist in alleviating the insomnia. For example, in depressed patients with early wakening a sedative antidepressant (e.g. mirtazapine) may be sufficient.

Certain drugs may produce insomnia, particularly the methylxanthines (theophylline and caffeine), the amphetamines and selegiline. Sleep disturbance is likely to be experienced in the early stages of treatment, and medication may need to be reviewed if problems persist.

Three main types of insomnia have been identified according to their duration.

- Transient insomnia. This may occur in those who normally sleep well, due to factors such as jet lag, shift work or acute stress, and lasts for only a few days. Only one or two doses of a hypnotic should be given.
- Short-term insomnia. This is usually related to an emotional problem such as bereavement, problems at work or marital relations. A hypnotic should not be given for more than 3 weeks (preferably only 1 week), omitting doses when not required.
- Long-term (chronic) insomnia. This can have many causes. Prescription of hypnotics in long-term insomnia is rarely beneficial.

NON-DRUG TREATMENT

A regular bedtime routine helps to induce sleep. Warm, milky drinks (not tea or coffee) can help. Relaxation exercises or relaxing with a book may be beneficial. An equable environmental temperature will be conducive to sleep.

DRUG TREATMENT

HYPNOTICS AND ANXIOLYTICS

Hypnotic drugs are thought to inhibit excitatory pathways in the brain. Benzodiazepines facilitate transmission of GABA, an inhibitory neurotransmitter.

Benzodiazepines

Benzodiazepines reduce the latent period and prolong the duration of sleep. Approximately 25% of total normal sleep time is REM sleep. This can be reduced by as much as 75% by the administration of benzodiazepines. When the benzodiazepine is stopped, there is a rebound increase in REM sleep as if the body requires to recover what has been lost. Nightmares occur with severe rebound, and it is at this point that many people resort to restarting the medication. The rebound increase in REM sleep does revert to normal over a period of weeks after ceasing

medication, but it is a major factor in the development of dependence on this group of drugs.

Benzodiazepines should be used to treat insomnia only when it is severe, disabling or subjecting the individual to extreme distress. Benzodiazepines may be divided into those with a short or longer duration of action. Shorter-acting benzodiazepines (temazepam and lormetazepam, half-lives of 6–15 h) are indicated for patients for whom residual effects are undesirable, and they are generally preferred when insomnia is not accompanied by daytime anxiety. They are also the most suitable benzodiazepine hypnotics for elderly people, although caution is still required. It should be noted that half-lives of benzodiazepines may be greatly extended in the elderly, as hepatic and renal function are known to deteriorate with age. The dosage should therefore be reduced accordingly. Benzodiazepines such as nitrazepam and diazepam, which have long half-lives, should be avoided; the same is true when the metabolites of benzodiazepines have long half-lives. Benzodiazepines have hangover effects such as drowsiness and lightheadedness the following day, confusion and ataxia, particularly in older people who are liable to fall and injure themselves. For this reason, they should be avoided in the elderly.

Interactions. Alcohol and benzodiazepines taken concomitantly may result in greater impairment of psychomotor function than either agent alone. The usual effect of the combination of alcohol and benzodiazepines is an increase in the sedative effects of the benzodiazepine.

Dependence. Dependence on benzodiazepines does occur and is now regarded as a serious problem, particularly with longer-term treatment and in patients with some types of personality disorder. Patients taking these drugs, even in therapeutic doses, may develop a physical withdrawal syndrome. The main symptom of this is anxiety, which usually subsides in 2–4 weeks but sometimes lasts longer, although many patients would have been prone to anxiety prior to treatment. In addition, depression, nausea, depersonalisation and perceptual changes such as intolerance of loud noises, bright lights or touch may occur. Insomnia may also be expected, but the symptoms are variable. Occasionally, epileptic seizures, confusion and visual hallucinations may occur.

Stopping treatment with short-acting benzodiazepines leads to withdrawal symptoms within about 2–3 days, whereas with longer acting drugs there may be a delay of 7 days. Patients being weaned from benzodiazepines need close supervision and support, and the drugs should be withdrawn slowly over weeks or even months.

Benzodiazepine withdrawal. The benzodiazepine is substituted with an equivalent dose of diazepam (e.g. diazepam 10 mg is equivalent to temazepam 20 mg or nitrazepam 10 mg). Diazepam is used because of its long half-life. The withdrawal symptoms from diazepam appear to be less severe, with little associated craving. However, there may be a problem with daytime sedation.

Once substitution has been achieved, a gradual reduction of the diazepam dosage should follow. Diazepam is available in 2-, 5- and 10-mg tablets, all of which can be halved, and in an oral solution of 2 mg in 5 mL and 5 mg in 5 mL. These reductions can be in steps of about one-eighth of the daily dose every fortnight. If withdrawal symptoms occur, the dose is maintained until symptoms improve. As the dose is reduced, small reductions are made, as it is better to reduce too slowly than too quickly.

Once the patient is at a dosage of 0.5 mg daily, the dose interval can be increased to every 2 or 3 days. Many long-term benzodiazepine users can successfully withdraw without experiencing significant withdrawal symptoms. A number of patients may find it extremely difficult to withdraw completely.

Zaleplon, zolpidem and zopiclone

Zaleplon, zolpidem and zopiclone are non-benzodiazepine hypnotics that act on the same receptors as benzodiazepines. They have a short duration of action with little or no hangover effect but, as with other hypnotics, they should not be used for long-term treatment. They are relatively expensive and offer little or no advantage over the short-acting benzodiazepines in terms of efficacy. The side-effect profiles, contraindications and precautions that must be observed with these drugs also differ little from established treatments.

They are rapidly absorbed and have a rapid onset of action, so that sleep is induced in about 30 min. They preserve normal sleep patterns and appear to be effective agents in inducing and maintaining sleep without adverse effects on daytime alertness or memory function.

Side-effects. These are as follows.
- Zaleplon: amnesia, paraesthesia, drowsiness, nausea, confusion, dizziness and hallucinations.
- Zolpidem: gastrointestinal disturbance, headache, daytime drowsiness, memory disturbances, ataxia, confusion and nightmares.
- Zopiclone: gastrointestinal disturbance, bitter or metallic taste, dry mouth, irritability, confusion, headache and dizziness.

Table 14.2 Half-lives and dosages of hypnotics[a]

Drug	Elimination half-life (h)	Hypnotic dose (mg)
Benzodiazepines		
Loprazolam	6–12	0.5–2
Lormetazepam	10–12	0.5–1.5
Temazepam	8–15	10–40
Non-benzodiazepines		
Zaleplan	1	5–10
Zolpidem	2.5–3	5–10
Zopiclone	5–8	3.75–7.5

[a]Doses are adult doses. Dosage should be reduced in older people.

The Committee on Safety of Medicines advises that zopiclone has the same potential for dependence as the benzodiazepines, and its use should therefore be subject to the same cautions.

Table 14.2 indicates the half-lives and dosages of commonly used hypnotics.

SUMMARY

The ideal hypnotic does not exist, and hypnotics should be reserved for people whose insomnia is debilitating. They should be prescribed for short courses and only when all underlying causes of insomnia have been investigated and treated.

ANXIETY

Anxiety is a normal reaction we all experience when faced with major events in our lives such as moving house and attending interviews. It becomes a medical problem only when it is excessive or inappropriate. The patient may describe a sensation of fear or dread, varying from mild to an overwhelming feeling of terror, the latter leading to panic attacks.

Physical symptoms include tremor, tensing of muscles, perspiration (particularly of the hands and forehead), hypertension, palpitations, gastrointestinal disturbances (such as frequency of defaecation), back pain, chest pain, dizziness and dyspnoea. These symptoms are very marked in panic attacks.

TREATMENT

Treatment of anxiety includes psychotherapy (relaxation, behavioural and reassurance techniques) as well as drug therapy. The decision whether to use psychotherapy, drug therapy or a combination of both is determined by the practitioner.

Drug treatment should be limited to the lowest possible dose for the shortest possible time. It relies mainly on the use of anxiolytics such as benzodiazepines and buspirone, but beta-blockers, antidepressants with a sedative action (such as clomipramine) and antipsychotics (such as zuclopenthixol) have also been used with varying degrees of success.

BENZODIAZEPINES

Benzodiazepines are anxiolytic, sedative and, in large doses, hypnotic. They also show muscle relaxant and anticonvulsant properties.

Benzodiazepines potentiate the effects of GABA, the major inhibitory transmitter in the brain, by binding with the receptor complex.

Pharmacokinetics. Compounds with a high potency at the receptor site and with a long half-life are best suited for use in anxiety, as they are less likely to cause withdrawal problems. For this reason, diazepam is suitable, with a half-life of 14–17 h and active metabolites. It is rapidly absorbed and quick-acting.

Chlordiazepoxide is also a long-acting benzodiazepine, and this type is most useful when a sustained action is required. Short-acting benzodiazepines (lorazepam, oxazepam) are used in intermittent anxiety such as episodes of panic, phobic disorders and acute stressful situations (e.g. public speaking, when a briefer action is required).

Table 14.3 gives dose ranges of benzodiazepines.

Table 14.3 Dose ranges of some benzodiazepines	
Drug	**Dose**
Chlordiazepoxide	10 mg three times daily, increased if necessary to 60–100 mg daily in divided doses
Diazepam	2 mg three times daily, increased if necessary to 15–30 mg daily in divided doses
Lorazepam	1–4 mg daily in divided doses
Oxazepam	15–30 mg three or four times daily

Reduced doses should be used in the elderly and in hepatic impairment.

Side effects. Benzodiazepines are generally well tolerated. However, sedation, ataxia, confusion, amnesia and dependence may occur.

BETA-BLOCKERS

Beta-blockers (e.g. propranolol, oxprenolol; see p. 200) do not affect psychological symptoms such as fear, worry and tension. They do, however, reduce autonomic symptoms such as palpitations and tremor.

BUSPIRONE

Buspirone has anxiolytic effects but lacks sedative, anticonvulsant and muscle relaxant properties. Buspirone is rapidly absorbed and undergoes considerable first-pass metabolism. It is eliminated by the liver and has a half-life of 2–11 h. Its anxiolytic effect occurs after 2 weeks of continuous therapy.

Initially, the dose is 5 mg two or three times daily, increased as necessary every 2–3 days; usual range 15–30 mg daily in divided doses; maximum 45 mg daily.

Side-effects. Common side-effects include drowsiness, dizziness, headache, lightheadedness, excitement and nausea, which occur most commonly at the beginning of treatment. No withdrawal symptoms have been reported on stopping treatment after 6 weeks to 6 months, and there is no evidence of tolerance. Buspirone does not appear to have an additive effect with alcohol. Diazepam remains the drug of choice for treatment of anxiety.

PSYCHOSES

Antipsychotic drugs, also known as neuroleptics, are used in the symptomatic treatment of psychoses, including schizophrenia and the manic phase of manic depressive illness. Antipsychotics can also be used to calm children with learning difficulties and agitated elderly patients.

SCHIZOPHRENIA

Schizophrenia is a severe mental illness affecting 1% of the population at some time in life. It can have a profound effect on a person's reasoning and thought processes, emotions and behaviour. Most people with schizophrenia are unable to hold down a job, have few friends and find it difficult to interact socially.

Schizophrenia can develop at any age but most commonly manifests itself in the late teens or early twenties. It affects both sexes equally, but women have a slightly later average age of onset. About 250 000 people are suffering from schizophrenia in Britain today, and each year about 35 000 patients with the condition are admitted to hospital. It involves the most basic attributes that give people a sense of individuality, uniqueness and direction in life. It causes a disintegration of the personality, with a wide range of symptoms and abnormal behaviour. These include delusions, often of persecution, hallucinations, usually of accusatory or abusive voices, incoherence of speech and thought, abnormal movements and a flattened affect. Hallucinations can, however, involve all senses including olfactory, tactile, visual and taste. During the illness, functioning at work, family life, social relations and self-care may deteriorate markedly. The symptoms are divided into two classes.

- Positive symptoms such as hallucinations, delusions and thought disorders.
- Negative symptoms, including marked social isolation or withdrawal, lack of volition, poverty of speech, anhedonia, failure in role functioning as wage earner or homemaker and marked lack of interests, motivation and energy. Some patients are predominantly disorganised in their behaviour and others mainly paranoid. The negative symptoms are often more prominent during the later stages of the illness, hampering rehabilitation and discharge into the community.

The disease frequently creates heavy burdens for the sufferer, often throughout the person's adult life. Furthermore, there is likely to be considerable impact on the patient's family and on society. The course of the illness varies. About 25% of people who present recover fully within a few months; another 50% recover but suffer recurring episodes of illness throughout their life. The remaining 25% are permanently disabled and provide the bulk of management problems and require constant intensive treatment. Table 14.4 provides prognostic indicators.

DRUG TREATMENT

The aim is to treat both positive and negative symptoms and to increase social functioning. Consent must be obtained for treatment unless there is a risk of significant harm to the patient or others by virtue of non-treatment of the illness, at which point the mental health legislation may require to be invoked to enable the patient to receive the appropriate treatment. Compulsory admission to hospital for treatment can be applied for under the terms of the relevant sections of the Mental Health (Care and Treatment) Acts if there is a significant risk of patients harming themselves or others as a result of their mental illness.

Conditions for compulsory detention and/or treatment orders are specified in the relevant Mental Health Acts. Patients retain the right of appeal against the imposition of such orders, and they are also protected by the involvement of the Mental Welfare Commission, the appointment of a mental welfare officer (usually a specially trained social worker) and the requirement to identify a named person to represent their interests.

The choice of drug treatment should be discussed with the multidisciplinary team. The choice of antipsychotic drug and the route of administration will depend on the individual circumstances of the patient. The dose will require to be titrated against clinical symptoms and side effects. Counselling and discussion with the patient of anticipated effects and side effects will create a better understanding, resulting in improved compliance and an increased likelihood of a positive outcome.

Mechanism of action of antipsychotic drugs. The mechanism of action is complex, and many details remain to be established. However, psychotic symptoms result from overactivity of the dopaminergic system. Antipsychotic drugs are believed to act by blocking dopamine receptors, especially D_2-dopaminergic receptors in the brain and, in this way, counterbalance the overactive dopaminergic system. While this will result in an antipsychotic effect, depending on the ability of the drugs to block the dopamine receptors, there may be extrapyramidal side-effects and parkinsonian symptoms.

Table 14.4 Prognostic indicators in schizophrenia

Good	Bad
No family history	Family history
Good premorbid personality	Shy, solitary
Functions well in work environment	Poor work record
Precipitating cause	No precipitating cause
Acute onset	Gradual onset
Prompt treatment	Delayed treatment

The antipsychotics may block other central neuro-transmitter pathways, and this may be clinically relevant.

- Cholinergic blockade is associated with dry mouth, blurred vision, constipation and urinary retention. Antipsychotic drugs with a significant antimuscarinic effect should not therefore be administered to patients with angle closure glaucoma or prostatism.
- Alpha-adrenergic blockade is associated with postural hypotension, particularly in the elderly.
- Histamine receptor blockade is associated with sedation, which may be desirable in some patients but not in others.

Pharmacokinetics. Oral antipsychotics generally show unpredictable absorption. Drug availability may be increased 4–10 times on intramuscular administration. Most antipsychotics have long elimination half-lives of about 20–40 h, which allow once-a-day dosage after stabilisation of the patient's condition. Older patients have a reduced capacity to metabolise and eliminate these drugs.

Administration of medication. The dose of anti-psychotic drugs must be individualised for each patient with respect to severity of illness, drug potency, route of administration, age, weight and liver function. A key factor is to ensure that the dose of medication is kept as low as possible. Treatment is usually initiated at low dose and increased gradually until symptom control is achieved or until side-effects limit further increases. Very large doses rarely improve response and usually increase the burden of side-effects. Because of slower metabolism and elimination rate, older people require much smaller doses.

Three main factors influence the choice of anti-psychotic medication:

- previous good response to an individual drug would point to use of the same drug on a subsequent occasion, and vice versa
- severity of the illness and the predominant symptoms
- side-effect profile.

Side-effects. Antipsychotics have a wide range of side effects, the severity varying between different groups and between individual drugs. These are grouped as follows.

- Behavioural:
  — depression
  — anxiety
  — agitation.

- Autonomic nervous system (anticholinergic):
  — dry mouth
  — blurred vision
  — nasal congestion
  — hypotension
  — urinary hesitancy.

Particular care is required in older people, because of the possibility of precipitating urinary retention or adversely affecting glaucoma. Postural hypotension associated with alpha-adrenergic blockade may also be troublesome in the elderly.

- Metabolic/endocrine:
  — weight gain
  — hyperprolactinaemia
  — galactorrhoea
  — gynaecomastia
  — amenorrhoea
  — hypo- or hyperthermia.

Neuroendocrine effects, which include gynaecomastia, galactorrhoea and amenorrhoea, occur less frequently. They are a consequence of a rise in prolactin (hyper-prolactinaemia) following dopamine blockade of the pituitary gland.

- Allergic/toxic:
  — cardiac arrhythmias
  — neuroleptic malignant syndrome
  — jaundice (chlorpromazine)
  — dermatitis
  — photosensitivity
  — blood dyscrasias.

All antipsychotic medications have the potential to cause blood dyscrasias. Clozapine has a much greater potential to cause agranulocytosis. Neuroleptic malignant syndrome is thought to occur in 0.5% of newly treated patients and to be greatly underdiagnosed. It is a potentially life-threatening complication of neuroleptic treatment. The main symptoms are hyperthermia, fluctuating consciousness, muscular rigidity, autonomic disturbance and extrapyramidal symptoms. The risk is greater the higher the starting dose of antipsychotic and the more rapidly it is increased. Antipsychotic symptomatic treatment should be stopped while the drug washes out. Intensive medical treatment is required when bromocriptine (a dopaminergic agonist) and dantrolene (a skeletal muscle relaxant) are usually administered.

- Central nervous system:
  — sedation
  — reduced convulsive threshold
  — extrapyramidal side effects.

Sedation may be useful when a patient is agitated. Antipsychotics lower the seizure threshold in a dose-dependent manner. The more potent, less sedative drugs tend to carry a greater risk than the less potent, more sedative drugs. Clozapine carries the greatest risk.

Extrapyramidal side-effects. Extrapyramidal reactions are well-recognised complications of antipsychotic medication. Clinical features are acute dystonia, akathisia, tardive dyskinesia and parkinsonism.

ACUTE DYSTONIA

Acute dystonias most commonly affect children and young adults. These frightening and sometimes painful conditions affect mainly the muscles of the face, jaw, neck and trunk. Typically, patients present with torticollis, facial grimacing and oculogyric spasm. Dystonias usually occur within 1–2 days of starting antipsychotic treatment but may also develop on drug withdrawal. Occasionally, persistent dystonias develop during prolonged treatment with antipsychotic drugs. Acute and subacute reactions will often improve or resolve rapidly on drug withdrawal. When this is not possible, reducing the dose of the drug or switching to another drug may improve symptoms. Acute dystonic reactions are treated with an antimuscarinic drug (e.g. procyclidine) given parenterally and continued by mouth, or with a benzodiazepine (e.g. diazepam).

AKATHISIA

This is characterised by restlessness and unease, which may be intense and distressing. Patients typically describe an inability to keep their legs still and feel a compulsion to move about. Akathisia usually occurs soon after starting drug therapy or after a rapid increase in dose. Persistent akathisia can develop in patients on long-term treatment with antipsychotics. Acute akathisia only rarely responds to treatment with antimuscarinic drugs, and these may exacerbate the problem, but a low dose of a beta-blocker or benzodiazepine may be helpful.

TARDIVE DYSKINESIA

This is most commonly seen in patients on chronic antipsychotic medication. It develops after months or years of treatment and is characterised by abnormal involuntary movements of the face (e.g. lip smacking, lateral jaw movements, fly-catching movements of the tongue) or trunk (e.g. rocking). Increasing age appears to be a risk factor. Withdrawal of long-term antipsychotics may unmask tardive dyskinesia. Symptoms may persist for an indefinite period after the drug has been discontinued. Concomitant administration of antimuscarinic drugs can worsen tardive dyskinesia, and these should be stopped if this can be done without precipitating severe parkinsonism. There is, however, no convincing evidence to support the idea that long-term antimuscarinics increase the risk of tardive dyskinesia. In severe cases, a specific antidyskinetic drug may be indicated (e.g. tetrabenazine may be worth trying). Benzodiazepines, baclofen and valproate have also been used with some success.

PARKINSONISM

This is the commonest extrapyramidal effect characterised by lack (akinesia) or slowness (bradykinesia) of movement, muscle rigidity and tremor. The patient has an expressionless face, speaks monotonously, develops a coarse tremor of the hands and can have difficulty in swallowing. It closely resembles the idiopathic form of the disease. Symptoms usually develop within days or weeks of starting antipsychotic treatment or after a recent increase in dose. Elderly patients are particularly susceptible to iatrogenic parkinsonism, especially those with dementia. The condition responds to lowering the dose of antipsychotic or treatment with an antimuscarinic drug (e.g. procyclidine or orphenadrine).

DRUGS ASSOCIATED WITH EXTRAPYRAMIDAL REACTIONS

Extrapyramidal reactions are associated with dopamine receptor antagonists, which include antipsychotic and antiemetic drugs (Table 14.5). High-potency (relatively high dopamine D_2 activity and low

Table 14.5 Some drugs associated with extrapyramidal reactions

Drug group	Example(s)
Antipsychotics	Chlorpromazine Flupentixol (flupenthixol) Fluphenazine Haloperidol Risperidone Trifluoperazine
Antiemetics	Metoclopramide Prochlorperazine
Antidepressants	Tricyclics (e.g. amitriptyline)
Selective serotonin reuptake inhibitors	Paroxetine

Table 14.6 Adverse effects of phenothiazines

Group	Adverse effects		
	Sedative	Antimuscarinic	Extrapyramidal
Group 1 (aliphatic phenothiazines) Chlorpromazine Levomepromazine (methotrimeprazine)[a] Promazine[a]	Pronounced	Moderate	Moderate
Group 2 (piperidine phenothiazines) Pericyazine[a] Pipotiazine	Moderate	Pronounced	Low
Group 3 (piperazine phenothiazines) Fluphenazine Perphenazine[a] Trifluoperazine	Low	Low	Pronounced

[a]Little or no antipsychotic action.

antimuscarinic activity) and depot antipsychotics have been particularly implicated. Tricyclic antidepressants and selective serotonin reuptake inhibitors (SSRIs) have also caused acute reactions. Other drugs occasionally reported to produce extrapyramidal reactions include anticonvulsants (carbamazepine) and methyldopa.

CLASSIFICATION OF ANTIPSYCHOTIC DRUGS

The phenothiazine group comprises a large proportion of the antipsychotics. This group can be divided into three subgroups with respect to the chemical side chain of the molecule. By altering the side chain, new molecules were formed, but this influenced the side-effect profile with particular regard to sedative effects, antimuscarinic effects and extrapyramidal side-effects (Table 14.6).

ALIPHATIC PHENOTHIAZINES (GROUP 1)

Chlorpromazine was the first antipsychotic to be introduced, in 1952. It is used for a wide range of indications, including control of disturbed behaviour and psychotic symptoms, and control and maintenance of schizophrenia and other psychoses. Chlorpromazine is also used to treat nausea, vomiting and intractable hiccup. Photosensitisation is more common with chlorpromazine than with other antipsychotics. Promazine is indicated for agitation, restlessness and anxiety, especially in the elderly. It is not sufficiently active by mouth to be used as an antipsychotic drug.

PIPERIDINE PHENOTHIAZINES (GROUP 2)

Pericyazine can be used for the control of disturbed behaviour, schizophrenia and other psychoses. Pipotiazine is available only as an intramuscular injection. It is fairly sedative, with a relatively low potential for causing extrapyramidal reactions, as it has pronounced antimuscarinic activity.

PIPERAZINE PHENOTHIAZINES (GROUP 3)

Fluphenazine is used as a depot formulation. Trifluoperazine is commonly used in paranoia, but its use is limited due to the high incidence of extrapyramidal side effects.

NON-PHENOTHIAZINES

The non-phenothiazines (Box 14.1) tend to have adverse effects similar to those of the phenothiazines group 3 (piperazine phenothiazines), i.e. they are generally characterised by fewer sedative and fewer antimuscarinic effects but more pronounced extrapyramidal effects.

Box 14.1 The non-phenothiazine antipsychotic drugs

- Butyrophenones:
  benperidol, haloperidol
- Diphenylbutylpiperidines:
  pimozide
- Thioxanthenes:
  flupentixol, zuclopenthixol

BUTYROPHENONES

Benperidol is used for the control of deviant anti-social sexual behaviour resulting from mental illness. However, its value has not been established. Haloperidol is a widely used antipsychotic and is possibly the drug of choice for acute mania. It is less sedating than chlorpromazine but has more pronounced extrapyramidal side effects.

DIPHENYLBUTYLPIPERIDINES

These are long-acting antipsychotics. Pimozide is long-acting and less sedating than chlorpromazine. An electrocardiogram (ECG) is required prior to commencing treatment and at regular intervals if doses greater than 16 mg daily are being prescribed.

THIOXANTHENES

These have activity similar to that of the piperazine phenothiazines. Flupentixol (flupenthixol) is indicated for schizophrenia and other psychoses, except when there is mania or motor hyperactivity or in confusional states; it is also useful in low doses in depression. It is used mainly as depot injections. Zuclopenthixol is indicated for schizophrenia, especially with agitated, aggressive or hostile behaviour. It too is used mainly as depot injections. Zuclopenthixol acetate injection is useful for the short-term management of acute psychosis and mania.

SUBSTITUTED BENZAMIDES

This is a structurally distinct group of drugs with a lower incidence of side-effects, particularly tardive dyskinesia. Sulpiride, at high doses, can control positive symptoms; at lower doses (less than 800 mg per day), it has an alerting effect useful for the treatment of negative symptoms.

Antipsychotics, type and dosage, are illustrated in Table 14.7.

ATYPICAL ANTIPSYCHOTICS

All conventional antipsychotics are targeted primarily at the D_2 receptor and are effective against positive symptoms (delusions and hallucinations) but have little impact on negative symptoms (e.g. lack of motivation and social withdrawal) and have potentially debilitating side-effects. These are very distressing for patients and contribute to poor compliance with treatment. It has been estimated that 40–65% of schizophrenic patients will discontinue oral antipsychotic therapy within 6 weeks of starting treatment, mainly because of extrapyramidal side effects.

In recent years, several new antipsychotic drugs, termed *atypical antipsychotics* because of their low propensity for causing extrapyramidal symptoms,

have been introduced. The first was clozapine, which differs from conventional antipsychotics in having a relatively weak affinity for D_2 receptors while affecting a number of other neuroreceptors (serotonergic, histaminergic, muscarinic, adrenergic). It improves both positive and negative symptoms and reduces hostile and aggressive behaviour and suicidality. Clozapine causes few extrapyramidal symptoms. However, the risk of neutropenia in the first year of treatment is 2–3%, and haematological monitoring is a mandatory condition of treatment. Initiation must be as a hospital in-patient. Leucocyte and differential blood counts must be normal before treatment commences and must be monitored weekly for the first 18 weeks, then fortnightly. Patients who have received clozapine for a year or more and have stable blood counts may have their blood monitoring reduced to every 4 weeks. Drugs that depress leucopoiesis (such as carbamazepine) should be avoided. Conventional antipsychotics should be tapered off before starting clozapine. The dose of clozapine should be titrated gradually upwards, with the patient being observed for side-effects, including:

- postural hypotension (due to α-adrenergic block)
- sedation (due to histaminergic block)
- tachycardia (due to muscarinic block)
- fever (may be due to neutropenia but usually unexplained and settles despite continued treatment).

Excess sedation sometimes responds to alterations in the timing of the daily dose. For example, early morning hangover may be reduced by giving the last dose of the day at 8 p.m. Care should be taken to distinguish true drug-induced sedation from lack of motivation, often seen in schizophrenia, or simple inactivity due to boredom. Hypersalivation can be alleviated by simple measures such as propping up the pillows at night, although antimuscarinic medication is usually required. When postural hypotension occurs, the patient should be advised not to stand up quickly. Dietary advice and exercise may be helpful to avoid constipation and weight gain. Seizures are dose-related, and the incidence may be increased by the rapid upwards titration of the dose – hence it is important to increase the dose slowly. Tachycardia, when persistent, can be alleviated by beta-blockers.

The dose regimen for clozapine is 12.5 mg once or twice on the first day then 25–50 mg on the second day, and then, if well tolerated, gradually increased in steps of 25–50 mg over 14–21 days to 300 mg daily in divided doses (larger dose at night, up to 200 mg daily may be taken as a single dose at bedtime). If

Table 14.7 Antipsychotics: type and dosage

Drug type	Drug	Oral dose
Butyrophenones	Benperidol	0.25–1.5 mg daily in divided doses
	Haloperidol	Initially 1.5–3 mg two or three times daily or 3–5 mg two or three times daily in severely affected or resistant patients; in resistant schizophrenia, up to 30 mg daily
Diphenylbutylpiperidine	Pimozide	2–20 mg daily
Phenothiazines	Chlorpromazine	Initially 25 mg three times daily; usual maintenance dose, 75–300 mg daily; maximum dose, 1 g daily
	Levomepromazine (methotrimeprazine)	Initially 25–50 mg daily in divided doses, increased as necessary to 1 g daily
	Promazine	100–200 mg four times daily; agitation and restlessness in the elderly, 25–50 mg up to four times daily
Piperazine phenothiazines	Fluphenazine	Initially 2–10 mg daily in two or three divided doses adjusted according to response to 20 mg daily
	Perphenazine	Initially 4 mg three times daily to a maximum of 24 mg daily
	Trifluoperazine	Initially 5 mg twice daily increased by 5 mg according to response
Piperidine phenothiazines	Pericyazine	Initially 75 mg daily in divided doses to a maximum of 300 mg daily
Substituted benzamide	Sulpiride	200–400 mg twice daily, maximum of 800 mg daily in patients with predominantly negative symptoms and 2.4 g daily in patients with mainly positive symptoms
Thioxanthenes	Flupentixol	3–9 mg twice daily, maximum 18 mg daily
	Zuclopenthixol	Initially 20–30 mg daily in divided doses to a maximum of 150 mg daily

necessary, there may be further increased steps of 50–100 mg once (preferably) or twice weekly. The usual antipsychotic dose is 200–450 mg daily (maximum 900 mg daily), with subsequent adjustment to usual maintenance of 150–300 mg. Lower doses should be used in the elderly and special risk groups. Other atypical antipsychotics include risperidone, olanzapine, quetiapine, amisulpride, zotepine, aripiprazole and sertindole.

Changing to an atypical antipsychotic is not necessary if a conventional antipsychotic controls symptoms adequately and the individual does not suffer unacceptable side-effects. The atypical antipsychotics should be considered:

- when choosing first-line treatment of newly diagnosed schizophrenia
- for an individual who is suffering unacceptable side-effects from a conventional antipsychotic
- for an individual in relapse whose symptoms were previously inadequately controlled.

There are subtle differences in the mode of action of the atypical antipsychotics. As a result, a patient who is doing less well while prescribed one of the atypicals may fare better when changed to another. Risperidone, for example, binds strongly to the 5-HT$_2$ receptor and less strongly to the D$_2$, histamine H$_1$, and α_1- and α_2-adrenergic receptors. The main clinical features of

Table 14.8 Atypical antipsychotics: dosages

Drug	Oral dose(s)
Amisulpride	400–800 mg daily in two divided doses for acute episode 50–300 mg for negative symptoms
Aripiprazole	15–30 mg daily
Clozapine	Titrated by 25-mg increments to 200–500 mg daily
Olanzapine	5–20 mg daily
Quetiapine	300–450 mg daily in two divided doses
Risperidone	4–6 mg daily
Sertindole	12–20 mg single dose
Zotepine	Up to 100 mg three times daily

Table 14.9 Equivalent doses of depot antipsychotics

Antipsychotic	Dose (mg)	Interval (weeks)
Flupentixol decanoate	40	2
Fluphenazine decanoate	25	2
Haloperidol decanoate	100	4
Pipotiazine palmitate	50	4
Zuclopenthixol decanoate	200	2

risperidone are thought to be due to its balance of 5-HT$_2$ and D$_2$ receptor antagonism. As a D$_2$ antagonist, risperidone relieves positive symptoms by countering the dopaminergic overactivity that causes them. 5-HT$_2$ antagonism may reduce negative and affective symptoms. Antagonism at 5-HT$_2$ receptors modifies dopaminergic transmission, reducing the effect of D$_2$ antagonism and lowering the risk of extrapyramidal side effects. α_1-adrenergic receptor antagonism may cause hypotension. α_2-adrenergic receptor antagonism may reduce the sedative effect.

Olanzapine and quetiapine bind to similar receptors as risperidone, whereas amisulpride, which also has a high affinity with dopaminergic receptors, has no affinity for serotonin and histaminergic receptors.

The atypical antipsychotics are well absorbed. Side-effects include weight gain, dizziness, postural hypotension (especially during initial dose titration) and extrapyramidal symptoms (usually mild and respond to dose reduction or an antimuscarinic drug), and occasionally tardive dyskinesia on long-term administration. Table 14.8 provides doses of atypical antipsychotic drugs.

ANTIPSYCHOTIC DEPOT INJECTIONS

Long-acting depot injections are used for maintenance therapy, especially when compliance with oral treatment is unreliable. Depot injections are esters of an antipsychotic molecule with a long-chain fatty acid, dissolved in vegetable oil. The oil retards the release of the depot drug and prolongs the duration of action. Once administered by deep intramuscular injection, the depot is slowly released into the bloodstream and is hydrolysed into the active drug and the inactive fatty acid. The rate at which the active drug is released depends on the concentration and volume of the injection. Intramuscular depot preparations are used for maintenance therapy for schizophrenia and other psychoses. The most significant clinical advantage of depot antipsychotics is that they avoid noncompliance. Depot injections are given every 1–4 weeks. When initiating therapy with sustained-release preparations of conventional antipsychotics, a test dose should be administered to assess the patient's sensitivity to drug and vehicle and susceptibility to side effects, which may be prolonged. Dose and dosage interval must be titrated according to the patient's response, as individuals respond very differently. Not more than 2–3 mL of oily injection should be administered at any one site. The Z-track technique should be used, and rotation of injection sites is essential.

SIDE-EFFECTS OF DEPOT PREPARATIONS

Depot antipsychotics have side-effects similar to those of oral antipsychotics. There tends to be a greater incidence of extrapyramidal side-effects, because a much higher dose is given as a single injection. All depot antipsychotics can cause weight gain. Erythema, swelling, nodules and pain at the injection site may develop.

Equivalent doses of depot antipsychotics are given in Table 14.9. As flupentixol has mood-elevating effects, it should be avoided in aggressive, agitated patients. Zuclopenthixol may have a specific indication for aggressive and agitated patients, as it does not have stimulant effects.

COMPLIANCE WITH MEDICATION

Poor compliance is a major problem and is due to factors that include:

- denial of illness
- time taken for therapeutic effect
- side effects of medication
- complexity of regimen
- poor social support
- poor relationship between patients and service providers
- meeting of patient's expectations
- level of professional supervision
- influence of family and friends.

Every effort requires to be made to improve compliance, such as:

- simple drug regimens
  — tablets organised in blister packs
  — the use of depot medications
- improved social support
- improved professional supervision of care
- patient and carer education and information.

MANIC DEPRESSIVE DISORDERS

The commonest disorder of mood is depression. Mania is much less common, but many patients with mania will also experience severe depression (although there is enormous variation in frequency, sequence and duration between patients). When the symptoms are serious or psychotic, the terms *manic depressive disorder* or *bipolar affective disorder* are used. Lifetime risk for bipolar disorder is less than one in 100, and the disorder is equally common in males and females. Cycle length refers to the length of time between the onset of one episode and the onset of the next. This can range from months to years. There is a high risk of recurrence in bipolar illness, and the severity tends to increase with successive episodes. Bipolar illness causes immense personal pain and disruption of families, and it carries a 10–15% lifetime risk of death by suicide.

CLINICAL FEATURES OF MANIA

The symptoms required for diagnosis of mania are as follows.

- Mood: there is an abnormally elevated mood characterised by euphoria, unwarranted optimism

and overconfidence, and the mood eventually changes from euphoria to irritability and aggressiveness.

- Talk: accelerated mental processes cause a flight of ideas with rapid speech; the patient jumps rapidly from subject to subject and may appear quite incoherent.
- Thought: inflated self-esteem, hyperactivity of thought with delusions of wealth, power and influence (counterpart of the depressive's delusions of worthlessness).
- Cognition: impaired concentration, short attention span.
- Behaviour: reduced sleep without tiredness; restless, demanding, loud; behavioural disinhibition with inappropriate laughter, dancing or singing; excessive libido; wearing of flamboyant clothes or make-up.

Attacks are extremely disruptive financially, socially and domestically. Overconfidence causes patients to undertake wildly ambitious commitments. The resulting impairment of judgement may cause business failure, excessive spending or generosity and sexual promiscuity.

MANAGEMENT

Patients may require compulsory admission to a psychiatric unit and detention under an appropriate section of the Mental Health (Care and Treatment) Act 2003 because of loss of judgement resulting in a risk to both themselves and others. Severe manic states used to be associated with significant mortality from exhaustion, dehydration and hyperthermia, but modern practice has reduced this risk considerably.

DRUG TREATMENT

The aims of treatment are to control behaviour, terminate the episode and minimise recurrence with prophylactic therapy. In an acute attack of mania, treatment with an antipsychotic drug is usually required. Mood stabilisers (e.g. lithium) may be given concurrently with the antipsychotic drug and treatment with the antipsychotic gradually tailed off as symptoms recede. If patients demonstrate a recurrent pattern, they must be assessed for maintenance lithium therapy.

LITHIUM

Lithium salts are used in the prophylaxis and treatment of mania, in the prophylaxis of manic depressive illness (bipolar affective disorder) and in the prophylaxis of recurrent depression (unipolar illness or unipolar depression). The body handles lithium in a manner very similar to that of sodium, and it is thought to enter neurones in the brain, decreasing their excitability.

Pharmacokinetics. Lithium is well absorbed from the gastrointestinal tract. It is not protein-bound and is distributed throughout the body water. Peak plasma concentrations are achieved within 1–2 h of oral ingestion (3–6 h with a controlled-release preparation). Elimination is by the kidneys.

Investigations prior to lithium treatment. Lithium has a narrow therapeutic index, and because it is almost completely renally excreted it is essential to have a baseline measure of renal function. Plasma urea and electrolyte levels should then be measured routinely, and creatinine clearance estimation is desirable in the elderly as lithium will be retained if the kidneys are not functioning properly. Hypothyroidism can present as depression, and lithium can induce clinical hypothyroidism, making it important to monitor thyroid function. A full blood count should be done, because anaemia can present as depression and lithium can induce a leucocytosis. An ECG should be carried out, as lithium should be avoided in cardiac disease.

Dose. The initial dose of lithium carbonate is 300–400 mg. Because the elimination half-life may be in excess of 24 h in some individuals, a serum lithium level (blood taken 12 h post dose) should be checked after 5–7 days. The dose is increased as necessary to achieve a serum level in the therapeutic range 0.6–1.0 mmol/L. Lithium levels should be determined weekly until they are stable. Thereafter, they should be checked every 3 months along with plasma creatinine and electrolytes. Thyroid function tests should be checked every 6 months. Lithium is widely prescribed in elderly patients, and levels in this group of patients should be monitored more frequently because an increased half-life can lead to increased levels of lithium.

Side-effects. The commonest clinical problems are gastrointestinal disturbances, tremor, polyuria, polydipsia and weight gain. It may be worth lowering the dose to try to reduce these symptoms, as they may all affect compliance. Lithium inhibits the response of the distal tubule to vasopressin (antidiuretic hormone), resulting in polydipsia and polyuria. Increased body weight may result from lithium-induced thirst and increased fluid intake. It is exacerbated by consumption of high-calorie drinks. Nausea and diarrhoea usually pass after 2–3 weeks' treatment but may be signs of impending intoxication.

Toxicity. Overdosage, usually with plasma concentrations over 1.5 mmol/L, may be fatal, and toxic effects include:

- early symptoms – nausea, vomiting, tremor, blurred vision, polyuria and polydipsia
- symptoms of severe toxicity or intoxication – convulsions, cardiac arrhythmias, impaired consciousness, coma, hyperextension of limbs.

If these potentially hazardous signs occur, treatment should be stopped and plasma lithium concentrations determined. Any predisposing condition that may have precipitated intoxication should be identified and treated. Appropriate supportive and corrective measures for complications of toxicity (e.g. continuous ECG, rehydration) should be instituted.

If there is acute poisoning, induced emesis with ipecacuanha is of benefit if carried out within 3 h of ingestion.

In mild to moderate intoxication, intravenous sodium chloride solution 0.9%, 1–2 L every 6 h, is given. This is of most benefit if the problem is volume depletion or hyponatraemia. If severe, (e.g. 4 mmol/L), haemodialysis should be initiated.

Drug interactions. Lithium toxicity is made worse by sodium depletion, therefore concurrent use of diuretics is hazardous and should be avoided. Lithium is reabsorbed in the proximal tubules in the same proportions as sodium and water. If anything occurs to produce sodium depletion in the body (e.g. use of diuretics, diarrhoea, vomiting), there is a compensatory attempt by the body to reabsorb sodium at the level of the proximal tubule. In someone taking lithium, this means a corresponding reabsorption of lithium and hence a raised serum lithium level. Caution is required when prescribing a diuretic to a patient stabilised on lithium. The severity of increase of lithium levels is greater with thiazides than with loop diuretics. Bendroflumethiazide, 2.5 mg daily, has been shown to increase lithium levels by 20–25%.

Dietary salt restriction can cause an increase in serum lithium as sodium and lithium ions are reabsorbed. Conversely, an excess of sodium can cause expansion of intracellular fluid and an excretion of sodium and hence lithium.

Some non-steroidal anti-inflammatory drugs (NSAIDs) are known to affect the control of lithium treatment by reducing the extent of elimination from the body and thus causing an increase in serum lithium level. Aspirin may be used safely, having no effect on plasma lithium levels.

Counselling of patients. Advice and information should be given to the patient on commencement of lithium therapy. This is essential to provide the patient with an understanding of the drug action and side effects and also to improve compliance. Advice and information given to the patient would be as follows:

- swallow tablets whole; do not chew (this would affect the modified-release mechanism)
- always take the same brand of lithium tablets (this will ensure consistent plasma levels); if in doubt, ask your pharmacist
- lithium will not have an immediate effect; it may be up to 14 days before benefits are apparent
- therapy may be lifelong, and it is important to keep taking lithium even though you may be feeling better
- information regarding common side-effects
- reason for monitoring levels/taking bloods and the importance of attendance at the lithium clinic when requested to do so
- importance of maintaining fluid intake, particularly in hot weather or following exercise – if weight gain is a problem, use low-calorie drinks
- dietary intake of sodium should not be subject to fluctuations
- over-the-counter drugs containing sodium or NSAIDs should be avoided
- sickness/diarrhoea due to risk of sodium depletion
- advice on contraception when appropriate.

Every patient taking lithium should have a lithium card (Fig. 14.3), provided by the pharmacist, which reinforces the advice and information given.

CARBAMAZEPINE AND VALPROIC ACID

Carbamazepine may be used for the prophylaxis of manic depressive illness in patients unresponsive to lithium. It seems to be particularly effective in patients with rapid-cycling manic depressive illness (four or more affective episodes per year).

Valproic acid may be used for the acute treatment of a manic episode associated with bipolar disorder.

DEPRESSION

About 60–70% of adults will, at some time, experience depression or worry of sufficient severity to influence their daily activities. Approximately 1.5% of the population in Britain is treated for depressive illness each year. Episodes of major depression are about twice as common among women as men, peak in middle age and are commonly associated with adverse social and economic circumstances such as unemployment, divorce or separation, inadequate housing and lower social class. Having a first-degree relative with depressive illness is associated with a fivefold increase in the risk of developing a similar illness. For the majority of people, episodes of depression are short-lived, but a minority experience a range of severe psychological and clinical symptoms that may persist.

MAJOR DEPRESSION

Criteria have been developed to identify people who are categorised as having a major depressive episode. Termed the *Diagnostic and Statistical Manual of Mental Disorders, third edition (revised)* (*DSM-III-R*) criteria, these are summarised in Box 14.2. The International Statistical Classification of Diseases and Related Health Problems 10 criteria are similar.

Major depression is diagnosed when at least five of the symptoms (which must include symptoms 1 or 2, or both) have been present over a minimum duration of 2 weeks.

The term *bipolar disorder* is used to indicate at least one episode of mania (i.e. manic depressive disorder). Depression may be further classified as mild, moderate or severe according to the intensity of the symptoms.

DIFFERENTIAL DIAGNOSIS

For depression to be diagnosed, certain other conditions may have to be ruled out:

- normal sadness
- anxiety neuroses with or without phobic or obsessional symptoms
- schizophrenia
- dementia (chronic organic brain syndrome)
- organic brain lesion
- other drug treatment (e.g. beta blockers).

TREATMENT

There is no evidence that very mild depressive symptoms respond to pharmacological treatment. Such symptoms are best managed with psychological support, encouragement and explanation to ensure that a clinical depression does not develop. Other psychological approaches include dynamic psychotherapy and cognitive therapy. Dynamic psychotherapy aims to change interpersonal dynamics that may contribute to an individual's vulnerability to developing depression, whereas cognitive therapy aims to alter cognitions, that is, the way in which an individual interprets adverse circumstances. For more severe symptoms, treatment with an antidepressant drug is the preferred option.

The choice of antidepressant is influenced by many factors, including the clinical presentation, response to treatment during previous episodes, side-effect profile and cost. Antidepressants with sedative properties may

THINKING ABOUT STARTING A FAMILY?

Because lithium can affect the unborn baby do NOT become pregnant without first talking to your doctor. If you are pregnant tell your doctor now.

PLEASE RECORD YOUR
BLOOD LEVEL OF LITHIUM

DATE TAKEN	BLOOD LEVEL	DAILY DOSE

LITHIUM TREATMENT CARD

CARRY THIS CARD WITH YOU AT ALL TIMES. SHOW IT TO ANY DOCTOR OR NURSE WHO TREATS YOU AND ANY PHARMACIST YOU BUY MEDICINES FROM

NAME ....

PREPARATION
OF LITHIUM ....

Should a different proprietary product be prescribed, the card must be suitably endorsed.

KEEP YOUR TABLETS IN
A SAFE PLACE WELL OUT
OF THE REACH OF CHILDREN

A

HOW SHOULD I TAKE THE TABLETS?

Swallow each tablet whole or broken in half, with water. Do NOT chew or crush it. Try to take the dose at the same time each day.

WHAT SHOULD I DO IF I MISS A DOSE?

Do NOT double your next dose. If you find you have missed a few doses, start taking your usual dose on the day you remember and tell your doctor.

WHY MUST I HAVE A BLOOD TEST?

This is to check the amount of lithium in your blood. It is very important to have the correct amount because too much can be dangerous. Take the blood test ABOUT 12 HOURS AFTER the last dose of lithium.

CAN I DRINK ALCOHOL?

It is safe to drink SMALL quantities.

B

CAN I TAKE OTHER MEDICINES WITH LITHIUM?

Some medicines can change the amount of lithium in the blood. These include diuretic (water) tablets and capsules, some pain killers and some indigestion mixtures and laxatives. So check with your doctor or pharmacist before taking other medicines.

Please note: it is safe to take paracetamol but not ibuprofen.

WHAT ELSE ALTERS THE LITHIUM LEVEL?

The level can be altered by the amount of fluids you drink, changes in the amount of salt in your food, sweating more than usual (in hot weather, fever or infection), severe vomiting, severe diarrhoea and a low salt diet. Check with your doctor if any of these things happen.

SIGNS OF A HIGH LITHIUM LEVEL

Vomiting, severe diarrhoea, unusual drowsiness, muscle weakness and feeling very giddy may mean that your level of lithium is too high. Stop taking the tablets and talk to your doctor IMMEDIATELY.

DOES LITHIUM HAVE SIDE-EFFECTS?

Some slight effects (such as sickness, shaking) may occur at first but they usually wear off if blood tests are normal. Discuss this with your doctor. Some patients may gain weight but this can be prevented with a sensible diet.

HOW LONG WILL I HAVE TO TAKE LITHIUM?

Lithium is a way of preventing illness so you may have to take it for many years. Never stop taking the tablets without asking your doctor.

Fig. 14.3 Lithium card.

be desirable in some patients but not in others (e.g. if retardation is marked). Previous good response to an antidepressant would make the same antidepressant a logical choice in subsequent episodes. Conversely, previous poor response would militate against the reuse of the same drug or one from the same class.

The side-effect profile should be borne in mind when there is pre-existing physical illness. For example, tricyclic antidepressants have a membrane-stabilising effect and should therefore be avoided in patients with cardiac conduction abnormalities. Antimuscarinic side- effects are also undesirable in those with angle closure glaucoma or prostatic hypertrophy.

CLINICAL MANAGEMENT PLAN

The choice of antidepressant drug and the starting dose should be tailored to the individual patient's needs. The dose should be titrated against both clinical symptoms and side-effects. Care should be taken to ensure that a therapeutic dose is reached. The patient should be counselled about both the anticipated effects and the side-effects of the drugs prescribed. Particular attention should be paid to the expected time of clinical effect and the overall duration of treatment.

TRICYCLIC AND RELATED ANTIDEPRESSANTS

Mode of action. Tricyclic antidepressants are thought to exert their clinical effect by blocking the reuptake of amines, for example noradrenaline (norepinephrine), serotonin and dopamine, into the presynaptic neurone, thus increasing the amounts available in the synaptic cleft.

Pharmacokinetics. Tricyclic antidepressants are rapidly absorbed and extensively metabolised in the liver. They have a long action and may need to be given only once a day. Patients differ widely in the extent to which they absorb or metabolise antidepressants, and dosage should always be adjusted to the individual's clinical response. There appears to be some evidence of a 'therapeutic window'.

Response. A patient is unlikely to experience any improvement in mood for at least 2 weeks. Treatment should be monitored at the optimum dose or maximum tolerated dose for at least 4–6 weeks to allow for a full therapeutic trial. The typical pattern of response to an antidepressant is:

- sleep pattern may start to improve after a few days and concentration after about a week
- lifting of mood may be delayed 2 weeks or more
- when response commences, good days will be followed by bad but after several weeks there will be more good days than bad ones.

Adverse effects (Table 14.10). The patient should be reassured that mild antimuscarinic side-effects are common initially, but if these are found to be intolerable they should be discussed rather than treatment discontinued. Patients who experience blurred vision need to know that this effect is reversible. It is not the time to buy new glasses. Patients should also be advised to stand up slowly if they feel dizzy and let their doctor know if they develop a rash. Patients with depression have very poor concentration, so it is important that they receive written information to support verbal advice.

Other antimuscarinic side-effects may be dry mouth and constipation. More serious and occurring less frequently are failure to pass urine, closed angle glaucoma, jaundice, depression of the white blood cell count, convulsions, arrhythmias and tachycardia.

Many tricyclic antidepressants have sedative properties so that they can be prescribed at night to help treat insomnia in the short term. This also helps to alleviate the antimuscarinic side-effects. The return of a more normal sleep pattern results as depression is alleviated. Taking more than one tricyclic antidepressant at the same time is not recommended. There is no

Table 14.10 Adverse effects of tricyclic antidepressants

Antidepressant	Average dose (mg/day)[a]	Relative side-effects				
		Antimuscarinic	Cardiac	Nausea	Drowsiness	Danger in overdose
Amitriptyline	75	XXX	XXX	XX	XXX	XXX
Clomipramine	75	XXX	XX	XX	XX	X
Dosulepin (dothiepin)	75	XX	XX	–	XXX	XXX
Doxepin	75	X	XX	X	XX	XX
Imipramine	75	XX	XX	XX	X	XX
Lofepramine	140	XX	X	XX	X	–
Maprotiline	75	XX	XX	XX	X	XXX
Mianserin[b]	90	X	–	–	XXX	X
Trazodone	150	X	X	XXX	XX	X

XXX, high incidence/severity; XX, moderate; X, low; –, very low/none.
[a]Higher doses may be required for severe depression.

evidence that side-effects are minimised. Examples of tricyclic and related antidepressants are listed in Table 14.10.

If a therapeutic response is obtained, an average course of antidepressants would be for 6 months to 1 year and should be given for at least 3 months after recovery. Care must be taken in withdrawing antidepressants following treatment. Reduction in dosage should be carried out gradually over a period of about 4 weeks, otherwise withdrawal symptoms will be experienced. These include gastrointestinal symptoms of nausea, vomiting and anorexia accompanied by headache, dizziness and insomnia. Panic, anxiety and motor restlessness may also occur.

A tricyclic or related antidepressant should not be started until 2 weeks after stopping a monoamine-oxidase inhibitor (MAOI). Conversely, an MAOI should not be started until at least a week after a tricyclic or related antidepressant has been stopped.

Choice of drugs. All tricyclic antidepressants have approximately equal clinical efficacy, and the choice of which tricyclic to use in a particular patient is determined by the side-effect profile. Agitated and anxious patients tend to respond best to more sedative products, whereas withdrawn and apathetic patients will obtain more benefit from less sedating compounds.

Clomipramine is useful in the treatment of depression linked with anxiety and is used in obsessional compulsive disorders, phobic anxiety states and panic disorder. Lofepramine is useful in the elderly. Mianserin has been reported for serious bone marrow suppression leading to leucopenia, agranulocytosis and aplastic anaemia. This would normally occur in the first 6 weeks of treatment and is more common in the elderly, requiring regular blood counts to be carried out. Weight gain is common with all tricyclic antidepressants.

MONOAMINE-OXIDASE INHIBITORS

Monoamine oxidase has a variety of isoenzymes, which have been classified as type A (present in the gut and liver) and type B (present in the brain). The different isoenzymes have different selectivities for amine substrates:

- MAO-A metabolises serotonin and noradrenaline (norepinephrine)
- MAO-B metabolises phenylethylamine and benzylamine
- dopamine and tyramine are metabolised to both the type A and type B enzymes.

Monoamine-oxidase inhibitors (MAOIs) inhibit the action of MAO, resulting in an accumulation of

263

monoamines such as serotonin, noradrenaline and dopamine within the synapse. It is this effect that is thought to be the primary action of MAOIs in relieving depression. The MAOIs are used much less frequently than other antidepressants, because of dietary and drug interactions. They are used to treat atypical depression with associated anxiety and obsessional, hysterical or hypochondriacal symptoms. They can also be used to treat resistant depressions.

Pharmacokinetics. The MAOI anti-depressants are readily absorbed from the gut, extensively metabolised and excreted mainly as metabolites in the urine and faeces.

Response. The dose needs to be gradually built up to a therapeutic level. There will be a time lag of 4–6 weeks to achieve a full antidepressant effect.

Choice. The drugs of choice are phenelzine or isocarboxazid, which are less stimulant and therefore safer than tranylcypromine. The dose of phenelzine is 15 mg three times daily, increased when required up to four times daily after 2 weeks (hospital patients, maximum 30 mg three times daily) then reduced gradually to lowest possible maintenance dose. Isocarboxazid is given initially up to 30 mg daily in single or divided doses, increased after 4 weeks if necessary to a maximum of 60 mg daily for up to 6 weeks under close supervision, and then reduced to a maintenance dose of 10–40 mg daily.

Side-effects. The MAOIs, especially tranylcypromine, can cause antimuscarinic side-effects. They are very alerting, causing sleep disturbance. To avoid this, the last dose can be taken in the early afternoon. Other side effects include weight gain, sexual dysfunction, dizziness, postural hypotension, liver damage, dry mouth, constipation, headache, tremor and ankle oedema.

Interactions. Hypertensive crisis is rare but severe. It is due to MAOIs preventing metabolism of tyramine in tyramine-rich food or drink. A hypertensive crisis may also arise with sympathomimetic drugs.

Tyramine. Irreversible MAOIs block the ability of MAO to inactivate tyramine in the gastro-intestinal tract and liver for a long period of time. The tyramine is present in foods such as cheese, salted fish, broad bean pods, Bovril, Oxo, Marmite, shrimp paste, pâté and drinks including red wine, beer, ale, and non-alcoholic beers and lagers. Excess tyramine enters the bloodstream and releases noradrenaline (norepinephrine) from its storage sites located in the sympathetic nerve endings. This can cause vasoconstriction and an increase in blood pressure, which can result in a potentially fatal reaction characterised by severe hypertension associated with

---

> **TREATMENT CARD**
> *Carry this card with you at all times. Show it to any doctor who may treat you other than the doctor who prescribed this medicine, and to your dentist if you require dental treatment.*
>
> **INSTRUCTIONS TO PATIENTS**
> Please read carefully
>
> While taking this medicine and for 14 days after your treatment finishes you must observe the following simple instructions:-
> 1. Do not eat CHEESE, PICKLED HERRING OR BROAD BEAN PODS.
> 2. Do not eat/drink BOVRIL, OXO, MARMITE, or ANY SIMILAR MEAT OR YEAST EXTRACT.
> 3. Eat only FRESH foods and avoid food that you suspect could be stale or 'going off'. This is especially important with meat, fish, poultry or offal. Avoid game.
> 4. Do not take any other MEDICINES (including tablets, capsules, nose drops, inhalations or suppositories) whether purchased by you or previously prescribed by your doctor, without first consulting your doctor or your pharmacist.
> NB *Treatment for coughs and colds, pain relievers, tonics and laxatives are medicines.*
> 5. Avoid alcoholic drinks and de-alcoholised (low alcohol) drinks.
>
> **Keep a careful note of any food or drink that disagrees with you, avoid it and tell your doctor.**
>
> **Report any unusual or severe symptoms to your doctor and follow any other advice given by him.**

Fig. 14.4 Monoamine-oxidase inhibitor treatment card.

severe headache, sweating, flushing, nausea, vomiting and palpitations. Patients on MAOIs are restricted to a low-tyramine diet. They are given a treatment card and counselled (Fig. 14.4).

Sympathomimetics. Sympathomimetics such as pseudoephedrine and phenylpropanolamine, which release noradrenaline (norepinephrine) at nerve endings, may be potentiated by MAOIs. A severe hypertensive crisis may result. An early warning symptom may be a throbbing headache. Sympathomimetics are present in many cough mixtures and decongestant nasal drops, and patients must be warned not to use these medicines. The danger of the reaction persists for up to 14 days after treatment with MAOIs has been discontinued.

Dopamine receptor agonists. Levodopa may cause similar hypertensive reactions in patients taking non-selective MAOIs and should be avoided.

Tricyclic antidepressants. Because tricyclic antidepressants inhibit noradrenaline (norepinephrine) reuptake by nerve endings, the combination of tricyclics with MAOIs is hazardous. MAOIs should not be started until at least 2 weeks after tricyclics and related antidepressants have been stopped and 2 weeks after cessation of Selective serotonin re-uptake inhibitors (SSRIs) (5 weeks for fluoxetine). Similarly, other antidepressants or another MAOI should not be given to patients for 14 days after treatment with a previous MAOI has been discontinued.

SELECTIVE MONOAMINE OXIDASE INHIBITORS

Because the transmitters considered to play a role in depression are serotonin, noradrenaline (norepinephrine) and dopamine, the antidepressant effects are thought to depend largely or exclusively on inhibition of MAO-A.

Drugs that reversibly affect mainly MAO-A are known as reversible inhibitors of MAO-A (RIMAs), as distinguished from the previously discussed irreversible MAOI. A RIMA, which preferentially inhibits MAO-A, interferes less with the metabolism of tyramine. Reversible inhibition of a MAO-A does not provoke an increase in blood pressure for two reasons. First, by preferentially inhibiting MAO-A, it leaves MAO-B free to metabolise ingested tyramine. Second, when an excess of tyramine is ingested, the RIMA inhibitor will dissociate with MAO-A, allowing the enzyme to metabolise the excess. Patients should avoid ingesting large quantities of tyramine while prescribed a RIMA, but they do not have to adhere to MAOI diet. An example of this type of drug is moclobemide.

MOCLOBEMIDE

Moclobemide is comparable in its effect with the tricyclic antidepressants and the MAOIs. The usual dosage range is 300–450 mg daily in two or three divided doses. There is 95% absorption, but extensive first-pass metabolism results in an oral bioavailability of 45–60%. The half-life is 1–2 h.

Moclobemide is well tolerated, largely devoid of antimuscarinic effects, postural hypotension or weight gain. The main side-effects include dizziness, headache, dry mouth, tremor, insomnia and nausea.

Withdrawal. Moclobemide can be stopped almost immediately without the requirement to reduce the dose slowly over a number of weeks.

When transferring from other antidepressants to moclobemide, the washout period depends on the

Table 14.11 Washout periods of antidepressants

Drugs	Washout period
Monoamine oxidase inhibitors	14 days
Amitriptyline	4–5 days
Imipramine	3–4 days
Selective serotonin reuptake inhibitors (except fluoxetine)	14 days
Fluoxetine	5 weeks

half-life of the parent drug or the active metabolite, as shown in Table 14.11.

SELECTIVE SEROTONIN RE-UPTAKE INHIBITORS

Selective serotonin re-uptake inhibitor (SSRI) antidepressants inhibit the neuronal reuptake of serotonin by blocking the action of the uptake pump, allowing the serotonin to remain longer in the synaptic cleft, therapy enhancing its action. SSRIs differ from tricyclic antidepressants in having a more selective action in the uptake of serotonin, producing less muscarinic receptor blockade and being free from membrane-stabilising effects in the heart. As a result, they are less likely to cause antimuscarinic and cardiotoxic effects.

Selective serotonin re-uptake inhibitors are rapidly absorbed, and food has little effect on absorption. Peak plasma concentrations are reached within 8 h and steady state concentrations within 2 weeks (2–6 weeks in the case of fluoxetine). SSRIs are metabolised in the liver, the metabolites having little or no activity, with the exception of N-desmethylfluoxetine, the main metabolite of fluoxetine. Metabolites are excreted mainly in the urine. Fluoxetine has a half-life of 1–3 days and that of desmethylfluoxetine is 1–2 weeks. The half-lives of the other SSRIs are less than 24 h.

SELECTION OF SSRIS

The dose range for each single SSRI is the same for all groups of patients. Fluoxetine and paroxetine are generally administered as a single dose in the morning. Fluvoxamine and sertraline, at therapeutic doses, tend to be given in two divided doses. Citalopram can be given as a single dose either in the morning or in the evening. Table 14.12 gives details of doses.

Table 14.12 Serotonin re-uptake inhibitors

Drug	Average daily dose/range (mg)
Citalopram	20–60
Fluoxetine	20–40
Fluvoxamine	100–200
Paroxetine	20–40
Sertraline	50–100

All SSRIs appear to be clinically equivalent, but they differ in their half-lives and thus have differing lengths of action. They may be considered as a first-line choice for those patients with heart disease, those at increased risk of overdose, the elderly and for those unable to tolerate tricyclic antidepressants.

Patients with impaired hepatic and renal function should be monitored when commenced on SSRIs. The drugs should be discontinued when dysfunction is severe. Care should be taken in patients with seizure disorders, and these drugs should be avoided in patients with unstable epilepsy.

Side-effects. The most common unwanted effects are nausea, dyspepsia, dry mouth, headache, somnolence, insomnia and dizziness. In general, the SSRI antidepressants have a much reduced incidence and severity of side-effects compared with the tricyclic antidepressants. They do not cause weight gain and there may even be a slight weight loss.

Withdrawal. Withdrawal of SSRIs should be undertaken slowly. An SSRI or related antidepressant should not be started until 2 weeks after stopping an MAOI. Conversely, an MAOI should not be started until at least a week after an SSRI or related antidepressant has been started (2 weeks in the case of paroxetine and sertraline, at least 5 weeks in the case of fluoxetine).

OTHER ANTIDEPRESSANTS

Other drugs used to treat depression include duloxetine, venlafaxine, mirtazapine, reboxetine, flupentixol and tryptophan.

Duloxetine and venlafaxine inhibit the re-uptake of both serotonin and noradrenaline (nor-epinephrine). The Committee on Safety of Medicines has recommended that because of concerns about toxicity in overdose, treatment with venlafaxine should be initiated and maintained under specialist

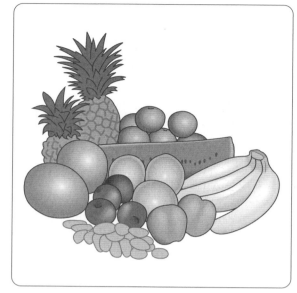

Fig. 14.5 Healthy foods.

supervision only. Flupentixol is given in low doses (1–3 mg daily) for depression. Mirtazapine enhances the neurotransmission of serotonin and norepinephrine but causes sedation during initial treatment. Reboxetine is a highly selective and effective inhibitor of norepinephrine reuptake. Tryptophan is initiated by hospital specialists for treatment-resistant depression after trials of standard antidepressant drug treatments.

OBESITY

Obesity is associated with many health problems, including diabetes mellitus and cardiovascular disease. The main treatment of the obese individual is a suitable diet and increased physical activity with appropriate support and encouragement. Drugs should never be used as the sole treatment of obesity; patients should be advised, for example, to eat five portions of fruit and vegetables per day (see Fig. 14.5) and avoid high-calorie fast foods (see Fig. 14.6). The individual should be monitored on a regular basis, and drug treatment should be discontinued if weight loss is less than 5% after the first 12 weeks or if the individual regains weight at any time while receiving drug treatment.

Drugs specifically licensed for the treatment of obesity include orlistat, sibutramine and rimonabant. Orlistat may be appropriate for those who have a high intake of fat, whereas sibutramine may be

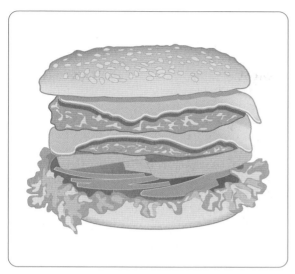

Fig. 14.6 Unhealthy foods.

selected for those who cannot control their eating. Orlistat is a lipase inhibitor that causes a reduction in fat absorption by increasing fat excretion. Orlistat or sibutramine should be prescribed only as part of an overall treatment plan for the management of obesity in people aged 18–75 (orlistat) or 18–65 (sibutramine) who meet the following criteria:

- a body mass index (BMI) of 30 kg/m^2 or more without associated comorbidities
- a BMI of 28 kg/m^2 (orlistat) or 27 kg/m^2 (sibutramine) or more in the presence of significant comorbidities (e.g. type 2 diabetes, hypertension).

One hundred and twenty milligrams of orlistat is taken immediately before, during or up to 1 h after each main meal. The most common side effects are gastrointestinal (e.g. fatty stools, faecal urgency and flatulence).

The starting dose of sibutramine should normally be 10 mg/day. Continuation of this therapy beyond 4 weeks should be supported by evidence of a 2-kg weight loss, and beyond 3 months should be supported by evidence of a loss of at least 5% of initial body weight from the start of drug treatment. Dosage may be increased to 15 mg/day after 4 weeks. Sibutramine therapy should be stopped if there is an inadequate response.

Because the use of sibutramine may increase the blood pressure of some individuals, blood pressure must be checked regularly in all those for whom it is prescribed. If blood pressure increases, continuation of sibutramine must be reconsidered, taking into account the risks and benefits of the effects of treatment on cardiovascular risk profile for the individual. Sibutramine is not recommended for individuals whose blood pressure before the start of therapy is above 145/90 mmHg. Treatment is not recommended beyond 12 months.

It is important for patients taking obesity treatments that arrangements exist for appropriate health professionals to offer advice, support and counselling on diet, physical activity and behavioural strategies.

NAUSEA AND VERTIGO

NAUSEA AND VOMITING

Antiemetics relieve nausea and vomiting (see also Ch. 26) from a variety of causes. The group of nuclei known collectively as the vomiting centre is located in the medulla oblongata in the brain stem and can receive stimuli from various sources. The nausea response can be initiated when the upper gastrointestinal tract sends nerve impulses to the vomiting centre along the vagus and sympathetic nerves. This can be stimulated, for example, by irritation of mucosal receptors in the gastrointestinal tract, radiation therapy injury of the gastrointestinal mucosa or malignant disease of the gastrointestinal tract.

Another collection of nuclei called the chemoreceptor trigger zone (CTZ) is located in the area postrema. Activation of the CTZ can stimulate the vomiting centre, which in turn causes nausea or initiates emesis. Motion sickness results from stimulation of the vestibular apparatus of the ear, which activates the vomiting centre via the CTZ. People who know they may experience motion sickness under certain circumstances can use an antiemetic prophylactically to avoid this.

Labyrinthitis resulting from inflammation of the vestibular apparatus of the ear causes nausea, vomiting, dizziness and hearing loss. Ménière's disease, which involves dilatation of the endolymphatic channels in the cochlea, also produces nausea as well as dizziness, tinnitus and hearing loss.

Cancer chemotherapy can directly or indirectly (through the CTZ) stimulate the vomiting centre, causing severe nausea and vomiting. Narcotics can cause nausea and vomiting either by stimulating the CTZ or by sensitising the vestibular apparatus of the ear.

Nausea and vomiting are frequent and often distressing side effects connected with anaesthesia and surgery. Various factors may be involved, including inhalation agents, premedication, postoperative pain, opioid analgesia and movement.

The main neurotransmitters in the area postrema, thought to have a role in emesis are:

- acetylcholine
- histamine
- dopamine
- serotonin.

The actions of certain antiemetics indicate that acetylcholine and histamine are more important in motion sickness than in other types of emesis. Many antiemetics are antidopaminergic, and this may lead to the occurrence of extrapyramidal reactions.

DRUG TREATMENTS
Hyoscine

Hyoscine acts on the vomiting centre in the medulla, where it has an antimuscarinic action. Its efficacy in motion sickness is due to an effect on the vestibular apparatus. Hyoscine is available as tablets, slow-release tablets and a transdermal presentation.

Phenothiazines

The phenothiazines are dopamine antagonists and act centrally by blocking the CTZ. They are rapidly absorbed after oral administration. Rectal or parenteral administration is required if vomiting has already started. Prochlorperazine, perphenazine and trifluoperazine are less sedating than chlorpromazine. Long-term use is limited by side-effects, including extrapyramidal reactions and antimuscarinic effects. Patients should be advised about drowsiness and warned not to drive or operate machinery.

Metoclopramide

Metoclopramide blocks peripheral and central dopamine receptors when in high doses, and it also acts on peripheral and central 5-HT$_3$ receptors.

Metoclopramide also reduces oesophageal reflux and enhances gastric emptying, which is useful in treating gastric hypomotility found in migraine. Side-effects are usually mild, transient and reversible on discontinuation of therapy. Extrapyramidal symptoms may occur.

Domperidone

Domperidone acts on the CTZ and has antiemetic properties, and its effects on gastrointestinal motility are similar to those of metoclopramide. It causes little extrapyramidal side-effects and is less sedating than metoclopramide; it is therefore useful in treating patients with Parkinson's disease when nausea and

vomiting associated with levodopa or bromocriptine are troublesome.

Selective 5-HT$_3$ antagonists

The 5-HT$_3$ antagonists, including ondansetron, granisetron and tropisetron, block 5HT$_3$ receptors in the gastrointestinal tract and in the central nervous system. The lack of therapeutic activity on dopamine receptors indicates that, unlike metoclopramide, antiemetic activity can be achieved without dose-limiting extrapyramidal side-effects. These drugs are used mainly to treat nausea and vomiting in patients receiving cytotoxics and in postoperative nausea and vomiting. If vomiting is not adequately controlled, the drug should be continued orally or intravenously for up to 5 days. Side-effects of 5-HT$_3$ antagonists include constipation and headache.

DRUG TREATMENT OF NAUSEA AND VOMITING IN PARTICULAR SITUATIONS

Motion sickness. Hyoscine is the most effective drug for the prevention of motion sickness. It is available both in tablet form and as a transdermal patch providing a slow continuous absorption into the bloodstream. A 300-microgram tablet is taken 30 min before the start of the journey, or a 500-microgram patch is applied to a hairless area of skin behind the ear 5–6 h before a journey and replaced after 72 h if necessary. Side-effects such as drowsiness, blurred vision, dry mouth and urinary retention do not occur to any great extent at the doses used.

Antihistamines. Antihistamines act on the vestibular apparatus, the vomiting centre and the CTZ. Cinnarizine, cyclizine and promethazine are effective. The first dose should be taken 30 min before the journey commences (2 h for cinnarizine). The latter two are more sedating. They potentiate central nervous system depressants such as alcohol, phenothiazines and benzodiazepines. The sedative effect and the times of administration of these drugs are shown in Table 14.13.

Table 14.13 Administration and sedative effect of some antihistamines

Antihistamine	Taken before journey (h)	Sedative effect
Cinnarizine	2	Mild
Cyclizine	0.5	Mild
Promethazine	0.5	Moderate

Drowsiness may affect performance of skilled tasks such as driving or operating machinery. Effects of alcohol are enhanced.

Drug-induced nausea and vomiting. Lowering the dose or withdrawal of the drug should be considered. If the drug has to be continued, choice of treatment depends on drug-induced emesis. Local gastric irritation may be reduced by increasing dosage frequency and lowering the dose, and also by taking the drug with food. Central effects such as opiate-induced vomiting may be treated with haloperidol or metoclopramide.

Postoperative vomiting. Postoperative nausea and vomiting may cause electrolyte imbalance and dehydration. Patients may have difficulty with food and fluid intake, and oral drug therapy can be disrupted. Metoclopramide or a phenothiazine can be used. More recently, ondansetron has been used to treat nausea and vomiting.

Pregnancy. Drug therapy of vomiting in pregnancy should be reserved for severe cases and, when possible, treatment should be avoided during the first trimester. Vomiting is usually most troublesome during this period, reaching a peak at about 10 weeks. On rare occasions when vomiting is severe, short-term treatment with an antihistamine such as promethazine may be required.

Cytotoxic drug therapy. Nausea and vomiting occur frequently during the treatment of cancer with cytotoxic drugs or irradiation. Not all cytotoxic agents cause vomiting, but those that frequently do include cisplatin, dacarbazine, doxorubicin, cyclophosphamide and high doses of methotrexate. Metoclopramide in higher doses is effective, but dosage is limited by side-effects. Vomiting due to highly emetogenic drugs can often be alleviated by dexamethasone. Adding a sedative such as lorazepam may help. For patients at high risk of emesis or when other treatments are inadequate, $5-HT_3$ antagonists are effective. Dexamethasone has been shown to enhance the efficacy of these.

VESTIBULAR DISORDERS

Acute labyrinthine disorders are distressing for the patient and are associated with the symptoms of nausea, vomiting and vertigo. Antihistamines and phenothiazines may be helpful. Betahistine and cinnarizine are useful in treating Ménière's disease. In an acute attack, cyclizine or prochlorperazine may be given rectally or by intramuscular injection.

MIGRAINE

Migraine affects at least 10% of the population of the UK (Steiner et al. 2003). Attacks generally start in the teens or twenties. After puberty, migraine affects more women than men. During the reproductive period, about 20% of women suffer, particularly those in their early forties. Headache is only one symptom of migraine, which has been defined as episodic headaches lasting between 2 and 72 h, with each attack accompanied by visual and/or gastrointestinal disturbance. Migraine's most common accompanying symptoms are photophobia, nausea and vomiting.

Migraine is classified into two main types:

- migraine without aura (common migraine)
- migraine with aura (classic migraine).

Only 10% of attacks are preceded by an aura. Patients who experience an aura can start their migraine treatment during this phase. Visual aura takes the form of blind spots. Other symptoms are sensory disturbances such as 'pins and needles' in one arm, moving up to the face.

TRIGGERS

Several factors need to be present to trigger a migraine attack. The triggers are not the same for everyone. The triggers are as follows.

- Hormonal factors (women):
  — pregnancy
  — oral contraception
  — hormone replacement therapy
  — menstruation.
- Environmental factors:
  — bright or flickering lights
  — overexertion
  — travel.
- Emotional factors
- Head and neck pain
- Insufficient food: missed meals
- Specific foods
  — cheese
  — chocolate
  — caffeine
  — citrus fruits.

TREATMENT

Early treatment during attacks with effective drugs is of the utmost importance, as the efficacy of oral medication during migraine is impaired by gastric stasis. Patients should carry medication at all times. A drop in blood sugar precedes a migraine attack, and

Table 14.14 Drugs used in prevention of prophylaxis

Drug	Class	Dose (mg)
Amitriptyline	Tricyclic antidepressant	10–50 at night
Cyproheptadine	Antihistamine with serotonin antagonist and calcium channel–blocking properties	4 at night
Pizotifen	Antihistamine and serotonin antagonist	0.5–3 daily
Propranolol	Beta-blocker	10–40 three times daily

food is an important part of treatment. If patients feel too nauseous, the attack is being treated too late. For many, sleep is the best natural remedy, and applications of hot and cold compresses can help to ease the pain.

DRUG TREATMENT

This includes analgesics, antiemetics and the $5HT_1$ agonists (almotriptan, eletriptan, frovatriptan sumatriptan, zolmitriptan, naratriptan, rizatriptan). Simple analgesics such as paracetamol and aspirin may be insufficient. There are specific over-the-counter migraine preparations such as Migraleve (contains buclizine, paracetamol and codeine). When these are unsuccessful, an antiemetic with an effect on gastric motility is used with analgesics. Metoclopramide by mouth, or if vomiting is likely, by intramuscular injection, relieves the nausea.

Triptans should be taken as the headache starts. Seven different triptans are now marketed as tablets. Two are additionally available as nasal sprays (sumatriptan and zolmitriptan), three as dispersible tablets (rizatriptan, zolmitriptan and sumatriptan, the first two being orodispersible), and one as a self-administered subcutaneous injection (sumatriptan).

A number of principal criteria exist for choosing any of these. Patient preference may be for dispersible rather than swallowed tablets or for nasal spray. Early vomiters, who cannot take oral medication, should use either zolmitriptan nasal spray (not sumatriptan, as it requires ingestion to be absorbed) or sumatriptan injection. Those in whom rapid efficacy is important above all else may need sumatriptan injection.

Side-effects of the HT_1 agonists include sensations of tingling, heat, heaviness, pressure or tightness, including throat and chest – discontinue if intense, as it may be due to coronary vasoconstriction or anaphylaxis.

Tolfenamic acid is effective as an acute treatment for migraine attacks.

PROPHYLAXIS

Some patients require prophylactic medication taken daily to prevent migraine (e.g. if the patient has more than two migraine attacks per month; Table 14.14).

EPILEPSY

INTRODUCTION

Both seizures and epilepsy are common (Sanders and Shorvon 1996). Epilepsy is the most common serious condition of the brain. It develops in 30 000 people per year in the UK and affects more than 300 000 people at any one time. The diagnosis of epilepsy can be difficult and needs to be established by a trained specialist, usually a consultant neurologist or paediatrician. Up to one in seven of those with a diagnosis of epilepsy may not have epilepsy but a different condition that requires a different treatment (Scheepers et al. 1998). This can be an explanation for antiepileptic medication not controlling a patient's condition. There are different forms of epilepsy and many causes. Different medications are used for different forms of epilepsy and not diagnosing epilepsy accurately may lead to inappropriate medication being used.

The term *neurone* describes the nerve cells and their processes that are situated in the brain. These neurones behave like a small electrical source and, when nerve impulses are generated, the impulses pass along the axon to the neuromuscular junction and from there they energise the muscle fibres. During an epileptic seizure, the nerve impulses generated are greatly in excess of normal and are uncoordinated. An epileptic seizure can be defined as a sudden, brief abnormal discharge of cerebral neurones that is accompanied by a disturbance of behaviour, emotion, motor function or sensation.

The manifestation of a seizure depends on which neurones are involved and how far and how quickly the discharge spreads or extends. A generalised seizure is a seizure that occurs simultaneously throughout the cortex and, conversely, a partial seizure begins in a specific group of cortical neurones that may then spread. If a partial seizure spreads to involve the whole cortex, then this is referred to as a secondary generalised seizure. A seizure results from an imbalance of the excitatory and inhibitory mechanisms within the brain, either in one specific area or in a generalised fashion.

Although epilepsy may result from brain malformation, brain damage from infection/fever, scarring from a head injury, hormonal changes, biochemical disorders, drug or alcohol abuse (symptomatic epilepsy), in many cases there is no known cause (idiopathic epilepsy). Although seizures can appear dramatic and frightening to an observer, it is important to realise that the person affected normally feels no pain during a seizure and may have no memory of it afterwards.

Antiepileptics act to prevent the spread of neuronal excitation by exerting a stabilising effect on excitable cell membranes or by enhancing the activity of neurotransmitters such as gamma-aminobutyric acid, which inhibit the spread of seizure activity by blocking synaptic transmission.

CLASSIFICATION OF SEIZURES

Many different terms have been used to describe the various types of epilepsy. A classification has been produced by the International League Against Epilepsy (Commission on Classification and Terminology 1981). In this classification, seizures are divided into two types: partial and generalised.

PARTIAL SEIZURES

- *Simple partial seizures*. These seizures result from a focal epileptic discharge in a localised area of the brain. A simple partial seizure may be motor (e.g. abnormal movement of limb), sensory (e.g. abnormal sensation) or both. It is not accompanied by unconsciousness and is usually of short duration. The nature of the symptoms depends largely on the anatomical site of seizure discharge. A partial seizure is often preceded by abnormal symptoms (an aura), such as a brief feeling of fear, panic or a particular taste, sight or smell.
- *Complex partial seizure*. This type of seizure may have a simple partial onset followed by impaired consciousness as it spreads throughout the brain to become secondarily generalised. During a complex partial seizure, a person may experience strange and unusual feelings and lose their sense of time. People can become unresponsive to what is happening around them. They can start to perform inappropriate or automatic movements. These can include plucking at clothing, lip smacking, slurred speech, repeating words, head turning, wandering aimlessly, running or undressing. The person may become hostile if restrained.

GENERALISED SEIZURES

- *Absence seizures*. Some people have generalized seizures, in which they go into a blank, trance-like state that lasts for seconds. These absence seizures mostly affect children. During brief periods (a few seconds) of lost consciousness, the ability to absorb and memorise information may be affected. The person stops suddenly, looks blank and stares into space. The eyelids may twitch, flutter or blink. Absence seizures can occur in clusters, sometimes dozens of times a day.
- *Myoclonic seizures*. With a myoclonic seizure, the person experiences sudden jerks caused by brief muscle contractions affecting the arms, head and sometimes the whole body. They occur most commonly in the morning shortly after waking. Recovery can be quick.
- *Clonic seizures*. These are characterized by repetitive jerking of the limbs.
- *Tonic seizures*. Tonic seizures exhibit a phase of intense stiffness.
- *Tonic–clonic seizures*. The most widely recognised seizure is the tonic–clonic seizure. It may start with the person making a sudden cry, losing consciousness and falling to the ground. The person then starts to convulse – the body stiffens (tonic phase), then it jerks (clonic phase) for a minute or so.

Sometimes, the lips may turn blue or the mouth may fill with frothy saliva that might be bloodstained if the tongue or the inside of the cheek has been accidentally bitten. Occasionally, someone may wet or soil themselves during a seizure. Within minutes, the individual's breathing and colour return to normal. During recovery, the person might be confused, sleepy or have a bad headache.

TREATMENT

Drug treatment aims at suppressing seizures completely without producing troublesome side effects.

Box 14.3 Principles of antiepileptic drug use

- Construct a management plan with the patient
- Before commencing new drug treatments, discuss potential risks and benefits with the patient
- Monotherapy if possible
- Start treatment at low doses
- Increase dosage until seizures are controlled or side effects are experienced
- Beware potential drug interactions
- Beware the risks of seizure relapse on changing treatments
- Provide written information to patients to aid retention of facts

Anti-convulsants have a fairly narrow therapeutic index, and dosages must be carefully tailored in order to maximise efficacy while minimising adverse effects. Box 14.3 provides principles of antiepileptic drug (AED) use. A major cause of treatment failure is poor compliance. It is essential that the patient understands the importance of regular medication. For improved compliance, once-a-day dosage would be preferable, but this may not be possible due to too short a half-life. Most AEDs can be given twice daily at the most.

Medication should be initiated with a single drug and very often at reduced dosage, gradually increasing until the clinically effective level is reached. This is in order to minimise toxic effects. If this drug fails to provide adequate control of seizures, another drug will be substituted. A second drug should be added to the regimen only if seizures continue despite high plasma concentrations or toxic effects. In order to attain the correct dose, plasma drug concentrations should be monitored where appropriate (e.g. with phenytoin).

Drugs of choice in the treatment of particular types of epilepsy are listed in Table 14.15 and dosages in Table 14.16.

When a patient is established on a brand (formulation) of one epileptic drug, this should not be changed, as variations in bioavailability may increase the potential for reduced effect.

COUNSELLING OF PATIENT

It is important that patients are given clear, accurate and appropriate information to ensure an understanding of their medication. This must be communicated in a friendly manner and any questions answered clearly. Important information may need to be repeated.

- *Compliance*. Check that the patient is aware of the name(s) and strength(s) of medicines and how and

Table 14.15 Drug choice in treatment of particular types of epilepsy

Seizure type	First-line drugs	Second-line drugs
Generalised tonic–clonic	Carbamazepine Lamotrigine Sodium valproate	Levetiracetam Oxcarbazepine Topiramate
Partial with or without secondary generalisation	Carbamazepine Lamotrigine Sodium valproate	Levetiracetam Gabapentin Oxcarbazepine Topiramate
Typical absence	Ethosuximide Sodium valproate	Clobazam Clonazepam Lamotrigine Topiramate
Myoclonic	Sodium valproate	Clonazepam Levetiracetam Piracetam Topiramate
Tonic	Lamotrigine Sodium valproate	Clobazam Clonazepam Levetiracetam Topiramate
Atonic	Lamotrigine Sodium valproate	Clobazam Clonazepam Levetiracetam Topiramate

when to take these. Is the patient choosing not to take the medicine? If not, then enquire why. Explain the relative risks of recurrent seizures due to non-compliance and the importance of commitment to long-term medication.
- *Missed dose*. Advise the patient to take medication as soon as remembered. If the missed dose is remembered and taken within 2 h of the next scheduled dose, the next dose should be skipped and the patient should carry on taking the rest of the tablets as usual. A double dose of tablets to make up the missed dose should not be taken.
- *Efficacy*. Ask if the medicine is working! Are seizures controlled? If not, how frequent are seizures? Does the patient keep a diary of seizure frequency?
- *Vomiting* up to 3 h after taking an AED can interfere with absorption. The patient should be advised to take a second dose when the vomiting subsides, unless it is less than 2 h before the next due dose.

Table 14.16 Doses for some antiepileptic drugs

Drug	Typical starting dose	Typical maintenance dose
Carbamazepine	100–200 mg once or twice daily	0.8–1.2 g daily in divided doses (the modified-release product is taken twice daily)
Clobazam	–	20–30 mg daily
Clonazepam	1 mg at night	4–8 mg daily in three or four divided doses
Ethosuximide	500 mg daily	1–1.5 g daily
Gabapentin	Day 1: 300 mg Day 2: 300 mg twice daily Day 3: 300 mg three times daily, then according to response 1 g daily as single or divided dose	0.9–1.2 g daily in three divided doses

Lamotrigine
    Monotherapy
    Adjunctive therapy with valproate
    Adjunctive therapy with enzyme-inducing drug
	
	25 mg daily
	25 mg on alternate days
	
	50 mg daily
		
		100–200 mg daily (in 1–2 divided doses)
		100–200 mg daily (in 1–2 divided doses)
		
		200–400 mg daily in two divided doses

Levetiracetam	500 mg twice daily	Max. 1.5 g daily in two divided doses
Oxcarbazepine	300 mg twice daily	0.6–2.4 g daily in divided doses
Sodium valproate	300 mg twice daily	1–2 g daily in divided doses (the modified-release product may be taken once or twice daily)

Topiramate
    Monotherapy
    Adjunctive therapy
	
	25 mg daily
	25 mg daily
		
		100 mg daily in two divided doses
		200–400 mg daily in divided doses

- *Trigger factors*. Ensure that patients are aware of seizure triggers (e.g. lack of sleep, alcohol and recreational drugs, stress, photosensitivity). Provide advice and a leaflet for carers and family on first aid should a seizure occur.

ADVERSE EFFECTS

Some of the newer AEDs appear to cause fewer problems with adverse effects. Common adverse effects are mostly dose-related, and gradual increase in dosage helps to minimise these. Common adverse effects such as drowsiness, headache, fatigue, dizziness and nausea can occur with most of the drugs. Idiosyncratic drug reactions usually occur in the first weeks of treatment and are potentially serious. Rash is the most common, occurring in up to 10% of patients on carbamazepine, phenytoin or lamotrigine. Most rashes are mild and

resolve promptly on discontinuation of therapy, but severe cutaneous reactions can occur in up to 0.1% of patients (Tennis and Stern 1997). However, more specific concerns exist with a number of agents, some of which are as follows.

- Vigabatrin can cause irreversible visual field defects. Onset varies from a few weeks to several years after starting treatment. Visual field testing is essential before treatment is started and should be carried out regularly thereafter. Patients should be asked to report any visual symptoms urgently; however, development of visual field defects can be asymptomatic.
- Lamotrigine commonly causes skin rashes. These are usually not serious, but patients should always report them because life-threatening skin reactions, including Stevens–Johnson syndrome and toxic

epidermal necrolysis, can occur. Serious reactions are more common in patients who are receiving sodium valproate and those who are prescribed initial doses of lamotrigine higher than recommended.

- Sodium valproate can cause hepatic failure, and this has resulted in a number of deaths. Patients should be advised to report immediately symptoms that might indicate hepatic failure (loss of seizure control, malaise, weakness, lethargy, oedema, anorexia, vomiting, abdominal pain, drowsiness, jaundice). Sodium valproate can also have teratogenic effects and should be used in women of childbearing age only when there is no satisfactory alternative.

DRUG INTERACTIONS

The potential for drug interactions with AEDs is significant (Patsalos et al. 2002). Furthermore, interactions are sometimes complex and to some extent unpredictable.

Antiepileptic drugs not only interact with many other types of drug, but also interact with each other, for example phenytoin, carbamazepine and phenobarbital induce liver enzymes and thereby reduce levels of sodium valproate, topiramate, lamotrigine, tiagabine and oxcarbazepine, as well as reducing their own blood levels. Sodium valproate inhibits liver enzymes, which can result in increased levels of carbamazepine, lamotrigine and tiagabine.

ORAL CONTRACEPTIVES INCLUDING THE COMBINED CONTRACEPTIVE PILL AND THE PROGESTOGEN-ONLY PILL (MINI-PILL)

Some AEDs make the pill less reliable, increasing the chance of unplanned pregnancy. These are called enzyme-inducing AEDs. There are also AEDs that do not affect the reliability of the pill (non–enzyme-inducing AEDs) (see Box 14.4).

If a patient is taking an enzyme-inducing AED while on the combined pill, a higher dose of the pill is suggested. However, even on a higher dose it would be unwise to rely on this method of contraception alone, as some women still find it unreliable. It is therefore advisable to use barrier methods also, such as the condom, cap or diaphragm, to avoid an unplanned pregnancy. The mini-pill (progestogen-only pill) is not effective if a patient is taking an enzyme-inducing AED.

RISKS TO THE FETUS FROM ANTIEPILEPTIC DRUGS

Most women with epilepsy have normal healthy babies. However, major and minor fetal malformations occur more commonly in infants exposed to AEDs during pregnancy (Holmes et al. 2001). The overall risk of major fetal malformation in any pregnancy is approximately 2%. This increases two- to threefold in women taking a single AED. The risk with valproate may be higher than with carbamazepine or lamotrigine (Craig et al. 2002). Polytherapy, particularly with certain combinations of drugs, carries a much higher risk (up to 24% in women taking four AEDs).

The most common major malformations associated with established AEDs are neural tube defects (valproate 3%, carbamazepine 1%), orofacial defects, congenital heart abnormalities and hypospadias. There is a link between folate levels and the development of neural tube defects, and some AEDs reduce folate levels. Women with epilepsy who are planning pregnancy should take folic acid 5 mg daily starting preconception and continuing through pregnancy.

WITHDRAWAL OF ANTICONVULSANTS

Withdrawal of anticonvulsant medication must be done slowly and in a staged dose reduction manner. If the dose is reduced too quickly or the time between each reduction is too short, then the likelihood of withdrawal seizures is increased. Even with a very slow and gradual reduction and withdrawal of

---

Box 14.4 Interactions involving oral contraceptives

Enzyme-inducing antiepileptic drugs
These epilepsy drugs can make the pill less reliable.

- carbamazepine (Tegretol)
- oxcarbazepine (Trileptal)
- phenobarbital/phenobarbitone
- phenytoin (Epanutin)
- topiramate (Topamax)

Non–enzyme-inducing antiepileptic drugs
These epilepsy drugs do not affect the reliability of the pill.

- acetazolamide (Diamox)
- benzodiazepines
- ethosuximide (Zarontin)
- gabapentin (Neurontin)
- lamotrigine (Lamictal)
- levetiracetam (Keppra)
- sodium valproate (Epilim)
- tiagabine (Gabitril)
- vigabatrin (Sabril)

phenobarbital/primidone, withdrawal seizures may occur months after either of these drugs is actually stopped. The changeover from one AED regimen to another should be done with care, building up the second drug to a therapeutic range while gradually decreasing the first.

DRIVING

Epilepsy sufferers may drive a motor vehicle (not heavy goods or public service) provided that they have had a seizure-free period of 1 year or, if subject to attacks only while asleep, have established a 3-year period of asleep attacks without awake attacks. Patients affected by drowsiness should not drive or operate machinery.

STATUS EPILEPTICUS

Status epilepticus occurs when a seizure lasts for more than 30 min or there are recurrent episodes without recovery of consciousness between attacks. Status epilepticus may be precipitated by a variety of conditions, such as a brain tumour, infection (e.g. meningitis), alcohol, reduction in or non-compliance with anticonvulsant medication, trauma or some metabolic abnormality (such as hypoxia or ischaemia).

It is a medical emergency and requires urgent treatment aimed at stopping seizures as quickly as possible. A nurse must stay with the patient. An airway should be established, and patients should be in a physical environment in which they cannot hurt themselves. Status epilepticus should be treated initially with intravenous lorazepam (4 mg). Intravenous diazepam emulsion is effective (10–20 mg at a rate of 2.5 mg per 30 s). This is repeated in 30 min if necessary, which may be followed by intravenous infusion to a maximum of 3 mg/kg over 24 h. However, diazepam has a risk of respiratory depression. Small doses of diazepam can be administered by rectal solution.

Alternatively, in prolonged or recurrent seizures, a single dose of midazolam can be given by the buccal route (10 mg) or intravenously (200 micrograms/kg). Propofol may also be used (see Ch. 4).

To prevent recurrence of seizures after the initial diazepam injection, phenytoin may be given by slow intravenous injection in a dose of 15 mg/kg, with ECG monitoring in case of cardiac arrhythmias. Paraldehyde may be given when other agents have failed to control seizures. Some 5–10 mL should be given by deep intramuscular injection. The dose may be repeated after 1 h. Paraldehyde may cause muscle necrosis. Doses of 10 mL should be split into 2-,

3- and 5-mL doses in separate muscles. When preparing paraldehyde for administration, contact with rubber and plastics should be avoided.

Phenobarbital can be given (10 mg/kg) by slow intravenous injection (maximum 1 g) at a rate of not more than 100 mg/min. Prolonged sedation or respiratory depression may be a problem.

Once seizures have been abolished, an appropriate oral regimen should be instituted immediately and loading doses of the particular anticonvulsant may have to be given, particularly if non-compliance has been a precipitating factor.

PARKINSON'S DISEASE

Parkinson's disease is a degenerative condition that affects a large number of people, particularly older people. The deterioration of health and quality of life caused by Parkinson's disease has a major impact not only on the sufferers but also on their family and carers. There is insufficient knowledge about the causes of Parkinson's disease to develop widespread strategies to prevent the disease, and there is no known cure.

The key symptoms of idiopathic Parkinson's disease are as follows.

- Tremor: present when the patient is at rest and when severe 'pill rolling' may be seen.
- Rigidity: on standing, the patient may exhibit stooped posture, arms slightly bent, weight on ball of foot, knees flexed.
- Bradykinesia:
  — general slowness in daily activities
  — difficulty initiating movement, particularly walking
  — difficulty in rising from a chair.
- Walking problems:
  — the patient's weight is on the ball of the foot, and there appears to be a loss of heel strike
  — reduction in length of stride
  — the patient leans forwards before commencing to walk and flexes knees to prevent falling forwards.
- Balance problems:
  — frequent falls can occur
  — difficulty in turning.

Other features of Parkinson's disease include excessive salivation, dysphagia (frequently in older people), anxiety, depression and a fixed staring appearance.

Onset of Parkinson's disease is usually insidious and progression is slow. Many patients notice a resting tremor, usually affecting the hands initially. The tremor disappears on movement and during

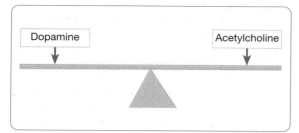

Fig. 14.7 Dopamine and acetylcholine in balance.

sleep, and may be worse under stress. Bradykinesia is reflected in immobile features and a fixed, staring appearance. Along with rigidity, it is responsible for the typical abnormalities of gait; difficulty in starting and finishing steps, with resultant shuffling; a stooped head, fixed neck, upper extremities and knees; and a lack of normal arm swing. Frequent falls may result from loss of postural reflex leading to postural imbalance.

Dopamine, working in balance with another chemical messenger, acetylcholine, is responsible for the mechanisms that control programmes of movements (Fig. 14.7). Imbalances in the neurotransmitters lead to movement disorders. In Parkinson's disease, degeneration of certain cells in the substantia nigra leads to a deficiency in the production of dopamine so that the normal balance between the neurotransmitters, dopamine and acetylcholine, is altered (Fig. 14.8).

The symptoms of Parkinson's disease do not appear until some 80% of the capacity to produce dopamine has been lost. The level of dopamine will continue to fall over subsequent years. However, each person with Parkinson's disease is very different, and the rate and character of the progression may vary greatly from one person to another. The disease usually presents in middle or old age.

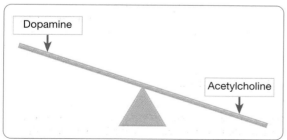

Fig. 14.8 Dopamine deficiency with resultant cholinergic overactivity leading to symptoms of the disease.

DRUG TREATMENT

The main aim of drug therapy is to restore the balance between dopamine and acetylcholine. This can be achieved by:

- replacing dopamine
- use of dopamine agonists to stimulate surviving dopamine receptors
- prolonging action of dopamine by inhibiting metabolism
- use of antimuscarinic drugs.

REPLACING DOPAMINE

Administration of dopamine is ineffective, because it cannot cross the blood–brain barrier into the brain cells where it is required to produce an effect. It is necessary to give its precursor, levodopa, which crosses the blood–brain barrier and is subsequently broken down to dopamine by the enzyme dopa decarboxylase. However, levodopa requires to be given in high concentrations, because over 90% is decarboxylated in the liver and gut before it reaches the brain. This results in peripheral side effects such as nausea, vomiting, anorexia and postural hypotension.

Levodopa is rarely given alone. It is usually given in combination with an inhibitor of extracerebral dopa decarboxylase, such as carbidopa (Sinemet) or benserazide (Madopar). This prevents the peripheral degradation of levodopa to dopamine and so increases effective brain levels. This allows the dose of levodopa to be reduced markedly, resulting in a reduction in side effects.

Levodopa is tolerated by most patients who experience considerable improvement for several years, especially when stiffness and slowness of movement are concerned. It is initiated at low doses (50–100 mg twice daily with benserazide), because some feelings of nausea are common due to stimulation of the dopaminergic receptors in the chemotherapy trigger zone (CTZ). These are usually mild and pass as the body adjusts to the drug. Taking levodopa with or after meals helps to minimise these effects.

Domperidone, a dopamine antagonist that does not cross the blood–brain barrier, may be useful in controlling nausea where this is severe (doses of 10–20 mg of domperidone 1 h before levodopa preparations are effective). The dosage regimen of levodopa is gradually increased, the final dose being a compromise between increased mobility and incidence of side effects.

The relatively short half-life of levodopa (2–3 h) has led to the development of controlled-release preparations that can be given less frequently and the use of which evens out the peaks and troughs associated with conventional levodopa therapy.

There is a small percentage of people who cannot tolerate levodopa because of severe sickness or other side effects, such as confusion, hallucinations and mood swings.

Levodopa usually provides very effective control of Parkinson's disease for a number of years, after which a deterioration in response often occurs. This is probably related to increasing degeneration of nigrostriatal neurones.

Interactions can occur with drugs that affect central monoamines, and MAOIs should be withdrawn at least 14 days before instituting levodopa treatment. Antipsychotic drugs, such as the phenothiazines, should not be administered concurrently, as they would exacerbate the disease. Caution should be exercised in patients with open angle glaucoma.

DOPAMINE AGONIST MONOTHERAPY

The long-term use of levodopa is associated with involuntary movements and response fluctuations that add to the complexities of later disease management. It is also suggested that levodopa is toxic to dopaminergic neurones. Trials have suggested that the modern dopamine agonists, such as cabergoline, pergolide, pramipexole and ropinirole, produce less dyskinesia compared with levodopa over 3–5 years' therapy (Clarke and Guthman 2002). There has been a move away from levodopa towards initial monotherapy with a dopamine agonist.

DOPAMINE AGONISTS

Dopamine agonists bromocriptine, cabergoline, lisuride, pergolide (ergot derivatives) and pramipexole and ropinerole (non-ergot derivatives) act by direct stimulation of surviving dopamine receptors. Sites of action are shown in Figure 14.9. The treatment of new patients is often started with dopamine receptor agonists. When used alone, dopamine receptor agonists cause fewer motor complications in long-term treatment compared with levodopa treatment, but their improvement on overall motor performance is slightly less. The dopamine receptor agonists are associated with more neuropsychiatric side effects than levodopa.

Doses of dopamine receptor agonists should be increased slowly according to response and tolerability. Also, they should be withdrawn gradually. The dopamine agonists are also used with levodopa in more advanced disease. They are usually used in conjunction with levodopa to smooth out control of symptoms in patients whose response to treatment is beginning to fluctuate. Treatment is begun at low dosage, taken with food and gradually increased to a maintenance dose. The use of dopa agonists allows a reduction in the levodopa dosage, and the effects of the combination should be carefully balanced. Drop-out rates can be high due to adverse effects. Gastrointestinal upset, postural hypotension, dizziness and headache are common. With bromocriptine, patients are best advised to refrain from excessive alcohol consumption, as alcohol may reduce tolerance of the drug and lead to increased side-effects.

MONOAMINE-OXIDASE-B INHIBITORS

Selegiline and rasagiline are drugs that prolong the action of dopamine at the receptor by inhibiting its enzymatic degradation. They are MAO-B inhibitors, and their use therefore does not involve dietary restriction. They can be used alone or in conjunction with levodopa for end-of-dose fluctuations. Selegiline can cause postural hypotension, nausea, constipation, diarrhoea, dry mouth and dyskinesia, and the side-effects of levodopa may be increased. Side-effects of rasagiline include dry mouth, dyspepsia, constipation, angina and headache.

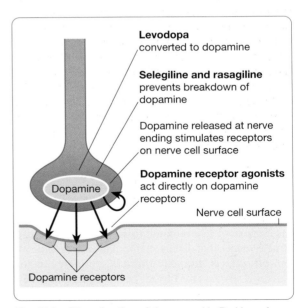

Fig. 14.9 Sites of action of drugs used in Parkinson's disease. (From Greenstein B, Gould D 2004 Trounce's clinical pharmacology for nurses. Churchill Livingstone, Edinburgh. With permission of Elsevier Ltd.)

CATECHOL-O-METHYL TRANSFERASE INHIBITION

Entacapone and tolcapone act by preventing the breakdown of levodopa due to inhibition of the enzyme catechol-O-methyl transferase. This results in an increase in the availability of levodopa to the brain and a reduction in the levels of the metabolite 3-O-methyldopa, which competes with levodopa for transport across the blood–brain barrier. They thus prolong the clinical response to levodopa.

Side effects experienced may include nausea, diarrhoea, abdominal pain and dyskinesia. The urine may be coloured brown.

Because of risk of hepatotoxicity, tolcapone should be prescribed under specialist supervision only.

'END-OF-DOSE' AND 'ON–OFF' EFFECTS

In excess of 50% of parkinsonian patients experience fluctuations in motor response after 5 years of levodopa treatment. Two of the most common side effects of levodopa therapy are the 'end-of-dose' deterioration and 'on–off' phenomena.

The duration of the beneficial response to each dose of levodopa becomes progressively shorter and may be reduced from an initial 4–6 h to as little as 30 min, with a return of symptoms towards the end of each dose, such as early morning immobility, dystonia and start hesitation. 'End-of-dose' effects are the result of failing levodopa plasma levels. This condition may respond to the administration of smaller doses of levodopa at more frequent intervals, with the first dose on waking and last dose at bedtime.

Adjunctive treatment may also be considered at this stage. Selegiline or rasagiline are both useful in conjunction with levodopa for smoothing out the effects of 'end-of-dose' deterioration. Controlled-release preparations of Sinemet or Madopar can also be used.

'On–off' effects are sudden fluctuations in disability that can occur, involving rapid and abrupt alterations between periods of good mobility and periods of hypokinesia, tremor and dyskinesia. This may last for only a few seconds or up to several minutes, or even hours, before normal function returns. Apomorphine has been used to overcome this effect. There is also some evidence that dietary manipulation may improve 'on–off' effects, because there is competition for transport across the blood–brain barrier between levodopa and certain dietary amino acids.

APOMORPHINE

Apomorphine can reduce and sometimes reverse these disabling 'off' period phenomena. The rapid and reliable onset of action of apomorphine can be used to advantage when oral doses of levodopa become progressively less effective and less predictable. The aim of treatment is to optimise the delicate balance between an effective response and minimal side effects. The complex nature of apomorphine therapy necessitates that it should be initiated in specialist centres.

Apomorphine is a directly acting dopamine agonist with no opiate or addictive properties. It is not used orally, because it undergoes extensive first-pass metabolism to an inactive metabolite. Treatment with apomorphine is usually administered either by intermittent subcutaneous injections or by continuous waking day subcutaneous infusion.

Following a single subcutaneous dose, apomorphine has an onset of action of between 5 and 15 min. The effect usually lasts for about 1 h.

Because apomorphine is a potent emetic, pretreatment with domperidone is necessary for at least 3 days before initiating therapy. A dose of 30 mg every 8 h is given. Domperidone is a peripherally acting dopamine antagonist, unlike metoclopramide or prochlorperazine, which have both peripheral and central effects. It does not cross the blood–brain barrier to act as an antagonist at central dopamine receptors with consequent detrimental effects on motor performance. Domperidone can usually be withdrawn gradually over several weeks to 6 months, although some patients may need to continue taking a low dose. In addition, it appears to counteract some of the other peripheral effects of apomorphine, such as postural hypotension.

After initiation of domperidone, all existing antiparkinsonian medication is stopped overnight to provoke an 'off' period. The lowest or 'threshold' dose of apomorphine that produces a definite motor response may be determined as follows.

- First, 1.5 mg of apomorphine is injected subcutaneously, and the patient is observed for 30 min for motor response.
- If there is no response, or a poor response, 3 mg is injected subcutaneously 40 min after the first dose, with increase in dose incrementally every 40 min until a response is seen. Patients not responding to a 7-mg dose are classified as non-responders. The maximum dose for a subcutaneous bolus injection is 10 mg.
- Finally, anti-Parkinson's therapy is started and continued using apomorphine at the dose determined above when required for 'off' periods.

The drug may be given by repeated single subcutaneous injections in doses of 3–30 mg daily titrated against response. The maximum total daily dose quoted in the data sheet is 100 mg.

If patients require many daily injections, apomorphine may be administered by continuous day-time subcutaneous infusion via syringe driver. The manufacturers recommend that infusions should start at a rate of 1 mg/h. Infusions may be increased in steps of not greater than 0.5 mg/h at intervals of not less than 4 h, to a maximum of 4 mg/h.

Side-effects. Stimulation of the CTZ by apomorphine commonly results in nausea and vomiting. Other side-effects include hypotension, bradycardia, sweating and respiratory depression. Drowsiness is common but usually resolves over the first few weeks of treatment.

Because apomorphine can cause hypotension, care should be taken in patients with pre-existing cardiac disease or in patients taking antihypertensive medication.

ANTIMUSCARINIC DRUGS

Antimuscarinic drugs (e.g., benzatropine, orphenadrine, procyclidine, trihexyphenidyl (benzhexol)) may be used in Parkinson's disease to reduce the relative excess of acetylcholine and, as a result, reduce to some extent the tremor, rigidity and sialorrhoea. All are given in gradually increasing doses until an optimal balance of efficacy and side effects is obtained (see Table 14.17).

The most common adverse reactions are dry mouth, constipation, blurred vision, tachycardia and dizziness. The antimuscarinics are contraindicated in urinary retention and glaucoma, and interactions may occur with antihistamines and tricyclic antidepressants. They can be useful for younger patients in the early stages when symptoms are mild. When treatment of mild symptoms is initiated with antimuscarinic drugs, levodopa is added or substituted as symptoms progress.

Table 14.17 Dosages of antimuscarinic drugs

Drug	Maintenance dose (mg)
Benzatropine	1–2
Orphenadrine	150–400
Procyclidine	10–30
Trihexyphenidyl (benzhexol)	5–15

DRUG-INDUCED PARKINSONISM

The features of drug-induced parkinsonism are the same as those of the idiopathic disease. There may be tremor, rigidity, bradykinesia, expressionless face, dysphagia and drooling. This occurs to some degree in all patients treated with conventional antipsychotic drugs, although there is a wide variation between patients. The following have a high propensity for causing extrapyramidal effects:

- piperazine phenothiazines (e.g. fluphenazine, trifluoperazine)
- butyrophenones (e.g. haloperidol)
- diphenylbutylpiperidines (e.g. pimozide).

Chlorpromazine has a lower propensity. Metoclopramide blocks dopamine receptors and also enhances the action of acetylcholine.

Drug-induced parkinsonism does not always require treatment and it is reversible on dose reduction or drug withdrawal. Severe cases may require treatment with antimuscarinics, but the routine use of these drugs should be avoided as they add to the antimuscarinic side effects of antipsychotic drugs. Because of the tendency of antipsychotics to accumulate, side-effects may be very prolonged, lasting days or weeks after the drug has been withdrawn.

CARE OF THE PATIENT WITH PARKINSON'S DISEASE

The symptoms of Parkinson's disease are fairly familiar to the general public. It follows therefore that when a diagnosis is made patients will be concerned and those involved must give every encouragement to patients and those who are close to them.

Education of the patient and participation in treatment are important from the outset, because treatment is likely to be prolonged and eventually problematic. Plans and objectives should be formulated in conjunction with the patient. Physiotherapy can assist in posture and walking, and regular exercise is important to maintain mobility. Occupational therapists can offer a wide range of helpful appliances. Constipation may be a concern for sufferers, but a high-fibre diet usually controls symptoms. In the UK, the Parkinson's Disease Society is recommended as a source of support.

SUBSTANCE DEPENDENCE

ALCOHOL DEPENDENCE

There are few drug treatments that reliably maintain abstinence in patients with alcohol dependence.

Disulfiram can help to reduce a patient's drinking but, in general, its use needs to be supervised (e.g. by the patient's partner) to help ensure adherence to therapy. Disulfiram gives rise to extremely unpleasant systemic reactions after the ingestion of even small amounts of alcohol, because it leads to accumulation of acetaldehyde in the body. This occurs because disulfiram inhibits the enzyme responsible for the oxidation of acetaldehyde, a metabolite of alcohol. Reactions can occur within 10 min and last several hours.

The dose is 800 mg as a single dose on the first day, reducing over 5 days to 100–200 mg daily. It should not be continued for longer than 6 months without review. Reactions include flushing of the face, throbbing headache, palpitations, tachycardia, nausea, vomiting and, with larger doses of alcohol, arrhythmias, hypotension and collapse.

Patients taking disulfiram should be instructed to avoid all substances containing alcohol, such as tonics, elixirs and gargles. They should also not apply alcohol-containing substances such as aftershave lotion, rubbing alcohol, and liniments, because the skin may absorb the alcohol. Alcohol should be avoided for at least a week after stopping disulfiram.

Benzodiazepines are also used in the management of withdrawal. Chlordiazepoxide or diazepam is given orally. The final dose should be determined by regular clinical monitoring of the patient's level of distress, the aim being a calm patient. Close monitoring is essential to avoid overdosage. Caution should be exercised in liver dysfunction, which is associated with reduced clearance of benzodiazepines, and airways dysfunction may be associated with respiratory depression.

Acamprosate is a newer preparation that, in combination with counselling, may be helpful in maintaining abstinence in alcohol-dependent patients. Therapy should be initiated as soon as possible after abstinence has been achieved. The recommended treatment period is 1 year.

The mechanism of action of acamprosate is uncertain. It has gamma-aminobutyric acid (GABA) agonist properties and glutamate antagonist properties. It is thought that, in chronic alcohol dependency, glutamate receptors increase and disrupt the excitatory–inhibitory balance between glutamate and GABA neurotransmission. Acamprosate may act by stimulating GABA inhibitory transmission and antagonise excitatory amino acids, particularly glutamic acid.

CIGARETTE SMOKING

Around one in four adults in the UK smokes cigarettes. It is notoriously difficult to stop smoking, but success rates are increased when nicotine products or amfebutamone/bupropion are used as an aid to smoking cessation in combination with motivational support.

BUPROPION (AMFEBUTAMONE)

Developed originally as an antidepressant, its mode of action in smoking cessation is not entirely clear. Bupropion (amfebutamone) may increase levels of dopamine and adrenaline (epinephrine) in the brain, thereby counteracting the reductions in these neurochemicals that result from nicotine withdrawal.

Pharmacokinetics. Bupropion (amfebutamone) is readily absorbed following oral administration, with peak plasma concentrations in 3 h. The elimination half-life is about 20 h.

Dose. It is recommended that treatment is started while the patient is still smoking and a target stop date set within the first 2 weeks of treatment, preferably in the second week. The initial dose is 150 mg to be taken daily for 6 days, increasing to 150 mg twice daily. If at 7 weeks abstinence is not achieved, treatment should be discontinued.

Side-effects. The most common side-effects are dry mouth and insomnia. Bupropion (amfebutamone) is contraindicated in patients with epilepsy.

NICOTINE REPLACEMENT

Several types of nicotine replacement are available in the UK, including chewing gum, transdermal patch, inhalator, a sublingual tablet, lozenges and a nasal spray. To use nicotine replacement, smokers are advised to set a date and a time for quitting smoking and from that point onwards to use the replacement product instead of cigarettes, generally for up to 3 months.

COUNSELLING

The effectiveness of smoking cessation initiatives is increased when counselling and support are provided in addition to the medication. In this way, the patient can be advised of the difficulties that will be experienced and the ways in which these can be anticipated and action taken to minimise their effect on the smoking cessation initiative. This can take the form of regular counselling both at the outset and during the course of the medication. A helpline may be available to deal with issues as they arise. A few examples of guidance are as follows:

- clean your home and car to get rid of the smell of cigarettes

- get a piggybank to save the money you currently spend on cigarettes
- get rid of smoking 'bits and pieces' (e.g. ashtrays, lighters)
- keep busy and plan your activities
- keep your hands active (e.g. doodle)
- change your routine around the times and places you normally smoke
- chew sugar-free gum or suck sugar-free sweets
- have a counsellor or friend you can ring for support
- take up a new hobby or activity
- reward yourself for no longer smoking
- if you have a lapse, try again – remember that you can still become a non-smoker.

OPIOID DEPENDENCE

Drug misuse, even with some degree of dependence, may not be in itself an indication to prescribe controlled drugs. Simple reassurance and the prescription of non-controlled drugs may be helpful and effective in alleviating the patient's anxiety about withdrawal.

Prescribing a substitute drug when appropriate can be a useful tool to change the behaviour of some misusers, either towards abstinence or towards intermediate goals such as a reduction in injecting or sharing of injecting equipment. A flexible plan should be agreed for stabilisation/maintenance, which may range from a week to many months. Important factors are length of use, stability of lifestyle and the patient's wishes and motivation. Goals for ultimate reduction/withdrawal and rate of reduction need to be discussed and regularly reviewed. An agreement or 'contract' should be established based on the agreed goals and when these will be reviewed.

METHADONE

Methadone mixture (1 mg/mL) can be substituted for opioids. It may be prescribed for daily dispensing of up to 14 days, allowing the client to collect medication from a community pharmacy on a daily basis. A 'drop in the mouth' arrangement entails the client consuming the dose in the pharmacy, supervised by the pharmacist. This avoids 'bingeing' and removes the opportunity for selling medication. The client should be seen every 2 weeks by a nominated GP or trained nurse and not given repeat prescriptions.

Methadone is a synthetic compound with properties similar to those of morphine. It is well absorbed from the gastrointestinal tract and has a bioavailability of 80–90%. The half-life is 1–2 days and once-daily dosing is sufficient. The initial dose is based on previous consumption. The dose is then titrated against signs of withdrawal, for example tachycardia, mydriasis, perspiration and sensations of discomfort. The ability to drive or operate machinery may be severely affected. Methadone is less sedating than the other opiates. Nausea may occur.

Interactions. Rifampicin, carbamazepine, phenobarbital and phenytoin accelerate the metabolism of methadone by induction of enzymes, leading to a reduced effect. Methadone may increase plasma concentration of zidovudine.

Contraindications. Methadone is contraindicated in respiratory depression, obstructive airways disease or during an acute asthma attack.

Urine testing. A urine sample should be taken before starting on methadone to establish whether the patient is using opiates – and also while on prescription for evidence of both taking methadone and not taking other drugs.

LOFEXIDINE

Noradrenergic neuronal hyperactivity is the pathway responsible for the signs and symptoms of opiate withdrawal. Lofexidine is an α-noradrenergic agonist that significantly reduces opiate withdrawal symptoms without the adverse sedative and hypotensive effects of clonidine.

NALTREXONE

Naltrexone is an opioid antagonist. It blocks the action of opioids such as diamorphine and precipitates withdrawal symptoms in opioid-dependent subjects. Because the euphoric action of opioid agonists is blocked by naltrexone, it is given to former addicts as an aid to prevent relapse. The patient should be narcotic-free 7–10 days prior to treatment as verified by urinalysis. Liver tests are required before and during treatment.

BUPRENORPHINE

Buprenorphine can be used as substitution therapy for patients with moderate opioid dependence. Administration is best managed through a 'consume on the premises' arrangement with a community pharmacist.

ALZHEIMER'S DISEASE

SYMPTOMS

Alzheimer's disease is characterised by an insidious onset with a gradual but relentless decline in memory and other aspects of cognitive function that is sufficient to impair activities of daily living. An early feature is memory impairment for recent events

Table 14.18 Drugs used in the treatment of Alzheimer's disease

Drug	Starting dose	Dose titration	Side-effects
Donepezil	5 mg once a day at bedtime	Reviewed after 1 month, increased to 10 mg daily if well tolerated	Diarrhoea, muscle cramps, fatigue, nausea, vomiting, insomnia
Galantamine	4 mg twice daily for 4 weeks	After 4 weeks, initial maintenance dose is 8 mg twice daily for at least 4 weeks, then consider increase to maintenance dose of 12 mg twice daily	Anorexia, dizziness, nausea, dyspepsia, vomiting
Memantine	5 mg in morning	Increased in steps of 5 mg at weekly intervals to maximum 10 mg twice daily	Constipation, headache, dizziness, drowsiness
Rivastigmine	1.5 mg twice daily	Increased in steps of 1.5 mg twice daily at minimum fortnightly intervals to 3–6 mg twice daily	Nausea, vomiting, diarrhoea, abdominal pain, dyspepsia, anorexia

and poor retention of new information. Memory for more distant events is usually preserved in the early stages. Language problems (aphasia) occur and are sometimes quite prominent even in the early stages of the disease. As Alzheimer's disease progresses, there are increasing changes in behaviour.

ACETYLCHOLINESTERASE-INHIBITING DRUGS (See Ch. 9)

Degeneration of cholinergic neurones and associated loss of cholinergic neurotransmission appear to contribute significantly to the cognitive decline seen in Alzheimer's disease. Acetylcholinesterase is the chemical that breaks down acetylcholine, and inhibition of this process results in a boost to the cholinergic system in Alzheimer's disease.

Donepezil, rivastigmine and galantamine are acetylcholinesterase inhibitors prescribed for patients with Alzheimer's disease (Table 14.18). Memantine affects glutamate transmission. Treatment should be initiated and supervised by a specialist experienced in the management of dementia. Benefit is assessed by repeating the cognitive assessment at around 3 months. Up to half the patients given these drugs will show a slower rate of cognitive decline.

ANAESTHESIA

INTRODUCTION

Detailed knowledge of individual anaesthetic drugs is necessary only for nurses working in the operating theatre or intensive therapy unit. However, all surgical ward nurses should have an appreciation of what comprises a modern anaesthetic. Most important of all is an understanding of the drugs used in the pre- and post anaesthetic treatment of the surgical patient.

Despite the technological complexity of modern anaesthetic practice, the exact mechanism of general anaesthesia has yet to be elucidated. The fact that compounds as diverse as inorganic gases, ethers and steroids can produce general anaesthesia suggests that their action is non-specific. In contrast, the mode of action of local anaesthetic drugs is well understood: transmission of peripheral nerve impulses is blocked by the reversible 'plugging' of sodium channels, preventing membrane depolarisation.

Both induction and maintenance of anaesthesia can be achieved by drugs given intravenously or by inhalation. Inhalation agents work by diffusing from the alveoli into the blood flowing through the lungs. However, in adults, induction is usually by the intravenous route and maintenance by inhalation. The intravenous dose depends on factors such as the patient's age, weight and general health. The needle-phobic adult can be offered inhalational induction with sevoflurane, which is smooth, rapid and not unpleasant. Once the patient is asleep, anaesthesia is usually maintained by a mixture of anaesthetic gases in oxygen.

Depending on the nature of the operation, patients may either breathe spontaneously or have their lungs mechanically ventilated while paralysed with a muscle relaxant (or neuromuscular-blocking) drug.

PREOPERATIVE MEDICATION

Sedative drugs are no substitute for explanation and reassurance by nursing staff. However, a benzodiazepine such as temazepam or lorazepam given orally helps patients to relax before going to theatre. Midazolam is an intravenous benzodiazepine used mainly to provide sedation for endoscopies. Flumazenil is a specific benzodiazepine antagonist that reverses its effect.

Many patients undergoing surgery will be taking medicines for conditions unrelated to their operation. Abrupt discontinuation can have adverse effects. For example, stopping beta-blockers (which slow the heart) can cause rebound arrhythmias and myocardial ischaemia or infarction. The nurse will be guided by the anaesthetist and should be prepared to administer certain drugs (particularly heart and blood pressure medication) as usual, with sips of water, even if the patient is 'nil by mouth'. On the other hand, oral hypoglycaemic agents should never be given to a fasting patient. Insulin will be administered with dextrose by intravenous infusion. The anaesthetist may prescribe additional medication, such as a nitrate patch (e.g. Transiderm-Nitro), for a patient with angina. Patients with asthma should have their salbutamol (or equivalent) inhalers available for use prior to induction of anaesthesia.

Regurgitation and aspiration of gastric contents (Mendelson's syndrome) is an important complication of general surgery, particularly emergency surgery. To increase the pH of gastric fluid, an H_2-receptor antagonist or a proton pump inhibitor can be taken 1–2 h or 12 h, respectively, before the procedure.

Patients who are pregnant or who have a hiatus hernia are at increased risk of inhaling gastric contents, which can cause a fatal pneumonitis. An H_2-receptor antagonist such as ranitidine is given before caesarean section to stop gastric acid secretion. Immediately before induction of anaesthesia, 30 mL of 0.3 molar sodium citrate solution is given by mouth to increase the pH of the stomach contents.

INHALATIONAL AGENTS

The desirable features of an 'ideal' inhalational agent are given in Box 14.5.

Nitrous oxide is supplied in blue cylinders. It is a weak anaesthetic and has to be administered with at least 30% oxygen. On the anaesthetic machine in the operating theatre, nitrous oxide and oxygen are directed to vaporisers, which are filled with potent liquid anaesthetic. Halothane, isoflurane, desflurane and sevoflurane are volatile liquid anaesthetics.

Box 14.5 Desirable features of an 'ideal' inhalational agent

- It should not form flammable mixtures with oxygen or other agents.
- The vapour should not be unpleasant to inhale.
- The drug should be insoluble in the bloodstream, allowing rapid induction and elimination.
- The drug should be free of organ-specific toxic effects (e.g. renal or hepatic failure) and should not undergo metabolism in the body.
- Depression of the cardiovascular and respiratory systems should be minimal.
- The drug should possess analgesic properties.

Box 14.6 Desirable features of an 'ideal' intravenous agent

- The drug should not cause pain on injection.
- Induction of anaesthesia should be rapid and smooth.
- Return of consciousness should also be rapid with no hangover, nausea, vomiting or unpleasant dreams.
- Depression of the cardiovascular and respiratory systems should be minimal.
- Serious adverse reactions should be extremely rare.

The depth of anaesthesia is varied by altering the concentration of vapour carried by the oxygen and nitrous oxide. A 50/50 mixture of oxygen and nitrous oxide is marketed as Entonox and Equanox. The cylinders have a blue body with a blue and white shoulder. The gas is carried by ambulances for use in emergency situations and is used for analgesia during labour and for short potentially painful procedures such as dressing changes. Some patients feel little effect from breathing the gas, yet others may lose consciousness. Therefore the mask should always be applied by the patient. Should loss of consciousness occur, the mask will fall away.

INTRAVENOUS AGENTS

The 'ideal' agent does not exist, but its features are shown in Box 14.6. Thiopental has been largely superseded by propofol. Propofol allows a rapid recovery without a hangover effect. In addition, anaesthesia can be maintained by continuous infusion, because recovery is rapid even after prolonged administration for total intravenous anaesthesia.

Box 14.7 Non-depolarising muscle relaxants

- Atracurium
- Cisatracurium
- Mivacurium
- Pancuronium
- Rocuronium
- Vecuronium

Box 14.8 Side-effects of opioids

- Respiratory depression
- Nausea and vomiting
- Dysphoria and hallucinations
- Cough suppression
- Constipation
- Pupillary constriction

MUSCLE RELAXANTS

Muscle relaxant drugs are used to paralyse a patient's muscles to allow passage of a tracheal tube, to maintain relaxation of the body's muscles for abdominal surgery, and to facilitate artificial ventilation. Suxamethonium chloride (depolarising muscle relaxant) is a particularly short-acting drug. It has a common, unique side-effect: pains in muscles not usually associated with strain after exercise (e.g. between the scapulae). The complaint is commonest in the muscular young patient who is up and about soon after the operation. A rarer problem is a genetic deficiency of the enzyme needed to break down the drug and terminate its action. A patient scheduled for a short procedure might have to be kept asleep with the lungs mechanically ventilated for a number of hours until the drug effect wears off. There are a number of other muscle relaxant drugs (Box 14.7) that differ in their onset and duration of action.

ANALGESICS

Short-acting synthetic opioids such as fentanyl, alfentanil and remifentanil are commonly used as components of the anaesthetic in small doses before or after induction to reduce the dose requirement of some drugs used during anaesthesia. They act within 1–2 min. Box 14.8 lists the side-effects common to opioids. The potential for causing slowing of breathing and respiratory arrest is by far the most important.

Postoperative analgesia has traditionally been prescribed as a fixed-dose intramuscular injection of opioid to be given no more frequently than 4-hourly. This regimen is unsatisfactory, because it does not allow for patients' enormous differences in analgesic requirements after the same operation. Some patients are reticent about asking for analgesia because of fear of the injection, demonstrating apparent failure to cope, or developing addiction. Moreover, drugs given intramuscularly are not well absorbed when patients are cold after lengthy surgery and skeletal muscle is poorly perfused. If injections are repeated in an attempt to control pain, there is a risk of absorption of dangerously large amounts when the patient warms up.

A major advance in the management of postoperative pain has been the development of patient-controlled analgesia (PCA; Fig. 14.10). In response to pressing a button, the patient receives boluses of opioid by the intravenous route. The key to understanding PCA is the 'lock-out interval'; this is the period after a bolus during which any further attempts by the patient to receive opioid will be turned down by the machine. A PCA system might initially be set to deliver a 1-mg bolus of morphine with a lock-out interval of 5 min. Because there are 12×5 min in an hour, the patient would be able to receive a maximum of 12×1 mg, i.e. 12 mg/h. Were this to prove inadequate, the anaesthetist would administer a further loading dose and increase the bolus setting. The safety of PCA relies on only the patient pressing the button. Dihydrocodeine 60 mg 4-hourly (maximum 240 mg/24 h) is an effective oral opioid for the patient being weaned from intravenous morphine.

Patients' pain, degree of sedation and respiratory rate should be evaluated and recorded as routinely as pulse and blood pressure. Whenever opioids are administered, naloxone, which is a specific antagonist, should be immediately available.

Non-steroidal anti-inflammatory drugs work by inhibiting enzymes involved in mediating pain from damaged tissue. Their advantage is that there is no risk of respiratory depression. They can be given in addition to opioids, improving the quality of postoperative analgesia and reducing the required dose of opioid with its concomitant side effects. However, there are important contraindications (Box 14.9).

Diclofenac suppositories are well absorbed. The rectal route avoids the potentially serious complications of intramuscular injection: nerve damage and abscess formation. Regular doses of paracetamol 1 g (orally or rectally, 6-hourly) can be given in addition to a NSAID. Both paracetamol and NSAIDs have an

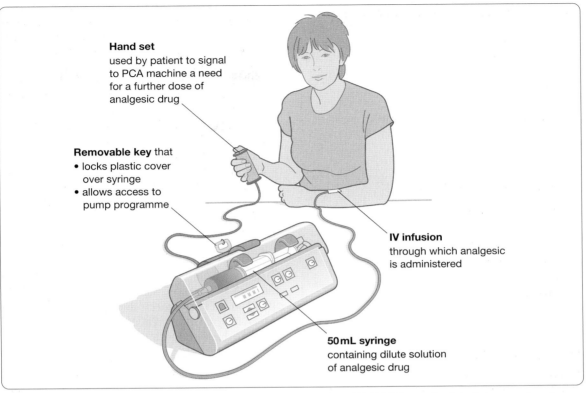

Hand set
used by patient to signal
to PCA machine a need
for a further dose of
analgesic drug

Removable key that
• locks plastic cover
  over syringe
• allows access to
  pump programme

IV infusion
through which analgesic
is administered

50 mL syringe
containing dilute solution
of analgesic drug

Fig. 14.10   Patient-controlled analgesia (PCA). (From Greenstein B, Gould D 2004 Trounce's clinical pharmacology for nurses. Churchill Livingstone, Edinburgh. With permission of Elsevier Ltd.)

Box 14.9 Contraindications to non-steroidal anti-inflammatory drugs

• Renal impairment, dehydration or hypovolaemia
• Bleeding abnormalities or risk of postoperative bleeding
• History of peptic ulcer or gastrointestinal bleeding
• Asthma known to be worsened by aspirin or non-steroidal anti-inflammatory drugs

Box 14.10 Factors contributing to postoperative nausea and vomiting

• Sex (women have higher incidence, greatest in weeks 3 and 4 of the menstrual cycle)
• History of motion sickness or vomiting after previous anaesthetic
• Whether antiemetics are given during anaesthesia
• Which anaesthetics/analgesics are used (opioids increase the incidence)
• Type of operation (e.g. laparoscopy, squint or middle ear surgery have high incidence)
• Adequacy of postoperative analgesia

---

opioid-sparing effect, i.e. they reduce the requirement for morphine.

ANTIEMETICS

Nausea and vomiting are frequent minor complications of surgery and anaesthesia. A number of factors contribute to its likelihood (Box 14.10).

Table 14.19 lists examples of antiemetic agents and their respective modes of action. Ondansetron is the most effective although more expensive than the others. It is therefore usually prescribed as a second-line drug.

LOCAL ANAESTHETICS

Local anaesthetics (Box 14.11) work by blocking conduction of nerve impulses conveying pain. The

Table 14.19 Antiemetic agents and their actions

Agent	Action
Cyclizine	Antihistamine
Hyoscine	Antimuscarinic
Metoclopramide	Dopamine antagonist (benzamide)
Ondansetron	5-HT$_3$ antagonist
Prochlorperazine	Dopamine antagonist (phenothiazine)

Box 14.12 Symptoms and signs of local anaesthetic toxicity

Symptoms
- Numbness of tongue or lips
- Lightheadedness
- Tinnitus
- Anxiety

Signs
- Slurring of speech
- Drowsiness
- Convulsions
- Cardiorespiratory arrest

Box 14.11 Local anaesthetics

- Lidocaine (lignocaine)
- Prilocaine
- Bupivacaine
- Levobupivacaine
- Ropivacaine

various agents have different durations of action and toxicity. They can be injected anywhere from the site of the incision (local infiltration) to the cerebrospinal fluid (spinal block). Local anaesthetics can contribute to analgesia following most operations. If catheters are inserted close to nerves running from the area of the operation (e.g. brachial plexus for hand surgery), analgesia can be maintained for as long as is necessary by topping up with local anaesthetic when pain returns. Bupivacaine acts longer than lidocaine (lignocaine), although it is more toxic in overdose. There is less risk of central nervous system or cardiac toxicity after inadvertent intravascular injection of levobupivacaine compared with bupivacaine. Epidurals are increasingly being used for postoperative analgesia following major abdominal, vascular and thoracic surgery. Drugs are injected via a catheter to bathe the nerves outside the spinal cord. Side effects of epidurals include hypotension (due to block of sympathetic nerves and treatable with ephedrine), urinary retention and block of motor nerves, causing inability to move the legs. The doses necessary for epidural use can be reduced by mixing the local anaesthetic with opioid. Prilocaine, the least toxic local anaesthetic, is used for Bier's block. This is a technique that facilitates hand or forearm surgery (a common procedure is reduction of Colles' fracture). The arm is held up in order to drain its blood, and a tourniquet is inflated. Local anaesthetic is then injected into a vein on the back of the hand. It is crucial that the tourniquet is not released for at least 20 min, in order to prevent a large toxic dose of local anaesthetic entering the circulation. The symptoms and signs of local anaesthetic toxicity relate to the drug reaching the brain and heart by either excessive absorption into the bloodstream or inadvertent injection into a blood vessel (Box 14.12).

SELF-ASSESSMENT QUESTIONS

1. Give the possible side-effects of hypnotics (long-acting).
2. Alcohol interacts with drugs acting on the central nervous system. Describe two main effects.
3. Name a muscle relaxant of the benzodiazepine class.
4. The centrally acting appetite suppressant sibutramine acts by inhibiting reuptake of noradrenaline (norepinephrine) and serotinin. True or false?
5. Give two advantages of ondansetron (5HT$_3$ antagonist) in the treatment of nausea and vomiting as compared with a phenothiazine (chlorpromazine).
6. Name an antimuscarinic used for premedication.
7. What are the possible side effects of the drug you named in answer to question 6?
8. Compound analgesics have disadvantages. Name two.
9. Give three side effects of morphine.

10. What are the advantages of diamorphine over morphine?
11. What name is given to a situation in which an epileptic seizure is prolonged and out of control?
12. What may be done to help people with Alzheimer's disease?
13. What drugs may be used to help a person who is dependent on one or more of the following substances?
    a. Cigarettes.
    b. Alcohol.
    c. Opioids.
14. How should the problem of obesity be tackled?
15. What is the main reason for epileptic patients continuing to have fits?
16. What is meant by 'end-of-dose' effects and 'on–off' phenomena?
17. How should anticonvulsant drugs be withdrawn?
18. Suggest how a patient may overcome his difficulty in sleeping.
19. Where is the vomiting centre?
20. What is migraine and what groups of drugs may be used to help to relieve an episode?

REFERENCES

Clarke CE, Guthman M 2002 Dopamine agonist monotherapy in Parkinsons' disease. Lancet 360:1767

Commission on Classification and Terminology, League Against Epilepsy 1981 Proposal for revised clinical and electroencephalographic classification of epileptic seizures. Epilepsia 22:489–501

Craig J et al. 2002 The UK pregnancy register: update of results 1996–2002. Epilepsia 43:abstract 079

Holmes LB, Harvey EA, Coull BA et al. 2001 The teratogenicity of anticonvulsant drugs. New England Journal of Medicine 344:1132–1138

Patsalos PN, Froscher W, Pisani F et al. 2002 The importance of drug interactions in epilepsy therapy. Epilepsia 43:365–385

Sanders JWAS, Shorvon SD 1996 The epidemiology of the epilepsies. Journal of Neurology, Neurosurgery and Psychiatry 61:433–443

Scheepers B, Clough P, Pickles C 1998 The misdiagnosis of epilepsy: findings of a population study. Seizure 7:403–406

Steiner TJ, Sacher AI, Stewart WF et al. 2003 The prevalence and disability burden of adult migraine in England and their relationship to age, gender and ethnicity. Cephalgia 22:519–527

Tennis P, Stern RS 1997 Risk of serious cutaneous disorders after initiation of use of phenytoin, carbamazepine or sodium valproate: a record linkage study. Neurology 49:542–546.

FURTHER READING AND RESOURCES

[Anonymous] 2004 What's wrong with prescribing hypnotics? Drug and Therapeutics Bulletin 42:89–93

[Anonymous] 2004 Which atypical antipsychotic for schizophrenia? Drug and Therapeutics Bulletin 42:57–60

[Anonymous] 2005 Drug treatments for bipolar disorder: 2. Maintenance, prevention and special situations. Drug and Therapeutics Bulletin 43:33–37

Allen S 2005 Insomnia and its management. Pharmaceutical Journal 274:243–246

Brooks D 2006 Rasagiline (Azilect®): new MAO-B inhibitor for Parkinson's disease. Prescriber 17:19–25

Cousins DA, Young AH 2005 Advances in the understanding of the treatment of bipolar disorder. Future Prescriber 6:11–14

Crawford P 2005 Guide to the withdrawal of antiepileptic drugs. Prescriber 16:43–47

Edwards G 2006 Withdrawing antidepressants: guide to patient management. Prescriber 17:29–33

Fallon R, Fraser C, Moriarty K 2005 Recommended management of nausea and vomiting. Prescriber 16:57–70

Fearnley J 2005 Current treatment options for Parkinson's disease. Prescriber 16:12–25

Ferguson B 2005 A recommended benzodiazepine withdrawal programme. Prescriber 16:20–27

Fontebasso M 2005 Migraine management: current preventive and treatment options. Prescriber 16:43–59

Fraser K, Martin M, Hunter R et al. 2004 Bipolar disorder: aspects of drug treatment. Hospital Pharmacist 11:135–145

Galloway A, MacGillivray S, Reid I 2006 Current approaches to the drug treatment of depression. Prescriber 17:41–53

Grace C 2004 Obesity management is essential for long-term health and fitness. Pharmacy in Practice June:138–142

Hart Y 2005 The multidisciplinary approach to epilepsy management. Prescriber 16:46–52

Liddy M 2005 Current treatments for Parkinson's disease. Pharmacy in Practice 15:299–304

Livingstone M 2006 Current recommended drug treatment of psychoses. Prescriber 17:43–58

Schapira AHV 2006 Rasagiline: a new drug for Parkinson's disease. Progress in Neurology and Psychiatry 10:8–12

Scottish Intercollegiate Guidelines Network 2003 Diagnosis and management of epilepsy in adults. SIGN, Edinburgh

Scottish Intercollegiate Guidelines Network 2005 Bipolar affective disorder. SIGN, Edinburgh

Scottish Intercollegiate Guidelines Network 2006 Management of patients with dementia. SIGN, Edinburgh

Simpson S, Leddy A, Neal J et al. 2006 Memantine for severe Alzheimer's: social benefits Progress in Neurology and Psychiatry 10:9–13

Sturrock A, Cockerell C 2006 Antiepileptic drugs: properties and recommended use. Prescriber 17:44–56

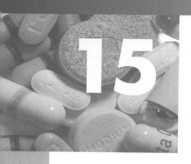

15

Drug treatment of infections

KEY OBJECTIVES

After reading this chapter, you should be able to:

- describe the role of the immune system in preventing infection
- identify the key principles in the management and control of infection
- distinguish between bactericidal and bacteriostatic activity

- discuss the main antibacterial, antifungal and antiviral drug groups
- discuss the importance of correct use of antibiotics
- explain the difficulty in eradicating so-called superbugs such as methicillin-resistant *Staphylococcus aureus* and *Clostridium difficile*
- describe the management of local and systemic candidiasis
- describe the management of HIV

- discuss the importance of careful handwashing in healthcare.

INTRODUCTION

Many bacteria have mutual relationships with humans, with both species benefiting in some way from their coexistence, for example many of the bacteria that live in the human gastrointestinal tract. These bacteria feed on nutrients from ingested food and in return carry out tasks such as producing enzymes involved in the breakdown of complex nutrients.

There are, however, bacteria that cause harm to humans, and these organisms are known as pathogens. Even some normally benign bacteria can cause harm to the human host in certain circumstances, for example when the host resistance is in some way compromised. This phenomenon is known as opportunism and the resulting infection as opportunistic infection.

The resistance of bacteria to antibiotics (p. 293) is increasingly becoming a very significant problem. The cost of resistance is measured not only in terms of failure of therapy but also in the increased costs of more expensive drugs needed to combat the resistant bacteria. In 1994, the World Health Organization Scientific Working Group on the Monitoring and Management of Bacterial Resistance to Antimicrobial Agents (Tenover and Hughes 1995) discouraged the unnecessary use of antibiotic prophylaxis in food animals and stated that 'antimicrobial agents should not be used as a substitute for adequate hygiene in animal husbandry'.

Many conditions for which antibiotics are prescribed are either of a self-limiting nature or are viral in origin and, as such, do not require antibiotics. The causes of this inappropriate prescribing by clinicians include insufficient training or knowledge, difficulty in selection of the appropriate drug, lack of microbiological information, fear of litigation and patients' expectations (Binyon and Cooke 2000).

HEALTHCARE-ASSOCIATED INFECTIONS

Approximately 9% of patients in UK hospitals suffer from an infection acquired during their hospital stay (Crowcroft and Catchpole 2002), many of which are due to multiresistant, Gram-positive and Gram-negative pathogens. The incidence of colonisation and infection with these pathogens continues to rise due to failures in hospital hygiene and selective pressures created by overuse of antibiotics.

Infection with these resistant pathogens can adversely affect clinical, microbiological and economic outcomes (Cosgrove and Carmeli 2003), and the costs

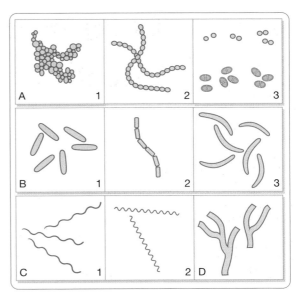

Fig. 15.1 Bacteria: examples of cell shapes. (**A**) Cocci (spherical bacteria): 1, staphylococci; 2, streptococci; 3, diplococci. (**B**) 1–3, Bacilli. (**C**) 1, 2, Spirochaetes. (**D**) Actinomyces.

associated with managing infections are considerable. In the UK, it has been estimated that costs increase threefold when hospital patients present with one or more healthcare-associated infections during an inpatient stay (Plowman 2000).

TREATMENT OF INFECTIONS

The discovery of sulphonamides in the 1930s, followed by penicillin in the 1940s, heralded a new era in the treatment of infections. Since then, a large number of drugs have been produced that either kill or inhibit the growth of bacteria, fungi or viruses. These drugs, in tandem with the patient's natural immunity, have cured many infectious diseases that previously often proved fatal. It should be noted that when immunity is impaired due to prolonged illness, old age or the use of cytotoxic drugs, infections are more difficult to eradicate. As organisms become resistant to chemotherapy, a continuing search is necessary for new drugs and modifications of those already in use.

CLASSIFICATION OF BACTERIA

Bacteria can be broadly classified according to cell shape (Fig. 15.1), that is:

Table 15.1 Classification of infectious bacteria

Cocci examples	Bacilli examples	Cocci examples	Bacilli examples
Gram-positive aerobes		**Gram-negative aerobes**	
Staphylococcus aureus	Corynebacterium diphtheriae	Neisseria meningitidis	Haemophilus influenzae
Staphylococcus epidermidis	Listeria monocytogenes	Neisseria gonorrhoeae	Klebsiella pneumoniae
Streptococcus pneumoniae			Escherichia coli
Viridans streptococci			Enterobacter spp. Proteus spp. Pseudomonas aeruginosa Legionella spp. Campylobacter spp.
Gram-positive anaerobes		**Gram-negative anaerobes**	
Peptococcus	Clostridium tetani Clostridium perfringens	Veillonella spp.	Bacteroides spp. Fusobacterium spp.

- cocci – spherical
- bacilli – straight rods
- vibrios – curved rods
- spirochaetes – spiral, flexible filaments
- spirilla – spiral, non-flexible filaments.

Subdivision of these categories is based on the Gram stain. This staining technique was developed by Christian Gram in 1884. A heat-fixed smear of bacteria undergoes a staining and counterstaining process. Gram-positive cells retain the deep purple conferred on them by the initial staining with crystal violet and iodine, whereas Gram-negative cells, which have been decolorised, exhibit the red colour of the counterstain. As a result, Gram-positive and Gram-negative cells can be readily distinguished under the microscope.

Micro-organisms are also classified as aerobes (those that can live and grow in the presence of oxygen) or as anaerobes (those that can live and grow without oxygen). These three factors:

- cell structure
- reaction to Gram stain
- aerobe/anaerobe

can be used in the classification of infectious bacteria (Table 15.1).

MICROBIOLOGY

Serious infections can be life-threatening, and decisions require to be made on the most appropriate therapy. For example:

- viral infections should not be treated with antibacterials
- samples should be taken for culture and sensitivity testing whenever possible
- knowledge of prevalent organisms (see Table 15.2) and their current sensitivity will help the selection of an antibacterial before bacteriological confirmation is available
- the dose should take account of age, weight, renal function and severity of infection
- life-threatening infections require intravenous therapy
- duration of therapy must be appropriate – a single dose of an antibacterial may cure uncomplicated urinary tract infections (UTIs), and in many cases a 5-day course is sufficient; however, in certain infections such as tuberculosis or chronic osteomyelitis, it is necessary to treat for prolonged periods.

Table 15.2 Causative pathogens in some common bacterial infections

Infection(s)	Bacterium or bacteria responsible
Respiratory infections	
Exacerbation of chronic bronchitis	Haemophilus influenzae Streptococcus pneumoniae
Pneumonia	Streptococcus pneumoniae Staphylococcus aureus Haemophilus influenzae
Urinary tract infections	Escherichia coli Proteus spp. Klebsiella spp. Streptococcus faecalis Pseudomonas
Venereal disease	
Gonorrhoea	Neisseria gonorrhoeae
Non-specific urethritis	Chlamydia
Skin/soft tissue infections	
Intravenous catheter site	Staphylococcus aureus Staphylococcus epidermidis
Surgical wound	Staphylococcus aureus Gram-negative rods
Furuncle	Staphylococcus aureus
Endocarditis	
Acute	Staphylococcus aureus Streptococcus pyogenes Gram-negative bacilli
Subacute	Streptococcus spp. Staphylococcus epidermidis Gram-negative bacilli
Septicaemia	Staphylococcus aureus Streptococcus pneumoniae Coliforms Enterobacter spp.
Meningitis (in adults; many organisms may cause meningitis in neonates)	Streptococcus pneumoniae Neisseria meningitides
Food poisoning	Salmonellae Clostridium perfringens

Other factors affecting the choice of antibiotic include:

- known allergies or hypersensitivities of the patient
- site of infection
- toxicity of chosen antibiotic
- cost.

It is advisable to obtain specimens for microbiological investigation before antimicrobial therapy is initiated, so that the antibiotic therapy can be reassessed or started after the organism is identified. Conventional laboratory techniques for identification require at least 18 h of incubation in appropriate media to allow detectable numbers of bacteria to grow. However, more rapid techniques help in diagnosis before culture results are available. The most valuable is a Gram-stained smear of blood or aspirate from the site of infection.

An identification of organisms from culture is followed by sensitivity tests. Filter paper discs impregnated with known concentrations of antibiotic are placed on to an agar culture plate containing the individual strain of organism isolated in the culture process. The degree of sensitivity of the organism to the antibiotic is assessed by the size of inhibition zones around the discs after further incubation. Results are reported back to the prescriber, indicating antibiotics effective in treatment.

ANTIBACTERIAL DRUGS

Antibacterial drugs act by a number of mechanisms (Fig. 15.2). They can be either bactericidal (kill bacteria) or bacteriostatic (arrest the growth of bacteria) (Box 15.1). Bacteriostatic agents, because they do not kill bacteria, rely on the host's immune and cell defence mechanisms to clear the bacteria. If these defence mechanisms are compromised, a bactericidal drug may be preferable.

MINIMUM INHIBITORY CONCENTRATION OF ANTIBIOTICS

As a guide to the sensitivity of a specific micro-organism to an antibiotic, the minimum inhibitory concentration (MIC) is utilised. This is the lowest concentration of antibiotic that will inhibit the growth of a given strain of micro-organism under controlled conditions. The lower the concentration, the more potent the antibiotic. However, the MIC is determined in laboratory conditions. In vivo, the drug may have to pass from the plasma into infected tissue to destroy bacteria. The penetration of antibiotics into

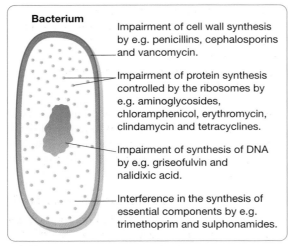

Bacterium

Impairment of cell wall synthesis by e.g. penicillins, cephalosporins and vancomycin.

Impairment of protein synthesis controlled by the ribosomes by e.g. aminoglycosides, chloramphenicol, erythromycin, clindamycin and tetracyclines.

Impairment of synthesis of DNA by e.g. griseofulvin and nalidixic acid.

Interference in the synthesis of essential components by e.g. trimethoprim and sulphonamides.

Fig. 15.2   Actions of antibacterial drugs.

Box 15.1 Some bactericidal and bacteriostatic drugs

Bactericidal drugs
- Aminoglycosides
- Cephalosporins
- Penicillins

Bacteriostatic drugs
- Tetracyclines
- Trimethoprim
- Erythromycin
- Chloramphenicol

---

abscess cavities may be poor, and surgical drainage is often necessary. In either case, higher doses would be required to achieve the MIC.

Minimum bactericidal concentration is the lowest concentration of antibiotic that will kill a given strain of bacterium under controlled conditions.

CONTROL OF ANTIBIOTIC USAGE

Because the rates of resistance are proportional to antibiotic use, the unnecessary use of antibiotics contributes to the spread of resistance. Most hospitals have adopted antibiotic policies and guidelines that are aimed at reducing the induction of resistance through controlling the range and use of anti-infective agents. Good antibiotic prescribing requires information about the probable cause and the antibiotic susceptibility of the infective agent. This can be obtained by taking appropriate specimens for culture and prescribing according to the results.

GENERAL PRINCIPLES

The objective of drug therapy in the treatment of infectious disease is to assist the body in overcoming the infecting organism. This is accomplished by the use of an anti-infective agent that is toxic to the causative organism while the normal biochemical functions of the patient are not seriously impaired.

When selecting the anti-infective agent, consideration must be given to the dose, route and frequency of administration. The dosage regimen for antibiotics excreted primarily by the kidneys will be decided according to the type of infection to be treated and the toxicity of the drug. The dose of antibiotics with a narrow therapeutic spectrum, such as the aminoglycosides, requires to be titrated according to the serum concentration. This is in order to maintain an effective therapeutic level but avoid toxic effects due to too high a level. Where renal dysfunction is present, which results in a longer half-life, dosage schedules should be lowered accordingly to prevent toxicity.

ROUTE OF ADMINISTRATION

If the infection is severe, the general condition of the patient may be poor. Oral absorption may therefore be ineffective due to nausea, vomiting or gastric stasis. In these instances, antibiotics are commonly administered by injection. After the infection is under control, appropriate concentrations will be maintained by the oral route, as this is more cost-effective and easier to administer.

Many antibiotic injections are presented as a sterile powder requiring reconstitution prior to administration. The nurse should refer to the manufacturer's product insert and to local policies in order to reconstitute the drug with correct diluent and the correct volume. Strict aseptic technique should be followed. It is advisable to discard any remaining solution after the dose has been withdrawn to avoid possible contamination or deterioration of the remaining solution.

ROUTINE PROPHYLAXIS

Routine antibiotic prophylaxis in surgical patients is needed only for those procedures associated with a high risk of postoperative infection (e.g. vaginal or colorectal surgery) or prosthetic insertions. Normally, prophylactic antibiotic treatment should not be extended beyond 48 h following surgery and should be given parenterally. Intravenous administration during induction, or intramuscular administration 30 min before surgery, usually ensures effective blood levels of antibiotic at the time when anticipated bacteraemia is likely to be highest. When gastrointestinal function is unimpaired during the postoperative period, oral administration of antibiotics provides an optimum non-invasive approach.

ALLERGIC RESPONSES

An accurate history of previous allergies is essential before antibiotics are administered. This applies particularly to penicillins with which anaphylactic shock occasionally occurs. Patients with a history of asthma, hay fever and eczema are more likely to experience severe reactions to penicillins. Some 10% of patients allergic to penicillins will also be allergic to cephalosporins. If patients are not allergic to penicillins, they are usually safe drugs.

MONITORING THE PATIENT'S RESPONSE

The patient's response to antibiotic therapy is monitored with regard to:

- controlling the infection
- adverse effects (e.g. temperature, white cell counts, erythrocyte sedimentation rate).

Specific toxic effects of antibiotics should be noted, for example hearing or renal impairment in patients receiving aminoglycosides (e.g. gentamicin). Phlebitis can occur on intravenous administration, and the nurse should monitor the patient's veins carefully for evidence of redness, swelling or pain, and report these to the doctor. When blood samples are taken, the doctor should ensure that times are recorded accurately so that maximum and minimum drug concentrations during the dosing interval can be accurately estimated.

SUPERINFECTION

Superinfection may occur as a result of the following.

- Proliferation of a resistant micro-organism following killing of a sensitive micro-organism at the site of infection.
- Proliferation of a resistant micro-organism in the alimentary tract due to suppression of the normal flora by antibiotic therapy. The broader the spectrum, the greater is the possibility of superinfection developing. Tetracyclines and ampicillin are examples. Pseudomembranous colitis results as an overgrowth of *Clostridium difficile* in the bowel presenting as watery diarrhoea, abdominal cramping, fever and leucocytosis. First-line antibiotic treatment is usually oral metronidazole: 800 mg initially then 500 mg every 8 h for 10 days (alternatively, oral

vancomycin 125 mg four times daily for 7–10 days). Vancomycin is not absorbed following oral administration and can achieve high concentration in the gut without risk of serious systemic adverse effects. Vancomycin is more expensive than metronidazole.
- Drugs interfering with the immune response of the body (e.g. corticosteroids and other immunosuppressive agents). Oral candidiasis, caused by *Candida albicans*, is the commonest example. This can be treated effectively with nystatin suspension.

BACTERIAL RESISTANCE TO ANTIBIOTICS

The resistance of bacteria to antibiotics is a problem that has continued to grow in parallel with the development of new antibiotics. Bacterial resistance reflects antibiotic use and is more of a problem when controls on antibiotic use are lax. The sensible use of antibiotics reduces this. There are several mechanisms by which resistance may emerge.

SELECTION

An antibiotic will eliminate the sensitive organisms within a bacterial population, and the resistant forms will proliferate.

MUTATION

Resistance to an antibiotic may develop as a result of a genetic change that converts a previously susceptible bacterium to a resistant one. This genetic change may be as a result of spontaneous randomly occurring gene mutation during the process of cell division. These mutants will then proliferate.

TRANSFERRED RESISTANCE

Resistance may be acquired by the exchange of genetic material between bacteria, which confers antibiotic resistance from one organism to another. Exchange of genetic material occurs primarily by the exchange of fragments of DNA known as plasmids. If these plasmids contain resistant genes, the genes are passed between bacteria conferring a survival advantage and promoting proliferation of resistant bacteria. This ability to share resistant genes has led to the rapid proliferation of bacterial resistance.

Transfer of plasmids is not confined to the same species, and they can be passed from, for example, *Escherichia coli* to *Salmonella*. Either way, new DNA enters the bacterium and codes for a mechanism that confers resistance. The real dilemma facing clinicians lies in the fact that many bacterial strains are resistant to multiple antibiotics, a phenomenon known as multiple resistance.

There are several mechanisms of antibiotic resistance.

- Enzymatic inactivation of the antibiotic. The bacterium produces enzymes that inactivate the antibiotic by altering its chemical structure. For example, the enzymes responsible for destroying penicillins and cephalosporins are called beta-lactamases; these enzymes are found in Gram-negative bacteria such as *Escherichia coli*, *Salmonella* species and *Pseudomonas* species and in Gram-positive bacteria (e.g. staphylococci). These enzymes open up the β-lactam ring of the penicillin, which is the portion responsible for antimicrobial activity. Aminoglycoside resistance is often due to a similar mechanism in which bacteria produce enzymes that alter the chemical structure of the aminoglycoside.
- Altered permeability of the bacterium to the drug. Some bacteria reduce the permeability of their cell membrane to antibiotics such as aminoglycosides or tetracycline so that less antibiotic is able to enter and bind to its target.
- Resistance occurs when bacteria alter the structure of the antibiotic target site and the antibiotic can no longer bind to it, rendering the antibiotic ineffective.
- Formation of alternative metabolic pathway. Sulphonamides and trimethoprim act by inhibiting the folate metabolic pathways within bacteria. If bacteria develop an alternative pathway for folic acid synthesis, resistance to sulphonamides and trimethoprim occurs.

The general spread of antibiotic resistance is most likely to occur in an environment in which there is a significant use of antibiotics and the opportunity to move from one host to another exists. In an environment where little use is made of antibiotics, there will be no selective advantage for the resistant bacteria. When antibiotics are used in low dose, there will be greater opportunity for resistance to develop and spread because strains will survive at low dose that would have been eliminated at a higher dose. An example of this is the huge increase in the level of resistance in *Salmonella* due to the use of low-dose antibiotics as growth enhancers in farm animals.

METHICILLIN-RESISTANT STAPHYLOCOCCUS AUREUS

Approximately 30% of the population carry the organism *Staphylococcus aureus*. This is a bacterium that is normally found in the nose and on skin. Although most healthy people are unaffected by it, it does have the potential to cause infection in those who have severely weakened immune systems (e.g. some ill patients in hospital).

Methicillin-resistant *Staphylococcus aureus* (MRSA) is a form of *Staphylococcus aureus*. It is transmitted in the same way and causes the same range of infections as other strains of *Staphylococcus aureus*. However, it has developed resistance to the more commonly used antibiotics. This makes infections caused by MRSA more difficult and costly to treat, and every effort should be made to prevent its spread.

The majority of individuals are *colonised* when the organism lives harmlessly on the body with no ill effects, as opposed to *infected*, which is when the organism penetrates tissue and causes disease.

In order to control and minimise the spread of MRSA, there must be compliance with the following:

- standard precautions (e.g. thorough hand hygiene; see p. 320)
- cleaning must be of an acceptable standard
- adherence to infection control policies (e.g. isolation, clinical waste, laundry)
- infection control training
- strict adherence to antibiotic policy
- minimal movement of patients and staff between wards, units and hospitals.

TREATMENT OF MRSA INFECTION

Patients who demonstrate clinical signs of infection will require treatment with the appropriate antibiotics. The agent used will depend on the site of infection (Table 15.3). Some of these organisms are sensitive only to vancomycin or teicoplanin. Strains may be susceptible to rifampicin, sodium fusidate, tetracyclines, aminoglycosides and macrolides. Treatment is guided by the sensitivity of the infecting strain. Swabs are taken from the nose and throat to establish a diagnosis (Figs 15.3 and 15.4).

Table 15.3 Decolonisation

Site	Treatment
Nasal carriage only	Nasal decolonisation only
Throat carriage	Nasal and throat decolonisation
Axilla or groin carriage	Nasal and body decolonisation

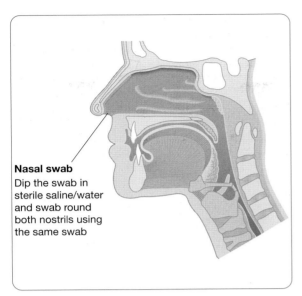

Fig. 15.3 Taking a nose swab.

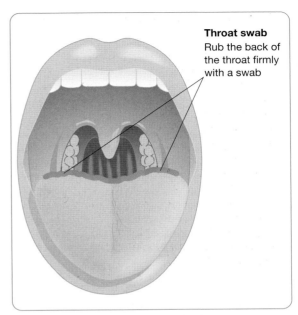

Throat swab
Rub the back of the throat firmly with a swab

Fig. 15.4 Taking a throat swab.

Nasal decolonisation

Nasal carriage treatment is to apply, with a cotton bud, mupirocin 2% nasal ointment three times daily to the inner surface of each nostril for 5 days. When mupirocin resistance is encountered, second-line treatment is with neomycin and chlorhexidine cream (Naseptin) provided that the organism is neomycin-susceptible.

Throat decolonisation

Oral hygiene is very important, as teeth and dentures may harbour MRSA. First-line treatment is oral trimethoprim (200 mg twice daily) and sodium fusidate tablets (500 mg three times daily) for 5 days. In the event of resistance or patient intolerance, an alternative is a combination of oral rifampicin (600 mg once daily) and trimethoprim 200 mg twice daily for 5 days. Rifampicin or sodium fusidate should not be used alone, because resistance may develop rapidly.

Skin decolonisation

Treatment consists of a direct application of 4% chlorhexidine to all skin using a damp disposable cloth daily for 5 days, using the chlorhexidine as a soap substitute and then rinsing it off. The hair should be washed twice during the 5-day period with 4% chlorhexidine. Alternatively, 2% triclosan or 7.5% povidone–iodine could be used. Hair conditioners and body lotions can be used after treatment if required.

Linezolid and quinupristin with dalfopristin

Linezolid and the combination of quinupristin and dalfopristin are active against MRSA, but these antibacterial drugs should be reserved for organisms resistant to other antibacterials or for patients who cannot tolerate other antibacterial drugs. Linezolid is available both orally (600 mg every 12 h) and by intravenous infusion. Thrombocytopenia, anaemia, leucopenia and pancytopenia have been reported, and weekly monitoring of full blood counts is recommended. Quinupristin with dalfopristin is available as an intravenous infusion. A novel broad-spectrum glycycline antibiotic (tigecycline) is active against Gram-positive, Gram-negative and anaerobic organisms including multidrug-resistant strains (see p. 301).

THE PENICILLINS

The penicillins are bactericidal and interfere with cell wall synthesis in growing and dividing bacteria. Lysis and cell death result from weakening of the cell wall. Penicillins are excreted in the urine in therapeutic concentrations.

The most significant and adverse effect of the penicillins is hypersensitivity, which manifests as rashes and, on occasion, anaphylaxis. Allergy to one penicillin indicates allergy to them all, because the hypersensitivity is related to the basic penicillin structure.

Excessively high serum levels due to either very high doses or to renal failure in patients given normal doses may give rise to encephalopathy, a rare but serious toxic effect due to cerebral irritation. The penicillins should not be given by intrathecal injection, as this can cause encephalopathy, which may be fatal. A second problem is accumulation of electrolyte, because most injectable penicillins contain either sodium or potassium.

Diarrhoea often occurs during oral penicillin therapy.

BENZYLPENICILLIN AND PHENOXYMETHYLPENICILLIN

Benzylpenicillin (penicillin G) is readily inactivated by gastric acid juice and is given by injection. It diffuses into most of the body tissues but does not pass the blood–brain barrier unless the meninges are inflamed; neither does it penetrate well into the pleural cavity nor into the synovial or ocular fluids. It is inactivated by bacterial beta-lactamases. Beta-Lactamases are enzymes that inactivate penicillin by attacking part of the penicillin molecule known as the beta-lactam ring. This structure is an essential part of penicillins and cephalosporins. Notable producers of beta-lactamases are staphylococci.

Benzylpenicillin is effective in a wide range of infections, including those shown in Table 15.4.

Phenoxymethylpenicillin (penicillin V) has a similar but less active antibacterial spectrum. It is indicated principally for respiratory infections in children, streptococcal tonsillitis and continued treatment following benzylpenicillin injection. It is used as a prophylactic against reinfection after recovery from rheumatic fever. Phenoxymethylpenicillin is not destroyed in the stomach and is quickly but unpredictably absorbed from the small intestine. Absorption is superior when administered on an empty stomach. Phenoxymethylpenicillin is not suitable for the treatment of severe conditions in which high blood levels of penicillin are necessary.

The dose range and side effects of benzylpenicillin and phenoxymethylpenicillin are shown in Table 15.5.

PENICILLINASE-RESISTANT PENICILLINS

Some organisms are resistant to penicillin because of their ability to produce the enzyme penicillinase, which destroys penicillin. Flucloxacillin is available for treatment of staphylococcal infections when resistant

Table 15.4 Infections for which benzylpenicillin is effective

Organism	Disease
Beta-haemolytic streptococci	Septicaemia, tonsillitis
Viridans streptococci	Subacute bacterial endocarditis
Streptococcus pneumoniae	Pneumonia
Neisseria meningitidis	Meningococcal meningitis
Clostridium tetani	Tetanus
Clostridium perfringens	Gas gangrene
Treponema pallidum	Syphilis
Neisseria gonorrhoeae	Gonorrhoea
Borrelia burgdorferi	Lyme disease

organisms are particularly common (see Table 15.6). Flucloxacillin is available in oral as well as injectable form and is well absorbed.

BROAD-SPECTRUM PENICILLINS

This group includes ampicillin and amoxicillin. The main difference between ampicillin and amoxicillin is in absorption from the gut. Less than half the dose of ampicillin is absorbed from the gut, and this is decreased by the presence of food. About 40% passes into the large bowel and diarrhoea, a common side-effect, is thought to be caused by a disturbance of the large bowel flora. Amoxicillin is better absorbed, producing higher plasma and tissue concentrations, absorption not being affected by the presence of food in the stomach. Both of these drugs are inactivated by β-lactamases, including those produced by almost all staphylococci, 50% of Escherichia coli strains and 15% of Haemophilus influenzae strains. They should not be used for hospital patients without checking sensitivity.

Co-amoxiclav is a combination of amoxicillin and beta-lactamase inhibitor, clavulanic acid. The clavulanate molecules penetrate the bacterial cell and combine with the beta-lactamase molecules. This inactivates the beta-lactamases, leaving the amoxicillin free to exert a full bactericidal effect. This makes the combination active against beta-lactamase-producing bacteria that are resistant to amoxicillin: Staphylococcus

Table 15.5 Benzylpenicillin and phenoxymethylpenicillin

Drug	Adult dose range	Onset of peak serum levels (min)	Side-effects
Benzylpenicillin	By IM or slow IV injection or by infusion: 2.4–4.8 g daily in four divided doses. Bacterial endocarditis – slow IV injection or by infusion: 7.2 g daily in divided doses. Meningitis – slow IV injection or by infusion: 2.4 g every 4 h.	15–30	Sensitivity reactions including urticaria, fever, joint pains, anaphylactic shock, diarrhoea
Phenoxymethylpenicillin	500 mg–1 g every 6 h half an hour before food.	30–60	As for benzylpenicillin

Table 15.6 Penicillinase-resistant penicillin

Drug	Adult dose range	Notes
Flucloxacillin	Oral: 250 mg 6-hourly at least 30 min before food. IM: 250 mg 6-hourly. Slow IV injection or infusion: 0.25–1 g every 6 h.	Side-effects as for benzylpenicillin; doses can be doubled in severe infections

aureus, *Escherichia coli* and *Haemophilus influenzae*, as well as many *Bacteroides* and *Klebsiella* species. The broad-spectrum penicillins are summarised in Table 15.7.

ANTIPSEUDOMONAL PENICILLINS

Ticarcillin is active against *Pseudomonas aeruginosa*, *Proteus* species and *Bacteroides fragilis* and, due to its combination with clavulanic acid, is active against beta-lactamase-producing bacteria resistant to ticarcillin.

Tazocin contains piperacillin with the beta-lactamase inhibitor tazobactam. Piperacillin has a broad spectrum and is more active than ticarcillin against *Pseudomonas aeruginosa*. These drugs are used in pseudomonal septicaemias. In those life-threatening conditions, it is preferable to give them in combination with an aminoglycoside such as gentamicin, as this combination is synergistic. This group of penicillins can be given only by injection.

The antipseudomonal penicillins are summarised in Table 15.8.

CEPHALOSPORINS

The cephalosporins were first obtained from a mould cultured from the sea near a Sardinian sewage outfall in 1945. The cephalosporins are related to the penicillins – both have a beta-lactam ring that confers on them a similar mode of action. They act, like the penicillins, by inhibiting bacterial cell wall synthesis.

The cephalosporins are broad-spectrum antibiotics. They are used in the treatment of septicaemia, pneumonia, meningitis, biliary tract infections, peritonitis and UTIs. All have a similar antibacterial spectrum, although individual agents have differing activity against certain organisms.

The principal side-effect of the cephalosporins is hypersensitivity, and about 10% of penicillin-sensitive patients will be allergic to cephalosporins. Allergic reactions include rashes, pruritus, urticaria, fever and anaphylaxis. Other side-effects include diarrhoea, nausea and vomiting.

Table 15.7   Broad-spectrum penicillins

Drug	Indications	Adult dose	Side-effects
Amoxicillin	As for ampicillin, plus *Helicobacter pylori* eradication and endocarditis prophylaxis	Oral: 250–500 mg every 8 h. IM: 500 mg every 8 h. IV: 500 mg every 8 h, increased to 1 g every 6 h.	As for ampicillin
Ampicillin	Urinary tract infections, otitis media, sinusitis, chronic bronchitis	Oral: 0.25–1 g every 6 h at least 30 min before food. IM, IV: 500 mg every 4–6 h.	Nausea, diarrhoea, rashes
Co-amoxiclav	Infections due to β-lactamase-producing strains (when amoxicillin alone not appropriate), including respiratory tract infections, genitourinary and abdominal infections, cellulitis, animal bites and severe dental infections	Expressed as amoxicillin 250–500 mg every 8 h. IV injection or infusion: 1 g every 8 h	As for ampicillin

Table 15.8   The antipseudomonal penicillins

Drug	Adult dose range	Side-effects
Piperacillin 2 g Tazobactam 250 mg	2.25–4.5 g by IV injection over 3–5 min or by IV infusion over 6–8 h	As for benzylpenicillin; also nausea, vomiting, diarrhoea
Ticarcillin with clavulanic acid	IV infusion: 10–20 g daily in divided doses	As for benzylpenicillin; also nausea, vomiting, coagulation disorders

ORAL CEPHALOSPORINS

The oral first-generation cephalosporins, cefalexin, cefradine and cefadroxil, and the second-generation cephalosporin, cefaclor have a similar antimicrobial spectrum. They are useful for UTIs that do not respond to other drugs or that occur in pregnancy, respiratory tract infections, otitis media, sinusitis, and skin and soft tissue infections. Cefaclor has good activity against *Haemophilus influenzae*, but it is associated with protracted skin reactions, especially in children. Cefadroxil has a long duration of action and can be given twice daily; it has poor activity against *Haemophilus influenzae*. Cefuroxime axetil, an ester of the second-generation cephalosporin cefuroxime, has the same antibacterial spectrum as the parent compound; it is poorly absorbed orally.

Cefixime has a longer duration of action than the other cephalosporins that are active by mouth. It is presently licensed only for acute infections.

Cefpodoxime is more active than the other oral cephalosporins against respiratory bacterial pathogens, and it is licensed for upper and lower respiratory tract infections.

Oral cephalosporins are listed in Table 15.9.

PARENTERAL CEPHALOSPORINS

In general, cefradine has been replaced by newer cephalosporins. Cefuroxime, a second-generation cephalosporin, is less susceptible than first-generation cephalosporins to inactivation by beta-lactamases and has greater activity against *Haemophilus influenzae* and *Neisseria gonorrhoeae*.

Table 15.9 Oral cephalosporins

Drug	Adult dose
Cefaclor	250–500 mg every 8 h.
Cefadroxil	0.5–1 g twice daily.
Cefalexin	250 mg every 6 h; 1–1.5 g every 6 or 8 h for severe infections.
Cefixime	200–400 mg daily as a single dose or in two divided doses.
Cefpodoxime	Upper respiratory tract infections: 100 mg twice daily with food (200 mg twice daily in sinusitis). Lower respiratory tract infections (including bronchitis and pneumonia): 100–200 mg twice daily with food.
Cefradine	250–500 mg every 6 h.
Cefuroxime axetil	250 mg twice daily.

Cefotaxime, ceftazidime and ceftriaxone are third-generation cephalosporins. They have a markedly increased activity against certain Gram-negative bacteria. However, they are less active than cefuroxime against certain Gram-positive bacteria, most notably *Staphylococcus aureus*, and superinfection may occur with resistant bacteria. Ceftazidime possesses good activity against *Pseudomonas* and is also active against other Gram-negative bacteria. Ceftriaxone requires only once-daily administration due to its longer half-life. It has potent bactericidal activity against a wide spectrum of Gram-positive and particularly Gram-negative organisms. Indications include serious infections such as septicaemia, pneumonia and meningitis.

Parenteral cephalosporins are summarised in Table 15.10, and some other β-lactam antibiotics are given in Table 15.11.

TETRACYCLINES

The most commonly used members of the tetracycline family are demeclocycline, doxycycline, lymecycline, minocycline, oxytetracycline and tetracycline.

Table 15.10 Parenteral cephalosporins

Drug	Indications	Dose
Cefotaxime	Infections due to sensitive Gram-positive and Gram-negative organisms	1 g every 12 h, increased for life-threatening infections up to 12 g daily in divided doses.
Cefradine	See cefotaxime; surgical prophylaxis	0.5–1 g every 6 h, increased in severe infections.
Ceftazidime	See cefotaxime; active against *Pseudomonas aeruginosa*	1 g every 8 h, increased in severe infections.
Ceftriaxone	See cefuroxime	1 g daily; severe infections, 2–4 g. Gonorrhoea: 250 mg as a single dose. Once-daily dosing facilitates a single dose in surgical prophylaxis: 1 g.
Cefuroxime	See cefotaxime	750 mg every 6–8 h, increased in severe infections.
	Surgical prophylaxis	1.5 g IV at induction followed by 750 mg, up to three further doses 8-hourly.
	More active against *Haemophilus influenzae* and *Neisseria gonorrhoeae*	Gonorrhoea: 1.5 g IM as single dose.

Table 15.11   Other β-lactam parenteral antibiotics

Drug	Indications	Side-effects	Dose
Aztreonam	Gram-negative infections, including *Pseudomonas aeruginosa*, *Haemophilus influenzae*, *Neisseria meningitidis*	Nausea, vomiting, diarrhoea, abdominal cramps, mouth ulcers, urticaria and rashes	1 g every 8 h or 2 g every 12 h.
Imipenem with cilastatin (cilastatin inhibits inactivation of imipenem by kidney enzymes)	Aerobic and anaerobic Gram-positive and Gram-negative infections, surgical prophylaxis	Nausea, vomiting, diarrhoea, fever, anaphylactic reactions, allergic reactions, blood disorders	IM: 500–750 mg every 12 h. IV infusion: 1–2 g daily in divided doses.
Meropenem	Aerobic and anaerobic Gram-positive and Gram-negative infections	Nausea, vomiting, diarrhoea, abdominal pain	500 mg–1 g every 8 h. Meningitis: 2 g every 8 h

Mode of action. The tetracyclines are generally bacteriostatic rather than bactericidal in action. They inhibit protein synthesis in bacterial ribosomes in susceptible organisms, thus preventing production of polypeptides.

Uses. Tetracyclines have a broad antimicrobial spectrum and demonstrate activity against most Gram-positive organisms that are sensitive to the penicillins and also against some Gram-negative organisms that are not susceptible to the penicillins. Table 15.12 lists some of the infectious diseases for which tetracyclines may be indicated. They are also used for the treatment of exacerbations of chronic bronchitis because of their activity against *Haemophilus influenzae*. Microbiologically, there is little to choose between the various tetracyclines. Minocycline is an exception, because it has a broader spectrum of activity. Tetracyclines may also be used in the treatment of acne vulgaris (p. 495).

Pharmacokinetics. The tetracyclines in general are reasonably well absorbed (about 70%), minocycline and doxycycline being absorbed to a greater extent (about 90%). The concomitant administration of milk, agents such as antacids containing aluminium, magnesium or calcium, and iron salts reduces absorption from the gastrointestinal tract because of the formation of insoluble chelates and should be avoided. The tetracyclines are widely distributed to body tissues and are taken up in teeth and bone, especially growing bone and teeth during the early stages of calcification. This can cause both discoloration and enamel hypoplasia in teeth and decreased growth of long bones. Tetracyclines should

Table 15.12   Main indications for the use of tetracyclines

Disease	Organism
Infections caused by chlamydia	
Psittacosis	*Chlamydia psittaci*
Lymphogranuloma venereum	LGV chlamydiae
Trachoma	*Chlamydia trachomatis*
Urethritis	*Chlamydia* and *Ureaplasma* spp.
Q fever	*Coxiella burnetii*
Typhus diseases	*Rickettsia* spp.
Mycoplasma pneumonia	*Mycoplasma pneumoniae*
Brucellosis (doxycycline with rifampicin)	*Brucella abortus*
Lyme disease	*Borrelia burgdorferi*

therefore not be given in pregnancy or to children under 12 years of age.

Approximately 50% of most tetracyclines are excreted in the urine unchanged. Renal failure causes decreased clearance and accumulation, resulting in toxicity. Minocycline and doxycycline are exceptions, being metabolised mainly in the liver, and doxycycline is the tetracycline of choice in compromised renal function.

Table 15.13 Dosages of tetracyclines

Drug	Dose
Demeclocycline	150 mg every 6 h
Doxycycline	200 mg initially then 100 mg daily
Lymecycline	408 mg every 12 h, increased in severe infection
Minocycline	100 mg twice daily
Oxytetracycline	250–500 mg 6-hourly
Tetracycline	250–500 mg 6-hourly

Adverse effects. Tetracyclines commonly produce gastrointestinal adverse effects (e.g. nausea, vomiting and diarrhoea). An increasingly occurring condition is superinfection with *Clostridium difficile*, resulting in pseudomembranous colitis. Oral superinfection with *Candida albicans* may result in thrush. Overgrowth in the bowel may cause diarrhoea. Treatment consists of stopping the administration of tetracycline and, in severe cases, treatment with nystatin. Minocycline, in addition, can cause dizziness, vertigo and severe exfoliative rashes.

Dosage. The dosages of the tetracyclines (see Table 15.13) vary, and this is partly accountable to different half-lives (e.g. oxytetracycline and tetracycline, 8 h; demeclocycline, 14 h; minocycline and doxycycline, 18 h).

TIGECYCLINE

Tigecycline is a recent introduction. It is a novel broad-spectrum glycylcycline antibiotic that has activity against a broad range of Gram-positive, Gram-negative and anaerobic organisms and many antibiotic-resistant bacteria (including MRSA, vancomycin-resistant *Enterococcus* and pencillin-resistant *Streptococcus pneumoniae* and multiresistant *Acinetobacter* species).

While exhibiting antibacterial activities typical of earlier tetracyclines or analogues such as minocycline, it has more potent activity against tetracycline-resistant organisms. Unlike existing tetracyclines, it is available only as an intravenous preparation administered twice daily.

It acts by preventing bacterial protein synthesis and growth. Nausea and vomiting are the most significant side effects. Tigecycline offers a therapeutic option in postsurgical wound infections or complicated skin and soft tissue infections.

AMINOGLYCOSIDES

This group of drugs includes amikacin, gentamicin, neomycin, netilmicin, streptomycin and tobramycin.

The aminoglycosides are bactericidal. The mechanism is not fully understood, but they inhibit the synthesis of bacterial protein by binding to ribosomes within the organism.

The aminoglycosides are active against some Gram-positive and many Gram-negative organisms.

Gentamicin is the most important aminoglycoside and is used for the treatment of serious infections, including septicaemia, meningitis, pyelonephritis and endocarditis. The main indication for amikacin is the treatment of serious infections caused by Gram-negative bacilli resistant to gentamicin. Amikacin, gentamicin and tobramycin are also active against *Pseudomonas aeruginosa*. Neomycin is not significantly absorbed following oral administration and is used for bowel sterilisation prior to bowel surgery. The aminoglycosides are effective agents for the local treatment of infections of the external ear and conjunctiva. Neomycin, which is too toxic for parenteral administration, framycetin and gentamicin are commonly used. Neomycin is also used topically, in combination with chlorhexidine, for attempted eradication of staphylococci in the nasal passage.

Pharmacokinetics. The aminoglycosides are poorly absorbed from the gastrointestinal tract and must be given by injection for systemic infections. They have a narrow therapeutic spectrum, and plasma concentration monitoring ensures that optimal therapeutic levels are maintained, thus preventing toxicity and ensuring efficacy. Plasma concentrations should be measured approximately 1 h after injection (peak level) and just before the next dose (trough level).

Parenterally administered aminoglycosides are excreted almost entirely by the kidneys. Care should be taken with dosage and, when possible, treatment should not exceed 7 days in order to minimise side-effects. Doses should be reduced in renal failure.

Adverse effects. The important side-effects are ototoxicity and, to a lesser degree, nephrotoxicity. These occur most commonly in the elderly and in patients with renal failure due to elevated serum levels, i.e. trough levels greater than 2 micrograms/mL and peak levels greater than 12 micrograms/mL (gentamicin).

Table 15.14 Dosages of aminoglycosides

Drug	Dose
Amikacin	IM, slow IV injection or IV infusion: 15 mg/kg daily in two divided doses
Gentamicin	IM, slow IV injection or IV infusion: 3–5 mg/kg daily in divided doses 8-hourly (monitor serum level, and creatinine clearance in renal impairment)
Neomycin	1 g every hour for 4 h then 1 g every 4 h for bowel sterilisation (for 2–3 days)
Netilmicin	IM, slow IV injection or IV infusion: 4–6 mg/kg daily; for urinary tract infection, 150 mg as single daily dose for 5 days; for gonorrhoea, 300 mg as a single dose
Tobramycin	IM, slow IV injection or IV infusion: 3 mg/kg daily in divided doses every 8 h; urinary tract infection, by IM injection 2–3 mg/kg daily as a single dose

Long duration of treatment is also a causative factor. Gentamicin tends to cause vertigo and ataxia, while neomycin causes deafness. Neomycin is too toxic for systemic use. Aminoglycosides should be avoided in pregnancy, as they cross the placenta and cause damage to the eighth nerve of the fetus. Aminoglycosides may impair neuromuscular transmission and should not be given to patients with myasthenia gravis.

Interactions. Aminoglycosides should not be given with furosemide, as these may potentiate the ototoxic and nephrotoxic effects.

Dosages. The dosages of aminoglycosides are summarised in Table 15.14.

MACROLIDES

This group of drugs includes erythromycin, clarithromycin, telithromycin and azithromycin.

Erythromycin is classified as a bacteriostatic drug, but it may be bactericidal in high concentrations or against highly susceptible organisms. Erythromycin inhibits protein synthesis in susceptible organisms by binding to ribosomes and inhibiting polypeptide synthesis. Resistance is rarely observed during successful short-term treatment.

Erythromycin has an antibacterial spectrum similar to that of benzylpenicillin and is used for infections in which benzylpenicillin would be the treatment of choice but where the patient is sensitive to penicillin. Erythromycin is indicated for respiratory infections, whooping cough, legionnaires' disease (*Legionella pneumophila*), chlamydia and mycoplasmas.

Erythromycin may be administered orally or by injection. Oral formulations containing the erythromycin base are enteric-coated, as the base is decomposed by gastric acid. The enteric coating breaks down in the higher pH of the duodenum, and the erythromycin is released and absorbed. The stearate and ethylsuccinate forms of erythromycin are not acid-labile. They dissociate in the duodenum, liberating active erythromycin, which is absorbed. Following absorption, erythromycin is widely distributed in the tissues. It penetrates the meninges only when they are inflamed. The drug is excreted primarily in the bile. Erythromycin may be given intravenously as the lactobionate.

The most common side-effects of the oral erythromycins are gastrointestinal and are dose-related. These include nausea, vomiting, diarrhoea and abdominal discomfort after large doses. Azithromycin and clarithromycin cause fewer gastrointestinal side effects than erythromycin. The intravenous injection of erythromycin causes venous irritation and thrombophlebitis, particularly in high doses. It is recommended that the drug be well diluted and infused slowly over 20–60 min to minimise these effects or, alternatively, to use clarithromycin.

Clarithromycin is a derivative of erythromycin with similar actions and uses. It is acid-stable and so has a greater degree of bioavailability.

Azithromycin is chemically related to erythromycin, but it is more acid-stable. It is well absorbed after oral administration, giving high tissue levels that decline slowly and so permit single daily doses. It is effective in many skin and soft tissue infections, respiratory tract infections, otitis media and genital chlamydial infections.

Telithromycin is indicated for community-acquired pneumonia, sinusitis and exacerbations of chronic bronchitis. See Table 15.15 for side effects and dosages.

CLINDAMYCIN

Clindamycin acts by inhibiting bacterial protein synthesis. It has restricted use owing to the significant side effects, in particular pseudomembranous colitis,

Table 15.15 Macrolides: side-effects and doses

Drug	Side-effects	Dose
Azithromycin	Gastrointestinal disturbances	500 mg daily for 3 days, 1 h before or after food.
Clarithromycin	Headache, rash and gastrointestinal disturbances	250 mg twice daily for 7 days, doubled for severe infections with treatment continued up to 14 days. By IV infusion: 500 mg twice daily.
Erythromycin	Gastrointestinal disturbances	250–1000 mg four times daily. IV: 25–50 mg/kg daily.
Telithromycin	Gastrointestinal disturbances, headache	800 mg daily for 5–10 days.

which may be fatal. The drug should be immediately discontinued if diarrhoea or colitis develops.

Clindamycin is active against Gram-positive cocci (including penicillin-resistant staphylococci) and also against many anaerobes, especially *Bacteroides fragilis*. Because of the adverse effects, clindamycin is generally reserved for staphylococcal bone and joint infections and endocarditis prophylaxis, and topically for severe acne.

Adverse effects. Adverse effects due to clindamycin include abdominal discomfort, nausea, vomiting, diarrhoea and pseudomembranous colitis, jaundice and altered liver function tests. It may cause thrombophlebitis following an intravenous injection.

Dosage. For oral therapy, the dose is 150–450 mg every 6 h; for deep intramuscular injection, 0.6–2.7 g daily in two to four divided doses. Single doses above 600 mg are administered by intravenous infusion only.

OTHER ANTIBACTERIALS

A number of other antibacterials are described in Table 15.16.

SULPHONAMIDES AND TRIMETHOPRIM

The first of the sulphonamides was used in the treatment of infections in the 1930s. However, the importance of sulphonamides in this role has decreased in recent years as a result of increasing bacterial resistance and replacement by more effective and less toxic antibiotics.

A combination of trimethoprim one part and sulfamethoxazole five parts (co-trimoxazole) has been used because of the synergistic activity of these drugs. However, co-trimoxazole is associated with rare but serious side-effects, including blood dyscrasias (notably bone marrow depression and agranulocytosis), especially in the elderly. Its use is therefore largely restricted to the treatment of *Pneumocystis* pneumonia. It is also indicated for toxoplasmosis and nocardiasis. Trimethoprim can be used alone for urinary and respiratory tract infections and for prostatitis, shigellosis and invasive salmonella infections. Although similar to co-trimoxazole, the side effects of trimethoprim are less severe and occur less frequently.

Mode of action. The sulphonamides are bacteriostatic and act by preventing the conversion of para-aminobenzoic acid to folic acid. Trimethoprim blocks bacterial folic acid synthesis at the stage immediately following that blocked by the sulphonamides.

Pharmacokinetics. Individual sulphonamides differ markedly in their absorption, distribution and excretion. Sulfamethoxazole and sulfadiazine are generally well absorbed. Trimethoprim is rapidly absorbed. It is excreted mainly in the urine, and dosages should be reduced in renal failure.

Adverse effects. Nausea, diarrhoea, headache, rashes and rarely depression of the blood count may occur. Special care should be taken when folate may be deficient (e.g. in the elderly, in the chronic sick and in those on prolonged treatment or high doses). Because of the possibility of jaundice and kernicterus (deposition of bilirubin in the brains of neonates), sulphonamides should not be given to pregnant women, particularly in the third trimester, or to newborn or premature infants.

Table 15.16 Other antibacterials

Indications	Pharmacokinetics	Adverse reactions	Dose
Chloramphenicol Only for life-threatening infections, because of toxicity (e.g. meningitis due to *Haemophilus influenzae*, typhoid fever). Eye drops useful for bacterial conjunctivitis.	Well absorbed from gastrointestinal tract.	Blood disorders, including aplastic anaemia caused by severe depression of bone marrow activity, nausea, vomiting, diarrhoea. 'Grey syndrome' in neonates, i.e. vomiting, respiratory depression, cyanosis and collapse associated with a reduced ability of the infant to metabolise and excrete chloramphenicol.	50 mg/kg daily in four divided doses.
Colistin Bacterial in action, it is active against Gram-negative organisms, including *Escherichia coli*, *Klebsiella* spp. and *Pseudomonas aeruginosa*.	Not absorbed from the gastrointestinal tract, so must be given IM or IV for treatment of systemic infections. However, it is toxic and seldom used systemically.	Nephrotoxicity is the most serious adverse effect. Allergic manifestations, paraesthesia, vertigo, apnoea and muscle weakness occur less frequently.	Oral for bowel sterilisation: 1.5–3 million units every 8 h. IM, IV injection or infusion: 2 million units every 8 h.
Sodium fusidate Infections due to penicillin-resistant staphylococci, particularly osteomyelitis, often in conjunction with a second antistaphylococcal antibiotic to prevent resistance (e.g. flucloxacillin).	Well absorbed, widely distributed in body tissues, including bone. Metabolised in liver and excreted in bile.	Nausea, vomiting, reversible jaundice.	Oral: 0.5–1 g every 8 h. IV infusion: 0.5 g over 6 h three times daily.
Teicoplanin Serious Gram-positive infections, including endocarditis, treatment of staphylococcal infections.	Longer half-life than vancomycin and requires only once-daily dosing.	No significant enhanced renal toxicity when used with aminoglycosides. Nausea, vomiting, diarrhoea, rash, fever, anaphylaxis, blood disorders, tinnitus, local thrombophlebitis.	By IM injection, IV injection or infusion: 400 mg initially, 200–400 mg daily.
Vancomycin Bactericidal activity against aerobic and anaerobic Gram-positive bacteria. In antibiotic-related pseudomembranous colitis (*Clostridium difficile*). Alternative to penicillins in infective endocarditis. Also used IV for other serious infections caused by Gram-positive cocci, including multiresistant staphylococci (e.g. methicillin-resistant *Staphylococcus aureus*).	Very poorly absorbed from the gastrointestinal tract. Widely distributed in body tissues following IV infusion. Almost completely eliminated unchanged in the urine. It has a long duration of action and can be given every 12 h. Accumulates in renal failure, necessitating a modified dosage schedule and serum concentration monitoring (below 30 micrograms/mL). Dose should be reduced in the elderly.	Ototoxic and nephrotoxic, which are dose-related. Extravasation causes necrosis and thrombophlebitis. After parenteral administration may get nausea, chills, fever, urticaria, rashes, tinnitus (discontinue use). It is important to administer as an infusion. Severe flushing of the upper body ('red man' syndrome) can occur if given as a bolus.	Oral: 125 mg 6-hourly. IV infusion: 500 mg every 6 h.

Table 15.17 Dosages of co-trimoxazole and trimethoprim

Drug	Dose
Co-trimoxazole	Two tablets twice daily. IM or IV infusion: 960 mg every 12 h
Trimethoprim	Oral: 200 mg twice daily

The dosages of co-trimoxazole and trimethoprim are summarised in Table 15.17.

TUBERCULOSIS

Tuberculosis is an infection caused by the bacterium *Mycobacterium tuberculosis*. In humans, the lung is the most common site of infection, although numerous other areas (meninges, bones, joints, peritoneum, genitourinary tract, skin) may also become infected.

Tuberculosis is spread by airborne droplets, from coughing and sneezing, which contain viable bacilli. These are inhaled and lodge in the alveoli, where the bacilli rapidly multiply. On primary infection, the bacilli multiply rapidly in the lungs and spread to the lymph nodes and to the bloodstream. The organism is thus distributed throughout the body, where it can remain viable but dormant for many years, particularly in the lungs, bones, lymphatic system and kidneys.

Primary infection is usually controlled by the host's immune system. The bacteria become engulfed by macrophages that coalesce to form a mass of cells – a tubercle or granuloma. The bacilli contained in the granuloma may survive and remain dormant for many years. The granuloma may break down in later years, leading to pulmonary or extrapulmonary clinical disease.

Widespread disease following primary infection is rare, although susceptible groups such as young infants, the immunocompromised, or malnourished and debilitated patients may be at risk (see p. 407 for vaccination against tuberculosis). In recent years, the incidence of tuberculosis has increased. Drug users and people with AIDS are very susceptible to this infection.

SIGNS AND SYMPTOMS

Primary tuberculosis is usually a mild asymptomatic illness that resolves spontaneously without problems. The onset of post–primary disease is slow. When symptoms occur, they include chronic cough, some-times with blood-streaked sputum (haemoptysis), malaise, weight loss, fever, night sweats, anorexia, anxiety and depression.

DIAGNOSTIC TESTS

The discovery of *Mycobacterium tuberculosis* by either microscopy of sputum smears or by culture is diagnostic of active tuberculosis. Tuberculin testing is an adjunct to diagnosis. The test used is as follows.

MANTOUX TEST

This consists of the intradermal injection of tuberculin purified protein derivative. The reaction is read 48–72 h after injection; a positive reaction, indicating the presence of antibodies, is demonstrated by an induration of 6 mm or more in diameter (see p. 407 for more details).

DRUG TREATMENT OF TUBERCULOSIS

The treatment of tuberculosis (Table 15.18) has two phases: an initial phase using at least three drugs, and a continuation phase with two drugs. Recommended regimens of the Joint Tuberculosis Committee of the British Thoracic Society for the treatment of tuberculosis in the UK are given below.

INITIAL PHASE

In order to reduce the population of viable bacteria rapidly and to prevent emergence of resistant bacteria, at least three drugs are given concurrently in the initial phase. This involves the daily use of isoniazid, rifampicin and pyrazinamide. Ethambutol is added when drug resistance to isoniazid is a possibility. This regimen should be continued for at least 8 weeks.

CONTINUATION PHASE

This follows the initial phase, and treatment with isoniazid and rifampicin is continued for a further 4 months.

METRONIDAZOLE AND TINIDAZOLE

Most bacteria can be divided into two groups: those that survive and grow in the presence of oxygen (aerobes), and anaerobes, which survive and grow in the absence of oxygen. Metronidazole is an antimicrobial drug with high activity against anaerobic bacteria and protozoa (see Table 15.19). Indications include treatment of urogenital trichomoniasis, invasive intestinal amoebiasis, extra-intestinal amoebiasis and giardiasis. It is also used for surgical and gynaecological sepsis in which its activity against colonic anaerobes, especially *Bacteroides fragilis*, is important. Metronidazole is also effective in the treatment of antibiotic-associated colitis (pseudomembranous colitis). Metronidazole by the rectal route is an effective alternative to the

Table 15.18 Drugs used in the treatment of tuberculosis[a]

Drug	Adult dosage	Adverse effects/interactions	Comments
Ethambutol	15 mg/kg daily	Optic neuritis, colour blindness and restriction of visual fields. These are related to plasma levels and are more common when excessive dosage is used. Therapy should be discontinued immediately when deterioration in vision develops.	Reduce dosage in renal failure. Patients should be advised to seek medical advice if they experience visual disturbance.
Isoniazid	300 mg daily	Well tolerated and side-effects not usually serious. Skin reactions may occur. Persistent nausea and vomiting may indicate liver damage. Peripheral neuropathy may occur, particular when diabetes, alcoholism, renal failure or malnutrition are present, in which case 10 mg of pyridoxine should be given daily.	Elimination by acetylation in the liver. Check hepatic function before commencing treatment.
Rifampicin	Under 50 kg, 450 mg daily; over 50 kg, 600 mg daily	Anorexia and nausea may occur. Hepatotoxicity is a serious side-effect and alcoholic patients, the elderly and patients with pre-existing liver disease are at risk. Concurrent administration of rifampicin with oral contraceptives increases the metabolism of oestrogen and progestogen, which may result in contraceptive failure. Alternative contraceptive methods should be used. Anticoagulant effects of warfarin are reduced by concurrent administration of rifampicin owing to increased metabolism of the anticoagulant.	Monitor liver function tests. Caution in pregnancy. Patients should be advised that rifampicin colours the urine, stools and tears. Soft contact lenses may become permanently discoloured.
Pyrazinamide	Under 50 kg, 1.5 g daily; over 50 kg, 2 g daily	Liver damage.	Monitor liver function tests. Readily absorbed and penetrates well into cerebrospinal fluid, making it particularly useful in tuberculous meningitis. Should not be given to patients with gout.

[a]Products are available containing various combinations of the above drugs, which may aid compliance.

intravenous route when oral administration is not possible. Intravenous metronidazole is used for the treatment of established cases of tetanus.

Metronidazole has no action against aerobic organisms and so, in mixed infections, combined treatment with an additional antibiotic is required. Metronidazole also has applications in the oral treatment of infected leg ulcers and pressure sores. It is also used locally as a 0.8% gel (Metrotop) in the control of malodorous fungating tumours associated with anaerobic bacteria, by application to the cleaned area once or twice daily.

Table 15.19 Metronidazole

Mode of action	Dosage in anaerobic infections[a]	Pharmacokinetics	Important adverse effects and interactions
Has high activity against anaerobic bacteria and protozoa. It is reduced to active metabolites that interfere with nucleic acid function of the organism.	Oral: treated for 7–10 days, 800 mg initially then 400 mg every 8 h. By rectum: 1 g every 8 h for 3 days then 1 g every 12 h. IV infusion: 500 mg every 8 h.	Well absorbed after oral and rectal administration. Effective serum concentrations are reached in 1–3 h and maintained for 8–10 h. Excreted mainly in the urine. Crosses placental barrier and appears in the milk of nursing mothers.	The most common reactions to metronidazole therapy are rash, nausea, furry tongue, dry mouth, metallic taste in the mouth. Patients are advised to avoid taking alcohol when receiving metronidazole as disulfiram-like reaction may occur, resulting in abdominal cramps, nausea, vomiting, headaches and flushing. Caution in pregnancy and breast-feeding.

[a]See British National Formulary for doses for bacterial vaginosis, leg ulcers and pressure sores, acute ulcerative gingivitis and surgical prophylaxis.

Tinidazole has similar actions, uses and side effects to those of metronidazole, with the advantage of a longer plasma half-life. The dose is 2 g initially, followed by 500 mg twice a day.

QUINOLONES

The original quinolone antibiotic is nalidixic acid, which has been available for over 30 years. More recently, molecular changes have produced fluorinated quinolones with a broader antibacterial spectrum and better pharmacokinetics. The quinolone antibiotics are bactericidal. They act by inhibiting the enzyme DNA gyrase, which is required by the bacterial DNA.

The spectrum of microbiological activity of the quinolone antibiotics is one of high activity against Gram-negative bacteria, slightly less activity against Gram-positive bacteria and little or no activity against anaerobes. Examples of the quinolones are summarised in Table 15.20.

Pharmacokinetics. The quinolones are well absorbed following oral administration. Antacids decrease their absorption. They are eliminated in three ways:

- secreted into the gut lumen and excreted in the faeces
- metabolised by the liver
- excreted as unchanged drug via the kidneys.

No differences have been found in serum half-lives in the elderly. Patients taking ciprofloxacin should ensure adequate fluid intake to minimise the risk of crystalluria.

Adverse drug reactions. Side-effects of the quinolones commonly involve the central nervous system: headache, dizziness, sleep disorders and less frequently restlessness, hallucinations, confusion. Patients should be advised of this, because performance of skilled tasks (e.g. driving) may be impaired. Because of these adverse reactions, the drugs should be used with caution in patients with a history of epilepsy. They may induce convulsions in patients with or without a history of convulsions. Gastrointestinal side effects including nausea, vomiting, abdominal pain and diarrhoea may occur.

Because weight-bearing joints of juvenile animals have suffered cartilage damage when quinolones were administered, caution should be exercised in children and adolescents. They can cause pain and inflammation in tendons, especially in older people. If tendinitis is suspected, the quinolone should be discontinued immediately.

Table 15.20   The quinolones

Drug	Indications	Dose
Ciprofloxacin	Particularly active against Gram-negative bacteria, including *Campylobacter*, *Neisseria*, *Pseudomonas*, *Salmonella*, *Shigella*. Less activity against Gram-positive bacteria such as *Streptococcus pneumoniae* and *Streptococcus faecalis*. Used for infections of the respiratory tract (but not for pneumococcal pneumonia), urinary tract, gastrointestinal system, gonorrhoea and septicaemia.	Oral: 250–750 mg twice daily. Gonorrhoea: 500 mg as a single dose. Available as IV infusion.
Levofloxacin	Greater activity against pneumococci than ciprofloxacin.	Oral: 250–500 mg daily for 7–14 days. IV infusion: 500 mg (over at least 60 min) once or twice daily for community-acquired pneumonia.
Nalidixic acid	Uncomplicated urinary tract infections	500 mg–1 g every 6 h.
Norfloxacin	Uncomplicated urinary tract infections	400 mg twice daily.
Ofloxacin	Infections of urinary tract, lower respiratory tract, gonorrhoea	200–400 mg daily. Gonorrhoea: 400 mg as a single dose. Available as an IV infusion.

URINARY TRACT INFECTIONS

Bladder urine is normally sterile, although transient small numbers of bacteria may be present after micturition or sexual intercourse. This occurs because of retrograde flow up the urethra. It is far more likely to happen with women, because of the length of the urethra and the increased number of organisms resident on the surfaces surrounding the orifice. The first step in the development of UTI is colonisation of the periurethral mucosa, commonly by *Escherichia coli* from faeces.

To initiate infection, bacteria present in the urine must adhere to the urothelial cells on the bladder surface. One of the more important host defence mechanisms is the continual renewal of the surface by shedding cells together with attached bacteria and mucus. Urine does not normally support the growth of bacteria because of the large variation in pH, osmolality and the antibacterial substances present.

In treating patients with UTI, the infection is often classified as simple (uncomplicated) or complicated. One way to define a complicated UTI is one that fails to respond to a short course of antibiotics. Symptoms commonly associated with lower UTIs (e.g. cystitis) include:

- urgency
- frequency
- pain or burning on micturition (dysuria)
- cloudy or malodorous urine
- suprapubic pain.

Patients with acute pyelonephritis may also present with loin pain, tenderness, fever, chills, nausea and haematuria (see Box 15.2).

Urinary tract infection is predominantly a disease of females from the age of one until about the age of 50, most neonatal cases of UTI occurring in boys. UTIs again become a problem for males after the age of 50,

---

Box 15.2 Terms associated with urinary tract infections

- Bacteriuria: presence of bacteria in the urine; asymptomatic bacteriuria exists if colony counts exceed 10^5/mL in a patient without urinary tract infection symptoms.
- Pyelonephritis: inflammation of the kidney, with pain, tenderness, bacteriuria, pyuria and fever.
- Pyuria: white blood cells in the urine.
- Urethritis: inflammation of the urethra, with dysuria.
- Prostatitis: inflammation of the prostate.

Table 15.21 Treatment of urinary tract infections[a]

Condition	Uncomplicated infection	Serious infection (pending culture results or in primary treatment failure)	Notes
Acute pyelonephritis	–	Cefotaxime, ciprofloxacin, co-amoxiclav, gentamicin, cefuroxime	Best treated initially by injection, especially if the patient is vomiting or severely ill.
Cystitis	Trimethoprim, cefradine, nalidixic acid, nitrofurantoin for 5–7 days	Ciprofloxacin, co-amoxiclav	Long-term therapy may be required in selected patients to prevent recurrence of infection. Trimethroprim, nitrofurantoin and cefalexin have been recommended for long-term therapy.
Cystitis on pregnancy	Cefradine, amoxicillin	Nitrofurantoin	–
Prostatitis	Trimethoprim	Ciprofloxacin, cefotaxime	Can be difficult to cure and requires treatment for several weeks with an antibiotic that penetrates prostatic tissue.

[a]Apart from nitrofurantoin, details of the drugs in this table have appeared in earlier pages.

when prostatic obstruction, urethral instrumentation and surgery influence the infection rate. In general, 10–20% of the elderly living at home have bacteriuria, and up to 40% in long-stay hospitals. The reasons for higher UTI rates in older people include the high prevalence of prostatitis in men, poor bladder emptying and faecal incontinence.

CAUSES

Most organisms involved are bowel commensals, the commonest being *Escherichia coli*. Less common causes include *Proteus* and *Klebsiella* species. *Staphylococcus epidermidis*, *Pseudomonas aeruginosa* and *Enterococcus faecalis* infection may occur following catheterisation or instrumentation. Whenever possible, a specimen of urine should be collected for culture and sensitivity testing before starting antibacterial therapy. The antibacterial selected should reflect local antibacterial sensitivity, which needs to be reviewed regularly.

TREATMENT

Table 15.21 outlines the drugs used according to the degree of infection being treated.

NITROFURANTOIN

Nitrofurantoin is bacteriostatic. It acts by inhibiting a number of bacterial enzymes essential for bacterial function.

Pharmacokinetics. Nitrofurantoin is rapidly and well absorbed following oral administration at a dosage of 50 mg four times daily with food. About 40% of the dose appears unchanged in the urine.

Adverse reactions. Nausea and vomiting are common, but this can be reduced by administering with food and lowering the dose. Mild allergic reactions may occur. Long-term therapy occasionally results in peripheral neuropathy, which is dose-related. It occurs as a result of renal failure, and patients with this condition should not be given nitrofurantoin. Alkalinisation of the urine may be undertaken with potassium citrate mixture to relieve the discomfort of cystitis.

FUNGAL INFECTIONS

Two general types of fungal infection exist:

1. topical infections affecting the skin and mucous membranes (e.g. vaginitis, oral thrush, athlete's foot)
2. systemic infections.

The patient's underlying condition may predispose to fungal infection, for example:

- a severely immunocompromised patient
- a patient receiving antibiotic therapy that eliminates normal flora.

Topical infections are more common and include candidiasis and infections by dermatophytes. The causative organism in candidiasis is usually *Candida albicans*, a yeast that may be found in up to 50% of healthy mouths and about one-third of adult vaginas. Hundreds of thousands of them live peacefully in our bodies. Infections are opportunistic and occur when the environment of the body becomes favourable for the organism to grow and spread. This can happen, for example, when someone is being treated with antibiotics. Infection caused by this organism is usually superficial, for example invasion of the superficial layers of the epidermis of the mouth or vagina, or very occasionally skin that has become damp and macerated, as in the nappy area. This condition is commonly referred to as thrush. Vaginal thrush is an opportunistic infection that affects women predominantly of childbearing age, because *Candida* thrives in the low pH and abundant glycogen present in the urine at this time. The initially harmless *Candida* is transformed into a pathogen either by local changes in the vagina or by lowered immune resistance. Pregnancy and diabetes are two predisposing factors.

Vulval pruritus and vaginal discharge are the usual presenting symptoms. Dysuria may be severe, especially when there is local excoriation and maceration due to scratching. Painful intercourse (dyspareunia) may occur and may be severe. When present, the discharge is usually thick and white or creamy.

Oral candidiasis presents in different forms, denture stomatitis being the most common. Acute pseudomembranous candidiasis is the form commonly referred to as oral thrush. The infected epithelium proliferates rapidly, producing the characteristic soft, creamy yellow plaques, and can occur on any mucosal surface of the mouth. Steroid inhalers are a common cause of thrush by thinning the oral mucosa and suppressing inflammatory reaction. Patients should be advised to rinse out the mouth following administration to help prevent this.

Fungi called dermatophytes cause many common infections that are named according to the affected part of the body:

- *Tinea pedis* – athlete's foot
- *Tinea capitis* – scalp ringworm
- *Tinea corporis* – body ringworm
- *Tinea unguium* – nail infection (onychomycosis).

Tinea versicolor is a fungal infection of the horny layer of the skin that shows as oval, light brown patches in fair-skinned people.

ANTIFUNGAL DRUGS

The treatment of fungal infections is outlined in Table 15.22. Clotrimazole, econazole, ketoconazole and miconazole are applied topically to treat fungal skin infections. Treatment should continue for 10–14 days after the lesions have healed.

Systemic fungal infections occur when fungi enter the bloodstream and may cause more serious conditions. Systemic fungal infections occur in a person with a weakened immune system through, for example, HIV or cancer chemotherapy.

VIRUSES

Viruses are much smaller than bacteria, consisting essentially of a core of nucleic acid in a protective protein envelope. They possess only one of the two classes of nucleic acids as carriers of their genetic information, either RNA or DNA. These organisms have no enzymes of their own such as are necessary for internal metabolism. It is for this reason that they are resistant to antibiotics that act by blocking some stage of microbial metabolism.

Viruses can be regarded as intracellular parasites. Because new proteins, not present in the normal cell, are synthesised in virus infected cells, this offers the possibility of selective inhibition of viral replication by chemical agents. The majority of virus infections resolve spontaneously in immunocompetent persons.

ANTIVIRAL AGENTS

Previously, the only therapeutic approach to viral illness was prevention by immunisation. Examples of vaccines include those against rubella, poliomyelitis and yellow fever. There are now a small number of therapeutic agents available to treat herpes viral infections (Table 15.23), including aciclovir, famciclovir and valaciclovir.

IMMUNE SYSTEM

The human immune system protects the body against foreign objects such as micro-organisms. It comprises many different cells that are spread throughout the body, each playing different roles and moving around the body as needed.

BLOOD CELLS

There are two major types of cell in the blood. The most common are red blood cells or erythrocytes, which carry oxygen to the body tissues and carry away

Table 15.22   Drugs used to treat fungal infections

Mode of action	Pharmacokinetics	Indications	Dose	Adverse effects
POLYENE ANTIFUNGAL DRUGS				
Amphotericin Alter permeability of cell membranes, resulting in loss of essential cell constituents.	Poorly absorbed from gastrointestinal tract. May be administered orally as lozenges for treatment of superficial candida infections. Administered by IV infusion to treat systemic infections.	Active against most fungi and yeasts (*Aspergillus*, *Candida* spp., *Cryptococcus*, *Coccidioides*, *Histoplasma*)	Lozenges given four times daily are used to treat oral candidiasis. IV infusion in glucose: 250 micrograms– 1 mg/kg daily. (It is precipitated from solutions containing cations such as sodium or potassium).	When given parenterally, toxicity is common and close supervision is necessary. Renal impairment occurs owing to renal vasoconstriction and a direct effect on the tubules, resulting in diminished renal plasma flow giving rise to acidosis and hypokalaemia. Other adverse reactions include nausea, vomiting, febrile reactions, headache, anaemia, blood disorders, rash, anaphylactoid reactions. Fever is common and may be reduced by IV hydrocortisone at start of treatment. Lipid formulations of amphotericin (Abelcet, AmBisome and Amphocil) are significantly less toxic and are recommended when the conventional formulation of amphotericin is contraindicated because of toxicity, especially nephrotoxicity.

Continued

Table 15.22 Drugs used to treat fungal infections *'cont ...'*

Mode of action	Pharmacokinetics	Indications	Dose	Adverse effects
Nystatin As for amphotericin.	Not absorbed after oral or topical administration. Too toxic for parenteral use.	Principally used for *Candida albicans* infections of gastrointestinal tract, skin, vagina and respiratory tract.	Oral: intestinal candidiasis, 500 000 units every 6 h.	Usually unimportant – may experience nausea, vomiting and diarrhoea at higher doses.
TRIAZOLE ANTIFUNGAL DRUGS				
Fluconazole Alters cell membrane permeability.	Absorbed by mouth. Effective parenterally.	Mucosal and systemic candidiasis; cryptococcal infections including meningitis.	Oral: single dose of 150 mg for vaginal candidiasis. 50–100 mg daily in oropharyngeal candidiasis. 200–400 mg daily orally or by IV infusion for systemic candidiasis or cryptococcal meningitis.	Gastrointestinal side-effects. Caution in pregnancy, breast-feeding and renal impairment.
Itraconazole As for fluconazole.	As for fluconazole.	Mucosal candidiasis and dermatophyte infections.	Oral preparations only. Oral candidiasis: 100 mg daily for 15 days. Vaginal candidiasis: 200 mg twice daily for 1 day. Tinea pedis and corporis: 100 mg daily.	Gastrointestinal side-effects. Caution in pregnancy and breast-feeding.
IMIDAZOLE ANTIFUNGAL DRUGS				
Ketoconazole Increases membrane permeability. Also inhibits cellular enzymes.	Poorly absorbed after local application. Widely distributed parenterally.	Systemic mycoses, serious candidiasis, resistant dermatophyte infections of skin and fingernails.	200 mg orally once daily with food until at least 1 week after symptoms have cleared.	Gastrointestinal side-effects, rashes, pruritus. Contraindicated in hepatic impairment. Avoid in pregnancy and porphyria. Monitor liver function.

Continued

Table 15.22 Drugs used to treat fungal infections *'cont ...'*

Mode of action	Pharmacokinetics	Indications	Dose	Adverse effects
Miconazole As for ketoconazole.	As for ketoconazole.	Oral, intestinal and systemic fungal infections.	5–10 mL in the mouth after food four times daily. Continue for 2 days after symptoms clear.	Nausea, vomiting.
OTHER ANTIFUNGAL DRUGS				
Flucytosine Penetrates certain fungal cells, where it is converted to fluorouracil and alters protein synthesis.	Well absorbed and widely distributed. Undergoes little metabolism.	Systemic yeast and fungal infections.	By IV infusion: 200 mg/kg daily in four divided doses. Reduce dose in renal impairment.	Gastrointestinal reactions, rashes. Caution in pregnancy and breast-feeding.
Terbinafine Interferes with fungal sterol biosynthesis at an early stage. This leads to deficiency in ergosterol and to intracellular accumulation of squalene, resulting in fungal cell death.	Well absorbed orally. Rapidly diffuses through dermis and concentrates in the stratum corneum. Distributed into nail plate within first few weeks of commencing therapy. Metabolites excreted predominantly in urine.	Dermatophyte infection of the nails. Ringworm infection.	250 mg daily up to 3 months or longer, depending on site of infection.	Gastrointestinal effects, headache, rash, arthralgia, myalgia.

carbon dioxide. The other group is the white blood cells or leucocytes. These are the immune cells.

Some white blood cells recognise specific foreign organisms to which the body has been exposed in the past. These specific immune cells are called lymphocytes. Other white blood cells are non-specific and can attack a range of different foreign organisms; these include neutrophils, eosinophils and natural killer cells (see Fig. 15.5).

LYMPHOCYTES

There are two different types of lymphocyte. B lymphocytes (sometimes just called B cells) produce antibodies. An antibody is a protein that can lock on to a distinctive part of a specific foreign organism. When this happens, the antibody signals to other immune cells to attack the organism.

T lymphocytes (sometimes just called T cells) are called different names depending on the molecules on their surface. They are white blood cells that play important roles in the immune system. There are two main types of T cell. One type has molecules called CD4 on its surface; these 'helper' cells orchestrate the body's response to certain micro-organisms such as viruses. The other T cells, which have a molecule called CD8, destroy cells that are infected and shut down the immune response once the infection has been dealt with.

OTHER IMMUNE CELLS

Natural killer cells attack tumour cells and virus-infected cells in a way similar to that of lymphocytes. However, while each lymphocyte can recognise and attack cells infected by only one specific virus, natural killer cells can attack a wider range.

Phagocytes are cells that attack and destroy foreign cells by engulfing them. There are two main different types of phagocyte.

Table 15.23 Drugs used to treat herpes infections

Mode of action	Use	Pharmacokinetics	Adverse effects	Dose
Aciclovir Aciclovir enters all cells. It is changed by a virus-specific enzyme, thymidine kinase, to the active derivative aciclovir triphosphate. This then inhibits DNA polymerase, an enzyme necessary for viral growth, and disrupts viral replication.	Active against herpes virus if started early. It is used IV for the treatment of systemic infections of herpes simplex and varicella zoster; topically for treating herpes infections of the skin and mucous membranes (including genital herpes); as an ointment in herpes simplex eye infections. Used in the immuno-compromised for prophylaxis and for prevention of recurrence.	15–30% absorbed orally, but this results in therapeutic serum concentration levels. Widely distributed throughout the body. There are a number of metabolites formed either in the liver or in cells infected by the herpes virus; the active aciclovir triphosphate is formed in the latter. The half-life increases as renal function deteriorates and dosage needs to be adjusted in patients with renal impairment.	Headache can occur with oral administration, as can gastrointestinal reactions such as nausea, vomiting and diarrhoea. Local reactions at the injection site, particularly with inadvertent extravasation, can occur. These include irritation, phlebitis, inflammation and pain.	Must be started at the onset of infection to be effective. Viral herpes simplex treatment: 200–400 mg five times daily. Herpes zoster (shingles): 800 mg five times daily for 7 days. By IV infusion over 1 h: 5–10 mg/kg every 8 h. Cream or eye ointment: to be applied every 4 h.
Famciclovir Converted in vivo to penciclovir triphosphate, which inhibits replication of viral DNA.	Treatment of herpes zoster and genital herpes.	Rapidly and extensively absorbed following oral administration.	Well tolerated. Headache and nausea have been reported.	Herpes zoster: 250 mg three times daily for 7 days.
Valaciclovir Converted in vivo to aciclovir.	Treatment of herpes zoster and herpes simplex.	Well absorbed orally and almost completely converted to aciclovir.	Headache, skin rashes, gastrointestinal disorders.	Herpes zoster: 1 g three times daily for 7 days. Herpes simplex: 500 mg twice daily for 5–10 days.

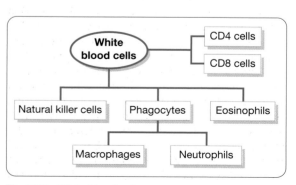

Fig. 15.5 White blood cells.

1. Macrophages roam the blood and the body tissues, killing organisms that can cause AIDS-related diseases and cells infected by viruses.
2. Neutrophils leave the blood to go to tissues in which infection or inflammation is developing. They mainly attack bacteria and fungi.

Eosinophils engulf organisms too large for phagocytes.

HUMAN IMMUNODEFICIENCY VIRUS

This virus is able to attach itself to the CD4 molecule, allowing the virus to enter and infect these cells. Even while a person with HIV feels well and has no symptoms, billions of CD4 T cells are infected by HIV and are destroyed each day, and billions more CD4 T cells are produced to replace them.

USES OF CD4 COUNTS

The number of CD4 T cells in a cubic millimetre of blood is used as a marker in HIV. A normal count in a healthy, HIV-negative adult can vary but is usually between 800 and 1500 CD4 T cells/mL.

Most people with HIV find that their CD4 count falls over time. This often happens at a variable rate, and so the count can still be quite stable for long periods. It is useful to have the CD4 count measured regularly for two reasons:

- to monitor the immune system and help decide whether and when to take anti-HIV drugs and treatments to prevent infections
- to help monitor the effectiveness of any anti-HIV drugs being taken.

If the CD4 count is persistently below 500 cells/mL, the immune system is slightly weakened and the patient is at a gradually increasing risk of infections the further it falls. If it drops below 200 cells/mL, there is increased risk from serious infections and the patient is diagnosed as having AIDS.

The HIV virus multiplies extremely rapidly, and this continues throughout the course of the disease. Initially, the virus is breeding at a rate of billions per day but is kept in check by the immune system. However, over time the virus slowly destroys the immune system's ability to produce the CD4 lymphocytes, and resistance to it falls. This takes around 10 years but varies – some people (about 20%) develop AIDS within 5 years of HIV infection, while others (about 5%) seem to resist the virus much longer than 10 years. Measurement of the number of viruses in the blood gives a good guide to the speed of progression. The higher the virus count per mL of blood, the faster the progression. During this very rapid multiplication, genetic 'errors' or mutations occur, and unfortunately this often leads to new strains that are resistant to drugs. Over time, the resulting immunosuppression permits the development of opportunistic infections. These are due to pathogens that cause asymptomatic infection or minor illness in the immunocompetent but can cause potentially life-threatening infection or malignancy in those who are immunosuppressed.

ANTI-HIV THERAPY

Anti-HIV drugs interfere with the way the virus tries to reproduce itself inside a human cell. Although anti-HIV drugs cannot kill the virus completely, they reduce the chance of infected cells producing new HIV particles that could go on to infect even more cells. There is currently no cure, only a slowing of the progression of HIV infection. Prescribing of antiviral therapy should provide at least three drugs acting at different stages of the HIV life cycle. *Combination therapy* and *highly active antiretroviral therapy* (*HAART*) are the terms used to describe three or more antiretroviral drugs used for treatment of HIV. The prognosis of those living with HIV has been dramatically improved by HAART, resulting in HIV being regarded as a chronic manageable disease.

The aim of HAART is to prolong and improve the patient's quality of life by suppressing viral replication, ideally to below the current level of detection of the virus (< 50 copies/mL) and to maintain this degree of viral suppression for as long as possible. In doing so, this should restore the immunological response and prevent the development of opportunistic infections.

The British HIV Association (2005) treatment guidelines provide healthcare professionals with evidence-based recommendations on the use of antiretrovirals. Because of increasing prevalence of transmitted resistance, the British HIV Association has recommended that all HIV-positive patients have a blood test to look for baseline resistance. The presence of specific virus mutations can identify patients who have been infected with a strain of HIV that is already resistant to certain drugs or classes. This can help the clinician choose initial therapy and maximise the chance of achieving viral suppression. The baseline resistance test should be performed as soon as possible after diagnosis. A resistance test is also recommended after treatment failure.

Following commencement of therapy, viral suppression should be achieved within 16 weeks. This is normally associated with an increase in the CD4 count. Viral suppression is dependent on the patient adhering to medication, but poor absorption, drug interactions, drug resistance (which can occur as a result of poor adherence) and inadequate drug levels can also be factors. Patients are described as being on 'stable' antiretroviral therapy when the viral load remains below the lower limit of detection of the available test (< 50 copies/mL) and there is a sustained increase in the CD4 count. Routine monitoring of CD4 count viral load, blood count, urea and electrolytes should be undertaken at 3- to 6-monthly intervals.

ANTIRETROVIRAL DRUGS

The antiretroviral drugs can be divided into four main classes:

- nucleoside (or nucleotide) reverse transcriptase inhibitors (NRTIs); tenofovir is the only nucleotide analogue
- non-nucleoside reverse transcriptase inhibitors (NNRTIs)
- protease inhibitors
- entry inhibitors.

NUCLEOSIDE REVERSE TRANSCRIPTASE INHIBITORS

Once HIV has locked on to and invaded a human cell, it uses an enzyme called reverse transcriptase to convert its genetic code into the same form as the genetic code of human cells (DNA). This viral DNA then merges with the human DNA, converting the cell into a factory for making the building blocks of new virus. The NRTIs target the enzyme reverse transcriptase, halting viral DNA synthesis. NRTIs include abacavir, didanosine, emtricitabine, lamivudine, stavudine, tenofovir, and zidovudine. Stavudine, especially with didanosine, is associated with a higher risk of lipodystrophy and lactic acidosis and should be used only if alternative regimens are not suitable. Patients should be counselled about the early warning symptoms of lactic acidosis, such as abdominal pain, nausea and vomiting. Lipodystrophy (which is also associated with regimens containing protease inhibitors) causes fat redistribution with loss of subcutaneous fat, increased abdominal fat, buffalo hump and breast enlargement.

Side-effects of the NRTIs include gastrointestinal disturbances, anorexia, pancreatitis, liver damage, central nervous system side-effects, blood disorders and rash.

NON-NUCLEOSIDE REVERSE TRANSCRIPTASE INHIBITORS

The NNRTIs act by binding directly to reverse transcriptase preventing the conversion of HIV RNA to HIV DNA. Efavirenz and nevirapine are NNRTIs.

Side effects include rash, gastrointestinal side effects, central nervous system side effects, impaired concentration and pruritus.

PROTEASE INHIBITORS

An HIV enzyme called protease cuts the long chains of HIV proteins into smaller individual proteins as part of the process of assembling a new virus particle. Protease inhibitors block this enzyme by selectively binding with it. Protease inhibitors include amprenavir, atazanavir, fosamprenavir, indinavir, lopinavir, nelfinavir, ritonavir, saquinavir and tipranavir. Ritonavir in low doses boosts the activity of most of the other protease inhibitors, although at these low doses the ritonavir has no intrinsic antiviral activity.

Protease inhibitors are associated with hypoglycaemia and should be used with caution in diabetics. The protease inhibitors are metabolised by cytochrome P450 enzyme systems and therefore have significant potential for drug interactions.

Side effects of the protease inhibitors include gastrointestinal disturbances, anorexia, hepatic dysfunction, blood disorders and rash.

ENTRY INHIBITORS

Enfuvirtide, which inhibits HIV from fusing to the host cell, is licensed for managing infection that has failed to respond to a regimen of other antiretroviral drugs. Enfuvirtide should be used in combination with other potentially active antiretroviral drugs.

The most common side-effect is rash, usually in the first 2 weeks. When mild or moderate, the rash usually resolves within a month. If the rash is severe, treatment should be discontinued. When severe depression or psychosis occurs, the doctor should be contacted. Gastrointestinal side-effects, sleep disturbances, impaired concentration and pruritus may also occur. Box 15.3 provides combination regimens.

DRUG THERAPY COMPLIANCE

Because antiretroviral therapy is a lifelong commitment for the patient, a balance must be achieved between using a highly effective drug combination that fits the patient's lifestyle while minimising the side-effects of these highly potent drugs. Lifestyle factors that influence patient choice include work patterns or nature of work.

High levels of adherence are crucial to the success of HAART and in order to prevent resistance, which can develop rapidly (within days for some drugs) when missed doses have occurred. The reasons patients

---

Box 15.3 Initial regimen choices

- Two nucleoside reverse transcriptase inhibitors (NRTIs) plus one non-nucleoside reverse transcriptase inhibitor (NNRTI) – efavirenz is the preferred first NNRTI option
- Two NRTIs plus boosted protease inhibitor – lopinavir boosted with ritonavir is the preferred first-option protease inhibitor

find taking HIV medicines difficult are multifaceted and include:

- fear of disclosure of HIV status
- intolerance to side-effects such as nausea and vomiting
- perceived harm from taking antiretrovirals
- forgetting to take them.

Because drug therapy for patients living with HIV is a lifelong commitment, adherence support and medication counselling are fundamental to ensure the best patient outcomes (See Box 15.4).

Predicting side-effects and coprescribing drugs to deal with them can help. It is common for patients to experience initial short-term side-effects such as nausea and vomiting, as well as headache and fatigue. Patients often require antiemetics, such as domperidone, for the first 6–8 weeks of therapy. Loperamide can be prescribed to counter diarrhoea.

POSTEXPOSURE PROPHYLAXIS

People may be exposed to HIV through their occupation (e.g. healthcare workers and needlestick injuries) as well as through high-risk sexual activity. Although drugs for postexposure prophylaxis are currently unlicensed, there is evidence to support their role in clinical practice. The Department of Health Expert Advisory Group on AIDS recommends that prophylaxis with combination antiretroviral therapy is initiated immediately (ideally within 72 h) on occupational exposure and continued for 1 month.

OPPORTUNISTIC INFECTIONS

There is a group of infections that the body normally easily controls but that can cause serious disease in people whose immune system is impaired by HIV (or other forms of immunosuppression, such as antirejection drugs after transplants). These are called cytomegalovirus (CMV) infections, and they particularly attack the eye (CMV retinitis) and can lead to blindness. Another infection seen commonly in AIDS is a form of pneumonia caused by *Pneumocystis carinii*. Different methods can be used to treat these infections, some of which are expensive.

The drugs used in opportunistic infections (HIV-positive patients) are described below.

PNEUMOCYSTIS PNEUMONIA

Pneumonia caused by *Pneumocystis carinii* occurs in immunosuppressed or severely debilitated patients. It is the commonest cause of pneumonia in AIDS. Co-trimoxazole (see p. 303) in high dosage is the drug of choice for the treatment of this condition.

Atovaquone is licensed to treat mild to moderate pneumocystis infection for patients who are intolerant of, or who do not respond to, co-trimoxazole. The dose is 750 mg twice daily with food. Pentamidine isetionate is an alternative to co-trimoxazole and is particularly indicated for patients with a history of adverse reactions or who have not responded to co-trimoxazole. Pentamidine isetionate is a potentially toxic drug that can cause severe hypotension during or immediately after administration. Other severe reactions include hypoglycaemia, pancreatitis and arrhythmias. It can be given by intravenous infusion but can also be administered by inhalation, which reduces side-effects.

CYTOMEGALOVIRUS

Ganciclovir, valganciclovir, cidofovir and foscarnet are used to treat CMV infection. Large doses are required to control the infection. Three have to be given intravenously at least twice a day (cidofovir weekly or biweekly). After the spread of infection has been halted, lower maintenance doses are given. No drug cures the CMV infection; they only suppress it. Resistance is inevitable over time. However, CMV retinitis is a late feature of AIDS.

These drugs have severe toxicity and side effects. Those of ganciclovir are less than those of foscarnet, but ganciclovir does affect the bone marrow, as does AZT, and the combination is often too toxic. Monitoring of blood counts and serum creatinine is required. Hydration and co-treatment with probenecid is required for cidofovir.

VIRAL HEPATITIS

Viral hepatitis B and C present a serious and increasingly widespread health hazard. Sharing of contaminated injection equipment ('works') in drug abuse, unprotected sex and contaminated blood or blood products can result in transmission of hepatitis B and C virus.

Interferon alfa is used in the treatment of chronic hepatitis B, but the response rate is less than 50%. It should be discontinued where no improvement occurs after 3–4 months. A combination of ribavirin and peginterferon alfa is used for the treatment of chronic hepatitis C.

INFLUENZA

Vaccination is the most effective way of preventing illness from influenza. This is recommended for the 'at risk' patients, who include those aged over 65 or who those have one or more of the following conditions: chronic respiratory disease, significant cardiovascular disease (excluding hypertension), chronic renal disease, immunosuppression or diabetes mellitus.

Oseltamivir and zanamivir reduce replication of influenza A and B viruses by inhibiting viral neuraminidase. To be most effective in the treatment of influenza requires commencement of therapy within a few hours of symptom onset (licensed for use within 48 h of the first symptoms). In otherwise healthy adults, the duration of symptoms is reduced by about 1–1.5 days.

MALARIA

There are four malaria parasites that infect humans, by far the most hazardous being *Plasmodium falciparum*, which causes malignant malaria; this can rapidly progress from an acute fever to severe multiorgan disease, leading eventually to cerebral malaria with coma and death. Falciparum malaria usually presents within 3 months of acquiring the infection and, once successfully treated, it does not relapse.

Infection with *Plasmodium vivax*, (benign malaria), can present many months after exposure and may relapse for years after the initial infection. It is a less severe illness than that caused by *Plasmodium falciparum*. Benign malaria is caused less commonly by *Plasmodium ovale* and *Plasmodium malariae*.

Most of Africa south of the Sahara is highly malarious, the risk decreasing in southern Africa. Many popular tourist destinations in South East Asia are low-risk. However, Vietnam, Cambodia and the Thai–Cambodian border are high-risk areas where multidrug-resistant falciparum malaria is transmitted. Melanesia and parts of South America are also malarious.

PROTECTION

It is important to reduce the chance of an infective bite as much as possible, for example travellers should sleep in screened accommodation and use aerosols or vaporisers to eliminate mosquitoes. See Figure 15.6 for the malaria life cycle.

CHEMOPROPHYLAXIS

Drug regimens should be started at least 1 week before departure and continued without interruption after return for a recommended period. This ensures therapeutic blood concentrations before travelling and enables unwanted effects to be dealt with before departure. The continued use of drugs after returning home will provide protection should infection have been contracted near the end of the trip. The drugs used in prophylaxis include chloroquine, proguanil, malarone and pyrimethamine, either alone or in combinations, depending on the risk factor and the emergence of resistant strains. Mefloquine or doxycycline used alone for short-term travellers is also an option for certain areas of the world.

For those intending travelling to areas where malaria is endemic, the most up-to-date information should be sought on the current chemoprophylaxis.

THREADWORMS (PINWORMS)

The only commonly occurring helminth infection in the UK is enterobiasis. This is caused by the threadworm *Enterobius vermicularis*, also known as pinworm, which is estimated to have affected up to 40% of children by the time they are 10 years old. It is also contracted by adults, but the incidence is lower. Threadworms are initially acquired through swallowing eggs, which hatch and mature in the small intestine. After copulating, the males die, and the females migrate to the caecum and anus at night to lay their eggs in the perianal area, attaching them to the skin with a sticky, highly irritant fluid. Some eggs hatch there and return to the rectum to mature. The intense itching caused by the sticky secretion provokes scratching by the host, and eggs are transferred on to the fingers.

Infestation is passed on or perpetuated through picking up eggs on the fingers and being transmitted

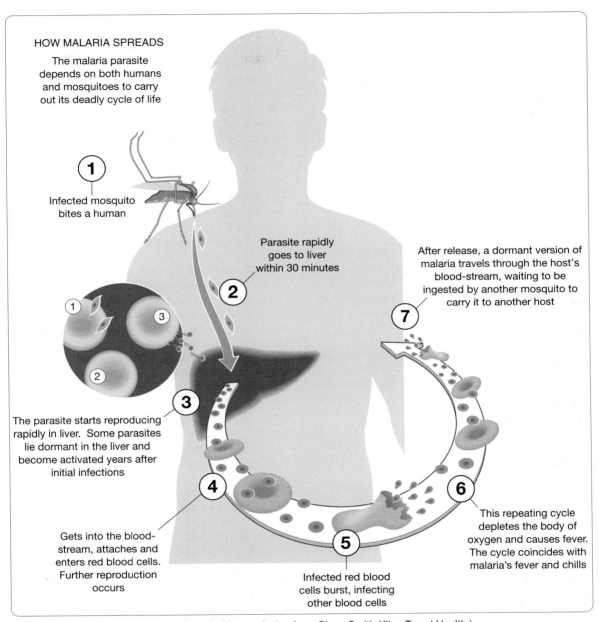

HOW MALARIA SPREADS

The malaria parasite depends on both humans and mosquitoes to carry out its deadly cycle of life

1 Infected mosquito bites a human

2 Parasite rapidly goes to liver within 30 minutes

3 The parasite starts reproducing rapidly in liver. Some parasites lie dormant in the liver and become activated years after initial infections

4 Gets into the blood-stream, attaches and enters red blood cells. Further reproduction occurs

5 Infected red blood cells burst, infecting other blood cells

6 This repeating cycle depletes the body of oxygen and causes fever. The cycle coincides with malaria's fever and chills

7 After release, a dormant version of malaria travels through the host's blood-stream, waiting to be ingested by another mosquito to carry it to another host

Fig. 15.6 Malaria life cycle. (Reproduced with permission from Glaxo Smith Kline Travel Health.)

on fingers to the mouth, often via food eaten with unwashed hands. Washing the hands and fingers with the aid of a nail brush before each meal and after each visit to the toilet is essential. Infection is transmitted either by direct contact between individuals or from contaminated surfaces or objects as, under suitable conditions, eggs can remain viable for several weeks outside the human host. Infection is recognised by sighting the whitish worms, about 10 mm in length,

on the stools after defaecation and sometimes around the anus, and also from the intense perianal itching that they cause.

Anthelmintics are effective in threadworm infections, and their use should be combined with hygienic measures to break the cycle of autoinfection. All members of the family require treatment.

Adult threadworms do not live longer than 6 weeks, and for development of fresh worms, ova must be swallowed and exposed to the action of digestive juices in the upper intestinal tract. A bath taken immediately after rising will remove ova laid during the night. Enterobiasis is treated with mebendazole or piperazine.

MEBENDAZOLE

Mebendazole irreversibly inhibits glucose uptake and causes immobilisation and death of the parasite within 3 days of administration. It also binds to tubulin, a protein required by the parasite for the uptake of nutrients. It is poorly absorbed from the human gastrointestinal tract, and the small proportion of a dose that is absorbed is almost entirely eliminated from the body following first-pass metabolism in the liver.

Adults and children over 2 years require a single dose of one 100-mg tablet. Treatment failures are rare, but reinfection is possible, in which case a second dose should be given after 2–3 weeks. Mebendazole is not recommended for children under 2 years.

PIPERAZINE

Piperazine acts by blocking the response of worm muscle to acetylcholine, and by interfering with the permeability of cell membranes to ions that regulate cell resting potential. Paralysis results and the paralysed worms are then expelled from the gut by peristalsis. Piperazine is readily absorbed from the gastrointestinal tract but is almost completely metabolised and excreted through the kidney within 24 h.

Piperazine phosphate is presented as a powder in sachets containing 4 g, together with standardised senna, which acts as a laxative to facilitate the expulsion of the paralysed worms. The dose should be stirred into a small glass of water or milk and drunk immediately. Because the life cycle of the threadworm is about 30 days, and some worms may be in the larval stage when the first dose is taken, a second dose should be taken after 14 days to eliminate the possibility of reinfection.

Piperazine citrate is available as a syrup containing the equivalent of 750 mg of piperazine hydrate per 5 mL.

HANDWASHING

The single most important measure in the prevention of cross-infection is handwashing. Depending on the procedure to be carried out, three levels of handwashing are employed in patient care:

- social
- hygienic hand disinfecting
- surgical.

In all cases, while working with patients, nurses should have short clean nails free of nail varnish and should not wear jewellery or a wristwatch.

The hands should be made *socially clean* by using soap and water, and drying with a paper towel *before* and *after* handling/serving food or working with patients.

Any procedure that requires to be carried out using an aseptic technique, such as the dressing of a wound or the insertion of a urinary catheter, involves hygienic hand disinfection.

Surgical handwashing, used prior to surgery, is not discussed.

Most handwash preparations are a formulation of chlorhexidine gluconate available in different strengths. They are considered suitable, as they combine detergency with antiseptic properties. They remove and kill transient organisms on the skin and also have some effect on bacteria in deeper layers of the skin. Organisms on the skin include Gram-positive ones such as *Staphylococcus aureus* and Gram-negative ones such as *Escherichia coli*, both of which are common causes of hospital infection. Regular use of an antiseptic handwash has a cumulative effect, and an extremely low level of resident organisms can be achieved. For each handwash (Fig. 15.7), the hands should be wetted first before the handwashing agent is applied, using an elbow dispenser. All surfaces are lathered, including the wrists. Particular attention should be paid to both the palms and the backs of the hands and to the thumbs and fingers, as well as between the fingers. Both hands should be cleaned thoroughly; right-handed people tend to clean the left hand more thoroughly and vice versa. Scrubbing the hands is not advocated, as this action creates disturbance to the resident flora and can cause trauma. The hands and wrists are rinsed under running water to remove lather and the taps turned off with the elbows or, if necessary, holding a paper towel. Careful drying of the hands with a paper towel is essential to protect the skin from possible breakdown, to make it harder for micro-organisms to thrive and to facilitate putting on gloves. The exact timing of handwashing prior to undertaking an aseptic procedure must be left to the discretion of the nurse. The wearing of gloves does not obviate the need for thorough handwashing.

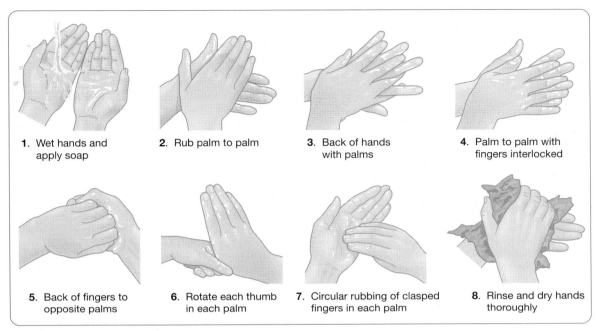

1. Wet hands and apply soap
2. Rub palm to palm
3. Back of hands with palms
4. Palm to palm with fingers interlocked
5. Back of fingers to opposite palms
6. Rotate each thumb in each palm
7. Circular rubbing of clasped fingers in each palm
8. Rinse and dry hands thoroughly

Fig. 15.7 Handwashing procedure.

SELF-ASSESSMENT QUESTIONS

A.

1. What would make you suspect that a patient has a urinary tract infection?
2. What immediate treatment may be prescribed?
3. How is the diagnosis confirmed?
4. What is a rigor and what causes it?
5. How would you nurse a patient through a rigor?

B. Quiz

1. Causes discoloration of the teeth
2. Active ingredient of most handwash preparations
3. Antibacterial that must never be given as a bolus
4. Caused by lax use of antibiotics
5. Tuberculin test
6. They can live and grow without oxygen
7. Route used for treating life-threatening infections
8. Growth in the bacteriology laboratory
9. They destroy foreign cells by engulfing them
10. Pathogen in the faeces that can cause urinary tract infection
11. Common helminth infection
12. Severest form of allergy to penicillin
13. Ketoconazole is one example
14. A complication of inhaling steroids
15. Penicillin G
16. *Tinea pedis*
17. Causes frequency of micturition and dysuria
18. Stain used to classify bacteria
19. Viral infection that can be caused by needlestick injury
20. Only controlled by adherence to infection control policy
21. Degree of response to an antibiotic as tested in the bacteriology laboratory
22. Kills bacteria
23. Organism which lives on or within another living organism and which benefits at the expense of the host

REFERENCES

Binyon D, Cooke RTD 2000 Restrictive antibiotic policies – how effective are they? Hospital Pharmacist 7:183–187

British HIV Association 2005 HIV treatment guidelines. BHIVA, London

Cosgrove SE, Carmeli Y 2003 The impact of bacterial resistance on health and economic outcomes. Clinical Infectious Diseases 36:1433–1437

Crowcroft NS, Catchpole M 2002 Mortality from methicillin resistant *Staphylococcus aureus* in England and Wales: analysis of death certificates. British Medical Journal 235:1390–1391

Plowman R 2000 The socio-economic burden of hospital acquired infection. European Surveillance 5:49–50

Tenover FC, Hughes JM 1995 WHO Scientific Working Group on monitoring and management of bacterial resistance to antimicrobial agents. Emerging Infectious Disease 1:37

FURTHER READING AND RESOURCES

Cheeseman M 2006 Antibiotic prescribing – a microbiology–pharmacy review. Hospital Pharmacist 13:177–178

Gompels M 2005 Current antiretroviral therapy for patients with HIV infection. Prescriber 16:14–25

Grosso A, Yogini J, Miniton J 2004 Tuberculosis chemotherapy in UK. Pharmaceutical Journal 273:385–388

Hand K 2006 How to best manage multidrug resistant bacterial infection in hospital wards. Pharmacy in Practice 16:12–18

Hand K 2006 Tuberculosis: pharmacological management. Hospital Pharmacist 13:81–85

Healy B, Barnes R 2006 Topical and oral treatments for fungal skin infections. Prescriber 17:30–43

Hill S 2006 Microbiology and antibiotic resistance of urinary tract infections. Trends in Urology Gynaecology and Sexual Health 11:26–31

Hunt K, Thomas S 2006 Recognition and treatment of pseudomembranous colitis. Prescriber 17:18–22

Minton J, Yogini J, Grosso A 2004 Treating drug-resistant tuberculosis. Pharmaceutical Journal 273:422–424

Nathan A 2006 Treatment of fungal nail infections Pharmaceutical Journal 276:597–600

Newsholme W 2006 Diagnosis and management of helminth infections. Prescriber 17:24–32

Rahman M, Anson J 2004 Peri-operative antibacterial prophylaxis. Pharmaceutical Journal 272:743–745

Storey A 2004 Tuberculosis: a general introduction. Pharmaceutical Journal 273:289–291

Weeks C, Jones G, Wyllie S 2006 Cost and health care benefits of an antimicrobial management programme. Hospital Pharmacist 13:179–182

Weston R, Portsmouth S, Benzie A 2006 An update on HAART: part 1. Pharmaceutical Journal 276:631–634

Weston R, Portsmouth S, Benzie A 2006 An update on HAART: part 2. Pharmaceutical Journal 276:693–696

Wickens H, Wade P 2004 The right drug for the right bug. Pharmaceutical Journal 274:365–368

Wickens H, Wade P 2005 Understanding antibiotic resistance. Pharmaceutical Journal 274:501–504

Williams S et al. 2005 A new approach to optimising hospital antimicrobial use. Hospital Pharmacist 12:321–324

Drug treatment of endocrine disorders

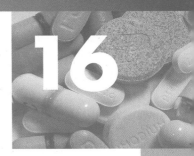

16

KEY OBJECTIVES

After reading this chapter, you should be able to:

- compare and contrast the clinical features associated with hyperthyroidism and hypothyroidism
- distinguish between the pharmacological actions of a mineralocorticoid and a glucocorticoid
- name the beneficial and adverse effects associated with glucocorticoids
- explain why patients on prolonged high-dose corticosteroids should carry a steroid card
- define diabetes mellitus (DM)
- state the normal fasting blood glucose range in mmol/L
- distinguish between type 1 and type 2 DM
- state five overall aims of treatment of DM

- give an example of a drug that may be used to treat (a) type 1 and (b) type 2 DM
- identify the clinical features of hypoglycaemia
- outline the action you would take if you suspected hypoglycaemia
- name three long-term effects of uncontrolled DM
- describe the action of calcitonin
- describe the action of bisphosphonates
- state how bisphosphonates should be taken and when they are contraindicated
- describe the immediate treatment of acute hypercalcaemia.

INTRODUCTION

Endocrine disorders due to under- or overproduction of hormones are a major cause of morbidity and mortality. Certain endocrine disorders are a particular feature of life in the twenty-first century. The increasing levels of obesity on a worldwide scale, especially in the prosperous economies of the world, are associated with very high levels of diabetes. People in the UK with diabetes have broken the 2 million mark. Although great progress has been made in the treatment of both types of diabetes (improved oral hypoglycaemic agents, parenteral and inhaled insulin, diagnostic procedures and management), major concerns remain. Diabetes may be underdiagnosed by as much as 25% (Health and Social Care Information Centre 2005). Underdiagnosis, together with poor management by patients, greatly increases the risk of serious complications developing (cardiac, renal, ophthalmic, neuropathy). There is a major need for public education on diet and related matters to ensure that the risks of being unhealthy are well known and understood. Specialist health professionals can do much both in the field of prevention and the improvement of outcomes for patients.

Excellent treatments are available for many conditions in which an endocrine deficiency has been diagnosed. Such treatments greatly improve the quality of life for many patients. Treatment with drugs that block the production of hormones are of great importance in the treatment of malignant disease. It is difficult to overestimate the value of corticosteroids in a wide range of conditions – from oral and parenteral use in life-threatening diseases to topical application for serious and debilitating skin conditions. Many older people have benefited from drugs used in the treatment of disorders of bone metabolism.

Nurses in all branches of the profession have an increasing role in the management of endocrine disorders, especially diabetes. All the indications are that this role will expand as the future burden of diabetes and even more frighteningly its complications increase (Diabetic Medicine 2002).

HORMONAL REGULATION

Although each ductless gland (Fig. 16.1) produces a hormone with specific functions, there is an integrated relationship between the activities of the glands. If these relationships are disturbed by a disease process, the consequences can be far reaching.

The hypothalamus and the pituitary gland together form the central control unit for the production and secretion of many hormones. The hypothalamus produces 'releasing' and 'inhibiting' hormones that influence the anterior lobe of the pituitary gland

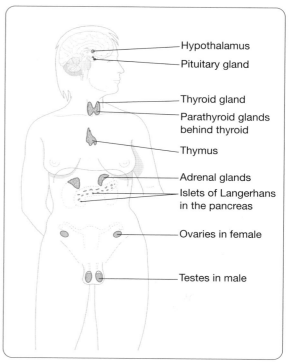

Fig. 16.1 The endocrine glands. (After Waugh A, Grant A 2001 Ross and Wilson anatomy and physiology in health and illness, 9th edn. Churchill Livingstone, Edinburgh. With permission of Elsevier.)

to release corresponding hormones, the trophic hormones, some of which affect target cells in the body directly while others do so through the intermediary of a second endocrine organ such as the thyroid, the adrenal cortex and the gonads. The second endocrine organ, in turn, produces a third specific hormone such as levothyroxine sodium (thyroxine sodium), corticosteroids or sex hormones, which influences various other body functions.

Chemoreceptors in the hypothalamus register the blood hormone level and react accordingly by either increasing or decreasing hormone production. If the blood hormone level is low, more hormone is secreted; if the blood hormone level is high, hormone production is reduced (negative feedback; see Fig. 16.2). Not all hormonal activities, however, follow this mechanism.

HYPOTHALAMUS AND PITUITARY GLAND

The hypothalamus forms the base of the brain (diencephalon). It is responsible for the coordination

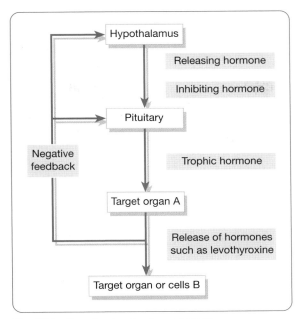

Fig. 16.2 Negative feedback mechanism.

of nervous and endocrine systems and therefore many basic life functions such as cardiovascular, respiratory and alimentary functions, sexual behaviour and reproduction. It is connected to the pituitary gland, a small endocrine gland of great importance, by the hypophyseal stalk or infundibulum. The pituitary gland lies almost completely surrounded by bone in the base of the skull. It consists of three parts: the anterior lobe (adenohypophysis), the median eminence and the posterior lobe (neurohypophysis).

The anterior pituitary (see Fig. 16.3) synthesises and releases seven known trophic hormones. These are somatotrophin, which is involved in prepubertal body growth; prolactin, which stimulates the growth and secretory activity of the female breasts during pregnancy; melanocyte-stimulating hormone, which causes an increase in cutaneous pigmentation; adrenocorticotrophic hormone (ACTH), which governs the secretions of some of the hormones by the adrenal cortex; thyrotrophin (thyroid-stimulating hormone, TSH), which stimulates thyroid activity; follicle-stimulating hormone or human menopausal gonadotrophin, which stimulates growth of ovarian follicles and secretion of oestrogen in the female and spermatogenesis in the male; and luteinising hormone, which stimulates the production of progesterone in the corpus luteum of the follicle (female) and activates androgen secretion by the Leydig cells of the testis (male).

The posterior pituitary (see Fig. 16.4) hormones vasopressin (antidiuretic hormone, ADH) and oxytocin are produced in the hypothalamus and secreted (neurosecretion) directly into the bloodstream of the infundibulum and posterior lobe of the pituitary gland, from where they can be released into the body.

Vasopressin controls the reabsorption of water by the kidney tubules. In large doses, it causes vasoconstriction of the smooth muscles with a concomitant rise in blood pressure. It also causes muscle contraction in the gastrointestinal tract and uterus.

Oxytocin causes the contraction of the uterine muscle towards the end of pregnancy and at parturition, and contraction of the mammary smooth muscle, which stimulates the release of milk into the ducts. The secretion of oxytocin from the pituitary gland is stimulated by the baby sucking at the mother's breast.

COMMON DISORDERS OF THE PITUITARY GLAND

HYPOPITUITARISM

Reduced secretion of pituitary hormones caused by tumour, trauma, etc. often results in a progressive loss of function of organs stimulated by trophic hormones, starting with growth hormone deficiency in children, then gonadotrophin deficiency, which causes amenorrhoea and anovulatory infertility in women and impotence and reduced spermatogenesis in men. At a later stage, levels of ACTH and eventually TSH decrease, resulting in hypothyroidism and Addison's disease.

HYPERSECRETION OF PITUITARY HORMONES

The excessive secretion of growth hormone (somatotrophin) leads to gigantism (excessive growth of the whole body) in prepubertal children and acromegaly in adults (increased size of tongue, lips and organs such as the heart and liver); both conditions are usually caused by a pituitary adenoma, and patients tend to have other problems associated with abnormal function of the pituitary gland, such as Cushing's syndrome caused by hypersecretion of ACTH.

Hyperprolactinaemia may be due to a variety of causes, such as prolactinoma (prolactin-secreting tumour), trauma and drugs. Hyperprolactinaemia causes infertility in women and impotence in men. Treatment usually consists of a combination of surgery,

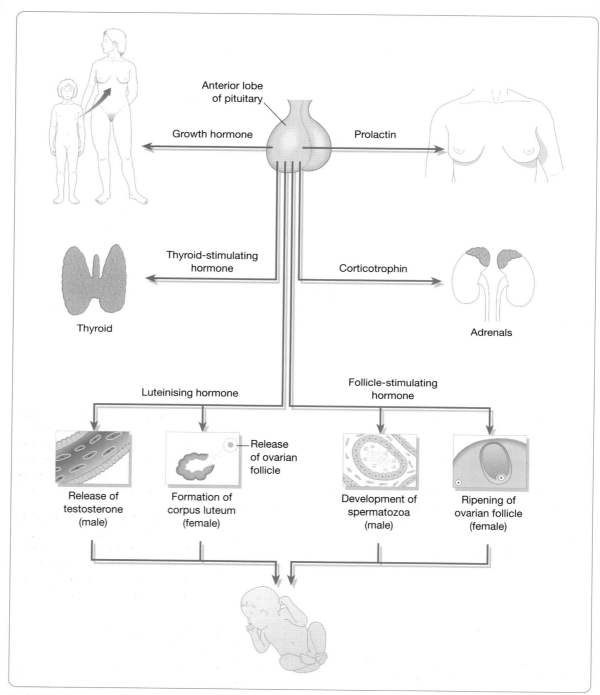

Fig. 16.3 Hormones released by anterior pituitary.

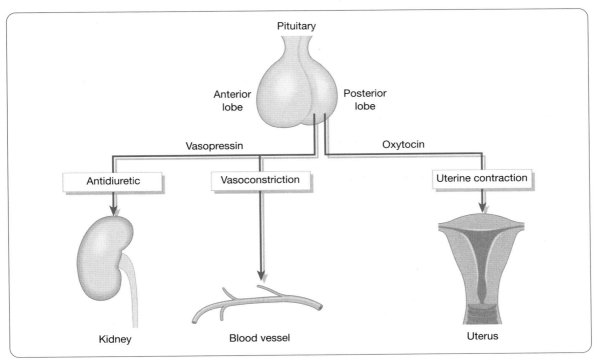

Fig. 16.4   Hormones released by posterior pituitary.

radiotherapy and drug treatment depending on the size of the tumour.

Diabetes insipidus occurs either when there is failure of secretion of ADH from the neurohypophysis (cranial diabetes insipidus) or when ADH secretion is adequate but the kidney fails to respond (nephrogenic diabetes insipidus). This causes a reduced reabsorption of water in the kidney tubules and an increased output of very dilute urine (up to 40 L/day). The loss of water has to be replaced by increased drinking (polydipsia).

MAIN DRUG GROUPS

HYPOTHALAMIC HORMONES AND ANTERIOR PITUITARY HORMONES

HYPOTHALAMIC HORMONES
Gonadorelin
Gonadorelin is the gonadotrophin-releasing hormone secreted by the hypothalamus.

Administration and dose. For the assessment of pituitary function in adults, 100 micrograms is given by intravenous or subcutaneous injection. Gonadorelin analogues are used in the treatment of endometriosis, infertility and anaemia due to uterine fibroids. Breast cancer and prostate cancer may be treated with gonadorelin analogues.

Protirelin (thyrotrophin-releasing hormone) stimulates the release of thyrotrophin from the pituitary. It is sometimes used to assess thyroid function in doses of 200 micrograms intravenously. Sermorelin is an analogue of the growth hormone-releasing hormone and is used as a diagnostic test for secretion of growth hormone.

ANTERIOR PITUITARY HORMONES
Corticotrophins
Tetracosactide is a synthetic anterior pituitary hormone and has the same physiological properties as ACTH (corticotropin) but a shorter duration of action. It stimulates the biosynthesis of glucocorticosteroids, mineralocorticosteroids and androgens in the adrenal cortex.

Use. Tetracosactide and its slow-release form are used for diagnostic purposes to investigate adrenocortical insufficiency. Tetracosactide (250 micrograms) is given as an intramuscular or intravenous injection for a 30-min test. The depot preparation is used for a 5-h test (1 mg by intramuscular injection) in cases in which the 30-min test has been inconclusive or the functional reserve of the adrenal cortex is being tested. Owing to the variable and unpredictable therapeutic response, tetracosactide is no longer used as a therapeutic agent. Corticosteroids are preferred in the treatment of such inflammatory conditions as Crohn's disease (see Ch. 11).

Contraindications and adverse effects. As a polypeptide, tetracosactide may cause allergic reactions and in severe cases anaphylactic shock.

SOMATROPIN (SYNTHETIC HUMAN GROWTH HORMONE)

Somatropin, a biosynthetic human growth hormone, has replaced growth hormone of human origin, which has been implicated as a cause of Creutzfeldt–Jakob disease. The infectious agent involved in Creutzfeldt–Jakob disease is a protein known as a prion.

Use. Growth hormone is used in the treatment of short stature in children with hypopituitarism whose epiphyses have not yet fused, and in short stature associated with Turner's syndrome. It is also used for the treatment of adults with growth hormone deficiency if the criteria established by the National Institute for Health and Clinical Excellence are met (British National Formulary no. 53).

Administration and dose. Like other peptides, somatropin must be given parenterally by subcutaneous or intramuscular injection. It is available as powder for reconstitution for subcutaneous or intramuscular injection.

The dose is determined on an individual basis depending on the condition being treated.

Contraindications and adverse effects. These are as follow:

- use of somatropin is contraindicated in children with fused epiphyses
- lipoatrophy at the injection site may occur; it can be prevented by varying the injection site
- somatropin may influence glucose tolerance, and patients with diabetes mellitus (DM) might have to change the dosage of their hypoglycaemic drugs.

A growth hormone receptor antagonist, pegvisomant (which is a genetically modified analogue of human growth hormone) is a highly selective growth hormone antagonist used for selected patients with acromegaly.

POSTERIOR PITUITARY HORMONES

VASOPRESSIN (ANTIDIURETIC HORMONE)

The use of vasopressin, a peptide with antidiuretic and vasoconstrictor properties, has declined since the development of more selective semisynthetic analogues desmopressin and terlipressin. Desmopressin has no vasoconstrictor effect, but it has an increased antidiuretic activity and a longer duration of action than vasopressin (synthetic porcine vasopressin); terlipressin is used for its vasoconstrictor effects.

Use. The uses are as follows:
- treatment of pituitary diabetes insipidus (desmopressin and vasopressin); for long-term treatment, desmopressin is preferred
- diagnosis of diabetes insipidus (desmopressin)
- primary nocturnal enuresis in adults and children (desmopressin)
- treatment of bleeding oesophageal varices (vasopressin, terlipressin).

Administration and dose. *Pituitary diabetes insipidus*. In acute cases, such as after a head injury, vasopressin or desmopressin are used as intramuscular or subcutaneous injection; because of its much longer duration of action, desmopressin has to be given only once a day (1–4 micrograms). For long-term maintenance treatment, desmopressin is available as nasal spray (10 micrograms/metered spray) or nasal solution (100 micrograms/mL). Oral treatment of diabetes insipidus (in adults and children) with desmopressin tablets (200 micrograms) requires careful monitoring and dosage adjustment.

Oesophageal varices

For the initial treatment of bleeding oesophageal varices in portal hypertension, vasopressin is given as an intravenous infusion (20 units diluted in 100 mL of glucose 5% w/v). Terlipressin is given as a single intravenous dose of 2 mg, which can be repeated every 4–6 h for up to 72h.

Contraindications and adverse effects. These are outlined as follows.

- Despite its reduced vasopressor effects, desmopressin, like all vasopressins, has to be used with extreme caution in patients with cardiovascular problems.
- Water retention and water intoxication may occur following large doses.

- In low doses, nausea, abdominal cramps and a rise in blood pressure may occur.
- Nasal preparations may cause nasal congestion and local ulceration.
- Patients on nasal preparations have to be counselled on the proper use of the device. Improper use will result in unsatisfactory response.

OXYTOCIN

See Chapter 17.

DOPAMINE RECEPTOR STIMULANTS (DOPAMINERGIC DRUGS)

Bromocriptine is chemically related to ergotamine and is a stimulant for dopamine receptors in the brain. It also inhibits the release of prolactin and growth hormone from the pituitary.

Use. The uses are outlined as follows:
- treatment of prolactin-secreting tumours of the pituitary gland (prolactinoma) and acromegaly alone or in conjunction with surgery and radiotherapy
- galactorrhoea, hyperprolactinaemic infertility
- suppression of painful lactation after childbirth (only if simple analgesia will not suffice)
- in the treatment of idiopathic Parkinson's disease
- cyclical breast pain and cyclical menstrual disorders.

Administration and dose. Bromocriptine is available as 1-mg and 2.5-mg tablets and 5-mg and 10-mg capsules. There is a great difference in the dosage range depending on the condition to be treated and the individual response to treatment. In most indications, apart from suppression and prevention of lactation, the optimum dosage is achieved by gradual introduction of bromocriptine. In this way, optimum response and minimum side effects can be properly balanced.

Contraindications and adverse effects. Bromocriptine is contraindicated in hypertension after childbirth, toxaemia of pregnancy and known hypersensitivity reactions to bromocriptine or ergot alkaloids. Adverse effects are numerous and dose-related and can usually be reduced by dose adjustment:

- gastrointestinal disturbance
- hypotensive reactions at the beginning of the treatment
- ovulation in hyperprolactinaemic women; this effect may be desired – as in the treatment of hyperprolactinaemic women; if the effect is undesired, patients should be advised on the use of contraception
- dry mouth, leg cramps, cardiac arrhythmias
- peptic ulceration in acromegaly patients.

Cabergoline has similar actions and uses to bromocriptine but may be better tolerated in some patients than bromocriptine. Quinagolide is a similar drug given in smaller doses than both bromocriptine and cabergoline.

These drugs may cause fibrotic reactions (pulmonary, retroperitoneal and pericardial). Dopaminergic drugs may also cause daytime sleepiness (sudden onset of sleep). Warnings regarding driving and operating machinery may need to be given.

THYROID GLAND

The thyroid gland is situated anteriorly in the lower part of the neck. It consists of two side lobes connected by a narrow region, the isthmus. The gland is made up of two types of secretory cell: the thyroid follicles secreting the hormones thyroxine (levothyroxine) and tri-iodothyronine (liothyronine), and the parafollicular cells, which secrete thyrocalcitonin (calcium-lowering hormone). Levothyroxine and liothyronine are derivatives of the amino acid tyrosine. They are formed in the thyroid follicles by incorporating circulating iodine, stored and transported in the plasma almost entirely bound to levothyroxine-binding globulin. After secretion, the minute unbound (free) hormone fraction diffuses into tissues and exerts its hormonal activity after conversion of levothyroxine into the more potent and more rapidly metabolised liothyronine.

Production of hormones is stimulated by TSH, which is released from the anterior pituitary gland in response to hypothalamic thyrotrophin-releasing hormone. The production is regulated by negative feedback through circulating concentrations of free liothyronine (Fig. 16.5).

Levothyroxine and liothyronine increase the oxygen consumption of almost all metabolically active tissues; this means an increase in the metabolic rate. They also affect growth and maturation, especially brain and skeletal development.

COMMON DISORDERS OF THE THYROID GLAND

HYPOTHYROIDISM (THYROID DEFICIENCY)

Hypothyroidism results from a reduced secretion by the thyroid gland, irrespective of the cause. The most common causes of primary hypothyroidism

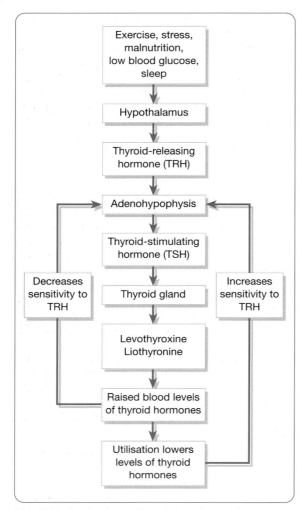

Fig. 16.5 Production and regulation of thyroid hormones.

anaemia, infertility, constipation and dermatological symptoms.

In children with hypothyroidism, the dominant features are reduction in growth and arrest of pubertal development.

Hypothyroid coma is the severest form of thyroid deficiency and a medical emergency. The patient has a reduced level of consciousness and a body temperature that may be as low as 25°C.

HYPERTHYROIDISM

Hyperthyroidism (thyrotoxicosis) results from exposure of the body tissues to excess circulating levels of free levothyroxine and/or free liothyronine. It is a fairly common disorder that affects women more than men.

It is very important to establish the cause of hyperthyroidism to be able to provide adequate treatment. The most common conditions are:

- Graves' disease
- toxic multinodular goitre
- toxic solitary nodule (autonomous thyroid hormone-secreting adenoma).

Hyperthyroidism causes an increase in the basal metabolic rate and affects almost every system in the body. It presents with a wide variety of symptoms and severity. Symptoms include:

- an increase in body temperature
- tachycardia
- restlessness
- vomiting and diarrhoea
- loss of libido and infertility
- pruritus
- ocular symptoms such as exophthalmos in Graves' disease
- goitre.

Thyrotoxic crisis ('thyroid storm') is a life-threatening increase in the severity of the clinical features of thyrotoxicosis and requires immediate treatment. It is very unusual but may occur after subtotal thyroidectomy, may occur within a few days after administration of radioactive sodium iodide-131, or may be precipitated by infection in a patient with hyperthyroidism that is inadequately controlled by antithyroid drugs.

Treatment includes intravenous fluids, hydrocortisone intravenously, propranolol (or nadolol) to control cardiac symptoms, oral iodine solution and an antithyroid drug such as carbimazole or propylthiouracil by nasogastric tube required.

are thyroid failure following radioactive sodium iodine-131 therapy and surgical treatment, thyroid failure associated with Hashimoto's thyroiditis or an autoimmune disease, and congenital thyroid failure (congenital hypothyroidism or cretinism). Hypothyroidism due to pituitary failure (secondary hypothyroidism) is much less common.

Hypothyroidism causes a reduction in the basal metabolic rate and affects most systems in the body, causing slow speech, lethargy, sensitivity to cold and mental impairment of hypothyroidism (myxoedema). Symptoms vary in range and severity. They may include goitre, bradycardia, depression, iron deficiency

NON-TOXIC GOITRE

Non-toxic diffuse goitre may be caused by iodine deficiency, drugs such as lithium carbonate, Hashimoto's thyroiditis or Graves' disease. It is usually straightforward to make the right diagnosis and provide adequate treatment. The simple goitre is of unknown aetiology and usually requires no treatment.

DRUGS AND THYROID FUNCTION

Drugs can influence thyroid function in different ways. Some drugs (e.g. androgens, oestrogens, salicylates) alter thyroid function tests. Some drugs may induce thyroid disease. Those that induce hypothyroidism include antithyroid drugs, lithium, sulphonylureas, amiodarone; those that cause hyperthyroidism include iodides and levothyroxine.

Thyroid disease can alter the distribution, metabolism and elimination of some drugs, such as digoxin. Thyroid disease may also alter the pharmacodynamic effects of some drugs, such as cardiac glycosides and warfarin.

MAIN DRUG GROUPS

THYROID HORMONES

Levothyroxine (thyroxine) and liothyronine are the naturally occurring thyroid hormones. Liothyronine, with a half-life of 1–2 days, has a much faster onset of action than levothyroxine, with a half-life of 7 days. Levothyroxine reaches its maximum effect after about 10 days. The difference in the onset of action is important for the therapeutic use of thyroid hormones.

Use. Because of its rapid and more potent effect, liothyronine is used in the treatment of acute hypothyroid states. In the treatment of hypothyroid coma, liothyronine as injection is the treatment of choice, usually in conjunction with other measures such as intravenous corticosteroids, intravenous fluids and slow rewarming using blankets and foil, with broad-spectrum antibiotic cover and oxygen.

Levothyroxine is normally the drug of choice for routine replacement therapy in hypothyroidism of any cause. In congenital hypothyroidism, treatment has to begin as soon as possible after birth to prevent irreversible brain damage and to promote normal development.

Thyroid hormones are also used to suppress the release of TSH from the pituitary gland in the treatment of non-toxic diffuse goitre, Hashimoto's thyroiditis and thyroid carcinoma, and in combination with antithyroid drugs to prevent the development of a goitre in hyperthyroid patients.

Administration and dose. A dose of 20 micrograms of levothyroxine sodium orally is equivalent to 100 micrograms of liothyronine. Dosage for replacement therapy is individual and is usually started slowly with a dose of 50 micrograms of levothyroxine sodium and then increased to a dose of 100–200 micrograms daily. In the elderly, and patients with ischaemic heart disease, the initial dose should be 25 micrograms/day.

When first treating severe hypothyroidism, liothyronine sodium is used as an initial dose of 5 micrograms, increased to 60 micrograms at weekly intervals. When a dose of 60 micrograms is reached, treatment should switch to low-dose levothyroxine sodium increased by 50 micrograms at 4-week intervals up to 200 micrograms if required.

The dose can be monitored by the clinical response of the patient, but serum liothyronine and TSH levels should be measured at intervals. The correct dose of liothyronine is that which restores serum TSH concentration to normal.

For the treatment of hypothyroid coma, 5–20 micrograms of levothyroxine sodium are given by slow intravenous injection, repeated at 12-h intervals or more frequently if necessary.

Contraindications and adverse effects. These are as follows.

- Thyroid hormones should be used with caution in older patients with cardiovascular problems, prolonged myxoedema or adrenal failure.
- Adverse effects are dose-related and usually disappear on reduction of dosage or withdrawal of treatment. Especially in the early stages of treatment, patients may suffer from anginal pain, cardiac arrhythmias or myocardial infarction. Patients with a pre-existing heart condition are especially at risk.
- Other side-effects include gastrointestinal disturbance, tremors, restlessness, excessive loss of weight and muscular weakness.

Interactions. Levothyroxine sodium (thyroxine sodium) increases the effects of anticoagulants, phenytoin, digoxin and adrenoceptor agonists such as salbutamol, accelerates the response to tricyclic antidepressants and also raises blood sugar levels. The dosage of antidiabetic agents may have to be adjusted.

Patients on replacement therapy should be advised that treatment has to continue for life and that follow-up is important, and that tablets should be taken regularly to ensure an adequate level of serum liothyronine and TSH. The outcome of treatment is usually very beneficial for patients, as the distressing symptoms are greatly eased.

ANTITHYROID DRUGS

CARBIMAZOLE AND PROPYLTHIOURACIL

Carbimazole and propylthiouracil prevent the conversion of iodide to iodine, the incorporation of iodine into the prehormonal stages and therefore the production of thyroid hormones.

Use. Carbimazole and propylthiouracil are used:
- in the long-term management of hyperthyroidism
- in the preparation for thyroidectomy in hyperthyroidism
- in the preparation for, and as concomitant therapy with, radioiodine treatment
- in combination with levothyroxine as a blocking replacement therapy to prevent the development of goitre and hypothyroidism.

Administration and dose. Carbimazole and propylthiouracil are both available as tablets only. The initial dose of carbimazole is 15–40 mg (propylthiouracil 200–400 mg) daily in two or three divided doses. Carbimazole is not effective until 10–14 days after the beginning of treatment, because the thyroid is still releasing its existing hormone reserves for a period of time. After about 3–4 weeks, the patient is usually clinically and biochemically euthyroid. The dose may then be reduced progressively to a maintenance dose of between 5 and 15 mg (propylthiouracil 50–150 mg) daily as a single dose. The dose should be determined by clinical status and ideally by the measurement of plasma thyroid hormone levels. Treatment should continue for 12–18 months. If a relapse occurs after discontinuation of treatment, further measures may have to be considered (see *Management of hyperthyroidism*).

Adverse reactions, side-effects and cautions. The most serious adverse effect of carbimazole and propylthiouracil is bone marrow depression, which can lead to agranulocytosis. This is almost always reversible following withdrawal of the drug. Because there is usually no cross-sensitivity between the antithyroid drugs, carbimazole may be successfully substituted by propylthiouracil and vice versa.

Common side-effects are skin rashes and pruritus, which are usually self-limiting and do not require withdrawal of the drug.

Both drugs may be used in pregnancy as long as the dose is in the standard range and the woman is monitored regularly. The blocking replacement regimen must not be used during pregnancy or lactation.

Both drugs are secreted in breast milk, but this should not preclude breast-feeding as long as neonatal monitoring is carried out and the lowest dose is used.

Patients should be advised to report sore throats, mouth ulcers, fever or rashes immediately, because these might be early signs of bone marrow depression, and to keep follow-up appointments, especially in the initial stages.

IODINE AND IODIDE (IN THE FORM OF POTASSIUM IODIDE)

Iodine and iodide act by inhibiting the release of levothyroxine and liothyronine from the thyroid into the plasma; iodine is not suitable as a long-term treatment, because the antithyroid action diminishes quite rapidly over time.

Use. Iodine and iodide are used to prepare a patient for thyroidectomy by reducing vascularity and friability of the thyroid and by reducing the risk of haemorrhage. The evidence for these benefits is sparse.

Administration and dose. Iodine and iodide are combined in Lugol's solution (aqueous iodine oral solution), which contains 5% iodine and 10% potassium iodide (total iodine 130 mg/mL).

Lugol's solution has to be given orally for 10–14 days in a dose of 0.1–0.3 mL well diluted three times daily prior to surgery.

Radioactive sodium iodide is increasingly used for the treatment of thyrotoxicosis at all ages, especially in older patients with cardiac disease when other treatments cannot be used. When radioiodine is given orally, it is taken up selectively by the thyroid gland. The short β radiation emitted affects only the thyroid follicle cells. Radioactive iodine is also used in diagnostic tests for thyroid disease.

Contraindications, adverse reactions and side-effects. Iodine is contraindicated in breast-feeding mothers, because it may cause goitre in the infant. Iodine can cause hypersensitivity reactions, conjunctivitis, pain in the salivary glands, bronchitis, gastroenteritis, insomnia and depression.

MANAGEMENT OF HYPERTHYROIDISM

Short-term treatment. Beta-adrenoceptor-blocking agents, propranolol or nadolol, are used to relieve acute symptoms such as tachycardia, tremor and anxiety in the latent period before antithyroid drugs become effective.

Long-term treatment. This involves three options:

- antithyroid drugs for 12–18 months
- radioactive sodium iodide (iodine-131) for those cases in which drug therapy fails

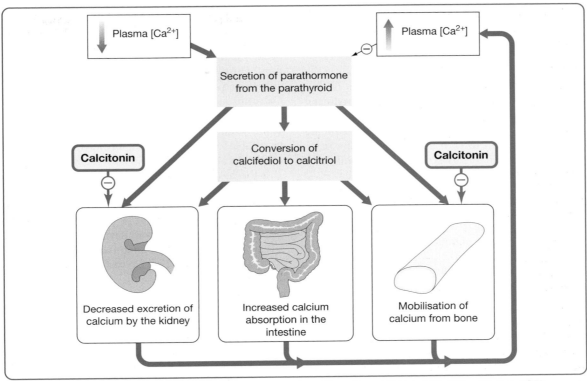

Fig. 16.6 Normal physiological response to fall in serum calcium. (From Rang HP, Dale MM, Ritter JM et al. 2003 Pharmacology. Churchill Livingstone, Edinburgh.)

- surgery in recurrent hyperthyroidism, a large goitre or a single adenoma.

PARATHYROID GLANDS

The parathyroids consist of four small endocrine glands that are situated behind the thyroid gland. They produce parathormone, which is essential for life. Parathormone regulates the metabolism of calcium and phosphorus in the body by action on the kidney, gut and bone (in a dual control mechanism with thyrocalcitonin). It also stimulates the formation of colecalciferol (vitamin D_3), which plays an important part in the mineralisation of bone. The release of parathormone from the parathyroid glands depends directly on the blood calcium level (Fig. 16.6).

COMMON DISORDERS OF THE PARATHYROID GLANDS

HYPOPARATHYROIDISM

Hypoparathyroidism is a deficiency in parathormone, which may be caused by surgical damage to the parathyroids after total or partial thyroidectomy. It results in a decrease of the blood calcium level (hypocalcaemia) and an increase in blood phosphorus (hyperphosphataemia). Hypocalcaemia causes tetany, which is characterised by increased tone of skeletal muscles with spasms of the hands, feet and larynx, and generalised convulsions.

HYPERPARATHYROIDISM

Hyperparathyroidism (primary) is an increased release of parathormone, usually due to a parathyroid adenoma. The presenting features are due mainly to the raised blood calcium level (hypercalcaemia).

Hypercalcaemia. The most common causes of hypercalcaemia are malignant disease and primary hyperparathyroidism, vitamin D intoxication, and immobilisation (paraplegia in the young and Paget's disease in the elderly). The main features include fatigue, weakness, polydipsia and polyuria, renal stones, nephrocalcinosis, bone changes (osteitis fibrosa), duodenal ulceration and chronic pancreatitis. Some drugs, such as the thiazides and lithium, can also cause hypercalcaemia. Severe hypercalcaemia is an emergency and requires urgent treatment.

MAIN DRUG GROUPS USED IN CONDITIONS AFFECTING BONE METABOLISM

CALCITONIN

Calcitonin lowers the blood calcium level by reducing the renal tubular reabsorption of calcium and increasing its deposition in the bone. By reducing the blood calcium level, it also relieves bone pain. Calcitonin is available as synthetic or recombinant salmon calcitonin (salcatonin).

Use. Calcitonin (salmon) is used for the treatment of:

- hypercalcaemia due to a raised bone turnover, such as in Paget's disease of bone and malignancies with bone metastases
- primary hyperparathyroidism
- vitamin D intoxication
- postmenopausal osteoporosis.

Administration and dose. Calcitonin (salmon) is currently available as an injection (subcutaneous or intramuscular). The dose depends on the condition treated and its severity. Dose adjustments should be made according to the patient's clinical and biochemical response. Dose regimens may range from 50 units of calcitonin (salmon) three times a week to 100 units daily in Paget's disease of bone, and may be as high as 400 units every 6–8 h in severe hypercalcaemia. A nasal spray (200 units/metered spray) is also available.

Adverse effects and cautions. Adverse effects of calcitonin (salmon) include nausea, vomiting, diarrhoea, flushing, paraesthesia and an unpleasant taste in the mouth. There does not seem to be other serious toxicity. However, calcitonin (salmon) should be used with caution in pregnancy and breast-feeding. Patients with a history of allergies should undergo a skin test before treatment is undertaken.

Teriparatide is a recombinant fragment of parathyroid hormone used for the treatment of postmenopausal osteoporosis. Cinacalcet (which reduces parathyroid hormone) is used to treat hypercalcaemia in malignant disease of the parathyroid glands, and secondary hyperparathyroidism in patients with end-stage renal failure on dialysis.

BISPHOSPHONATES

Bisphosphonates reduce bone turnover by inhibiting the growth and dissolution of hydroxyapatite crystals and retarding bone resorption and formation.

Osteoporosis occurs in postmenopausal women (see Ch. 17). Risk factors include low body weight, tobacco and alcohol abuse (alcohol is toxic to bone metabolism), low levels of physical activity and a family history. Treatment with long-term oral glucocorticoids (e.g. prednisolone) is a major risk factor. Calcium and vitamin D deficiency must be treated and any underlying hormonal problems (e.g. of the parathyroid gland) dealt with. Osteoporotic bones are very liable to osteoporotic fragility fractures, especially of the hip and vertebrae.

If the bisphosphonates cannot be tolerated or do not produce an adequate response, raloxifene may be used in postmenopausal women under 65 in whom the risk of vertebral fracture is high. The dose is 60 mg daily, but it is contraindicated in patients with a history of venous thromboembolism or hepatic or renal impairment (see specialist literature). In severe osteoporosis, combination therapy is also of value in the treatment of osteoporosis (Table 16.1). Oestrogens decrease the resorption of bone and can reduce the incidence of hip fracture. Idiopathic osteoporosis can affect young or middle-aged men. Testosterone deficiency may be linked with spinal osteoporosis and elderly men may suffer hip fractures. Male osteoporosis is treated with etidronate or alendronate.

The main indications and dosage regimens of bisphosphonates are outlined in Table 16.1.

Contraindications, adverse effects and cautions. Bisphosphonates are contraindicated in patients with known hypersensitivities to etidronate, pamidronate or clodronate. Because bisphosphonates are excreted by the kidney, they should be used with caution in patients with renal impairment. In higher doses, disodium etidronate causes demineralisation of bone, which can lead to spontaneous fractures. Patients may also experience increased bone pain during the first month of treatment. The adverse effects of bisphosphonates are nausea, diarrhoea and a metallic taste. The bisphosphonates may cause oesophageal reactions, and it is vitally important to ensure that the patient takes the tablet in the correct manner. Osteonecrosis of the jaw is a risk in patients receiving IV bisphosphonates and rarely in those taking them orally. Oral hygiene is essential.

TREATMENT OF SEVERE HYPERCALCAEMIA

The initial treatment consists of intravenous fluid replacement with sodium chloride 0.9% solution,

Table 16.1 Bisphosphonates

Drug	Preparation(s)	Main indications/dose	Notes
Alendronic acid	5-mg and 10-mg tablets.	Postmenopausal osteoporosis: 10 mg daily for treatment, 5 mg daily for prevention. Corticosteroid-induced osteoporosis: 5–10 mg daily.	Biochemical monitoring essential with all these drugs. Higher dose for women not receiving hormone replacement therapy. This drug is associated with oesophageal problems. Patients must be advised to take the tablets sitting upright with plenty of water for at least 30 min.
Disodium etidronate	200-mg and 400-mg tablets.	Paget's disease of bone: 5 mg/kg as a single daily dose for up to 6 months (higher doses may be given for shorter periods up to a maximum of 20 mg/kg daily). Also given with calcium carbonate in the treatment of osteoporosis.	Patients should be advised to avoid iron and mineral supplements, and antacids. Food should be avoided 2 h before and after treatment.
Disodium pamidronate	15-, 30- and 90-mg injection.	Hypercalcaemia of malignancy in dosage determined by serum calcium concentration, by slow IV injection into a large vein. Osteolytic lesions/bone pain: 90 mg every 4 weeks. Paget's disease of bone: various dosage regimens.	May be given to coincide with courses of chemotherapy in breast cancer.
Ibandronic acid	50-mg tablet and concentrate for IV infusion.	Reduction of bone damage in bone metastases in breast cancer: 50 mg daily by mouth *or* by IV infusion 6 mg every 3–4 weeks in the treatment of hypercalcaemia of malignancy.	Symptoms of oesophageal irritation should be reported, and patients should be advised to seek medical attention if dysphagia, pain on swallowing or retrosternal pain occur.
Risedronate sodium	5 mg and 30 mg. tablets	Paget's disease of bone: 30 mg daily for 2 months. Osteoporosis: 5 mg daily.	This drug should be avoided in patients with oesophageal abnormalities.
Sodium clodronate	400-mg capsules, 520-mg and 800-mg tablets, IV solution (for dilution) 30 mg/mL.	For osteolytic lesions and bone pain in malignant disease: 1.6 g daily in single or two divided doses up to a maximum of 3.2 g daily (orally). Slow IV administration in hypercalcaemia of malignancy: 300 mg daily for up to 10 days or a single infusion of 1.5 g.	Essential to maintain adequate fluid intake during treatment.
Strontium ranelate	Granules 2 g per sachet.	Postmenopausal osteoporosis to reduce risk of vertebral and hip fractures: 2 g daily in water at bedtime.	Patients to be advised to avoid food for 2 h before and after taking the drug. Antacids containing calcium and magnesium should also be avoided for 2 h after taking the drug.

Continued

Table 16.1 Bisphosphonates 'cont ...'

Drug	Preparation(s)	Main indications/dose	Notes
Tiludronic acid	200-mg tablets single dose for 12 weeks.	Paget's disease of bone: 400 mg daily as a single daily dose.	The drug is contraindicated in patients with moderate to severe renal impairment, and in pregnancy and breast-feeding.
Zoledronic acid	Concentrate for IV infusion and concentrate.	Paget's disease (single dose of 5 mg). Hypercalcaemia of malignancy (4mg every 3–4 weeks).	Calcium and vitamin D supplementation also given. As with all this group of drugs, it is important to monitor serum electrolytes, and renal and hepatic function.

Box 16.1 Hormones secreted by the cortex of the adrenal gland

- Outer zone (zona glomerulosa): mineralocorticoids
- Middle zone (zona fasciculata): glucocorticoids
- Inner zone (zona reticularis): glucocorticoids, sex hormones

---

4–6 L in 24 h as necessary. Intravenous potassium and magnesium may be needed to correct imbalances. Once the patient has been rehydrated adequately, intravenous furosemide (frusemide), which has a calciuretic effect, may be added. If these measures are insufficient, a bisphosphonate, or salmon calcitonin, may be used to lower the blood calcium level further (see also p. 334).

ADRENAL GLAND

Corticosteroids are secreted from the outer layer of the adrenal gland known as the cortex. It is regarded as a separate endocrine gland from the inner section, which is called the medulla. The cortex is divided into three different zones, each of which secretes different hormones, as shown in Box 16.1.

MINERALOCORTICOIDS

These hormones play an important part in regulating mineral salt (electrolyte) metabolism. The hormone with the most physiological importance is aldosterone. The release of aldosterone from the adrenal cortex is controlled by angiotensin, which is formed by renin. Renin is an enzyme released by the kidneys whenever the blood pressure in the afferent arterioles decreases to a certain level. Aldosterone facilitates the reabsorption of sodium by the kidney tubules. When there is an increase in the amount of aldosterone secreted, there is retention of sodium chloride and hence water, leading to oedema.

GLUCOCORTICOIDS

The main glucocorticoids are cortisol, also known as hydrocortisone, and corticosterone, which are essential to life. Glucocorticoids have a number of vital functions. They:

- accelerate the breakdown of cellular proteins to amino acids; the amino acids in turn circulate to the liver, where they are converted to glucose, a process referred to as gluconeogenesis
- accelerate the mobilisation and breakdown of fats; fat metabolism therefore tends to take over from the usual carbohydrate metabolism
- are essential for maintenance of the blood pressure
- increase their secretion in times of physical or emotional stress
- in high concentration, reduce the number of eosinophils and cause the lymphatic tissues to atrophy, reducing the number of lymphocytes and plasma cells
- have anti-inflammatory properties
- suppress calcium absorption and inhibit bone formation
- decrease sex hormone production, which may in the longer term cause osteoporosis.

Corticosteroids, like other hormones, are used in both replacement therapy and in the treatment of a wide range of conditions, such as inflammatory bowel disease (IBD), asthma, allergies, malignant diseases and skin diseases, both orally and topically. Some properties of corticosteroids are summarised in Table 16.2.

Table 16.2 Some properties of corticosteroids

Corticosteroid	Main properties/actions
Mineralocorticoids Fludrocortisone acetate	Fludrocortisone has only minimal anti-inflammatory action and is used solely for its mineralocorticoid activity in Addison's disease. The daily dosage range is 50–300 micrograms per day. If glucocorticoid activity is required, cortisone or hydrocortisone is given concurrently, especially at times of stress and severe illness. Adverse effects are broadly similar to those occurring with glucocorticoids but, as would be expected from the physiology, major problems are oedema, weight gain, hypertension and electrolyte disturbances. Biochemical monitoring is advised.
Glucocorticoids Betamethasone Cortisone Dexamethasone Hydrocortisone Methylprednisolone Prednisolone The above glucocorticoids have varying potencies in termsof the anti-inflammatory effects, e.g. 5 mg of prednisolone is equivalent to 20 mg hydrocortisone. Although all the above drugs have broadly similar properties, differences between them influence the choice of drug in particular conditions	*Beneficial properties* Anti-inflammatory action. Euphoria.[a] Stimulation of appetite.[a] Protect the body from effects of acute hypersensitivity reactions Immunosuppression. *Adverse effects* Cushing's syndrome (at higher doses over a prolonged period) Diabetes mellitus Infection risk in patients exposed to viral diseases (especially chickenpox) Insomnia/mental disturbances/euphoria Muscle wasting Osteoporosis (of particular concern in older patients) Peptic ulceration/dyspepsia Taste disturbances In children, corticosteroids may suppress growth The use of corticosteroids in pregnancy and in breast-feeding has been reviewed by the CSM and advice issued in the BNF It is vitally important to recognise that prolonged corticosteroid therapy may cause adrenal atrophy. Sudden termination of therapy may be catastrophic. Adrenal insufficiency, hypotension and even death can result (patients on corticosteroid therapy must be carefully assessed prior to surgery). Any changes in dosage levels must be carefully adjusted and a tapering regime adopted if dosage reduction in indicated

[a]In certain situations, these properties may cause problems in the treatment of patients.

USE OF GLUCOCORTICOIDS (OTHER THAN REPLACEMENT THERAPY)

The use of corticosteroids (glucocorticoids) in certain conditions is dealt with as follows (see appropriate chapters):

- emergency treatment
- eye diseases
- diseases of the gastrointestinal tract (treatment of IBD)
- malignant disease
- palliative care
- diseases of the respiratory tract
- skin diseases
- renal disease
- rheumatic disease.

Glucocorticoids in various forms bring great benefits to patients, although side-effects must be guarded against. The main properties of the commonly used glucocorticoid drugs are summarised in Tables 16.2 and 16.3. Adverse effects (see Box 16.2) are significant, but with careful dosage adjustment and other measures these can be minimised. Patient counselling is vitally important. All patients should be encouraged to read

Table 16.3 The glucocorticoids

Drug	Dose range^a/route	Properties/uses
Betamethasone	Oral: 0.5–5 mg daily. IM or IV: 4–20 mg 6-hourly.	Very high glucocorticoid activity. Insignificant mineralocorticoid activity (widely used topically as the valerate).
Cortisone	Oral: 25–37.5 mg daily in divided doses.	Has significant mineralocorticoid activity. Not suitable for long-term therapy. Useful for replacement therapy.
Dexamethasone	Oral: 0.5–10 mg daily. IV in cerebral oedema: 10 mg initially then 4 mg IM every 6 h.	As betamethasone. Also used to treat nausea and vomiting following cytotoxic therapy.
Hydrocortisone	Oral: 20–30 mg per day in divided doses. IM or IV: 100–500 mg three to four times daily. Rectal foam: 125 mg.	Hydrocortisone is produced by conversion of cortisone in the liver. Hydrocortisone is the active agent and is therefore often preferred to cortisone. Other properties similar to cortisone.
Prednisolone	Oral: 10–20 mg daily. IM: 25–100 mg weekly. Rectal foam: 20 mg.	Prednisolone is a derivative of hydrocortisone and has predominant glucocorticoid activity. It is the most commonly used oral glucocorticoid.

^aWide variation of dosage depending on condition. Doses must be reduced gradually (see BNF).

the patient information leaflet supplied and given a 'steroid' card (Fig. 16.7). Local therapy in respiratory and skin conditions has reduced the incidence of systemic side effects. However, it should be noted that absorption of active ingredient from a topically applied or inhaled product can occur, with resultant side effects (see p. 449).

Glucocorticoids are also used in replacement therapy when natural production of adrenal steroids is deficient due to Addison's disease (adrenal failure) or anterior pituitary disease.

Figure 16.8 illustrates the adverse effects of prolonged glucocorticoid in excessive doses.

SEX HORMONES

In both sexes, the adrenal cortex secretes significant amounts of both oestrogens (female hormones) and androgens. In the female, the ovaries produce oestrogens and progesterone – oestrogen from the graafian follicles and progesterone from a temporary structure known as the corpus luteum. In the male, testosterone is secreted by the testes.

TREATMENT USING FEMALE SEX HORMONES

Sex hormones are used in replacement therapy when natural secretions are deficient and for the treatment of certain tumours (see Ch. 19). Long-term therapy with oestrogens requires the addition of a progestogen to reduce the risk of endometrial cancer. The therapeutic use of female sex hormones is discussed in Chapter 17.

MALE SEX HORMONES AND ANABOLIC STEROIDS

The therapeutic uses of male sex hormones and the related anabolic steroids are outlined in Table 16.4.

THE PANCREAS

In addition to its predominantly exocrine function, the pancreas has two types of cell – α and β – that make up the remaining endocrine part of the gland, known as the islets of Langerhans. The α cells secrete the hormone glucagon; β cells secrete the hormone insulin. In health, insulin and glucagon work in harmony with each other, insulin decreasing the blood glucose level and glucagon increasing it.

When an excess of carbohydrate has been taken in, insulin promotes storage of glucose by accelerating the transport of glucose through the cell membrane. Insulin also converts glucose to glycogen, which is stored in the liver and muscles. It also has the capacity to synthesise protein and to convert glucose to fat. The secretion of insulin is stimulated by a rise in blood glucose reaching the islet cells.

The glucocorticoids in Table 16.3 have varying potencies in terms of the anti-inflammatory effect (5 mg of prednisolone is equivalent to 20 mg of hydrocortisone). Although all these drugs have broadly similar properties, differences between them influence the choice of drug in particular conditions.

- Cushing's syndrome (at higher doses over a prolonged period)
- Diabetes mellitus
- Infection risk in patients exposed to viral diseases (especially chickenpox) and other infections, because the response to infection (natural defence system) is suppressed
- Insomnia/mental disturbances, euphoria
- Muscle wasting
- Osteoporosis (of particular concern in older patients)
- Peptic ulceration/dyspepsia
- Taste disturbances

In children, corticosteroids may suppress growth. The use of corticosteroids in pregnancy and in breast feeding has been reviewed by the Committee on Safety of Medicines and advice issued in the British National Formulary.

It is vitally important to recognise that prolonged corticosteroid therapy may cause adrenal atrophy. Sudden termination of therapy may be catastrophic. Adrenal insufficiency, hypotension and even death can result (patients on corticosteroid therapy must be carefully assessed prior to surgery). Any changes in dosage levels must be carefully adjusted and a tapering regimen adopted if dosage reduction is indicated (see also Fig. 16.8).

When the blood glucose level is low because of an insufficient intake of carbohydrate or an excessive amount of exercise having been taken, glucagon acts by mobilising the glycogen stores in the liver, converting them into glucose and thus raising the blood glucose level. Glucagon also has the capacity to convert amino acids to glucose in the liver and to increase the conversion of fat to glucose.

DIABETES MELLITUS

In diabetes mellitus (DM), there is an elevation of the blood glucose (normal fasting level 2.9–6.4 mmol/L) with consequent glycosuria resulting from an absolute or relative deficiency of insulin. The factors that predispose to the condition are:

- genetic
- coxsackievirus
- autoimmunity (leading to destruction of islet cells)
- pregnancy
- endocrine disorders (e.g. Cushing's syndrome)
- pancreatic disease
- stress
- obesity, dietary excess, lack of exercise, high alcohol intake
- drugs (e.g. corticosteroids, thiazide diuretics, thyroid hormones and phenytoin).

There may be interaction between the above factors and social and environmental factors.

There are two types of diabetes. Type 1 diabetes is due to a severe lack of insulin, whereas type 2 diabetes is due to a reduced secretion of insulin or the peripheral resistance to the action of insulin. The main characteristics of each type are indicated in Table 16.8. Other types of DM will not be discussed here.

Diabetes mellitus is a major challenge to all those involved in the care of patients in hospital or increasingly in the community. It is a multisystem disease that, if not properly controlled, can cause serious renal, neurological, ophthalmological, cardiovascular, gastrointestinal, metabolic and biochemical disorders. The human toll of the disease is massive, as is the economic burden. DM in children and in pregnancy presents difficult management problems. Diabetic patients facing surgery also need special care (see BNF).

Diabetes mellitus is characterised by hyperglycaemia and glycosuria. Glycosuria occurs when the glucose concentration in the blood exceeds the capacity of the renal tubules to reabsorb it. The presence of glucose in the glomerular filtrate increases the osmolality, which prevents the reabsorption of water. This considerably increases the volume of urine produced, leading to polyuria. Loss of water and minerals leads to thirst and polydipsia. If the fluid and mineral (electrolyte) loss is not corrected, significant complications can ensue. Poor utilisation of glucose triggers the compensatory mechanisms of glycogenolysis (breakdown of glycogen) and gluconeogenesis (breakdown of protein). Lipolysis (breakdown of fats) also occurs, leading to a raised fasting plasma concentration of non-esterified fatty acid (NEFA). In severe insulin deficiency, high levels of NEFA lead to the accumulation of ketone bodies and the dangerous condition of ketoacidosis. The chain of events leading to ketoacidosis is summarised below.

1. Lipolysis plasma concentration of NEFA rises.
2. Fatty acids are normally broken down in the liver to give acetyl-coenzyme A.

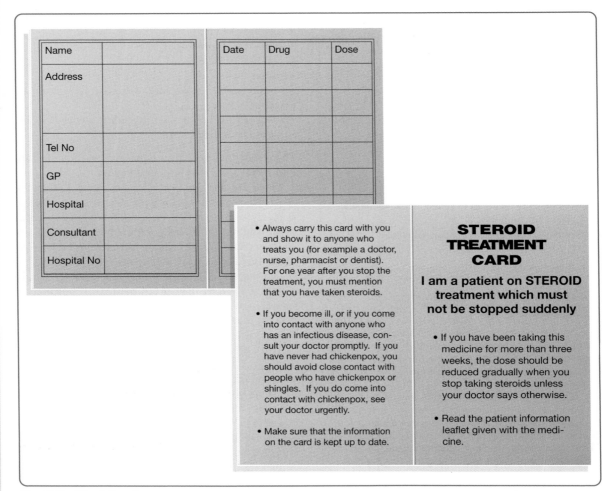

Name			Date	Drug	Dose
Address					
Tel No					
GP					
Hospital					
Consultant					
Hospital No					

- Always carry this card with you and show it to anyone who treats you (for example a doctor, nurse, pharmacist or dentist). For one year after you stop the treatment, you must mention that you have taken steroids.

- If you become ill, or if you come into contact with anyone who has an infectious disease, consult your doctor promptly. If you have never had chickenpox, you should avoid close contact with people who have chickenpox or shingles. If you do come into contact with chickenpox, see your doctor urgently.

- Make sure that the information on the card is kept up to date.

STEROID TREATMENT CARD

I am a patient on STEROID treatment which must not be stopped suddenly

- If you have been taking this medicine for more than three weeks, the dose should be reduced gradually when you stop taking steroids unless your doctor says otherwise.

- Read the patient information leaflet given with the medicine.

Fig. 16.7 'Steroid' card.

3. Levels of acetyl-coenzyme A exceed the body's ability to clear it.
4. Acetyl-coenzyme A forms acetoacetic acid.
5. Acetoacetic acid is converted into acetone (ketone bodies).
6. Normally the ketone bodies are metabolised, but in DM levels accumulate, causing a fall in the pH of body fluids.
7. The fall in pH is countered to some extent by naturally occurring bicarbonate.
8. Bicarbonate levels fall and ketoacidosis results.
9. Hydrogen ion concentration increases, as does P_aCO_2. Clinically, this may be seen as hyperpnoea.

DIAGNOSIS OF DIABETES MELLITUS

Although DM is characterised by an elevated blood glucose (fasting level over 7 mmol/L and over 11 mmol/L after a meal) and glycosuria, it is essential to differentiate it from other conditions, such as renal glycosuria caused by a low renal threshold for glucose. Estimation of the fasting blood glucose concentration and random blood glucose concentrations will normally be sufficient to confirm the diagnosis of DM.

The oral glucose tolerance test is seldom used in the diagnosis of DM; it is still used to establish the presence of gestational diabetes (see British National Formulary).

AIMS OF TREATMENT OF DIABETES MELLITUS

The overall aims of treatment can be summarised as follows:

- to keep blood glucose levels for most of the day between 4 and 9 mmol/L (4–7 mmol/L before meals and not more than 9 mmol/L after meals)
- to achieve and maintain a normal metabolic state
- to avoid hyperglycaemia

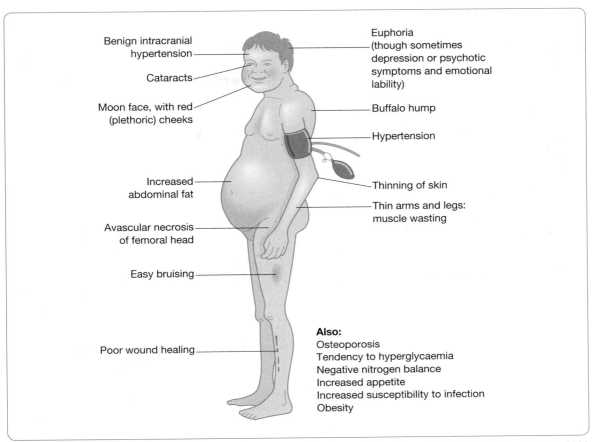

Fig. 16.8 Adverse effects of prolonged glucocorticoid in excessive doses. (From Rang HP, Dale MM, Ritter JM et al. 2003 Pharmacology. Churchill Livingstone, Edinburgh. With permission of Elsevier Ltd.)

Table 16.4 Anabolic steroids and male sex hormones (androgens) and anti-androgens

	Therapeutic use
Anabolic steroid(s)	
Nandrolone Stanozolol	Related to androgens but have much less virilising effects. These drugs have limited use in medicine in osteoporosis and aplastic anaemia. Illegal use by athletes has been well documented. Side-effects are similar to those seen with testosterone and are a growing cause for concern.
Male sex hormones	
Testosterone (available in a number of forms for use orally or by slow-release IM injection; a transdermal patch and gel are also available).	In deficiency states, 120–160 mg daily by mouth as the undecanoate compound. Testosterone enantate is given IM 250 mg every 2–3 weeks. In breast cancer, 250 mg IM every 2–3 weeks. Side-effects are as would be expected from the physiology (e.g. virilism in women and precocious sexual development in men). Caution must be exercised in patients suffering from candida or from renal or hepatic impairment. Fertility is not enhanced by testosterone administration.
Antiandrogens	
Cyproterone acetate Finasteride Duasteride	Cyproterone is used in male hypersexuality (50 mg orally twice daily). These drugs act to reduce the potency of naturally occurring testosterone. They are of value in benign prostatic hyperplasia (see p. 362).

- to avoid hypoglycaemia
- to avoid the complications of the disease (see p. 342)
- to avoid acute illness (e.g. ketoacidosis)
- to involve the patient fully in the management programme
- to enable the patient to lead a normal life.

With generally increasing life expectancy, complications are of particular concern in the older patient, because ischaemic changes may lead to serious morbidity (e.g. diabetic gangrene). Apart from drug treatment, particular attention must be paid to diet, personal hygiene (especially the feet), exercise and other aspects of lifestyle such as intake of alcohol, smoking and avoiding hot baths and saunas.

MEASURING GLYCAEMIC CONTROL

Fasting blood glucose levels are critically important in the diagnosis of DM (measurements are in mmol/ L). Fasting levels of 6.1–6.9 indicate impaired glucose tolerance, which may be amenable to treatment by diet and exercise. Levels of 7–7.8 indicate diabetes, but again diet/exercise may be adequate treatment. However, if levels of 7.8–11.1 are found, diet/exercise and drugs will be required. Above 11.1, oral drugs or insulin coverage will be needed to provide a 24-h control of blood glucose.

A measure of the total glycated haemoglobin (HbA$_1$; glucose 'sticks' to haemoglobin over the life of the red blood cell by a process known as glycosylation) or a specific fraction HbA$_{1c}$ provides a good indication of glycaemic control related to the risk of complications. A concentration of between 6.5 and 7.5% HbA$_{1c}$ is ideal. To achieve this target, blood glucose levels of 4–6 mmol/L fasting, 4–7 mmol/ L preprandial and 7–9 mmol/L after meals are likely to be required. Blood glucose concentration should not fall below 4 mmol/L, to avoid the risk of hypoglycaemia.

A combination of routine blood glucose self-monitoring together with a measure of glycated haemoglobin at suitable intervals provides a good overview of glycaemic control.

MAJOR COMPLICATIONS OF DIABETES MELLITUS

If not properly controlled, DM can result in highly significant morbidity. High concentrations of glucose in the blood are very damaging, due to a range of adverse effects on cells, proteins and fats. Tissue repair is inhibited and artery walls become 'sticky', encouraging deposits and clots. A combination of these damaging actions results in eye (retinal) problems, renal damage,

neuropathies and increased risk of heart attacks and other cardiovascular problems.

In addition to the neuropathies, hyperglycaemia, ketoacidosis and hypoglycaemia require prompt and effective treatment. Patients with DM may have a lowered resistance to infection. Hyperlipidaemia (elevated cholesterol) is a major risk factor for cardiac death in diabetic patients. Cholesterol-lowering therapy may be required (see p. 220).

DIABETIC NEPHROPATHY (SEE ALSO CH. 18)

In order to minimise the risk of renal deterioration, careful control of blood pressure is required using an angiotensin-converting enzyme inhibitor or angiotensin-II receptor antagonist (see p. 205). The presence of protein/microalbuminuria is a key diagnostic sign.

DIABETIC NEUROPATHY

A basic requirement in the treatment of diabetic neuropathy is optimal diabetic control with suitable drugs to relieve pain. Tricyclic antidepressants (see p. 262) such as amitriptyline or nortriptyline are preferred for painful neuropathic conditions. Anticonvulsants (see Ch. 14) such as gabapentin, carbamazepine and phenytoin are used for shooting pains. Opioid analgesics may be needed, and codeine phosphate is helpful in diabetic diarrhoea. Neuropathic positional hypotension is treated by a mineralocorticoid (fludrocortisone) and increased salt intake. Patients with neuropathic oedema may benefit from oral ephedrine hydrochloride 30–60 mg three times daily. Duloxetine may be used for neuropathic pain.

HYPOGLYCAEMIA: ACUTE AND CHRONIC

A hypoglycaemic patient (blood glucose less than 3 mmol/L) is pale and may appear different from usual – acting oddly, possibly aggressive or seeming to be intoxicated. Such patients feel dizzy and begin to tremble, and their vision becomes blurred. Beads of sweat appear on the brow and upper lip. Hypoglycaemic attacks are more likely to occur before the midday meal and at night. If hypoglycaemia does occur, whatever the cause, prompt action is required. Diabetics are taught to recognise the onset of hypoglycaemia and to take glucose appropriately. People who are conscious may be given a cup of tea or coffee with one spoonful of sugar and a couple of biscuits.

Alternatively, they may chew Dextrosol tablets. GlucoGel contains 9.2 g glucose in 23 g of gel. The gel is applied to the buccal mucosa, followed by external massage of the cheek. The method has been shown to enhance absorption, providing a more rapid rise in blood glucose (5 min) than if taken orally (10–15 min). The gel is available as an oral ampoule. Non-diet drinks such as Lucozade and original Ribena may also be useful.

Hypoglycaemia may cause unconsciousness. In such cases, glucagon is given by intramuscular or subcutaneous injection. This is a valuable method for those patients troubled by recurrent hypoglycaemia and for whom a trained family member can give the injection. A kit complete with vial containing the glucagon powder and syringe (with needle attached) containing 1 mL of water for injections is available.

If the patient does not respond to oral glucose or to glucagon (within 10 min), or if the patient is discovered unconscious, 50 mL of glucose 20% or 25 mL of glucose 50% should be given intravenously. Strong glucose solution is highly irritant to the tissues and must be injected carefully into the vein to avoid extravasation. Larger volumes of a 10% glucose solution may also be used. The dose may have to be repeated. The nurse should remain with the patient and be ready to provide reassurance and support as the patient regains consciousness.

TREATMENT OF TYPE 1 DIABETES MELLITUS

The aims of treatment of DM (types 1 and 2) are essentially the same (see p. 339). Replacement therapy is essential in type 1 diabetes. Natural secretion of insulin provides control of blood glucose on a minute-by-minute basis. This cannot be achieved by currently available regimens. Delivery of insulin by specially designed pumps may be used in patients in whom there is intractable hyperglycaemia. This delivery method can achieve satisfactory basal levels of insulin but is sadly not practicable for widespread use. Efforts are being made now to improve insulin administration/delivery systems. Inhaled insulin has recently been licensed (subject to NICE guidance).

In the majority of cases, adequate control of blood glucose can be achieved by a combination of mealtime and basal requirement. It is important to keep the regimen as simple as possible. Typical regimens are illustrated in Table 16.5. As insulin (a protein) is destroyed by gastric enzymes, the parenteral route must be used. In addition, attention must be paid to diet and appropriate levels of exercise.

Table 16.5 Typical insulin regimens

Insulin type	Before meal times				Notes
	B	L	EM	B/T	
Short-acting insulin with intermediate-acting insulin	√		√		Convenient for patients
Short-acting insulin with Intermediate-acting insulin	√				Involves the use of three preparation
Short-acting insulin Intermediate-acting insulin			√	√	
Short-acting insulin Intermediate-acting insulin	√	√	√	√	Suitable for acute-onset diabetes
Intermediate-acting insulin	√			√	Before breakfast OR at bedtime. May be useful for patients with type 2 diabetes who need insulin
Intermediate-acting insulin with short-acting insulin	√			√	As above

All these regimes require careful monitoring and adjustment of doses of insulin on an individual basis. Presence of other non-medical conditions, stress and trauma will influence requirements. Management of patients who are pregnant requires special skills.
Key: B = breakfast, L = lunch, E/M = evening meal, B/t = bedtime

There is a particular need to ensure good control of blood glucose levels in pregnancy. Poor glucose control is associated with fetal malformation and other problems. Joint (obstetric and diabetic) care is essential, as is regular monitoring, together with special care during delivery (blood glucose monitoring and glucose and insulin infusions). Failure to diagnose insulin-dependent DM can have very serious consequences for the patient and health professionals involved. A case of multiple failures to measure blood and urinary glucose by both GP and hospital and therefore failure to diagnose DM led to a patient suffering permanent damage to body systems (urinary tract and gastrointestinal tract symptoms). The outcome of the case was the award of £1 million damages to the patient (Casebook Medical Protection Society 2006).

INSULINS

Great progress has been made with the development of sophisticated insulins (Table 16.6) designed to achieve optimal control of blood glucose levels. Physiological insulin requirements vary according to food intake, exercise and metabolic stress. It is very difficult to achieve optimal replacement therapy,

owing to the need to give insulin subcutaneously and erratic absorption into the circulation. In addition, it is necessary to limit the number of times daily insulin is administered for reasons of patient convenience. Insulin analogues, produced by genetic engineering, retain their biological activity but have been engineered to achieve differing lengths of action following subcutaneous injections. As the range of insulins develops, it will become possible to mimic more closely the actions of naturally secreted insulin. It should be remembered that, once given, there are no means to adjust insulin absorption.

ADMINISTRATION OF INSULIN

In many cases, subcutaneous administration using a disposable insulin syringe will meet the patient's needs. The use of a pen injector system and a cartridge of insulin is helpful for many patients.

Pen injector systems have the advantage of portability, greater social acceptability and flexibility of lifestyle. Disadvantages of this means of administration must be appreciated. Patients may be lulled into a false sense of security, because of the ease of use. This may lead to poor control of diet.

Table 16.6 Classification of insulins (for full range, see BNF)

Official name/source	Length of action (can also be given IM and IV infusion)		Notes, clinical uses (not including emergency treatment), doses adjusted on individual patient basis
	Subcutaneous	Intravenous	
Soluble (neutral)/insulin (bovine, porcine, human)	Onset: 30–60 min. Peak: 2–6 h. Duration up to 8 h.	Half-life: 5 min. Duration: 30 min.	Administer 30 min before a meal if possible (onset slower than physiological insulin). Dangers of hyperglycaemia after a meal and, because the action may last several hours, there is a risk of hypoglycaemia later on.
Insulin aspart (recombinant human insulin analogue)	Onset: 15 min. Peak: 30–90 min. Duration: 3.5 h.	Can also be given by SC infusion, IV infusion and IV injection	The molecule forms smaller monomers than soluble insulin and as a result acts more rapidly. The action is closer to the physiological action of naturally produced insulin. Administered immediately before a meal.
Insulin lispro (recombinant human insulin analogue)	Similar to above.	Can also be given by SC infusion, IV infusion and IV injection.	As with insulin aspart.
Insulin detemir (recombinant human insulin analogue)	Up to 24 h.	–	Administer once or twice daily in combination with meal-related short- to rapid-acting insulin.
Insulin glargine (recombinant human insulin analogue)	Up to 24 h.	–	Administer once or twice daily at same time each day. (See NICE guidance in BNF)

Continued

Table 16.6 Classification of insulins (for full range, see BNF) 'cont...'

Official name/source	Length of action (can also be given IM and IV infusion)		Notes, clinical uses (not including emergency treatment), doses adjusted on individual patient basis
	Subcutaneous	Intravenous	
Insulin zinc suspension lente (bovine, porcine or human in a complex with a suitable zinc salt particle size 10–40 microns)	Onset: 1–2 h. Peak: 6–10 h. Duration: 12–14 h.	–	Twice daily injections required. Even so, nocturnal hypoglycaemia is a cause for concern to patients and their carers. Important to mix well before using to ensure homogenicity of suspension.
Isophane insulin. (Isophane protamine insulin; Isophane insulin (NPH) – intermediate acting)	Onset: 30 min–2 h. Peak: 3–6 h. Duration: 8–14 h.	Useful for twice-daily regimens. Can be mixed with soluble insulin in syringe or ready-mixed preparations are more convenient.	–
Protamine zinc insulin	–	–	Now rarely. used (see British National Formulary).
Biphasic insulin aspart, 30% insulin aspart, 70% insulin aspart protamine	The profiles of the action of the biphasic insulins is as would be expected from the components.	–	Available in cartridge form for pen injection. Given 10 min before a meal or soon after.
Biphasic insulin lispro, 25% insulin lispro including lispro protamine or 50% of each insulin	As above.	–	As above. Given up to 15 min before or soon after a meal.
Biphasic insulin isophane, porcine or human insulin complexed with protamine sulphate in a solution of insulin from the same species (see BNF for detail of available forms)			A number of different combinations is available in cartridgea or prefiled disposable injection devices. These are much more convenient for patients than using a vial and a syringa. In using these biphasic insulins, it is vitally important to check with the patient and to ensure the proportions of the components are clearly stated on the prescription.

Patients need to understand the adjustment of dosage, taking into account blood glucose levels. Cartridges of mixed insulins may not always be appropriate, especially for younger, brittle diabetics whose requirements are more likely to fluctuate. Pens are available in disposable as well as reusable forms.

The constant quest to achieve control of blood glucose levels corresponding to those of a well non-diabetic continues to challenge all those involved in providing care for diabetic patients. Four to six injections daily of a small dose of soluble insulin is an option that would achieve good control, but this is not often practicable. Controlled continuous subcutaneous infusion of insulin may be administered using a pump system. Additional doses can be administered to cover meals by the activation of a mechanism incorporated into the pump. A highly sophisticated implantable device that releases insulin in response to blood glucose level fluctuations remains an objective for researchers.

INSULIN REGIMENS

Insulin regimens (Table 16.5) will vary widely, taking into account many factors, such as the patient's preferences, lifestyle and delivery device preferred. The regimens include once-daily injections that do not give good control and are rarely used. Twice-daily injections are the most suitable for new patients. A combination of short- and intermediate-acting insulins is injected before breakfast and the evening meal. Premixed preparations are widely used. Multiple injections (up to four daily) can give good control in well-motivated patients who are able and willing to do frequent and regular blood glucose tests. An insulin analogue or soluble insulin is injected before each meal, and an intermediate or a long-acting insulin is injected to provide background cover. In each case, the dose of insulin in units is highly specific to the individual patient's needs.

SOME PROBLEMS OF INSULIN THERAPY

Hypoglycaemia is always a potential problem. Although many insulin preparations have similar basic characteristics, inadvertent changes may result in severe problems for the patient. Conditions in which insulin requirements are reduced include diseases of the adrenal, pituitary or thyroid gland. Reduced doses are also required when there is renal or hepatic impairment, or by the concurrent administration of drugs that have a hypoglycaemic action.

Insulin lispro and insulin aspart are genetically engineered insulins with an immediate onset of action, which means that they must be administered closer to mealtimes than is required for soluble insulin. They are therefore more convenient in use. In addition, their duration of action is short and, as a result, hypoglycaemia may occur less often than with conventional insulins.

Local side effects of insulin therapy include local hypersensitivity reactions, lipodystrophy and insulin resistance. Reactions to human insulin are claimed to be less than with insulins of animal origin, but in trials no demonstrable advantage has been found.

TREATMENT OF TYPE 2 DIABETES

Diet is the first line of treatment in type 2 diabetes. Emphasis is placed on weight reduction when indicated

Table 16.7   Some oral antidiabetic drugs

Class/mode of action	Examples	Notes/dose[a]
Sulphonylureas (act by stimulating insulin secretions for 12–24 h; some β-cell activity required)	Chlorpropamide Glibenclamide	Not recommended. Risks of hypoglycaemia due to prolonged action are significant.
	Gliclazide Glimepiride Glipizide	40–80 mg daily up to 160 mg depending on response. 1 mg daily adjusted according to response up to 4 mg. 2.5–5 mg daily before breakfast or lunch. Adjust according to response. Up to 15 mg as a single dose. Higher doses up to 20 mg given in divided doses.
	Gliquidone	15 mg daily before breakfast. Adjust to 45–60 mg daily in divided doses.
	Tolbutamide	500 mg–1.5 g daily in divided doses.
Biguanides (decrease gluconeogenesis and increase peripheral utilisation of glucose; endogenous insulin must be present)	Metformin (the only available biguanide)	Contraindicated in renal impairment. Can cause lactic acidosis (withdraw treatment if this occurs). May be combined with other agents if a combination of strict diet and metformin fail to achieve adequate control (see British National Formulary). 500 mg with breakfast for 1 week, then 500 mg with breakfast and evening meal for 1 week, then add 500 mg with lunch. Also used for polycystic ovary disease; this is an unlicensed indication.
α-Glucosidase inhibitor (inhibits the intestinal α-glucosidases; delays the digestion of starch and glucose)	Acarbose	May be used as an adjunct with other agents. 50 mg daily increasing to 50 mg three times daily. Side effects include gastrointestinal disturbances (see British National Formulary).

[a]Doses given are illustrative. Individual regimens are required depending on the patient's needs.

Table 16.8 Types of diabetes mellitus: a comparison[a]

Type 1 diabetes (insulin-dependent diabetes)	Type 2 diabetes (non-insulin-dependent diabetes)
Genetic predisposition	Genetic predisposition
Caused by destruction of islet cells of the pancreas (autoimmunity)	Caused by resistance to insulin and inadequate secretion of insulin
Dependent on insulin for life and prevention of major complications	Not dependent on insulin for survival
Behavioural/social factors have significant impact on the development and management of the condition	As Type 1
Affects younger age group (usually lean people)	Affects older age group (usually obese people)
Prone to ketosis	Resistant to ketosis
Associated with hypertension, hyperlipidaemia and atherosclerotic heart disease	As Type 1
Acute lack of insulin: condition does not deteriorate over time as with type 2 diabetes	Progressive disorder: becomes more difficult to treat; should not be considered as 'mild' diabetes

[a]Other types include diabetes due to glucocorticoid therapy, pancreatic destruction, recognised genetic syndromes and gestational diabetes.

and otherwise a 'healthy' high-fibre, low-sugar, low-fat, low-salt diet evenly distributed throughout the day. For many, adherence to the diet is sufficient.

Oral antidiabetic drugs are widely used in the treatment of this condition, especially in older, obese patients and when dietary restriction alone has failed. Younger patients or patients with brittle diabetes cannot be treated with oral agents. The range of drugs available is described in Table 16.7.

Many patients with type 2 diabetes may not exhibit any overt symptoms, but their hyperglycaemia may be causing vascular damage without the awareness of either doctor or patient. Particular attention needs to be paid to patients with a family history of ischaemic heart disease and blood lipid abnormalities. Hypertension is another major risk factor, as is smoking. Regular screening and well-managed therapy can help patients (especially older patients) achieve a better quality of life with reduced incidence of morbidity. Patients with type 2 diabetes who have reached the maximum level of oral therapy and are still hyperglycaemic should be considered for insulin therapy.

A new range of oral antidiabetic compounds has recently been introduced. The thiazolidinediones, pioglitazone and rosiglitazone, reduce blood glucose levels by reducing the peripheral resistance to insulin. These drugs are used in combination with metformin

or, if metformin is contraindicated, a sulphonylurea is used (see BNF for NICE guidance).

A comparison of type 1 and type 2 DM is given in Table 16.8.

BLOOD GLUCOSE TESTING

Whenever possible, self-monitoring of the blood glucose in diabetics is to be encouraged to allow the patient to be independent and to reduce the risk to staff of blood-borne infection. Admission to hospital provides an opportunity for the nurse to check the patient's technique, especially when there is some concern over diabetic control. Some hospital patients are, of course, not well enough to perform this procedure, and so the responsibility temporarily falls on the nurse.

A sample of capillary blood may be obtained from the pinna of the ear or from the side of the thumbnail, the former being the more vascular.

Apart from reasons of cleanliness, the patient's ear/hand should be washed with soap and warm water and dried before carrying out the blood test, so as to improve the circulation and allow blood to be more easily obtained. An alcohol swab is not used to clean the skin, as the alcohol from the swab may create a false reading. Because the maintenance of an optimum blood glucose level is highly dependent on the use of biochemical tests,

Table 16.9   Areas to cover in a teaching programme for new diabetic patients

Subject area	Details
Anatomy and physiology	A clear understanding of: • the pancreas, the blood and the tissues • carbohydrate metabolism.
The disorder itself	What has gone wrong with the pancreas and why treatment is essential.
Controlling the blood glucose level	Administration of insulin or oral antidiabetic agent as appropriate: • prescriptions • supplies • storage (especially insulin) • equipment • aids to administration • dosages • timing • frequency • sites of administration • technique.
Controlling the diet	An understanding of the different classes of food and the need to avoid pure sugars. Knowledge of dietary exchanges. The need to eat regularly, including snacks between meals and before bedtime. Importance of trying to eat, even if feeling unwell.
Monitoring the disorder	The importance of keeping careful records of: • blood glucose readings • urinalysis • insulin administered • hypoglycaemic episodes and action taken.
The patient's self-care	How to recognise hypoglycaemic reactions. The importance of meticulous care of the feet. The importance of attending clinics as arranged: • diabetic clinic • dietetic clinic • eye clinic • chiropody Encouragement of healthy lifestyle with adequate sleep, minimisation of stress and reduced exposure to infections when possible. Advice and encouragement to allow the continuation of normal activities such as schooling, work, sport, travel. The benefits of carrying some indication that the patient is diabetic, (e.g. card, medical pendant/bracelet). What to do when feeling unwell. Sources of help: • medical • nursing • dietetic • pharmaceutical • financial.

it is essential to follow the manufacturer's instructions implicitly.

Reagent strips used for measuring plasma glucose levels may be read against a colour chart or by using a meter specially designed to record the result accurately. Because colour vision may be impaired in diabetics, the glucometer is a considerable advantage for self-monitoring. There are several different kinds of glucometer. Each type has its own reagent strip.

ROLE OF THE NURSE IN THE MANAGEMENT OF DIABETES MELLITUS

Nurses play a vital role at all stages in the management of diabetes. The routine screening of patients attending any clinic is performed with a view to identifying previously undiagnosed diabetes. Assisting in the assessment and diagnosis of suspected diabetes, including carrying out the oral glucose tolerance test if needed, is another important part of the nurse's role. Once diabetes is diagnosed and treatment agreed, the day-to-day management of the condition and the education of patients (and their families) is left largely in the hands of nurses. On no other occasion are the nurse's teaching skills more greatly drawn on than during the period between confirmation of the diagnosis and discharge from hospital. The challenge for nurses is to have patients who are both competent and confident in managing their condition. Such an opportunity lends itself to a planned programme of teaching using different teaching methods, including explaining, demonstrating with the help of visual aids,

supervising practice and providing suitable written information. Subject areas to be covered are detailed in Table 16.9.

In any clinical setting at any time, the nurse may be involved with the diabetic patient, and so it is essential that all nurses have a grasp of the condition and an understanding of the aims of treatment. Nurses in accident and emergency departments and acute medical wards will, from time to time, have to care for the acutely ill diabetic patient. Especially with the insulin-dependent diabetic, the need to be observant, adhere to correct procedures, maintain high standards of hygiene and keep meticulous records cannot be overemphasised. Diabetic prescribing and recording sheets should reflect an accurate diabetic 'picture'. This can be achieved by combining, into a single document, blood glucose and glycosuria test results as well as ketonuria if relevant. The document must give details of the hypoglycaemic agent(s) (oral or parenteral) prescribed and a record of administration.

CASE STUDY

Time scales (approximate):

1932–1979	no significant illness
End of 1979	IBD – ulcerative colitis
1980	discharged on salazopyrine; DM diagnosed – oral hypoglycaemic agent begun (not known which one)
1983	insulin therapy begun
1988	salazopyrine replaced by budesonide
Early 2006	unwell; insulin dose adjusted
Mid 2006	coping reasonably well.

Mr S. is a retired farmer aged 74 years. He lives happily with his wife of 40 years. They are comfortably off and enjoy life despite the limitations of Mr S.'s illnesses.

In 1979 (during a busy and stressful period on his farm), he developed ulcerative colitis, which resulted in hospital admission. He lost 4 stones in weight and felt that his problems were not well managed, especially his diet. He was discharged after some weeks, still feeling unwell. Oral salazopyrine was prescribed for his colitis. On returning home, he felt very lethargic and lost interest in his farm work. Blood tests showed that he had DM, which Mr S. felt should have been detected during his hospitalisation. There was no previous family history of either condition.

During the first few months of 2006, he has not enjoyed life, because of difficulties managing his conditions. His medication for the IBD had been changed to oral budesonide and rectal budesonide.

His insulin regimen is 13 units of rapid-acting insulin before his main meals (three) and 58 units of an intermediate-acting insulin at bedtime (using a pen injector). In mid 2006, his condition is generally quite good 'but could be better'.

In a general discussion with Mr S., his views and some concerns on his medication were identified.

He has significant problems retaining the rectal budesonide and is not sure why his salazopyrine was changed. He felt quite happy on salazopyrine.

Mr S. made it clear that he 'knows how it feels' and does not see the need to perform his regular blood tests. His dietary habits are not ideal, and he regards his insulin as a means to facilitate occasional overindulgence. He feels that the prescribed insulin dosage is excessive, despite assurances that many more fellow patients are receiving much higher dosages. As a farmer, his views on food are predictable, i.e. 'If you can eat, there can't be much wrong with you'. He has seen no benefit in joining a patient support group. Mr S. is still able to drive. He has no marked eye deterioration and only minimal signs of neuropathic changes. Following minor day surgery, he experienced a hypoglycaemic episode at home. This was dealt with promptly with oral sugar but gave him 'quite a fright'. No other episodes have occurred since.

Mr S. accepts his condition and welcomes the benefits of his medications. Overall, he has a positive attitude to his life. His IBD gives him more day-to-day problems than the DM.

QUESTIONS

1. Why would his medication for IBD have been changed?
2. Should he have been informed about the reasons for a change?
3. What approach would you take to Mr S.'s attitude to his diet and insulin regimen?
4. Describe how you would approach Mr S.'s erratic blood glucose testing.

ANSWERS

1. *Probably to reduce the likelihood of side-effects.*
2. *Yes, a non-alarmist explanation about side-effects.*
3. *This requires a fairly fundamental retraining with a clear explanation of the risks he is running.*
4. *The benefits of regular testing and meaning need to be explained.*

The aim for nurses in primary care is to maximise quality of life for the diabetic, prevent long-term diabetic complications and increase longevity. Increasingly, health authorities are utilising the skills of nurses specialising in care for diabetics. The importance of close liaison between diabetic clinic and GP cannot be overstressed. Similarly, good communication between nurses and doctors is paramount.

In summary, nurses play an especially full part in the diagnosis, treatment and care of the diabetic patient. It is, however, in their teaching role that there is the greatest potential to contribute to maximum independence and otherwise good health for diabetics.

SELF-ASSESSMENT QUESTIONS

SECTION A

What advice should be given to a patient who is to start oral levothyroxine for thyroid failure?

SECTION B

1. What clinical features might a young patient suspected of having diabetes mellitus present with?
2. What are the differences between type 1 and type 2 diabetes?
3. Name a group of drugs that may produce glycosuria.
4. What is the normal blood glucose range?
5. How would you recognise a hypoglycaemic attack?
6. At what times of the day are such attacks most likely to occur?
7. What action should you take?
8. What type of diet should a person with diabetes take?
9. Insulin is secreted by the β cells of the pancreas. True or false?
10. What type of insulin would be administered to a patient in diabetic coma, and what route would be used?
11. How is insulin stored?
12. What are the long-term complications of diabetes?

SECTION C

Complete the following statement using words from the word bank below.

Diabetes _____ is a _____ disorder of carbohydrate, fat and _____ metabolism caused by a _____ or complete lack of _____ secretion by the _____ cells situated in the islets of Langerhans in the _____.

relevant   pancreas   complicated   insipidus

glucose	α	nitrogen	β
spleen	complex	protein	mellitus
insulin	relative		

SECTION D

Unscramble the following table.

Hyperglycaemia	Hypoglycaemia
Thirst	Slurred speech
Facial sweating	Glycosuria
Slow onset	Raised blood glucose
Smell of ketones on breath	Dehydration
Treat with glucose	Treat with insulin
Polyuria	Rapid onset
Change in behaviour	Tachycardia
Lack of food	Low blood glucose

SECTION E

Consider a patient you have cared for who has diabetes mellitus. (No answers given.)

- What type of diabetes did the patient have?
- How was his or her diabetes controlled?
- Why was it necessary to carry out blood glucose testing?
- What other recordings were taken and why?
- What dietary restrictions were there?
- Was the patient's diabetes the primary complaint?
- Were any long-term effects evident?
- How well did the patient understand his or her diabetes and its treatment?
- Given the patient's age and other conditions and circumstances, how normal a life was he or she able to lead?
- What improvements, if any, were or could have been made to the overall management of the condition?

	Oral hypoglycaemic agent	Short-acting insulin	Long-acting insulin
Example			
Indication			
Contraindications			
Side effects			
Patient instruction			

SECTION F

Diabetes is increasing in the western world. Consider the factors contributing to this situation and suggest how nurses may play their part in reducing the incidence of diabetes.

SECTION G

Using the British National Formulary, if necessary, complete the table above.

REFERENCES

[Anonymous] 2002 Incidence of diabetes in the UK population. Diabetic Medicine 4(suppl):1–5

Casebook Medical Protection Society 2006 Volume 14, issue 3. Medical Protection Society, London

Health and Social Care Information Centre 2005 National diabetes audit. Sponsored by the Health Care Commission, London

FURTHER READING AND RESOURCES

Harrison PTC 2001 Endocrine disrupters and human health. British Medical Journal 323:1317–1318

Harvey JN 2002 Diabetic nephropathy [editorial]. British Medical Journal 325:59–60

Hindmarsh P 2002 Commentary: exogenous glucocorticoids influence adrenal function, but assessment can be difficult. British Medical Journal 324:1083

Mason P 2002 Diet and diabetes. Pharmaceutical Journal 268:499

Murray JS, Jayarajasingh R 2001 Deterioration of symptoms after start of thyroid hormone replacement. British Medical Journal 323:332–333

National Institute for Clinical Excellence 2002 Management of type 2 diabetes; management of blood pressure and blood lipids. NICE, London

National Institute for Clinical Excellence 2003 Guidance in the use of glitazones for the treatment of type 2 diabetes. Technology appraisal 63. NICE, London

National Institute for Health and Clinical Excellence 2004 Type 1 diabetes in adults. NICE, London

Pickup J, Keen H 2001 Continuous subcutaneous insulin infusion in type 1 diabetes. British Medical Journal 322:1262–1263

Pollock AM, Sturrock A 2001 Thyroxine treatment in patients with symptoms of hypothyroidism but thyroid function tests within the reference range: randomised double blind placebo controlled crossover trial. British Medical Journal 323:891–895

Sackey GH 2000. Recurrent generalised urticaria at insulin injection sites. British Medical Journal 321:1449

Sexton J, Vincent M 2004 Remedying calcium and phosphate problems in chronic kidney disease. Pharmaceutical Journal 274:561–564

Tannan N 2005a Osteoporosis and its prevention. Pharmaceutical Journal 275:521–548

Tannan N 2005b Osteoporosis and its treatment. Pharmaceutical Journal 275:581–584

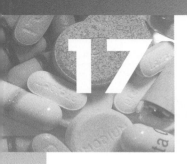

17 Drugs used in obstetrics, gynaecology and urinary tract disorders

CHAPTER CONTENTS

KEY OBJECTIVES

After reading this chapter, you should be able to do the following.

Obstetrics and gynaecology:

- list the dangers of prescribing in pregnancy
- name the constituents of routine oral contraception
- state what constitutes emergency hormonal contraception
- identify the symptoms arising from the menopause
- name the constituents of hormone replacement therapy (HRT)
- describe the risks associated with HRT
- discuss the reasons why there is an increased risk of vulval infection in older women.

Urinary tract disorders:

- label a diagram of the female urinary tract
- describe the clinical features of benign prostatic hyperplasia
- give examples of drugs used to treat urinary frequency and incontinence

- give examples of drugs used to treat erectile dysfunction
- discuss the general principles of bladder irrigation
- name the preparations that may be used to maintain patency of indwelling urinary catheters.

INTRODUCTION

Modern drug treatment of the distressing disorders of the genitourinary system in both women and men has significantly improved the quality of life for many people. Older people have greatly benefited from drugs that help to achieve improved bladder control, hormone replacement therapy (HRT) and drugs to treat sexual dysfunction. The scourge of cancer of the prostate is still a major cause of morbidity and mortality, but progress is being made. Medical treatment of male lower urinary tract symptoms (poor stream, hesitancy and urgency) is now standard, although surgical interventions may still be required. α-Blockers and suppression of androgen stimulation of prostate growth are cornerstones of treatment.

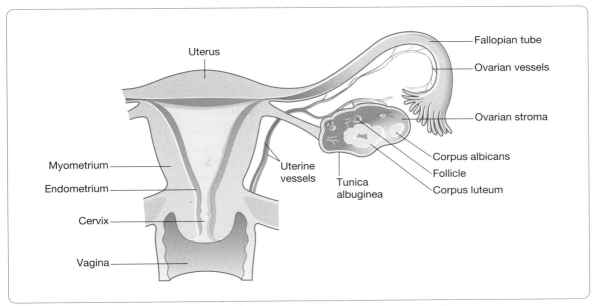

Fig. 17.1 The female reproductive system. (From Page CP, Hoffman BF, Curtis M et al. 2006 Integrated pharmacology. Mosby, Edinburgh. With permission of Mosby.)

Sexual health services have been developed to meet the greatly increased demands placed on them. Many specialities are involved in providing sexual health services, and there needs to be an effective working relationship between genitourinary medicine and family planning services. Changes in lifestyle leading to an increase in the number of sexual partners of both men and women have led to a massive increase in sexually transmitted infections. Early diagnosis, tracing of sexual partners and effective antimicrobial therapy must be made available to all who need this care. The spread of HIV and other blood-borne viral diseases is an increasing cause for concern. In the developed world, retroviral drugs are normally available, but issues relating to the lack of availability of these drugs in some parts of the world where the need is great remain largely unresolved.

Prescribing in pregnancy requires careful consideration on a case-by-case basis. Although drugs are given in pregnancy for the benefit of the mother, drugs can pass to the fetus via the placenta. The aim must be to eliminate any risk of structural or functional damage to the fetal organs.

Nurses and all those involved in the care of patients with genitourinary tract disorders need to be aware of the need to work in an effective and coordinated way. Many disorders of the genitourinary tract have causes that can be ameliorated by sensible changes in lifestyle.

These need to be put in place sooner rather than later if long-term consequences are to be avoided.

OBSTETRICS AND GYNAECOLOGY

ANATOMY AND PHYSIOLOGY

The female reproductive system consists of two ovaries, two fallopian/uterine tubes, the uterus, the vagina and external genitalia (Fig. 17.1). The ovary contains ovarian follicles, each of which contains an ovum. Under the influence of the gonadotrophic hormones, follicle-stimulating hormone and luteinising hormone from the pituitary, the ovarian hormones oestrogen and progesterone, respectively, are produced. If the ovum is fertilised, it embeds itself in the uterine wall, where it grows and develops into an embryo; if not, the corpus luteum degenerates, menstruation follows and the cycle begins again. Oestrogen is secreted in the first phase of the cycle and prepares the reproductive system for possible pregnancy; progesterone is produced if the ovum is not fertilised and is produced in the second (secretory) phase of the cycle. Hormonal control of the female reproductive system is complex and depends on a hormonal inter-relationship that is illustrated in Figure 17.2.

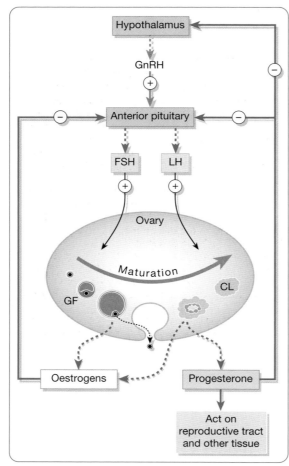

Fig. 17.2 Hormonal control of the female reproductive system. CL, corpus luteum; FSH, follicle-stimulating hormone; GF, Graafian follicle; GnRH, gonadotrophin-releasing hormone; LH, luteinising hormone. (From Rang HP, Dale MM, Ritter JM et al. 2003 Pharmacology. Churchill Livingstone, Edinburgh. With permission of Elsevier Ltd.)

DRUGS USED IN OBSTETRICS

The main drugs used in obstetrics are the oxytocics and the prostaglandins. These drugs are used to induce abortion, induce or augment labour and minimise blood loss. A summary of the main products is given in Table 17.1 and Boxes 17.1 and 17.2. All these drugs act by inducing uterine contractions. Such contractions are accompanied by pain, depending on the strength of the contractions induced. Whenever these drugs

are used, the importance of monitoring fetal health cannot be overemphasised.

Drugs are also used to postpone premature labour and are used to reduce harm to the child. The delay can be used to administer therapy or take measures designed to improve perinatal health. The drugs used are outlined in Table 17.2.

PREMATURE LABOUR

β_2-adrenoceptor stimulants are used in uncomplicated premature labour to inhibit premature delivery. Following successful preventive therapy, oral therapy may be used for maintenance of the situation. The drugs available have significant side effects, and there are potential drug interactions. The oxytocin receptor antagonist antobisan has fewer side effects and may be preferred to the β_2 agonists.

HORMONAL CONTRACEPTION

ORAL CONTRACEPTIVES

Oral contraception has proved to be a very acceptable and convenient method of contraception for many women. Despite some problems and contraindications, well-managed hormonal contraception is relatively safe and highly effective. Two basic types of routine oral contraceptive products are available: a combined pill containing both an oestrogen and a progestogen, and a progestogen-only pill (Table 17.3). Hormonal emergency oral contraception may be required for women who have had unprotected intercourse or experienced failure of a contraceptive barrier device (Table 17.4). The key points relating to the prescribing and contraindications of oral contraceptives are summarised in the tables.

MODE OF ACTION OF ORAL CONTRACEPTIVES

The mode of action of the oral contraceptives is mainly based on the joint actions of oestrogen and progestogen. Oestrogen inhibits secretion of follicle-stimulating hormone and thus suppresses the development of the ovarian follicle. Progestogen inhibits luteinising hormone secretion and thus prevents ovulation. Progestogen has an action on the cervical mucus, making it less suitable for the passage of sperm. Together, oestrogen and progestogen act to discourage implantation. Fertilisation and implantation are also inhibited by interference with the coordinated contraction of the cervix, uterus and fallopian tubes.

Table 17.1 Prostaglandins

Product	Main indications
Carboprost	Used for the treatment of postpartum haemorrhage when the patient is unresponsive to ergometrine and oxytocin. It is given by deep IM injection 250 micrograms, repeated if necessary at intervals of $1\frac{1}{2}$ h. Total dose should not exceed 2 mg (8×250 micrograms). The side-effects include gastrointestinal effects, bronchospasm, respiratory disturbances and pain at injection site.
Dinoprostone	Available as vaginal tablets, pessaries and gel for the induction of labour. Care must be taken to use the correct product, as the gel and vaginal tablet are not bioequivalent. Doses: pessary 5 mg over 12 h; vaginal gel 1 mg followed by 1–2 mg after 6 h. The injection is seldom used. The side-effects are similar to those of other prostaglandins.
Gemeprost	Induction of abortion. By vaginal pessary – the dose will depend on the procedure being undertaken and the stage of pregnancy. A dose of 1–3 mg softens and dilates the cervix, which facilitates surgical procedures. In second-trimester abortion, 1 mg every 3 h for five administrations. A second course 24 h after the start of the first treatment may be given. In second-trimester uterine death, 1 mg is given every 3 h up to a maximum of 5 mg. Side-effects include vaginal bleeding; uterine pain; central nervous system, respiratory and flu-like symptoms; and cardiovascular disturbances. Mifepristone, an antiprogestogenic steroid, sensitises the myometrium to prostaglandin-induced contractions, and it softens and dilates the cervix. It is given in a dose of 200–600 mg orally prior to the gemeprost.

[a]These are potent drugs with significant side-effects. Please consult specialist literature for further information on the use of these important drugs.

Box 17.1 Actions and uses of oxytocin

Main actions

Oxytocin is a hormone that regulates myometrial activity. Oxytocin contracts the uterus. Oestrogen sensitises the oxytocin receptors. At term, the uterus is highly sensitive to oxytocin. The amplitude and frequency of the contractions depend on dose. In low-dose infusion, the uterus relaxes completely between doses. At higher doses, there is an increased frequency of contractions. Higher doses can cause sustained contractions, with the risk of fetal distress or death.

Oxytocin has other actions, including contraction of the myothelial cells in the mammary gland, a vasodilator action that may cause hypotension and a weak antidiuretic action that may cause water retention. Patients with renal or cardiac disease may be especially at risk from side effects of oxytocin.

Clinical outline of applications

- Administration. By intramuscular or intravenous route. Normally by intravenous infusion. Oxytocin is inactivated by an enzyme (oxytocinase).

- Contraindications. When there is a mechanical obstruction to delivery or fetal distress, and in the presence of severe cardiac disease, pre-eclamptic toxaemia and other conditions (see specialist literature). Careful uterine and fetal monitoring is essential. In the presence of fetal distress, the infusion is discontinued.

- Induction of labour. Intravenous infusion, maximum 5 units/day.

- Caesarean section. Slow, intravenously, immediately after delivery, 5 units. A similar dose is used to prevent postpartum haemorrhage. It may be necessary to give a slow intravenous infusion of 5–30 units in 500 mL in severe cases.

- Oxytocin is also used in combination with ergometrine (see Box 17.2).

Box 17.2 Actions and uses of ergometrine maleate

Main actions
Ergometrine contracts the uterus, being especially active on an inappropriately relaxed uterus. Strong contractions are induced, which reduce bleeding from the raw surface of the placental bed. It has a vasoconstrictive action, having actions on the α adrenoreceptors and serotonin receptors.

Note: great care must be taken to distinguish ergometrine from ergotamine.

Outline of clinical applications
- Postpartum haemorrhage: 250–500 micrograms by intravenous injection. This dose is given between 5 and 10 units of oxytocin intravenously and an infusion of oxytocin of 5–30 units in 500 mL of fluid. The infusion is regulated to control uterine atony.
- For the routine management of the third stage of labour: a concentration of ergometrine (500 micrograms) and oxytocin 5 units is used intramuscularly.

At all stages of labour, the importance of careful monitoring cannot be overstated. The use of drugs that contract the uterus is highly specialised, and the above is for general guidance only.

The side-effects of ergometrine are potentially serious and include nausea, vomiting, central nervous system symptoms, cardiac disturbances, vasoconstriction, stroke and myocardial infarction.

MENSTRUAL PROBLEMS

AMENORRHOEA

Primary amenorrhoea (the failure to establish menstruation) occurs in 0.3% of women. Secondary amenorrhoea (the absence of menstruation for 6 consecutive months in a woman who has previously had regular periods) occurs in 3% of women (Khalaf 2003).

Numerous underlying conditions may explain the occurrence of these conditions. Congenital anatomical and hormonal abnormalities must first be excluded.

Lack of oestrogen produces features similar to the menopause, and oestrogen replacement therapy may be useful in making the woman feel more comfortable. In those who wish to become fertile, clomifene 50 mg daily is used. Patients taking clomifene should be monitored for signs of ovulation, ovarian enlargement and pregnancy. The drug should not be used in pregnancy.

DYSMENORRHOEA

Lower abdominal pelvic pain radiating to the back or thighs that occurs before or during menstruation is well known to women of reproductive age and accounts for much incapacity (Auld and Sinha 2004). This pain, in the absence of any obvious underlying disease, is known as primary dysmenorrhoea; secondary dysmenorrhoea results from some underlying cause, either congenital or endometriosis.

Table 17.2 Drugs used in the management of premature labour

Drug	Mode of action	Dose and notes
Antobisan	Oxytocin receptor antagonist	IV 6.75 mg over 1 min. Then used to delay labour in uncomplicated premature labour between 24 and 33 weeks of gestation. This drug may be preferred to the β_2 agonists, because cardiovascular problems are fewer.
Nifedipine (unlicensed indication; see p. 211)	Calcium-channel blocker	20 mg initially, then 10–20 mg three or four times daily according to response. May have fewer side-effects than β_2 agonists.
Ritodrine hydrochloride	β_2 agonist (see p. 144)	Given by IV infusion, initially 50 micrograms/min every 10 min (see specialist literature). The side-effects of this drug, especially on the cardiovascular system, are potentially serious. It is essential to avoid fluid overload.
Salbutamol Terbutaline	β_2 agonist β_2 agonist	Similar indications to the above (uncomplicated premature labour). Also similar side-effects. See specialist literature.

Table 17.3 Hormonal contraception

Product, strength and dose	Notes and precautions
Low oral Ethinylestradiol 20 micrograms with norethisterone 1 mg. Ethinylestradiol 20 micrograms with desogestrol 150 micrograms. One tablet daily for 21 days, repeated after a 7-day tablet-free interval.	With these products, withdrawal bleeding occurs in the tablet-free interval. With *all* oral contraceptives, care must be taken to evaluate the risk factors for venous thromboembolism and arterial disease. Smoking is to be avoided. Side-effects such as nausea and vomiting, headache, breast tenderness, body weight changes, water retention and thrombosis may occur (see specialist literature). Worsening of migraine may be a reason for discontinuation of a combined oral contraceptive. Oestrogen-containing contraceptives should be discontinued 4 weeks before major elective surgery (suitable alternative contraceptive device should be used). Great care is needed if the surgery involves prolonged immobilisation (see specialist literature). Changing from one combination to another requires care and full cooperation of the patient (see specialist literature).
Oral Progestogen-only contraceptives. A range of products is available, for example containing: • desogestrel 350 micrograms • norethisterone 350 micrograms • levonorgestrel 30 micrograms.	These products are useful when oestrogens are contraindicated (in patients with a history of venous thrombosis; older women; smokers; those with cardiac disease, diabetes mellitus and menstrual irregularities). The progestogen-only contraceptives are less reliable than the combined oral contraceptive. Side-effects include menstrual irregularities, nausea, vomiting, headache, dizziness, weight changes and changes in libido
Parenteral Progestogen-only contraceptives include: • medroxyprogesterone acetate 150 mg (aqueous suspension) deep IM • norethisterone enantate (200 mg/mL oily) deep IM • implant containing 68 mg of etonogestrel. See specialist literature for details of doses, etc.	These are long-acting products that provide contraception for some weeks, and in the case of the implant the effect lasts for up to 3 years. In women with a certain body mass index, lower blood concentrations of etonogestrel are present. The implant may provide effective contraception for only 2 years. Medroxyprogesterone carries risks of reduction in bone mineral density. Osteoporotic fractures have been reported.
Low Transdermal patches containing ethinylestradiol and norelgestromin. The patches are designed to release the active ingredients at a controlled rate. One patch is applied weekly for 3 weeks, followed by a 7-day patch-free interval.	Useful in women who have a history of poor compliance with oral therapy. Withdrawal bleeding occurs during the patch-free interval.
Standard The combinations available are: • ethinylestradiol with levonorgestrel • ethinylestradiol with norethisterone • ethinylestradiol with norgestimate • ethinylestradiol with desogestrel • ethinylestradiol with disirenone • ethinylestradiol with gestodene. The dose range is the same, i.e. one tablet daily for 21 days followed by a tablet-free interval of 7 days.	A range of different strengths is available (see British National Formulary for details). If starting on day 4 of the cycle or later, additional contraceptive precautions must be taken (barrier method). The dosage regimen is the same, i.e. one tablet daily for interval of 7 days. Some products have 'dummy' (inactive) tablets to be taken during the 7-day intervals. This may aid compliance, because there are no 'tablet-free' days. The regimen is normally started on day 1 of the cycle.

Table 17.4   Emergency contraception

Product, strength and dose	Notes and side-effects
Levonorgestrel 1.5-mg tablet A single dose of 1.5 mg is given as soon as possible after coitus. The ideal time is within 12 h but no later than 72 h.	This product can be sold by pharmacists without prescription and in accordance with Royal Pharmaceutical Society of Great Britain guidelines. The 'morning after' pill is widely used but should be regarded as an emergency measure and in no way as a substitute for basic contraceptive measures. Side-effects include nausea, low abdominal pain, fatigue, headache, breast tenderness and vomiting. It is important that when supplying the product (on prescription or otherwise), suitable advice and guidance be given to the woman on such aspects as changes in period dates and the need to use a barrier method of contraception until the next period. If lower abdominal pain occurs, medical advice should be sought without delay, as this could indicate ectopic pregnancy. Enzyme-inducing drugs (see p. 133) can reduce the effectiveness of the hormonal method of emergency contraception.

Many women will endure the discomfort and resort to mild analgesics only when necessary. Those whose lives are disrupted by the pain, sometimes for as long as 3 days every month, will require thorough investigation.

INFERTILITY TREATMENT

Infertility treatments have been developed during the past 20 years to enable a very high level of success to be achieved. All treatment programmes must be preceded by a full investigation of both partners. Problems identified in the male partner must be referred to a urologist or an endocrinologist. For the female partner, a number of baseline hormonal levels are determined (progesterone, prolactin, oestradiol, follicle-stimulating hormone and luteinising hormone). Having determined these levels, it is then necessary to decide on the ovarian stimulation regimen. Screening for viruses such as rubella, hepatitis B and HIV is normally carried out. Common infections such as chlamydia are also screened for. Ultrasound scans are used to identify problems such as fibroids, polyps, or ovarian cysts.

Laparoscopic assessment of disease of the ovaries is also carried out as required. Counselling of both partners is an integral part of the treatment, but a key factor in success or otherwise is the woman's age and her ovarian age as determined by the hormone level measurements. Clomifene and tamoxifen (antioestrogens) are used in the treatment of female infertility due to oligomenorrhoea (see specialist literature).

HORMONE REPLACEMENT THERAPY

The distressing symptoms arising from the hormonal changes associated with the menopause can be alleviated with hormone replacement therapy (HRT). Menopausal symptoms include hot flushes, night sweats, sleep disturbances, mood changes, joint aches and pains, and genitourinary problems. Menopausal women, especially those with work and domestic responsibilities, will benefit significantly from HRT. Postmenopausal osteoporosis (see p. 334) is also treated with HRT. HRT does have detractors, who rightly highlight the risks involved. HRT involves therapy with a small dose of an oestrogen with a progestogen for women with an intact uterus. The progestogen is needed to reduce the risk of cystic hyperplasia and similar complications. The benefits of treatment of menopausal symptoms are significant, but it is generally felt that treatment should be short term. Risks identified include endometrial and breast cancer, venous thromboembolism and stroke (see specialist literature).

Hormone replacement therapy, like all the therapies using sex hormones, must be carefully managed on an individual basis taking into account the balance between risk and benefit. The British National Formulary (BNF) contains important information on such aspects as the need to stop HRT 4–6 weeks before surgery (risk of venous thromboembolism).

Preparations for use in HRT include patches containing estradiol and tablets containing various combinations of estradiol and a progestogen. Implants (estradiol), a nasal spray and a topical gel are also available. If the patient cannot tolerate hormonal therapy (or other reasons preclude hormonal therapy), alternatives may be suitable, such as clonidine or venlafaxine. The value of these treatments lies in the ability to reduce hot flushes. However, side-effects of these treatments (cardiotoxicity) may preclude their use.

Tibolone is a compound that has oestrogenic, progestogenic and weak androgenic activity. It is used to treat postmenopausal symptoms and osteoporosis (dose 2.5 mg daily). Side-effects include weight changes, dizziness, nausea and abdominal pain.

ENDOMETRIOSIS

Endometriosis is regarded as a puzzling condition that creates problems for both GPs and specialists. Essentially, the condition can be defined as the presence of endometrial tissue at ectopic sites, which may be at a number of sites in the abdomen. The causes of the condition are not fully understood, but a genetic disposition has been confirmed. A factor of significance is the role of endogenous oestrogens. The condition affects mainly women in their thirties and forties, but it can affect women at any time during their reproductive years. No major racial or class factors have been identified. Endometriosis is associated with premenstrual soiling and infertility. The condition often presents as dysmenorrhoea and pelvic pain. Where extrapelvic sites are involved, there may be soreness, swelling and bleeding.

Treatment options include the improvement of fertility and pain relief. Surgery may be indicated if medical therapy fails. Hormonal treatments are also used and have additional contraceptive effects. If a woman is trying to achieve a pregnancy, dydrogesterone may relieve symptoms without reducing fertility. In the treatment of endometriosis, there is clearly a major risk–benefit aspect to be considered, especially when treating subfertile women suffering from a debilitating condition. Medical management should not be used in the asymptomatic or infertile patient. Where drug therapy is indicated, the following drugs may be useful:

- progestogens (e.g. norethisterone)
- gonadotrophin release inhibitors
- gonadotrophin-releasing hormones
- goserelin (by implantation)
- danazol, which acts by inhibiting pituitary gonadotrophins; it also has androgenic activity with antioestrogenic and antiprogestogenic activity
- gestrinone, which is similar to danazol, having an antiprogestogen action.

For the relief of pain associated with endometriosis, non-steroidal anti-inflammatory drugs are useful.

ADMINISTRATION OF VULVAL AND VAGINAL MEDICATIONS

The treatments are mainly used to treat menopausal atrophic vaginitis and infections (see Ch. 15). Locally applied oestrogens, in the form of a cream, vaginal tablets or an impregnated vaginal ring, are used. Systemic oestrogens are not used, owing to the hazards associated with their use (endometrial hyperplasia and carcinoma; see BNF for details).

Gynaecological conditions are judged by many women to be a source of extreme embarrassment and fear. Patients express these feelings in different ways. Some are hesitant to ask for further explanation of their condition or treatment, showing a natural reservation about intimate matters. Others fear being thought of as unclean, embarrassed by odour, itching and perhaps staining of underclothes from vaginal discharge. Patients may fear discovery of a malignant condition or that they have developed an infection that has been sexually transmitted. Knowledge of anatomy and physiology of the female genital tract in some instances may be scant, and attitudes to bodily functions may have been influenced by folklore.

Nurses working in gynaecological wards and clinics become accustomed to carrying out intimate procedures and discussing very personal issues with their patients. Sensitivity to the feelings of each new patient is important. General ward nurses and district nurses are required to care for patients with gynaecological disorders from time to time and must be ready to turn their attention to the special needs of these patients.

In all cases, embarrassment or attitude on the part of the nurse should never be allowed to interfere with establishing and dealing with the full nature of the problem. Tact, patience and gentleness are essential at all times.

Vulval and vaginal preparations that contain a drug should be prescribed, administered and recorded according to local policy. The genital area should be clean, and traces of previously applied cream should

---

Box 17.3 Insertion of vaginal pessaries

Documentation
- Prescribing and recording sheet

The medicine
- Pessary as ordered, with applicator

The environment
- Privacy, warmth, comfort

The nurse and the patient
- Patient identified
- Patient given explanation of what is involved and advised to empty bladder
- Patient assisted if necessary into supine position, with knees flexed and thighs abducted, or left lateral position with buttocks at edge of bed

Technique
- Nurse attends to own hand hygiene and applies disposable gloves
- Pessary inserted, using applicator, as high as possible along posterior vaginal wall in an upwards and backwards direction for the full length of the vagina
- Patient's vulval area wiped dry and sanitary pad applied to prevent staining of clothes (tampons should not be used in the presence of infection)
- Applicator washed in warm, soapy water, rinsed and dried

Hazards
- Pessary can easily be dislodged and so is best inserted on retiring to bed

---

be removed. Whenever possible, the patient should apply the preparation herself. Nurses must guarantee privacy for patients, whether they are explaining self-administration or actually carrying out the treatment. It is important to explain to which particular area the treatment is to be directed, the recommended times of administration and the need to complete the course. Disposable gloves should be worn by the nurse when administering vulval and vaginal preparations, to protect the patient and nurse from acquiring infection or the nurse from absorbing any of the medication. Whether nurse or patient carries out the procedure, the hands should be washed before and after. Applicators should be washed in warm soapy water, rinsed and dried. A separate treatment kit should be assigned to the individual patient (Box 17.3).

URINARY TRACT DISORDERS

INTRODUCTION

It is important to note that while drug treatment plays an important role in treating disorders of the genitourinary tract, a combination of treatment strategies may be required. Surgery and/or the use of various appliances may be required in addition to drug therapy. The skills of specialist nurses are increasingly used in the care of patients with urinary problems.

Products used following surgical procedures on the genitourinary tract and other irrigations appear in Table 17.5. Conditions for which patients may derive benefit from drug therapy are discussed below.

ANATOMY AND PHYSIOLOGY

Following production by the kidneys, urine is conveyed via the two ureters to the bladder through a tunnel that functions as a valve to prevent backflow. The bladder serves as a collection and temporary storage organ for urine before it is discharged via the urethra. The middle layer of the ureters and the bladder consists of muscle fibres that assist in propulsion and expulsion of urine. The bladder is capable of considerable distension. The urethra is the passage for elimination of urine and, in the male, semen. It too has a muscular layer with an internal sphincter under autonomic control and an external sphincter under voluntary control. The prostate gland is located underneath the bladder. It usually enlarges with age and as a result interferes with the flow of urine.

URINARY INCONTINENCE

Urinary incontinence in adults is a common condition that may significantly damage the person's quality of life. Following careful assessment and accurate diagnosis, both drug and non-drug treatment can be very valuable. Non-drug treatment will not be considered here but is often a vital part of patient care.

Urinary incontinence in women arises because of detrusor instability and stress incontinence. In men, urinary incontinence is less common. Causes include detrusor instability and bladder disorders. The presence of infection should always be excluded.

BENIGN PROSTATIC HYPERPLASIA

Benign prostatic hyperplasia (BPH) is a common disease in older men. Figure 17.3 shows the position

Table 17.5 Sterile solutions used for bladder irrigation catheter patency*

Name	Strength[a]/composition	Pack or presentation	Uses, indications and precautions
Amphotericin	50 micrograms/mL	50-mg vial (powder) made up before use into a solution	Fungal infections.
Chlorhexidine*	1 in 5000 (0.02%)	100-mL Uro-Tainer (other pack sizes are available)	Used for its mechanical effect. Also has a bacteriostatic action on organisms commonly found in the urinary tract. Inactive against *Pseudomonas* species.
Glycine	1.5%	3-L plastic bag	Used in transurethral resection of the prostate gland. Non-haemolytic, weakly ionised. Any glycine absorbed is metabolised; ammonia may be produced, which has toxic effects. Cases of hyponatraemia have been reported, but these are rare.
Sodium chloride*	0.9%	500-mL or 3-L plastic bag	Used for its mechanical effect. It is also used as a vehicle for certain drugs instilled into the bladder.
Sodium citrate	3%	500 mL	Used primarily for the dissolution of blood clots.
Solution G (Suby G)	3.23% citric acid, other ingredients (see BNF)	100-mL Uro-Tainer	Use between twice daily and twice weekly to prevent the formation of encrustations. Should not be used for a period of 10–14 days following prostatic surgery, owing to absorption of salts, leading to electrolyte imbalance.
Solution R*	6% citric acid, 0.6% glucono-lactone, 2.8% magnesium carbonate, 0.01% disodium edetate	100-mL Uro-Tainer	Used to dissolve existing catheter encrustations. Use between twice and four times a week for 2 weeks, before reverting to solution G. Should not be used for a period of 10–14 days following prostatic surgery, owing to absorption of salts, leading to electrolyte imbalance.

[a]All percentages given are w/v.

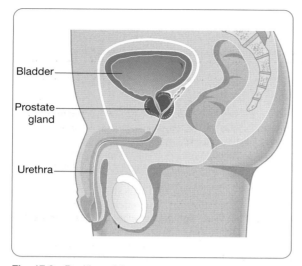

Bladder

Prostate
gland

Urethra

Fig. 17.3   Position of the prostate gland.

of the prostate gland. Autopsy studies have shown histological evidence of BPH in 50% of 51- to 60-year-olds, increasing to 90% in 85-year-olds (Taylor et al. 2004). The condition presents with frequency, urge incontinence and poor urinary stream. The treatment is based on selective alpha-adrenoceptor antagonists (alpha-blockers) that relax the smooth muscles of the bladder neck and prostate. Bladder outlet resistance is decreased and urinary flow is facilitated.

Drugs that inhibit the enzyme 5-α-reductase, which metabolises testosterone into the more potent androgen dihydrotestosterone, are also available for the treatment of BPH. Dutasteride 500 micrograms and finasteride 5 mg are given daily (orally) on a long-term basis. Urinary flow is improved as the prostate is reduced in size. Six months' treatment may be needed before a benefit is achieved. A combination of both a selective α antagonist and a 5-α-reductase inhibitor may be required if the gland is grossly enlarged.

The drugs used to treat BPH are summarised in Table 17.6.

URINARY RETENTION

Acute urinary retention results from prostatic obstruction or urethral stricture. In women, a possible cause is meatal stenosis. Catheterisation may be required to reduce the risk of renal damage (see Ch. 18). Given that the treatment of urinary frequency involves the use of antimuscarinic (atropine-like) drugs, it follows that the treatment of urinary retention may involve the use of parasympathomimetics for their muscarinic effects (see p. 145). Parasympathomimetics

used include carbachol and bethanechol (now seldom used). Catheterisation is preferred. These drugs have potentially dangerous side effects, such as bradycardia and intestinal colic. Patients with asthma or susceptibility to asthmatic attacks must not be treated with parasympathomimetic drugs, owing to the danger of precipitating an acute episode of bronchoconstriction (see p. 142).

Another parasympathomimetic is distigmine, which is given orally (5 mg half an hour before breakfast) or by intramuscular injection 500 micrograms 12 h after surgery to prevent urinary retention. This drug acts by inhibiting the breakdown of acetylcholine (anticholinesterase; see p. 145). Distigmine is a long-acting drug and should be used with care, especially after surgery, particularly when bowel anastomosis has been carried out.

DRUG TREATMENT OF URINARY INCONTINENCE

Drug treatment for incontinence in adults is usually managed by a combination of drug therapy and physical means, such as pelvic floor exercises and bladder training. Stress incontinence may be managed by non-drug methods. The addition, however, of a drug such as duloxetine may be beneficial. Antimuscarinic drugs (see p. 145) may be useful but must be avoided in patients with certain conditions, notably myasthenia gravis, angle closure glaucoma, bladder obstruction and gastrointestinal conditions such as ulcerative colitis and gastrointestinal obstruction. The main drugs used are summarised in Table 17.7.

ERECTILE DYSFUNCTION

Reasons for failure to produce a satisfactory erection include psychogenic, vascular, neurogenic and endocrine abnormalities. Many drugs are also liable to induce impotence. Drugs for the treatment of erectile dysfunction may be prescribed on the NHS only in accordance with official guidelines (see BNF).

Alprostadil is a prostaglandin given by intra-cavernosal injection for the management of erectile dysfunction. The first dose must be given by medically trained personnel. Self-administration may be undertaken only after proper training. The first dose is 2.5 micrograms, which is increased depending on response in steps of 5–10 micrograms to obtain a dose suitable for producing an erection lasting not more than an hour. Patients should be instructed to report an erection lasting more than 4 h, which may require treatment by aspiration initially and, if unsuccessful, cautious intracavernosal injection of a sympathomimetic drug (e.g. phenylephrine) with

Table 17.6   Drugs used in benign prostatic hyperplasia

Drug (action)	Dose	Notes
Alfuzosin (selective alpha-blocker)	2.5 mg three times daily	As with all these drugs, when treating older patients the lowest possible dose should be used.
Doxazosin (selective alpha-blocker)	1 mg daily	Possibility of hyposensive effect. Must be considered carefully, especially in older patients and/or those taking antihypertensive therapy.
Dutasteride (inhibitor of 5-α-reductase)	500 micrograms daily	May require 6 months' treatment to achieve a benefit.
Finasteride (inhibitor of 5-α-reductase)	5 mg daily	As above. A low-strength preparation is available to treat male pattern baldness. These drugs should not be prescribed until a diagnosis of benign prostatic hyperplasia has been made, because the drugs increase the concentration of prostate-specific antigen (a marker for prostate cancer). Side effects include impotence, decreased libido and ejaculation disorders.
Indoramin (selective alpha-blocker)	20 mg twice daily, increasing by 20 mg every 2 weeks to 100 mg daily in divided doses; 20 mg at night may be adequate for an older patient	Renal and hepatic impairment may be contraindicated to the use of these drugs.
Prazosin (selective alpha-blocker)	500 micrograms twice daily for 3–7 days, adjusting according to response	Side-effects include hypotension, gastrointestinal tract disturbances, erectile disorders, cardiovascular system side effects and hypersensitivity reactions.
Tamsulosin (selective alpha-blocker)	400 micrograms as a single dose	–
Terazosin (selective alpha-blocker)	1 mg at bedtime, slowly adjusting to 5–10 mg daily	–

action on α-adrenergic receptors (see p. 144). If such a drug is used, cardiovascular monitoring may be required. The side-effects of alprostadil include penile pain, prolonged erection and reactions at the injection site. A urethral gel of alprostadil is also available. The injection of papaverine into the corpus cavernosum has been used as a treatment for erectile dysfunction, but its use is not licensed. Alprostadil, sildenafil and related drugs are the main drug treatments of erectile dysfunction. Careful physical examination must be undertaken before any treatment for erectile dysfunction is initiated, because the side-effects are a cause of concern, especially in patients with cardiovascular disease.

Sildenafil, the first oral treatment for erectile dysfunction, is available for the treatment of erectile dysfunction in men. The dose is 50 mg 1 h before sexual activity. Subsequent doses should be adjusted according to response. The maximum single dose is 100 mg in a 24-h period. There are a number of contraindications to the use of this drug, especially cardiovascular disease and deformation of the penis. Tadalafil and vardenafil are similar drugs. Apomorphine, given as a sublingual tablet (dose 2–3 mg) is another treatment for erectile dysfunction.

URINARY TRACT INFECTIONS

Most infections of the genitourinary tract are treated with systemic antibiotics (see p. 298). In certain conditions, local instillation of antimicrobial agents may be used but are of limited value. Bladder instillations (irrigations or washouts) are of some

Table 17.7 Drugs used in urinary incontinence and frequency

Drug	Dose and route	Notes and cautions
Duloxetine (inhibition of serotinin and noradrenaline [norepinephrine] uptake)	Moderate/severe stress incontinence: 40 mg twice daily orally, reducing to 20 mg twice daily depending on side-effects.	Cautions include cardiovascular diseases, raised intraocular pressure and bleeding disorders. Hepatic impairment is a contraindication, as is pregnancy and breast feeding. Side-effects are varied. Gastrointestinal tract and central nervous system symptoms predominate. Care should be taken if considering prescribing this drug for patients with a history of depression or suicidal thoughts.
Flavoxate hydrochloride (selective urinary tract spasmodic)	Frequency, incontinence, dysuria, urgency, nocturia: 200 mg three times daily orally.	Less side-effects than duloxetine but similar cautions etc. apply. Because the drug is an antispasmodic, it must be avoided in patients with glaucoma.
Oxybutinin hydrochloride (urinary smooth muscle relaxant)	Frequency and incontinence, neurogenic bladder instability: 2.5–5 mg two or three times daily, increasing to 5 mg four times daily. Reduced dose for older patients. A modified-release form is available as is a transdermal patch.	The patch or modified-release form may reduce side-effects that may limit the use of this drug in some patients.
Propantheline bromide	Adult enuresis: 15 mg three times daily.	An antimuscarinic drug. Cautions apply.
Propiverine hydrochloride	Frequency, urgency, incontinence and neurogenic bladder instability: 15 mg three daily.	See above.
Solifenacin succinate	Frequency, urgency and urge incontinence: 5 mg daily increasing to 10 mg daily.	See above.
Tolterodine tartrate	Frequency, urgency and incontinence: 2 mg twice daily, reducing to 1 mg twice daily to reduce side-effects.	See above.
Trospium chloride	Frequency, urgency and incontinence: 20 mg twice daily before food.	See above.

value, but risks of cross-infection, poor antimicrobial action and local irritancy limit their use. Whenever possible, systemic therapy, based on the results of microbial sensitivity tests, is preferable.

HAEMATURIA

Blood in the urine should always be a matter of concern and be thoroughly investigated to exclude malignancy or other serious conditions (Box 17.4).

MALIGNANT DISEASE OF THE URINARY TRACT (SEE CH. 19)

Instillation of locally acting cytotoxic drugs may be indicated in the treatment of superficial bladder tumours. Doxorubicin, epirubicin, mitomycin and

Box 17.4 Causes of haematuria

In the kidney
- Cysts
- Tumour
- Vascular malformation
- Glomerular disease
- Inflammatory disease
- Degenerative disease
- Interstitial disease
- Infarction
- Clotting disorders

In the ureter
- Tumour
- Ureteric calculi

In the bladder
- Infection
- Tumour

In the urethra
- Trauma

thiotepa are used, made up in sterile water or sodium chloride solution. Any evidence of absorption must be taken into account in selecting the concentration of drug in the irrigating fluid and the period of treatment.

PAIN IN THE URINARY TRACT

Pain in the urinary tract may be due to a number of conditions. The acute pain of ureteric colic is treated with pethidine or diclofenac (see p. 517). Lidocaine chlorhexidine in the form of a 1% or 2% gel may be useful for urethral pain and prior to male and female catheterisation. Discomfort caused by cystitis may be relieved by alkalinisation of the urine using potassium citrate or sodium bicarbonate. Hyperkalaemia and hypernatraemia are possible side effects of this treatment. Pain due to metabolites of the cytotoxic drugs cyclophosphamide and ifosamide can be relieved using mesna. In prescribing for patients experiencing urinary tract pain, care should be taken to establish if the patient is using an over-the-counter medicine that may contain potassium citrate.

ADMINISTRATION OF MEDICATIONS INTO THE BLADDER

The main reasons for instilling medication into the bladder are the treatment of bladder infection,

dissolution of blood clots, and the treatment and prevention of bladder cancer.

BLADDER INFECTION

Indwelling catheters, even when introduced into the bladder under the most rigorous aseptic conditions, are an important source of urinary tract infection. In the course of time, crystallisation and debris around and within the eye of the lumen of the catheter further increase the risk of infection by obstructing the flow and causing stasis of urine. Bypassing of urine then follows, leading to discomfort, embarrassment and skin breakdown.

Depending on the organism being treated, chlorhexidine or sodium chloride solution 0.9% may be used. For fungal infections, amphotericin may be used.

DISSOLUTION OF BLOOD CLOTS

Patients who produce haematuric urine can also develop severe drainage problems and discomfort, especially when the catheter is blocked by blood clots. Clot retention is usually treated by irrigation with sterile sodium chloride solution (0.9% w/v), although, when clots prove to be obstinate, alternative methods of irrigation may have to be employed. Sterile sodium citrate solution 3% may also be used to break up clots.

METHODS USED FOR BLADDER IRRIGATION OR INSTILLATION

The methods most commonly used for introducing fluid into the bladder are:

- intermittent, either using an irrigation device such as the Uro-Tainer or by mechanical irrigation using a form of suction
- continuous.

The method used will depend on the reason for carrying out the irrigation or instillation.

INTERMITTENT IRRIGATION (Box 17.5)
THE URO-TAINER SYSTEM
This ready to use irrigation device involves a simple technique that is quick and can be mastered by patients or their relatives for use at home. A range of solutions for maintaining patency of a catheter is available.

- Sodium chloride solution 0.9% may be all that is needed for the management of infection.
- Aqueous chlorhexidine solution (0.02% w/v) has a bacteriostatic action against many of the common

---

> **Box 17.5** Intermittent bladder irrigation
>
> **Documentation**
> - Standard prescribing and recording sheet
> - Fluid balance chart
>
> **The medicine**
> - Sterile irrigating solution in either Uro-Tainer or 500-mL bag
> - Solution as prescribed, visibly clear and at room temperature
>
> **The environment**
> - As for any aseptic procedure
> - Privacy
>
> **The nurse and the patient**
> - Patient identified as corresponding to prescription
> - Explanation as to what is involved
> - Patient assisted into relaxed position with only catheter exposed; patient kept warm
> - Clothes and bedding protected
> - Patient made comfortable on completion of procedure
>
> **Technique**
> - Aseptic (gloves not required with Uro-Tainer)
> - Observation of returned fluid
> - New drainage system attached to catheter after irrigation completed
> - All urine measured and recorded
> - Administration recorded
>
> **Hazards**
> - Infection

urinary tract pathogens, although ineffective against *Pseudomonas* species. Some clinicians recommend routine use of chlorhexidine solution immediately prior to the removal of all urinary catheters. The solution is left in the bladder until such time as the patient wishes to void.

- Solution G is weakly acidic and is used for flushing out and for preventing crystal formation, or for dissolving crystals already formed in the catheter. The volume of solution in each Uro-Tainer is 100 mL, although the amount instilled into the bladder is not critical, rather the time the solution is left in the bladder, which may be up to half an hour. Gloves are not necessary when this method of irrigation is used. However, thorough handwashing is essential, and care must be taken to connect the catheter and irrigation tubing without contaminating them. A regimen in current use for patients with

long-term catheters involves alternate use of a urinary antiseptic, such as chlorhexidine (0.02% w/v), with a decrystallising solution twice a week; for example, one solution every Tuesday, the other every Friday.

MECHANICAL IRRIGATION USING SUCTION

In the event of a catheter becoming completely blocked by blood clots, the catheter may be washed out in an effort to break down the clots by a form of suction using a catheter-tipped syringe and sterile irrigating solution. When blood clots are especially troublesome, a large volume of sterile sodium chloride solution (0.9% w/v) will be required. This method is based on first introducing approximately 50 mL of solution, which is left in the bladder. This acts as a physical buffer to allow further volumes of fluid to be instilled under pressure, then withdrawn by suction through the catheter, depending on the severity of the blockage. The nurse wears gloves for this procedure, because of the many manipulative processes involved. It may take a considerable time until the catheter drains freely. Patients, who may already be in pain and be losing blood into the bladder, can find this a tedious and uncomfortable experience. They should therefore be kept warm and as comfortable as possible. As with all such procedures, the encouragement and support of the nurse are vital throughout. To minimise the deposition associated with long-term catheterisation, consideration should be given to the choice of catheter (latex versus silicone) and it should be changed every 6 weeks.

CONTINUOUS IRRIGATION

Continuous irrigation of the bladder may be employed following prostatic surgery to rid the bladder of blood clots and prostatic debris. A three-way catheter, or alternative combination of catheters, is inserted in theatre. This allows one inlet for inflating the catheter balloon and another for the entry of irrigating solution, and an outlet for drainage of the bladder contents. Sodium chloride solution (0.9% w/v) is introduced into the bladder from a 3-L bag suspended from an infusion stand, via an administration set connected to the catheter. In the immediate postoperative period, the control clamp is left open fully to allow for continuous flushing of the bladder and of the eyes of the catheter. After several hours, depending on the degree of haematuria, the rate may be decreased. Volumes of irrigating solution ranging from 15 to 45 L may be required to treat the patient during the first 24 h. The flow of such large volumes of fluid demands frequent attention by the nurse in maintaining input, discarding output and keeping records of both. In urological wards, anticipating needs and finding adequate storage space for large volumes of irrigation solutions can present problems. To some extent, these may be alleviated by active involvement of the ward pharmacist who can, among other things, help to ensure that supply keeps pace with demand.

It should be remembered that hypertension (resulting from absorption of sodium) and perforation of the bladder may each result from this form of irrigation. Nurses in urology wards have particular responsibility therefore to ensure that close monitoring of the blood pressure and pulse (every half-hour at first), fluid balance and pain is carried out. If the patient complains of pain, no matter how mild, irrigation should not proceed without seeking further advice. While it is important not to alarm junior nursing staff, and hence patients, at this time, the possibility of perforation, especially following transurethral resection of the prostate gland, must never be forgotten.

GENERAL PRINCIPLES OF BLADDER IRRIGATION

When using any form of bladder washout, the broad principles of medicine administration apply. The details of the solution are checked against the prescription and the fluid visually examined before use to make sure that it is free from any particulate matter. Any container whose contents are not clear should be rejected. In view of the high risk to the patient of microbial contamination, all procedures are carried out using a strictly aseptic technique. Ideally, solutions should be warmed to body temperature before use in a solution-warming cabinet. Improvised methods of warming solutions are not recommended, because control of the solution temperature is impossible to achieve. In the absence of a solution-warming cabinet, it is probably best to use the solution at room temperature.

Patients with an indwelling catheter that has been on continuous drainage for weeks or months may have difficulty in tolerating the instillation of volumes of solutions in excess of 50 mL, because of reduced bladder capacity or bladder irritability. When the bladder is irritated by infection or is reduced in capacity by tumour, it may be possible to tolerate only very small volumes of fluid. On occasion, a volume as small as 10 mL is as much as the patient can hold. Infected fluid is never reinjected. When the patient indicates that the bladder feels uncomfortable and as though it cannot take in more fluid, then this must be taken as the maximal amount that can be instilled. As soon as possible following any manipulations of

a catheter, the catheter should be attached to a sterile closed drainage system. The drainage tubing should be stiff enough to reduce the likelihood of kinking, and the drainage bag should be adequately supported on a floor stand positioned for ease of observation of the colour, consistency and volume of urine drained. Bag holders can become distorted, for example when lowering the height of the patient's bed. This increases the risk of the tubing becoming kinked. Also, the drainage tap may come into contact with the floor, with obvious risk of contamination.

Details of sterile solutions used in bladder irrigation and some of the drugs used in bladder instillations are given in Table 17.5.

SELF-ASSESSMENT QUESTIONS

1. Complete the following table.

Pituitary hormone	Ovarian hormone	Uses in obstetrics and gynaecology
Follicle-stimulating hormone		
	Progesterone	

2. A fit 70-year-old gentleman is admitted with acute retention of urine. He is pyrexial and dehydrated. On examination, the prostate is enlarged but smooth. A catheter is passed with difficulty and a leg bag attached. He is prescribed alfuzocin 10 mg daily oral and ciprofloxacin 500 mg twice daily oral and discharged 48 h later. What advice would you give to this patient?

3.a. Urinary retention has been treated with parasympathomimetic drugs (muscarinic agonists). Why is this approach seldom followed today?

b. Name two selective alpha-blockers (antagonists) that are used to treat benign prostatic hyperplasia.

c. Which β_2 agonists are used to treat premature labour.

d. Name two solutions that can be used to maintain catheter patency.

e. Describe a possible side-effect of prolonged irrigation of the bladder with sodium citrate solution.

f. Give two side-effects of finasteride.

g. What drug-based alternatives are available to oral contraception?

REFERENCES

Auld B, Sinha S 2004 Dysmenorrhoea: diagnosis and current management. Prescriber 15:42–55

Khalaf Y 2003 Managing primary and secondary amenorrhoea. Prescriber July:39–42

Taylor C, Foley C, Kirby R 2004 Safe and effective management of BPH in primary care. Prescriber February:30–37

FURTHER READING AND RESOURCES

Barnes J 2005 Herbal medicinal products for treating gynaecological women. Pharmaceutical Journal 275:515–516

Barry MJ, Roehrborn CG 2001 Benign prostatic hyperplasia. British Medical Journal 323:1042–1045

Clark C 2004 Erectile dysfunction and other problems. Pharmaceutical Journal 272:608–610

Clark C 2004 Prostatitis, BPH and prostate cancer. Pharmaceutical Journal 272:511–513

Gulliford G, Bidmead J 2001 Management of incontinence. Pharmaceutical Journal 267:230–232

Lawton V 2003 Management of female urinary incontinence. Prescriber March:38–40

McVeigh E 2004 Today's medical management of endometriosis. Prescriber August:18–22

Shakir SAW, Wilton LV 2001 Cardiovascular events in users of sildenafil: results from first phase of prescription event monitoring in England. British Medical Journal 322:651–652

Speakman MJ, Kirby R 2004 Medical treatment of male lower urinary tract symptoms. Trends in Urology, Gynaecology and Sexual Health Sep–Oct:21–28

Drugs used in kidney diseases

18

CHAPTER CONTENTS

KEY OBJECTIVES

After reading this chapter, you should be able to:

- outline the main functions of the kidney
- name the hormones produced by the kidney
- name the hormones that influence renal activity
- list the main risk factors in the development of renal disease
- describe two conditions other than renal failure that may adversely affect the functioning of the kidneys
- discuss the importance of the control of high blood pressure in patients with renal disease
- discuss the importance of the control of diabetes mellitus in patients with renal disease
- explain the risks to kidney function caused by obstructions in the urinary tract
- outline the essential differences between haemodialysis and continuous ambulatory peritoneal dialysis
- name two drugs that must be taken by patients undergoing haemodialysis.

INTRODUCTION

The kidney has several vitally important functions, including the excretion of waste products and the maintenance of fluid and electrolyte balance. In addition, the kidney is an important producer of hormones, renin, vitamin D in an active form,

erythropoietin and prostaglandins. Several hundred litres of plasma pass through the kidneys each day, with about 1.5 L of filtered fluid being voided as urine. Despite the fact that the kidney is a very robust organ, kidney disease is a significant and growing cause of morbidity and mortality. Kidney function deteriorates with age, but kidney disease can develop throughout life. Major risk factors are cardiovascular disease, hypertension and diabetes mellitus. Such conditions must be treated effectively in order to minimise the risk of renal damage. Early identification of kidney disease (and associated impairment) and effective treatment are essential if complications are to be avoided or at least minimised.

Certain drugs are nephrotoxic and must be either avoided altogether or given in reduced doses to patients who have a degree of renal impairment.

Although effective drugs are available for the treatment of some kidney diseases, end-stage renal failure will require some form of dialysis or perhaps renal transplantation. Renal failure has a massive impact on both the patient and his or her family due to the treatment impacting on the patient's lifestyle (e.g. time taken up with dialysis treatments and dietary restrictions). Men are more likely to present with kidney failure than women. Black and Asian people are more likely to suffer kidney failure than white people. While some causes of kidney failure are well understood, in a number of cases (in up to 30% of patients) the cause of kidney failure cannot be found. In preventing kidney disease, there can be no doubt about the importance of keeping to a healthy lifestyle, with particular emphasis on obesity, with a consequent increased risk of developing diabetes mellitus.

Although major strides have been made in the management of kidney diseases, much remains to be done to improve the quality of life for patients with kidney failure. The kidney is a remarkable organ that has an amazing capacity to cope with many different stresses. In helping to preserve kidney function, it is essential to encourage patients to eat a healthy diet, to take suitable exercise and to stop smoking. Compliance with prescribed treatment, for example for elevated blood pressure, is extremely important. The treatment of kidney disease is essentially a team effort; it is vital to ensure the patient is a full member of the team.

ANATOMY AND PHYSIOLOGY

The prime function of the kidneys is to form and excrete urine. In so doing, water and electrolyte balance are maintained and the waste products of metabolism, urea, uric acid and creatinine are excreted. The structure of the urinary system is illustrated in Figure 18.1.

A longitudinal section of the kidney (see Fig. 18.2) indicates the structures visible to the naked eye, namely a fibrous capsule, the cortex and the medulla.

At the microscopic level, the kidney is made up of nephrons (see Fig. 18.3). The nephrons are responsible for maintaining fluid and electrolyte balance.

PRODUCTION OF URINE

Urine is produced in the kidney within the nephron, of which there are over 1 million in each kidney. Each nephron is a functional unit that consists of:

- Bowman's capsule, the cup-shaped mouth of the nephron
- proximal tubule
- loop of Henle
- distal tubule
- collecting tubule, a straight tubule ultimately leading to the bladder (see Fig. 18.3).

The glomerulus within Bowman's capsule and the tubules lie in the cortex of the kidney; the loops of Henle and collecting tubules lie in the pelvis of the kidney.

The tubule walls are one epithelial cell thick and at certain points are flattened to allow them greater permeability. Lying within each capsule in close

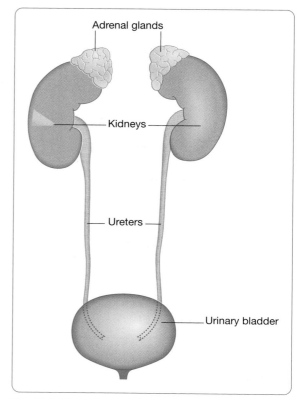

Fig. 18.1 The urinary system.

proximity to the capsule wall is a cluster of intertwining arterial capillaries known as the glomerulus. Arterial blood enters the glomerulus via the afferent arteriole and leaves via the efferent arteriole. Essentially, there are three phases in urine production.

GLOMERULAR FILTRATION

Water and most small molecules filter through the semipermeable walls of the glomerulus and the glomerular capsule, because the blood pressure in the glomerulus is greater than the pressure of the filtrate within the glomerular capsule. In health, large molecules and large cells (e.g. erythrocytes) and plasma proteins remain in the capillaries.

TUBULAR REABSORPTION

Most of the water, glucose, sodium and potassium, which have filtered through the glomerulus into the tubules but which the body still requires, are reabsorbed in the proximal tubule. This process ensures that fluid and electrolyte balance and blood pH are maintained. Selective reabsorption is regularised by both the autonomic nervous system and hormones.

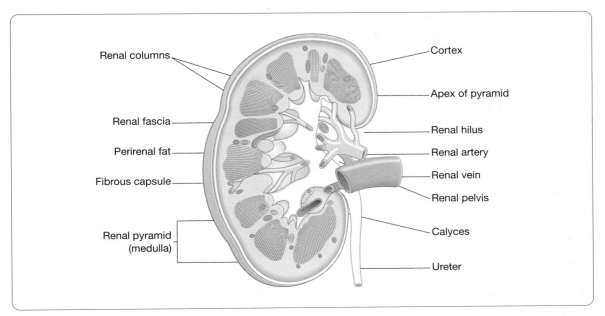

Fig. 18.2 Longitudinal section of kidney.

The hormones are:

- parathormone from the parathyroid and calcitonin from the thyroid, which regulate the reabsorption of calcium and phosphate
- aldosterone from the adrenal cortex, which influences the reabsorption of sodium and the excretion of potassium
- antidiuretic hormone (vasopressin) from the pituitary, which regulates water reabsorption from the distal and collecting tubules.

TUBULAR SECRETION

Substances that were not given sufficient time to filter through the glomerular wall are cleared from the body by secretion into the proximal tubules. Some drugs are excreted in this way.

EXCRETION OF URINE

From the collecting tubule, the urine is received into the renal pelvis before passing into the ureter and thence to the bladder. The smooth muscle of the bladder wall comes under the influence of the autonomic nervous system. The external urethral sphincter is under voluntary control, and only when it is released will micturition occur. Depending on fluid intake and other factors, a healthy adult will pass 1–2.5 L of urine daily.

WATER BALANCE

The amount of water excreted in the urine is influenced by the antidiuretic hormone and the level of waste material to be removed from the blood. Antidiuretic hormone is released as part of a feedback mechanism involving the hypothalamus and the posterior pituitary (see p. 328).

ELECTROLYTE BALANCE

Sodium, potassium, calcium and magnesium ions are present in body fluids. For the body to maintain a constant internal environment, the concentration of each electrolyte in the body fluids must be maintained (see p. 432). Changes in concentration of electrolytes may result from changes in the amount of water or electrolytes. The amount of sodium and potassium in the urine is regulated by a feedback mechanism dependent on the blood flow through the kidneys (see Fig. 18.4).

DIURETICS

These drugs have a profound effect on the excretion of urine and electrolytes. Diuretics are used for the treatment of retention of water and sodium chloride in the tissues (oedema). These drugs are discussed in detail in Chapter 12.

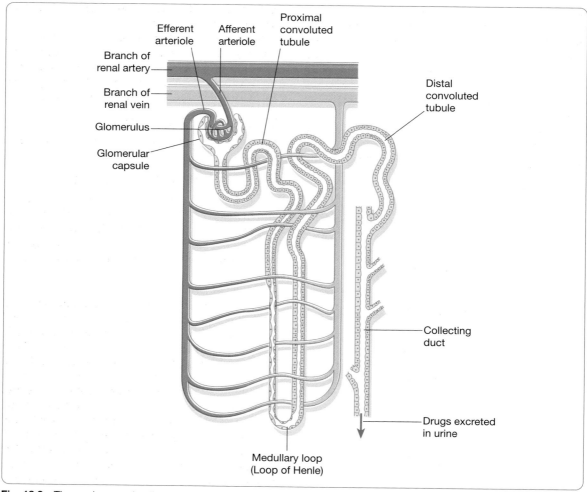

Fig. 18.3   The nephron and collecting ducts.

OTHER FUNCTIONS OF THE KIDNEY

The kidney is an important hormone producer as well as a responder to hormones secreted elsewhere in the body. The hormones produced by the kidney are summarised in Table 18.1.

These hormones are of considerable physiological importance in many conditions. These are discussed in more detail in other chapters.

KIDNEY FAILURE

Given the important functions performed by the kidney, it follows that any malfunctioning of the

kidneys will have serious consequences for the patient. Kidney function does deteriorate with age (see p. 369), but the kidneys are very adaptable organs and some degree of failure may not be very obvious unless diagnostic tests are undertaken. However, some signs of chronic kidney failure are readily observed.

Oedema, frequency of passing urine, frothy urine (due to protein in the urine), pain, anaemia (due to lack of erythropoietin), increased tiredness and falling off in the ability to perform physical tasks may be seen. The skin may be itchy, and bone problems may develop. Night cramps are a distressing problem, as are 'restless legs'. Elevated blood pressure may cause kidney damage or may arise as a result of kidney damage. The presence of blood in the urine (haematuria) requires urgent and full investigation, but the cause of this may be unrelated to kidney failure. For example, urinary tract infection or tumour may be the cause. Pain on passing (or attempting to pass) urine may be an indication of an obstruction to the flow of urine. Changes in the volume of urine produced may also be seen. Such pain is increased if large volumes of fluids (especially alcoholic fluids) are drunk by the patient. Some drugs are toxic to the kidneys (see p. 128), and in any investigations of suspected renal failure a careful drug history must be taken. Blood tests may reveal abnormalities in lipid levels and elevated blood glucose levels, as well as high levels of toxic waste products.

The grades of renal impairment can be defined in terms of glomerular filtration rate, usually measured by creatinine clearance calculated on a 24-h urine sample. The British National Formulary includes a grading system of renal impairment from mild to severe.

CAUSES OF KIDNEY FAILURE

There are many causes of kidney disease, the most important of which are listed in Table 18.2.

TREATMENT OF RENAL FAILURE

Failing kidney function can be replaced by a number of means, notably by a form of dialysis or by renal transplantation. Detailed discussion of these procedures is beyond the scope of this text. The general principles of dialysis are illustrated in Figure 18.5.

HAEMODIALYSIS

Blood-containing waste products (urea, uric acid and creatinine) are treated with heparin (to prevent blood clotting) and passed across an artificial semipermeable membrane. This process must be continued for about 4 h on about three occasions per week. As the blood flows continuously through the dialyser, more waste products are eliminated. The washing fluid (dialysate) is charged so as to maintain a gradient in the concentration of waste matter across the membrane.

A number of drugs will be needed by patients on haemodialysis. Iron, vitamins and phosphate binders (to remove phosphate from the blood) will be required. In addition, a vitamin D preparation (see p. 333) and erythropoietin will be needed. Conditions such as

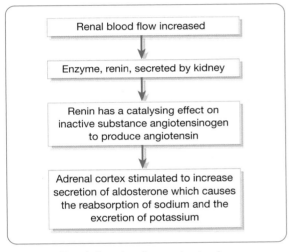

Fig. 18.4 Regulation of sodium and potassium.

Table 18.1	Hormones produced by the kidney	
Name of hormone	**Site of production**	**Main action(s) and notes**
Erythropoietin	Juxtatubular cells	Promotes the formation of red blood cells (see p. 430)
Prostaglandins (group of compounds)	All parts of the kidney	Regulate blood flow, sodium excretion and blood pressure
Renin (a proteolytic enzyme)	Cells beside glomerular apparatus	Produces angiotensin (see p. 207), which constricts blood vessels and raises blood pressure
Vitamin D (active form)	Liver; converted into active form in the kidney	Essential for the formation and maintenance of healthy bone (see p. 333) by regulating calcium metabolism

Table 18.2 Causes of kidney disease

Cause	Notes	Treatment
High blood pressure	A major risk factor.	Lower blood pressure using suitable regimen (see p. 205), especially angiotensin-converting enzyme inhibitors.
Diabetes mellitus	A major risk factor.	Control of blood glucose levels essential and other measures (see Ch. 16).
Heart failure	–	See Chapter 12.
Glomerulonephritis	Progressive glomerulonephritis is a major problem in young adults. Damage to the glomerulus may be caused by infection, malignant disease, sarcoid, hepatitis B and some drugs.	See treatment of renal failure (p. 373). There is no specific treatment for this condition, but not all forms of glomerulonephritis lead to kidney failure.
Urinary tract infection	Younger people may suffer from recurrent urinary tract infections that may be associated with vesicoureteric reflux, which damages the nephrons by the reverse flow of urine (see also chronic pyelonephritis).	See also Chapter 15.
Other infections	If an infection results in sepsis, kidney failure can result.	Antimicrobial therapy and dialysis.
Inherited disorders (e.g. polycystic disease)	Cysts develop within Bowman's capsule and at other places in the nephron. These cysts disrupt normal kidney function by displacing renal tissue.	No effective treatment. It will be necessary to treat the resulting kidney failure with dialysis.
Obstruction of the urinary tract	May be accompanied by infection.	Early detection and treatment are essential to reduce or avoid further renal damage.
Congenital stones within the ureter	–	See treatment of ureteric colic (p. 376).
Prostatic enlargement	A common cause of kidney failure in older men.	See page 360.
Haemorrhage	Hypovolaemia/shock.	–
Drugs	Gentamicin and other aminoglycosides. non-steroidal anti-inflammatory drugs. Many other examples could be given. See British National Formulary's section on renal impairment.	
Nephrotic syndrome	This is caused by glomerulonephritis due to diabetes mellitus, viral infections, non-steroidal anti-inflammatory drugs and other causes. Protein is present in the urine, and there is generalised oedema. There are low levels of albumin in the plasma. Not all forms of nephrotic syndrome lead to kidney failure. It can occur at any age.	Diuretics, high protein diet or treatment of kidney failure.

Continued

Table 18.2 Causes of kidney disease *'cont …'*

Cause	Notes	Treatment
Malignant disease of the kidneys	May cause an obstruction of the urinary tract (see above).	See also Chapter 19.
Infection with *Escherichia coli* 0157:H7	In susceptible people at extremes of age, this infection can cause a haemolytic uraemic syndrome. Red blood cells are destroyed and kidneys may fail.	Antimicrobial therapy and dialysis.
Chronic pyelonephritis	The tissue around the glomeruli becomes inflamed, possibly due to repeated infections in early life. Renal tissue becomes scarred. This condition is linked to reflux.	Dialysis for the renal failure.
Renal artery stenosis	Narrowing of the major blood vessels supplying the kidneys and associated renal hypertension is an increasingly common cause of kidney failure in older people. Smoking is a risk factor.	Healthy lifestyle, aspirin and control of high blood pressure. Surgery may be used.
Immunoglobulin A nephropathy	Possibly caused by an antibody immunoglobulin A found in the core of the glomerular filters (see also Ch. 20).	If this condition eventually leads to kidney failure, dialysis will be required.
Sickle cell disease	An inherited condition seen in people from West Africa or people descended from West Africans.	May cause kidney failure due to anoxia in the medulla. Dialysis may be required.

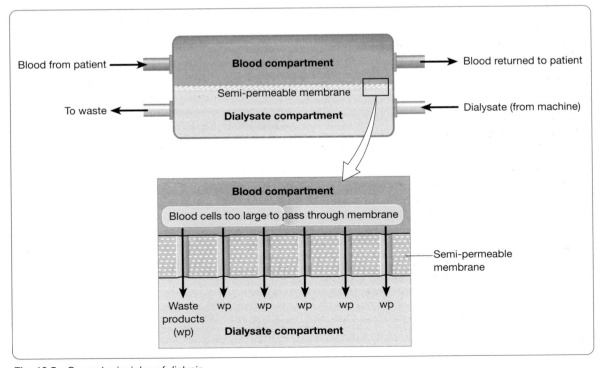

Fig. 18.5 General principles of dialysis.

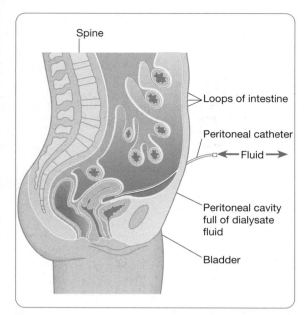

Spine

Loops of intestine

Peritoneal catheter

← Fluid →

Peritoneal cavity
full of dialysate
fluid

Bladder

Fig. 18.6 Continuous ambulatory peritoneal dialysis.

hypertension and diabetes mellitus must continue to be treated. Constipation may be troublesome; laxatives should be prescribed rather than purchased over the counter. Diet and fluid intake must be controlled, and specialist advice will be required.

Viral diseases (notably hepatitis and HIV) are a risk to patients receiving haemodialysis. Special procedures are needed to protect both patients and staff if there is any history of viral disease. Careful testing for the presence of hepatitis is essential at all stages. Patients with HIV infection will require the use of a designated machine or have their dialysis at home.

CONTINUOUS AMBULATORY PERITONEAL DIALYSIS

As with haemodialysis, continuous ambulatory peritoneal dialysis (CAPD) will not cure renal failure but will maintain the patient in reasonable health. In CAPD, the membrane used is the natural peritoneal membrane that has a large surface area and a rich blood supply (see Fig. 18.6). Specially formulated sterile solution is introduced into the peritoneal cavity. The solution contains salts and importantly glucose, usually in a concentration of 1.5, 4.5 or 6.5%, which by a process of osmosis removes water and waste products at the same time. It is important to manage fluid balance during this process. The stronger the glucose solution used, the more water will be removed.

The strength chosen will be in accordance with the needs of the patient so as to ensure that the fluid balance is maintained.

Generally, about four exchanges are needed each day. Between 1.5 and 3 L of fluid is normally run in and left in situ for 4–8 h before it is drained off. The importance of sterile procedures and aseptic technique cannot be overstated. Drugs needed by patients undergoing CAPD are similar to those for patients undergoing haemodyalisis.

An automated process is an alternative to CAPD.

RENAL TRANSPLANTATION

This a major plank in the treatment (probably the most successful) of end-stage renal failure. Many patients throughout the world owe their lives to this procedure. Choice of patients for this treatment is a complex matter, and the availability of suitable donors remains problematical. Great progress has been made with antirejection therapy (see Ch. 20; see also specialist literature).

CHRONIC RENAL FAILURE

Unless treatment is successfully carried out, progressive deterioration of renal function leads to uraemia (an excess of urea and other waste products in the blood) and death. Gastrointestinal, cardiovascular system, respiratory, central nervous system, metabolic, personality, skin, anaemia, and fluid and electrolyte disturbances make a miserable picture. In the terminal stages of the illness, coping with 'simple' problems such as drowsiness, demanding behaviour, pruritus, hiccup and oedema provide a significant challenge for the nurse.

OTHER DISEASES OF THE KIDNEY

RENAL STONES AND URETERIC COLIC

Stones may be caused by a number of conditions. Hypercalcaemia, dehydration and renal tubular acidosis may cause the formation of calcium stones. Uric acid stones result from low urine pH, hyperuricaemia, gout and a high purine diet. Stones made up of calcium phosphate and magnesium ammonium phosphate may result from urinary tract infection, high urinary pH and urinary stasis.

A major part of treatment is the relief of the pain and spasm. Depending on the location of the stone, pain may be felt in the loins (kidney stone) or the ureter, causing the excruciating pain of ureteric colic. Pain may be relieved by pethidine or diclofenac. Lidocaine and chlorhexidine gel may be useful for urethral pain.

Surgery and ultrasonic dissolution may be required to remove the stone.

Large stones ('staghorn' calculi) may develop in association with urinary infection. Such stones may damage the kidney without the patient suffering any pain. Surgery may be needed to remove this type of stone.

SELF-ASSESSMENT QUESTIONS

SECTION A

Define the following terms:

1. glomerular filtration
2. dialysis
3. ureteric colic
4. electrolyte.

SECTION B

True or false?

1. In diabetic nephropathy, it is important to ensure effective control of common cardiovascular risk factors.
2. Obstruction is a potentially reversible cause of worsening renal failure.
3. Target blood pressure in all patients with renal disease is more than 130/85 mmHg.
4. Hyperlipidaemia is not a risk factor for chronic renal disease.
5. It is vitally important to treat chronic renal failure early to reduce the progress of complications and comorbidities.

SECTION C

1. Define: dialysate
   diuretic

2. Why is Vitamin D deficiency found in patients with renal failure?

3. Name three causes of renal failure.

4. The kidneys are an important site for the production of hormones. True or false?

5. How is the kidney linked to the formation of erythrocytes?

6. Name the two anti-rejection drugs used in connection with renal transplantation.

7. Name two conditions relating to renal diseases where compliance with drug therapy is vitally important.

FURTHER READING AND RESOURCES

British Medical Association and Royal Pharmaceutical Society of Great Britain 2006 Appendix 3. Renal impairment. British National Formulary, no. 53. BMA and RPSGB, London, pp. 759–772

Calne RY 1985 Organ transplantation from laboratory to clinic. British Medical Journal 291:1751–1754

Calne RY 1998 The ultimate gift. Headline, London

Page C, Curtis M, Walker M et al. 2006 Integrated pharmacology, 3rd edn. Mosby, London

Parmar SP 2002 Chronic renal disease. British Medical Journal 325:85–90

Parsons F 1989 Origins of haemodialysis in Great Britain. British Medical Journal 299:1557–1560

Sexton J 2003 Drug use and dosing in the renally impaired adult. Pharmaceutical Journal 271:744–746

Sexton J, Vincent M 2004 Remedying calcium and phosphate problems in chronic kidney disease. Pharmaceutical Journal 274:561–564

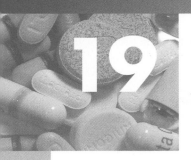

19 Drug treatment of malignant disease

KEY OBJECTIVES

After reading this chapter, you should be able to:

- outline the key roles of the nurse in the care of patients with malignant disease
- describe three categories of cytotoxic medicines and give an example of each
- understand and discuss key aspects in the safe handling of cytotoxic medicines
- outline the management of the common side effects of cytotoxic medicines.

INTRODUCTION

Despite the fact that survival rates for many cancers have considerably improved over the past decades, malignant disease remains a major cause of morbidity and mortality. Cancer has existed for thousands of years. It can occur in infants but is more commonly associated with increasing age. Certain cancers show an increased incidence in lower socio-economic groups, and different cancers can affect different populations. Cancer is not one disease; indeed, over 200 different cancers have been identified. In fact, there are as many cancers as there are types of human cell.

Nowhere in drug management is the nurse required to be more vigilant than in the care of the patient receiving cytotoxic drug therapy. Nurses must also have a clear grasp of the principles of cytotoxic drug therapy and the likely effects that the main drug groups will have on the patient. In this way, they will know how to advise the patient, what to look out for and what action to take if required. They must act calmly, be available at those times when they are most required by the patient and take on the roles of teacher and counsellor. Extreme care is required in correctly identifying the patient and maintaining accurate records. With additional instruction, nurses are increasingly involved in the administration of parenteral chemotherapy. The skills required are of a technical nature and call for an understanding of how the various factors interact.

AETIOLOGY

There is no known single cause of cancer, although a number of predisposing factors have been incriminated. These include:

- chemical factors (e.g. tars in tobacco, asbestos, cytotoxic drugs)
- physical factors (e.g. sunlight, radiation, chronic trauma or infection)
- viruses
- poor diet, low in fruit and vegetables, high in red meat or processed meat products
- genetic factors (e.g. increased incidence in Down's syndrome)
- familial factors (e.g. polyposis coli in families leading to colonic cancer)
- geographical factors (e.g. Japanese women who go to live in the USA go from a low risk of developing breast cancer to high risk, and have as great a chance of developing it as American women; bowel cancer is almost unknown on the African continent, probably owing to dietary factors).

CLASSIFICATION OF CANCERS

Cancers may be classified in different ways. They may be considered as solid tumours (e.g. lung, liver, or 'liquid' tumours, i.e. of the blood or lymph). Alternatively, they may be classified according to their tissue of origin (Table 19.1).

SPREAD OF CANCER

Cancer spreads either by direct infiltration of adjacent tissues or by cells from the primary tumour being transported to another often distant site (or sites) in the body, where they become established and grow. These secondary deposits are known as metastases. The pathways taken by the metastasising cells include the lymphatic system, the blood, serous cavities and cerebrospinal fluid pathways. Different primary tumours tend to show preference for particular secondary sites (Box 19.1).

Some patients develop a second primary tumour.

Table 19.1 Classification of tumours according to tissue of origin

Tissue of origin	Type of tumour
Epithelial tissue	Carcinoma (e.g. of breast, of lung)
Connective tissue	Sarcoma (e.g. of bone, of muscle)
Lymphatic tissue	Malignant lymphoma (e.g. Hodgkin's lymphoma, non-Hodgkin's lymphoma)
Bone marrow	Leukaemia (e.g. myeloblastic leukaemia)
Pigment cells	Malignant melanoma

Box 19.1 Spread of some primary tumours

- Bronchus to brain
- Breast to bone
- Testis to lung
- Colon to liver

PRESENTATION

A malignancy may be an incidental finding when some other condition is being investigated or at a routine check. It otherwise presents in many different ways, ranging from bleeding, swelling and loss of function to anaemia and general malaise depending on the type of tumour and its location. Pain tends to be a feature of more established disease when there is tissue erosion or pressure from metastases.

DIAGNOSIS AND TREATMENT OPTIONS

The diagnosis of cancer is arrived at through careful history taking, physical examination, cytological and pathological examination, and various imaging techniques. Treatment mainly takes the form of surgery, radiotherapy or chemotherapy, or combinations of these. Much will depend on the stage the cancer has reached, the condition and wishes of the patient, and

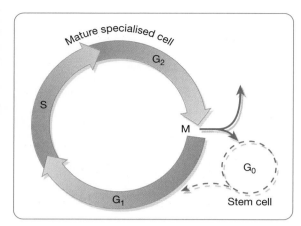

Fig. 19.1   The cell life cycle.

The synthesis (S) and mitosis (M) phases are the main points of activity. The G_1 and G_2 phases occupy the gaps between these phases and allow nutrients to be gathered in to supply energy for the immediately following S and M phases, respectively.

Once the two new cells have been formed, one will mature and differentiate to become a specialised cell, while the other remains a stem cell that will go into a resting (only from replication) phase known as the G_0 phase. There it will remain until it is stimulated to undergo cell division.

Some cells therefore are 'cycling' and some are resting. Of those cycling, at any point in time the cells of any given tissue may be at any stage of the cycle. The time taken for the completion of the cycle varies depending on the type of tissue. Although malignant cells replicate in exactly the same way as normal cells, their cell cycle time is often shorter.

the sensitivity/resistance of the tumour. Cancer cells, like other living organisms, develop resistance to toxic drugs, which may result in treatment failure.

CELL BIOLOGY

In order to appreciate how cancer chemotherapy affects cellular function, it is necessary to have a basic understanding of cell biology. Present in the nucleus of every cell is DNA, which provides the blueprint or template for the chromosomes that carry our genetic characteristics in the form of genes. Also in the nucleus is another acid, RNA, which transmits genetic instructions from the nucleus to the cytoplasm. A cell is stimulated to reproduce in response to the death of another cell. It does this by means of the cell cycle.

CELL CYCLE

The cell cycle is a continuous process during which some cells are replicating while others are resting. The cycle comprises four discrete phases of activity resulting in the production of two identical daughter cells (Fig. 19.1).

- G_1: RNA synthesis occurs in preparation for DNA synthesis
- S: DNA synthesis occurs in preparation for supplying two new cells
- G_2: RNA synthesis occurs in preparation for cell division
- M: Cell mitosis occurs (i.e. production of two new cells)
- G_0: resting phase.

CHARACTERISTICS OF CANCER

Cancer is a problem of abnormal cell growth resulting from an interaction between the causal factor and DNA in a normal cell. The result is that normal control mechanisms are lost and the cancer cells reproduce uncontrollably, invading the surrounding tissues and eventually metastasising to sites distant from the primary tumour.

Malignant cells are therefore not new cells. They are an alteration of existing cells, a change that may have taken place as many as 15 years previously as the result of some insult or combination of effects on the body. The malignant cell behaves in a delinquent way, with no respect for the normal patterns of cell differentiation, growth and control. It is a parasite to the body and as such harms the host, which may ultimately lead to death (Fig. 19.2).

CANCER CHEMOTHERAPY

Cancer chemotherapy is directed towards controlling abnormal cell growth and reducing the number of actively dividing cells. Cytotoxic drugs are used to kill cancer cells, but they kill healthy cells as well. All cells, whether they are normal or malignant, are in different stages of the cell cycle at any time or they may be resting (G_0 phase). Chemotherapy drugs are described as being either phase-specific, i.e. they act more powerfully in one specific phase of the cycle, or cycle-specific, i.e. they work equally well killing cells in any or all phases of the cycle. Chemotherapy drugs

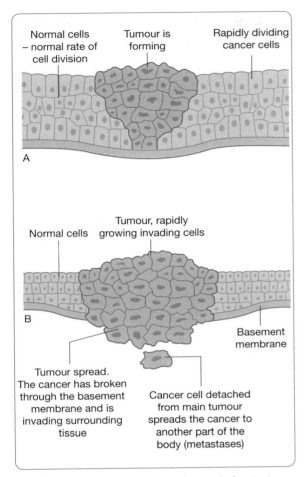

Fig. 19.2 Formation of tumour and spread of metastases.

A

Normal cells – normal rate of cell division

Tumour is forming

Rapidly dividing cancer cells

B

Normal cells

Tumour, rapidly growing invading cells

Basement membrane

Tumour spread. The cancer has broken through the basement membrane and is invading surrounding tissue

Cancer cell detached from main tumour spreads the cancer to another part of the body (metastases)

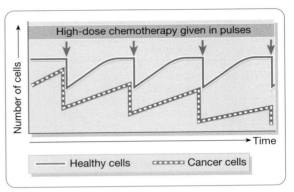

Fig. 19.3 The effect of chemotherapy on normal and cancer cells.

will not kill cells in the G_0 phase. They are also more effective when the number of cancer cells is small. It is for this reason that chemotherapy is used as adjuvant therapy, i.e. following surgery and/or radiotherapy. High individual doses of chemotherapy will kill a high percentage of cancer cells. Although healthy cells will be destroyed, they will repair themselves quickly and regrow to normal numbers far more quickly than cancer cells following chemotherapy (Fig. 19.3). Intervals between doses are needed to allow normal cells to recover. Repeat doses at intervals are needed to kill those cells that were in the resting phase and therefore protected from chemotherapy. By combining different chemotherapy drugs (e.g. in some cases using four drugs together), remission rates in many situations are hugely increased. Cancer chemotherapy is therefore at its most effective when used:

- when the tumour is small or has been surgically removed or reduced in size with radiotherapy
- in high doses
- intermittently
- in appropriate combinations, often according to internationally agreed protocols (see Table 19.2).

The initial letters of cytotoxic drugs may be used to represent a regimen forming an acronym. For example, CHOP stands for cyclophosphamide, doxorubicin (formerly known as hydoxyrubicin), vincristine (Oncovin) and prednisolone. Here, a proprietary name is being used as well as a change in name to form the acronym.

The timing of each pulse of treatment is critical to achieving success in eradicating the malignant cells. However, it must always be borne in mind that the patient's normal cells, especially the rapidly dividing ones, are also being damaged. To ensure that the patient can withstand the treatment, regular haematological monitoring is essential. The tissues that are most chemosensitive are the:

- bone marrow
- epithelial lining of the gastrointestinal tract
- skin and hair
- ovaries and testes.

CYTOTOXIC DRUGS

SIDE-EFFECTS OF CYTOTOXIC DRUGS

Cytotoxic drugs tend to have a common side-effect profile, as listed below. Each individual class of medicine will also have its own characteristic profile. For individual drugs, the manufacturer's product

Table 19.2   Cancer chemotherapy regimens[a]

Regimen	Components	Indication(s)
ABVD	Doxorubicin, bleomycin, vinblastine, dacarbazine	Hodgkin's lymphoma
BEP	Bleomycin, etoposide, cisplatin	Advanced teratoma and seminoma
ChlVPP	Chlorambucil, vinblastine, procarbazine, prednisolone	Hodgkin's lymphoma
CHOP	Cyclophosphamide, doxorubicin, vincristine, prednisolone	Non-Hodgkin's lymphoma
CMF	Cyclophosphamide, methotrexate, fluorouracil	Breast cancer
CVP	Cyclophosphamide, vincristine, prednisolone	Non-Hodgkin's lymphoma
FMD	Fludarabine, mitoxantrone, dexamethasone	Follicular and indolent lymphoma and chronic lymphoid leukaemia
VAD	Vincristine, doxorubicin, dexamethasone	Multiple myeloma
MVP	Mitomycin, vinblastine, cisplatin	Lung cancer

[a]Consult specialist literature for details of dosage/route of administration etc. Many other regimens are quoted in the literature.

literature should always be consulted for current side-effect details.

Bone marrow suppression. All cytotoxic drugs with the exception of vincristine and bleomycin cause bone marrow suppression; haematological monitoring is essential especially prior to initiating the next course of treatment.

Effects on reproductive function. The majority of cytotoxic drugs are teratogenic and are therefore contraindicated during pregnancy. Some have an effect on gametogenesis and can therefore affect fertility.

Nausea and vomiting. Drugs vary in their ability to induce emesis, and there is also differing individual patient susceptibility. Cisplatin, dacarbazine and high-dose cyclophosphamide are particularly emetogenic.

Hyperuricaemia. Rapid destruction of a large number of leukaemia cells may cause a rise in blood uric acid or urea and lead to the development of hyperuricaemia (see p. 393).

Extravasation. Many cytotoxic drugs will cause severe local tissue necrosis if leakage occurs into the extravascular compartment.

Oral mucositis. Sore mouth is a common complication most associated with fluorouracil, methotrexate and the anthracyclines.

Hair loss. Reversible hair loss is a common problem, varying between the drug and the individual patient's susceptibility.

CYTOTOXIC DRUG GROUPS

Cytotoxic drugs fall into a number of classes, each with characteristic antitumour activity, sites of action, and toxicity:

- alkylating drugs
- antimetabolites
- cytotoxic antibiotics
- vinca alkaloids
- other antineoplastic drugs.

It is important to be aware of the metabolism and excretion characteristics, as weakened drug metabolism as a result of disease is not unusual and could result in increased toxicity. The chemotherapy of cancer is complex and should therefore be restricted to specialists in oncology. The National Institute for Health and Clinical Excellence (NICE) has examined many of these drugs and their application in specific cancers/leukaemias and has made recommendations on their use. Details can be found on the NICE website (http://www.nice.org.uk).

ALKYLATING DRUGS

These drugs are among the most widely used in cancer chemotherapy. They are phase-specific (M phase) and act by causing breaks in, and cross-linking on, the strands of DNA, resulting in inhibition of, or inaccurate, replication and finally cell death. In addition to the side effects common to many cytotoxic drugs, there are two major problems associated with use: gametogenesis is often badly affected, and prolonged use of these drugs, particularly when combined with extensive irradiation, is associated with an increased incidence of acute non-lymphocytic leukaemia.

Cyclophosphamide is used in the treatment of chronic lymphocytic leukaemia, lymphomas and some soft-tissue solid tumours. It can be given orally or by intravenous infusion, but it is inert until activated in the body by microsomal enzymes in the liver. One of the metabolites of cyclophosphamide is acrolein, which can cause haemorrhagic cystitis, a serious side effect. As a consequence, when high-dose therapy is used mesna can be given to prevent this. A high fluid intake should be maintained for 24–48 h after intravenous injection. Ifosfamide is similar to cyclophosphamide but given only by intravenous infusion.

Chlorambucil is used to treat chronic lymphocytic leukaemia, non-Hodgkin's lymphoma, Hodgkin's lymphoma and ovarian cancer. It is given orally and, apart from bone marrow suppression, side effects are not common, yet some patients develop a widespread rash that can lead to Stevens–Johnson syndrome or to toxic epidermal necrolysis. Lung damage has been reported.

Melphalan is used to treat multiple myeloma, ovarian adenocarcinoma, breast cancer and, by regional arterial perfusion, localised malignant melanoma. As the drug is unstable in infusion fluids, it must be administered via the port of a freely running infusion system. Busulfan is given for the palliative treatment of chronic myeloid leukaemia. Excessive myelosuppression can result in irreversible bone marrow aplasia, and so careful monitoring of blood counts is especially important.

Carmustine is used intravenously in the treatment of multiple myeloma, non-Hodgkin's lymphoma and brain tumours. Renal damage and delayed pulmonary fibrosis can occur. Lomustine is given orally to treat Hodgkin's lymphoma, brain or lung tumours and malignant melanoma. Bone marrow suppression can be delayed, and permanent damage can occur with prolonged use. Estramustine is a combination of estradiol and normustine used in cases of prostatic cancer responsive to other therapies. It has both an effect on cell division and a hormonal effect.

Thiotepa is mainly used to treat malignant effusions or bladder cancer when used as an intracavity drug. It has been used intravenously in the treatment of breast cancer. Treosulfan is given either orally or intravenously in the treatment of ovarian cancer. Skin pigmentation is a common side-effect, and allergic alveolitis, pulmonary fibrosis and haemorrhage cystitis can also occur rarely.

ANTIMETABOLITES

These are cycle-specific. They are substances that substitute for, or compete with, intracellular metabolites and become incorporated into the nucleic acids, DNA and RNA, preventing DNA synthesis and leading to cell death.

Methotrexate is used to treat a wide range of conditions, such as leukaemia, lymphoma, breast cancer, lung cancer, head and neck cancer, bladder cancer and osteogenic sarcoma. It acts during the S phase of cell division. It inhibits the enzyme dihydrofolate reductase, which in turn interferes with DNA production. It is a folic acid antagonist. It can be given by all main routes, including intrathecal; as a result, a wide range of doses are used. It is excreted primarily via the kidneys, therefore use is contraindicated in severe renal disease. It can cause, among other side-effects, myelosuppression, stomatitis, hepatic toxicity, photosensitivity, central nervous system symptoms, abdominal distress, rashes and genitourinary toxicity. It interacts with a significant number of drugs, leading to possible toxicity.

CALCIUM FOLINATE RESCUE FOR PATIENTS RECEIVING METHOTREXATE

Calcium folinate is chemically related to the essential coenzyme for nucleic acid synthesis. It is used to diminish the toxicity of folic acid antagonists such as methotrexate. The dose of calcium folinate will depend on the dose of methotrexate previously administered. As an example, up to 120 mg would be given in divided doses over 12–24 h by intramuscular injection, intravenous bolus or intravenous infusion. Following the initial doses, 12–15 mg intramuscularly or 15 mg is given orally every 6 h for the next 48–72 h. Steps should be taken to increase the rate of excretion of the methotrexate (e.g. by alkalinisation of the urine and maintaining the urinary output at a high level).

Fluorouracil inhibits cell division by interfering with DNA and RNA synthesis. It is usually given by intravenous infusion, or injection, to treat colon and breast cancer, as absorption after oral administration is unpredictable. In addition, it can be used locally as a topical cream to treat premalignant and malignant skin lesions. Side effects include haematological damage, gastrointestinal haemorrhage, stomatitis, diarrhoea, nausea and vomiting. Capecitabine is metabolised to fluorouracil and is given by mouth. It is used alone to treat metastatic colorectal cancer or as adjuvant treatment of advanced colon cancer following surgery. It is also used as second-line treatment of locally advanced or metastatic breast cancer, either alone or in combination with docetaxel. Tegafur, a prodrug of fluorouracil, is given orally with calcium folinate in the management of metastatic colorectal cancer.

Cytarabine acts by inhibiting pyrimidine synthesis. It is given subcutaneously, intravenously or intrathecally. It is mainly used in the induction of remission of acute myeloblastic leukaemia but can also be used in the treatment of acute lymphoblastic and acute non-lymphoblastic leukaemia. Fludarabine can be given orally, by intravenous injection or infusion, to treat advanced B-cell chronic lymphocytic leukaemia or after first-line treatment in patients with sufficient bone marrow reserves. Cladribine is given by intravenous infusion for the treatment of hairy cell leukaemia. Cytarabine, cladribine and fludarabine have potent immunosuppressive effects, therefore regular haematological monitoring is essential.

Gemcitabine is used intravenously to treat non-small cell lung cancer and pancreatic cancer. In combination with cisplatin, it is also used in the treatment of advanced bladder cancer. It may cause mild gastrointestinal side-effects, rashes, renal impairment and pulmonary toxicity. Influenza-like symptoms and haemolytic uraemic syndrome have also been reported.

Pemetrexed and raltitrexed both inhibit thymidylate transferase and other folate-dependent enzymes. Pemetrexed is given by intravenous infusion to treat unresectable malignant pleural mesothelioma, and it is also used in the treatment of locally advanced or metastatic non-small cell lung cancer that has previously been treated with chemotherapy. Raltitrexed is given intravenously for palliation of advanced colorectal cancer when fluorouracil and calcium folinate cannot be used. Common adverse effects include myelosuppression, gastrointestinal toxicity and skin disorders.

Mercaptopurine acts by interfering with synthesis of nucleic acid in proliferating cells. It is used as maintenance therapy in the treatment of acute leukaemias. Tioguanine, used in the treatment of both acute and chronic leukaemia, acts by inhibition of purine synthesis.

CYTOTOXIC ANTIBIOTICS

These are phase-specific (S phase) and act by binding to the DNA helix, inhibiting its synthesis and replication, and disrupting RNA synthesis. Many of the cytotoxic antibiotics act as radiomimetics, and therefore the concurrent use of radiotherapy should be avoided, as this may cause enhanced toxicity. Daunorubicin, doxorubicin, epirubicin and idarubicin are anthracycline antibiotics.

Doxorubicin is used in the treatment of acute leukaemia, lymphoma, soft-tissue and osteogenic sarcoma, and breast and lung cancer. It is given by intravenous injection through a freely running intravenous infusion. Extravasation can cause severe tissue damage. Supaventricular tachycardia can arise from drug administration, and cumulative doses are associated with cardiomyopathy. Above a maximum dose of 450 mg/m^2, symptomatic and potentially fatal heart failure is common. Account must also be taken of treatment with other cardiotoxic drugs. Electrocardiogram monitoring is required both before and after treatment. A formulation of doxorubicin inside liposomes provides a delivery system that may reduce the incidence of cardiotoxicity and lower the potential for local necrosis. However, infusion reactions, sometimes severe, can occur. Hand–foot syndrome occurs commonly with liposomal doxorubicin and may occur after two or three treatment cycles. It may be prevented by cooling hands and feet and by avoiding socks, gloves, or tight-fitting footwear for 4–7 days after treatment. Doxorubicin can also be given by intra-arterial injection and bladder instillation (bladder tumours).

Epirubicin is structurally related to doxorubicin and is used in the treatment of breast, ovarian, gastric and colorectal cancers; lymphomas; leukaemia; and multiple myeloma. A maximum cumulative dose of 0.9–1 g/m^2 is recommended to avoid cardio-toxicity. Like doxorubicin, it is given intravenously and by bladder instillation. Idarubicin and daunorubicin have properties similar to those of doxorubicin. Idarubicin is available as a capsule for oral administration when intravenous therapy is not practicable.

Mitoxantrone is structurally related to doxorubicin; it is used for metastatic breast cancer, non-Hodgkin's lymphoma and adult non-lymphocytic leukaemia. It is given intravenously; myelosuppression and dose-related cardiotoxicity can occur. Cardiac examinations are recommended after a cumulative dose of 160 mg/m^2. Careful technique is essential when diluting the drug for intravenous infusion, as it is very irritant.

Bleomycin inhibits cell growth and DNA synthesis in tumour cells and is used to treat squamous cell carcinoma of the mouth, nasopharynx, oesophagus and external genitalia or skin. It can be given intravenously, intramuscularly or by intracavity injection. It can cause increased pigmentation, particularly affecting the flexures, and subcutaneous sclerotic plaques may occur. Mucositis, Raynaud's phenomenon and hypersensivity reactions have all been reported. The main problem with the use of bleomycin is progressive pulmonary fibrosis. This is dose-related, occurring more commonly at cumulative doses greater than 300 000 units and in the elderly. Basal lung crepitations or suspicious chest x-ray changes are an indication to stop therapy.

Dactinomycin inhibits cell proliferation by combining with DNA and interfering with RNA synthesis. It is mainly used to treat paediatric cancers; it is given intravenously through a freely running intravenous infusion. While its side effects are similar to those of doxorubicin, cardiac toxicity is not a problem. Mitomycin has an alkylating action, forming a complex with DNA in cancer cells. It is given intravenously to treat stomach, pancreatic, colonic, rectal and breast cancers and by bladder instillation for superficial bladder tumours. It causes delayed bone marrow toxicity, and therefore it is usually administered at 6-weekly intervals. Prolonged use may result in permanent bone marrow damage. It may also cause lung fibrosis and renal damage.

VINCA ALKALOIDS

These are phase-specific (M phase) and bind to the microtubular proteins that are needed for formation of the mitotic spindle. Because the cell is unable to divide, it dies. The vinca alkaloids, vinblastine, vincristine, and vindesine, are used to treat the acute leukaemias, lymphomas, and some solid tumours such as breast, renal and lung cancer. Vinorelbine, a semisynthetic vinca alkaloid, is used for advanced breast cancer and for advanced non-small cell lung cancer. They must only be given by intravenous administration as intrathecal administration can cause severe neurotoxicity that is usually fatal. Neurotoxicity, usually as peripheral or autonomic neuropathy, occurs with all vinca alkaloids. Myelosuppression is the dose-limiting side effect of vinblastine, vindesine and vinorelbine. The vinca alkaloids may cause alopecia and can cause severe local irritation, and so care must be taken to avoid extravasation.

Etoposide is a mitotic inhibitor classed along with the vinca alkaloids. It may be given orally or by slow intravenous infusion, the oral dose being double the intravenous dose. It has been used to treat small cell lung cancer, the lymphomas, and non-seminomatous testicular cancer. Side-effects include alopecia, myelosuppression, nausea and vomiting. Hypotension may occur due to a rapid infusion rate.

OTHER ANTINEOPLASTIC DRUGS

The exact mechanism by which dacarbazine acts is unknown; it inhibits pyrimidine synthesis and it may have some alkylating action. It is used intravenoulsy in the treatment of malignant melanoma and soft tissue sarcoma, and in combination therapy to treat Hodgkin's lymphoma. Nausea and vomiting can be intense, but it can be restricted by reducing intake of food and drink 4–6 h prior to therapy. Temozolomide is structurally related to dacarbazine and is used as a second-line treatment for malignant glioma.

Hydroxycarbamide acts by interfering with DNA synthesis. It is used orally in the treatment of chronic myeloid leukaemia and in combination with radiotherapy to treat cervical cancer. The mechanism of action of procarbazine is not known. It is mainly used orally, in the treatment of Hodgkin's lymphoma (as in MOPP).

Imatinib is a protein tyrosine kinase inhibitor used in the treatment of chronic myeloid leukaemia when bone marrow transplantation is not considered first-line treatment. It is also used for chronic myeloid leukaemia in the chronic phase, after failure of interferon alfa, in accelerated phase or in blast crisis. Side effects of imatinib are nausea, vomiting, diarrhoea, oedema, abdominal pain, fatigue, myalgia, headache and rash. Gynaecomastia, because of reduced testosterone levels, has been reported.

Platinum compounds include carboplatin, cisplatin and oxaliplatin. They are platinum-containing compounds that have an alkylating action. All can cause nephrotoxicity, ototoxicity and neurotoxicity to varying degrees. They are given by the intravenous route. Cisplatin therapy requires intensive intravenous hydration. Carboplatin is used in ovarian and small cell lung cancer, and cisplatin for the treatment of metastatic germ cell cancers and bladder and lung cancers. Oxaliplatin, in combination with fluorouracil and folinic acid, is used to treat metastatic colorectal cancer. Careful monitoring of renal function is required with all these drugs.

The taxanes exert their antineoplastic effects by disrupting the microtubular network in cells, causing disruption of mitotic and other cellular functions. Docetaxel is used (in combination with doxorubicin) in advanced metastatic breast cancer when there is resistance to other agents and/or relapse. Paclitaxel is used in the treatment of ovarian cancer, given in combination with either cisplatin or carboplatin. Routine pretreatment with a corticosteroid, an anti-histamine and an H_2 antagonist is recommended to prevent severe hypersensitivity reactions. Side-effects include myelosuppression, peripheral neuropathy and cardiac conduction defects with arrhythmias.

Irinotecan and topotecan are both inhibitors of topoisomerase-1, an enzyme involved in DNA replication. Irinotecan is recommended by NICE as a possible treatment for patients with advanced colorectal cancer, when used with fluorouracil and calcium folinate in those who have not had previous chemotherapy, or given as monotherapy when chemotherapy has failed. Topotecan should be considered as one of the treatment options for women with advanced ovarian cancer if first-line chemotherapy has not been successful. Myelosuppression can be dose-limiting for both these drugs; gastrointestinal effects, asthenia, alopecia and anorexia may also occur.

Trastuzumab in combination with paclitaxel is an option for women with advanced breast cancer who have tumours expressing human epidermal growth factor receptor-2 (HER-2), scored at levels of 3+, who have not previously received chemotherapy for metastatic breast cancer and in whom anthracycline treatment is inappropriate. Monotherapy with trastuzumab is also an option in patients with HER-2-positive tumours (3+) who have received at least two chemotherapy regimens for metastatic breast cancer. Prior chemotherapy must have included at least an anthracycline and a taxane when these treatments are appropriate. It should also have included hormonal therapy in suitable oestrogen receptor-positive patients. Trastuzumab is a recombinant humanised monoclonal antibody that specifically targets the HER-2 protein. Preliminary results from trials using trastuzumab in early breast cancer show some promising outcomes. However, use may be limited by cardiotoxicity. It is given by intravenous infusion, which carries a risk of infusion-related side-effects such as chills, fever and hypersensitivity reactions including anaphylaxis and angioedema.

There are other antineoplastic drugs used in the treatment of malignant diseases, including amsacrine (acute myeloid leukaemia), bexarotene (cutaneous T-cell lymphoma), bortezomib (multiple myeloma), cetuximab (metastatic colorectal cancer), crisantaspase (acute lymphobalstic leukaemia) and tretinoin (acute promyelotic leukaemia). Rituximab is a monoclonal antibody used in non-Hodgkin's lymphoma and advanced chemotherapy-resistant follicular lymphoma. Alemtuzumab is also a monoclonal antibody used for chronic lymphocytic leukaemia.

OTHER DRUGS USED IN THE TREATMENT OF MALIGNANT DISEASES

Malignant disease is treated by a range of drugs in addition to the cytotoxic drugs previously described. Table 19.3 lists the range, together with a brief description of clinical indications. Table 19.2 outlines some combination regimens designed to overcome resistance to therapy with a single agent.

KEY ELEMENTS OF THE TREATMENT OF MALIGNANT DISEASE WITH CYTOTOXIC DRUGS

The treatment of malignant disease with cytotoxic drugs presents many challenges for clinicians, nurses and pharmacists. In order to achieve the best outcome for the patient and to protect the staff involved, it is vitally important that all those involved in providing anticancer treatment work together within the following framework.

- The importance of discussing the full implications of the treatment with the patient and/or the patient's relatives cannot be overstated.
- Only clinicians having specialised experience and access to full back-up services should initiate and control cytotoxic therapy.
- When treatment is provided on a shared-care basis with the patient's GP, communications and flow of information must be well managed and clearly understood by all involved.
- All personnel involved in providing the drug therapy must observe the regulations designed to prevent chronic exposure to cytotoxic drugs. These regulations are intended to minimise the risk to handlers of cytotoxic drugs from the known hazards (e.g. teratogenicity). Guidance on the safe handling of cytotoxic drugs is given later in this chapter.
- Particular attention must be paid to all aspects of drug management, such as drug selection, dosage determination, calculation, prescribing, presentation of the drug, route of administration and timing of the administration of individual doses within a course of therapy.
- Every effort must be made to reduce the impact on the patient of foreseeable adverse effects of the therapy. It will often be important to provide advice and support to relatives and carers.

Table 19.3 Other drugs used in malignant disease

Drug(s)	Indications
Antiandrogens Cyproterone, flutamide, bicalutamide	Treatment of prostate cancer.
Antibacterial agents	Antibiotic cover due to immunosuppression.
Aromatase inhibitors Anastrozole, letrozole, exemestane	Treatment of metastatic breast cancer.
Corticosteroids (especially prednisolone)	Treatment of leukaemia, breast cancer, Hodgkin's lymphoma, palliation in terminal conditions.
Granulocyte-colony stimulating factor Filgrastim, lenograstim, pegfilgrastim	Reduction in duration of neutropenia from cytotoxic chemotherapy.
Gonadorelin analogues Buserelin, goserelin, leuprorelin, triptorelin	Treatment of metastatic prostate cancer. (Goserelin also used for advanced breast cancer in premenopausal women).
Interferons Interferon alfa, peg-interferon alfa-2a, peg-interferon alfa-2b	Various lymphomas and solid tumours (e.g. chronic lymphocytic leukaemia, hairy cell leukaemia, malignant melanoma).
Oestrogens Ethinylestradiol	Palliative treatment of prostate cancer.
Interleukin Aldesleukin (recombinant interleukin-2)	Treatment of metastatic renal cell cancer.
Oestrogen receptor antagonists Tamoxifen, fulvestrant, toremifene	Treatment of breast cancer.
Progestogens Medroxyprogesterone acetate, megestrol	Treatment of endometrial cancer.
Somatostatin analogues Octreotide, lanreotide	Relief of symptoms associated with neuroendocrine tumours. Reducing vomiting in palliative care. Treatment of thyroid tumours.

- Without causing unnecessary alarm among staff or patients, a respect for cytotoxic drugs should be engendered in much the same way as is required for radioactive materials. Provided that staff make themselves fully conversant with the guidelines laid down on the safe handling of these drugs and are seen to incorporate the practical measures into their day-to-day work, protection for the user, the patient and all other personnel working near treatment areas should be guaranteed.

DRUG MANAGEMENT IN CYTOTOXIC DRUG THERAPY

The general principles of drug management are discussed in detail in Chapter 3. However, in view of the special importance of drug management in cytotoxic drug therapy, the following additional guidance is offered. All the factors listed are not of equal importance but nevertheless must be given full consideration in patients' particular circumstances. Factors in drug selection include:

- condition being treated, stages of disease and prognosis
- regimen to be followed – single or combination therapy
- cost–benefits of the therapy (the escalating cost of newer forms of therapy is of major concern)
- back-up resources available locally
- general condition of the patient – any previous exposure to cytotoxic drugs and/or radiotherapy
- current guidance – consider advice from NICE, the Scottish Intercollegiate Guidelines Network and the Committee on Safety of Medicines
- any coexisting condition that could affect treatment and/or cause complications for the patient
- reproductive status of the patient
- possibility of drug interactions.

DOSE DETERMINATION

Many factors are involved in dosage determination, and it is the responsibility of the clinician to take all factors into account in arriving at the actual dosage and frequency of administration. All the above factors will be considered, along with the following:

- patient's age, sex, body weight and other physical parameters (e.g. body surface area)
- nutritional status
- full haematological profile
- renal and hepatic function
- neurological status
- pharmacokinetics of the drug.

Doses are determined according to generally well-defined regimens, being modified according to the factors outlined above. The main approaches are based on two parameters: body weight and surface area.

DOSAGE DETERMINATION BASED ON BODY WEIGHT

Melphalan is used as an example. The dosage range in multiple myeloma is 150–300 micrograms/kg of body weight daily, by mouth, for 4–6 days. The course is repeated after 4–8 weeks. Given that the patient has some degree of renal impairment, it may be decided to begin the course of therapy at the lower end of the dosage range. Blood counts will enable the effect of this dose to be monitored.

For a patient of body weight 68 kg, the dose would be 150×68 micrograms/day for, say, 5 days, i.e.:

10 200 micrograms

$$= \frac{10\ 200}{1000\ mg}$$

$$= 10\ mg\ (to\ nearest\ mg)$$

The number of 2-mg tablets to be administered each day is $(10 \div 2)$ five tablets per day.

It is important to realise that the patient's 'true' body weight must be taken into account. In a patient suffering from fluid retention or obesity, the actual weight on the scales should be treated with some caution, because this is not generally a good indication of the patient's ability to metabolise the drug. Reference to standard height and weight tables may be required. The main factor to take into account is the patient's lean body mass.

DOSAGE DETERMINATION BASED ON BODY SURFACE AREA

This parameter is felt to be a more accurate indicator than body weight of the patient's ability to metabolise the drug. The patient's surface area is derived from tables. Given the patient's height (in cm) and body weight (in kg), the patient's body surface area can be determined from a nomogram (Fig. 19.4). Nomograms are available for both adults and children.

PRESCRIBING

Prescribing cytotoxic drug therapy is more complex than the prescribing of more routine therapy. Great care must be taken to ensure that all personnel involved in the treatment of the patient have information that is complete and accurate. Special prescription forms have usually been developed, because it is not possible to provide all the necessary information on the standard form. Clinical management guidelines, drawn up by a multidisciplinary professional group, should be in place for all common tumour types (Scottish Executive 2005).

A separate cytotoxic prescription should be used for ordering chemotherapy drugs from the pharmacy for each individual patient. Details of the patient's identity; diagnosis; height, weight and surface area; and blood count should be provided. The required regimen; the names of the drugs included in the regimen; the dose, route and method of administration; the diluent; and the final volume should be entered and signed for by the prescribing doctor.

Chemotherapy regimens should be initiated by an appropriately trained and accredited oncologist or haematologist familiar with the use of cytotoxic medicines. The decision and the proposed plan

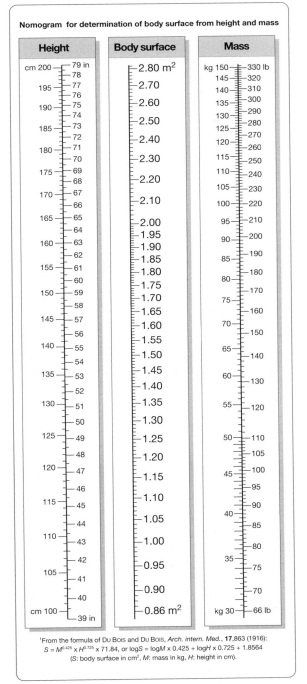

Nomogram for determination of body surface from height and mass

Height	Body surface	Mass
cm 200 — 79 in	2.80 m²	kg 150 — 330 lb

[^1]From the formula of Du Bois and Du Bois, *Arch. intern. Med.*, **17**,863 (1916):
$S = M^{0.425} \times H^{0.725} \times 71.84$, or $\log S = \log M \times 0.425 + \log H \times 0.725 + 1.8564$
(S: body surface in cm², M: mass in kg, H: height in cm).

Fig. 19.4 Nomogram (adult).

should be clearly recorded in the patient's notes. It is good practice to use a preprinted prescription sheet (Fig. 19.5) or predefined electronic prescribing system. Chemotherapy protocols should be in place for all cytotoxic chemotherapy regimens detailed in the clinical management guidelines. These can be paper-based or within an electronic prescribing system.

ROUTES OF ADMINISTRATION

ORAL

Although cytotoxic drug therapy is very often given parenterally, there are nevertheless a number of effective oral cytotoxic preparations. These formulations are no less toxic in tablet or capsule form, and the same attention to care in their administration is required. In the interests of safety, tablets of cytotoxic medicines should be swallowed whole, and only in very exceptional circumstances should they be crushed (advice should be taken from pharmacy). When nausea and vomiting are known side-effects, an antiemetic may need to be given in advance. Patients who are to take cytotoxic drugs while at home should be given clear written instructions in their use.

SUBCUTANEOUS AND INTRAMUSCULAR

Because of the risk of damage to the tissues, only a few cytotoxic drugs are administered by these routes. Care should be taken to select an area with adequate subcutaneous or muscle tissue and to give the injection with a needle of the smallest possible calibre.

INTRAVENOUS

Absorption is more reliable by the intravenous route, and hence it is the one most commonly used. Drugs with vesicant properties must always be given intravenously. The need for strict asepsis is paramount, because chemotherapy patients will have some degree of immunosuppression. A chemotherapy infusion administration record should be maintained throughout the infusion that reflects its ongoing progress in detail. Of particular importance are the infusion device number and which line is being used. The volume of fluid already infused and still to be infused should be checked after the first 15 min and hourly thereafter. The rate of the infusion and the expected time of completion should be recorded at each check.

A central venous catheter (e.g. Hickman catheter) may be used to provide long-term access to the patient's circulatory system, thus obviating the need for repeated venepuncture and injections, and avoiding damage to veins. It may be single, double or triple lumen. Either under general anaesthetic or under sedation and local anaesthetic, an incision is made just below the right clavicle and the cephalic vein isolated.

Cisplatin 50 mg/m^2 over 2 hours

CHEMOTHERAPY PRESCRIPTION SHEET
REGIMEN: CISPLATIN single agent, 50 mg/m^2

PROTOCOL CHECKED BY: _____ (Consultant)

DATE:

Cycle no.	Day number	Total no. of cycles	Interval between cycles
Weight	Height	Surface area	Max S.A.

Hb.	PLAT.	WCC.	NEUT.	UREA.	CREAT.	CrCl.

Note: 1. If urine output is less than 100 mL/hour, call Dr. to give IV Furosemide 10 mg.
2. IV fluids may be stopped 3 hours after cisplatin if patient can maintain oral intake of 1–2 litres for 6 hours after IV fluids discontinue.
3. Discharge supply of antiemetics should be started at 6 pm on day of chemotherapy

IF AN INFUSION DEVICE IS BEING USED PLEASE ENTER PUMP ID/MP No. ....

	Day/ Date/ Time	Fluid / Additive medicine	Volume / Dose	Route of Admin.	Duration of Admin.	Prepared by pharmacy Sig.	Date	Code no. Serial no. Batch no.	Start time	Given by
A		**Furosemide**	20 mg	Oral	Stat					
B		Sodium chloride 0.9% Potassium chloride 20 mmol Magnesium sulphate 8 mmol	1000 mL	IV	2 hours					
C		**Ondansetron**	8 mg	IV	Slow bolus					
D		**Dexamethasone**	8 mg	IV	Slow bolus					
E		Sodium chloride 0.9% Potassium chloride 10 mmol Mannitol 10 g **Cisplatin 25 mg/m^2**	450 mL	IV	1 hour					
F		Sodium chloride 0.9% Potassium chloride 10 mmol Mannitol 10 g **Cisplatin 25 mg/m^2**	450 mL	IV	1 hour					
G		Sodium chloride 0.9% Potassium chloride 20 mmol Magnesium sulphate 8 mmol	1000 mL	IV	2 hours					
H		Sodium chloride 0.9%	500 mL	IV	1 hour					

Doctor's signature .... Date ....

Fig. 19.5 Example of a preprinted chemotherapy prescription sheet.

A skin tunnel is then formed, starting at a point between the nipple and the sternum. The catheter is drawn through the tunnel under x-ray control and inserted into the subclavian vein before reaching the cephalic vein and the superior vena cava, where it is positioned at the entrance to the right atrium. Both veins are sutured. A Dacron cuff plugs the tunnel in the subcutaneous tissues, which gradually become fibrosed, thus reducing the risk of ascending infection from the catheter exit point. A transparent dressing is applied and a cap placed on the protruding end. Patients and/or their families are taught to heparinise the line to keep it patent. This may be daily for the first 3 months and then twice weekly thereafter. A daily shower is encouraged. Patients should be encouraged to report any signs of discharge, pain or redness round the catheter or any movement of the catheter. The wound should be dressed and the cap renewed on a weekly basis. If the dressing becomes dislodged or there is evidence of infection, the dressing must be changed. A bacteriological swab should be taken if indicated.

SAFE HANDLING OF CYTOTOXIC DRUGS

The widespread use of cancer chemotherapeutic agents has led to an increased number of employees being exposed to potential contamination by them. The dangers that may be encountered fall into two categories. Certain cytotoxic drugs produce a local irritant effect, causing immediate damage to the skin and eyes. Others are, in addition, known to be mutagenic, carcinogenic and teratogenic agents. These long-term consequences resulting from absorption of substances via the skin, the lungs or the gastrointestinal tract warrant energetic implementation of policies by health authorities to reduce to the minimum risks to their staff.

PERSONNEL

Doctors, nurses and pharmacists involved in the handling of cytotoxic drugs should be instructed in the dangers, precautions and techniques of administration. Training may be given by a suitably experienced senior member of medical, nursing or pharmacy staff, and *only* those so trained should be responsible for the handling of these drugs. All personnel involved in the handling of cytotoxic drugs should be familiar with the written guidelines on the handling of cytotoxic drugs and be given a personal copy. A departmental register of those staff involved in

such procedures should be maintained. In the event of an accident involving cytotoxic drugs, staff must report to their head of department. Such measures comply with the code of practice for Control of Substances Hazardous to Health Regulations. Staff, including those of childbearing potential, are not at risk when involved in the administration of cytotoxic drugs provided that they adhere to the guidelines.

PREPARATION

In view of the well-recognised hazards of manipulating cytotoxic drugs, their preparation for use should take place in a specially designated area within the pharmacy. This helps to ensure the protection of staff, accuracy of compounding and reconstitution, and best presentation in a ready to use form, fully labelled with all the necessary details. Particular care is required in the labelling of the vinca alkaloid drugs, which must carry a warning that the drug is not for intrathecal use. Only pharmacy staff trained and validated in aseptic and cytotoxic chemotherapy reconstitution should be involved in the preparation of chemotherapy in a pharmacy or pharmacy-controlled area. A negative-pressure ducted isolator should be used for preparing solutions of cytotoxic chemotherapy. All staff involved in the preparation of cytotoxic drug solutions must wear suitable protective clothing.

Only in very rare circumstances should cytotoxic drugs have to be prepared outside a centralised area (e.g. when a particular drug has a very short half-life). In such cases, every effort should be made to segregate drug preparation from other ward or clinic activities, and compliance with local protocols should be followed. Procedures should be undertaken only by staff who are suitably trained and experienced. The same applies in hospitals in which cytotoxic drugs are used infrequently and there is no centralised service. However, in this situation consideration should be given to purchasing drugs prepared by another hospital or commercially.

PROTECTION AGAINST OCCUPATIONAL EXPOSURE

Protection against exposure to cytotoxic drugs (or their metabolites) must be available for, and utilised by, all staff involved in the preparation of cytotoxic drugs. Protective clothing must be of the correct specification to ensure adequate protection of the skin and eyes and to prevent inhalation of aerosolised drug particles. It should consist of the following.

- A long-sleeved gown or one-piece sterile suit.
- Plastic apron.

- Disposable gloves, which should be powder-free, made of latex or nitrile and designed for handling cytotoxic chemotherapy. For all procedures, two pairs of gloves should be worn (double-gloved). Should spillage of a cytotoxic medicine on to the glove or damage to the glove occur during a procedure, the gloves must be discarded immediately and replaced. The outer gloves used within the isolator should be changed at the start of each day that the isolator is to be used. The inner gloves (the operator's gloves) should be changed at the start of each session of chemotherapy preparation.
- Safety glasses. It is advisable to wear protective glasses or goggles complying with BS2092C, which provide all-round protection whether or not ordinary spectacles are worn; these should be washed thoroughly in soap and water after use.
- Face mask. A good-quality disposable surgical mask should be worn when reconstituting dry powder, especially if presented in an ampoule.
- Suitable hat and overshoes, depending on the environment in which the isolator is situated.

Every effort should be made to reduce aerosolisation. Ampoules, including those containing diluents, should be opened with care using a file if necessary and plastic ampoule breaker to avoid cuts and scratches. They should be held away from the face when being opened or drawn up from. Care should be taken when adding diluent to allow it to run slowly down the side of the ampoule. The exact volume of drug required should be drawn into a syringe and the remainder discarded or used immediately for another patient. Air from the syringe should be expelled into the empty ampoule over sterile cotton wool or a gauze swab. A new sheathed needle must be placed on the syringe before the final expulsion of air bubbles.

Drugs in powder form must be reconstituted with particular care, as they may be released as a fine spray through the needle hole if excess pressure is produced in the vial. This may be avoided by removing an appropriate amount of air from the vial before injecting the diluting fluid, or by the use of a special venting needle (Fig. 19.6).

Filled syringes should be suitably labelled and placed in a receiver ready for use. They should also carry a biohazard or cytotoxic-drug warning label.

DISPOSAL OF SURPLUS DRUGS AND CONTAMINATED EQUIPMENT

The use of disposable equipment is recommended whenever possible. Items of waste should be disposed of in accordance with local procedures for discarding of cytotoxic waste. This may be as follows.

- Unused solution: double bag and seal ampoule or vial in polythene bags and place bag in sharps container and send to pharmacy for destruction.
- Syringes, needles, empty ampoules, infusion sets: double bag and seal in polythene bags then place in sharps container marked CYTOTOXIC MATERIAL.
- masks, gloves, apron, foil trays, towels, swabs, infusion bags without administration set attached: seal in polythene bag and place in yellow incinerator bag.

All these items are incinerated at 1000°C.

Safety glasses should be washed thoroughly in soap and water, dried and hung up. The hands must be thoroughly washed on completion of any procedure involving cytotoxic drugs. Time-expired cytotoxic drugs should be returned to the pharmacy for disposal.

ADMINISTRATION OF CYTOTOXIC DRUGS

Very careful attention must be paid to the route of administration. While the use of an inappropriate route of administration is always hazardous,

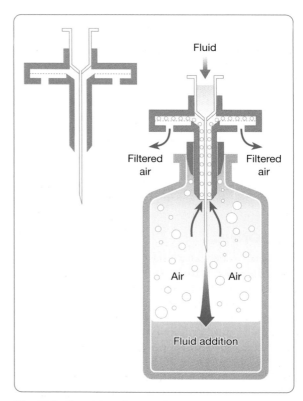

Fluid

Filtered air   Filtered air

Air   Air

Fluid addition

Fig. 19.6   Special venting needle.

the consequences of using an incorrect route of administration for cytotoxic drugs can be catastrophic. Most notably, there have been tragic cases in which a vinca alkaloid was given by the intrathecal route instead of intravenously. Most cytotoxic drugs are highly irritant to the tissues and, if extravasation occurs, local tissue damage and/or necrosis can occur. Most parenteral cytotoxic drugs are given intravenously either as a bolus into a freely running solution or as an infusion. As with all parenteral administration, the diluent used must be compatible with the drug and all expiry dates and storage instructions of reconstituted solutions observed. It is also important to ensure that the time taken to inject or infuse the drug is in accordance with the prescription. Intravenous infusions containing cytotoxic drugs should be controlled with the help of an infusion pump.

Cytotoxic chemotherapy administration should be prescribed to coincide with times when appropriately trained staff are available to administer the medicines. Cytotoxic chemotherapy should be administered only during normal working hours or in specialist units in which support and expert advice are available. Patients should receive chemotherapy in designated wards or outpatient clinics that are equipped to deal with any emergencies that may arise.

PARENTERAL ADMINISTRATION

An assessment of the patient and a peripheral blood count are carried out prior to the administration of cytotoxic drugs to ensure that the patient is fit to withstand the treatment. Monitoring is also essential throughout the course of treatment. The patient's weight and height are measured in order to calculate the dose of drug(s) to be given. The calculation of the dose, volume and concentration should be checked and recorded.

Each syringe should be clearly labelled with the name and dose of the drug. The used vial or ampoule should be placed with the loaded syringe(s) in a receiver bearing the patient's name and/or prescription to allow a final check to be made.

Prior to administration of the drug, the prescription should be compared with the patient's name, the labelled syringes and the used ampoules or vials. When the person administering the drug is the one who prepared it, a check should be made by a second qualified person and recorded appropriately. For intramuscular and subcutaneous injections, two nurses must be involved, one of whom is registered, and the checking procedure followed in the standard way.

Particular care must be taken when assisting a doctor with the administration of drugs using the intrathecal route that the drug is intended for intrathecal use (see British National Formulary).

In any event, it is particularly important to check that the correct patient is identified to receive the drug and that the correct route of administration is established. The prescription sheet must be signed by the person administering the chemotherapy.

Risks of contamination are still present during administration, and therefore precautions should be continued. Gloves that provide protection for the person administering the cytotoxic drug must be worn.

The area round the injection site should be protected by an absorbent, disposable towel. A butterfly needle is convenient when drugs that require a dilution intravenous infusion are being given. If there is any doubt about the siting of the needle, whether for infusion or direct bolus administration, the procedure should be abandoned and begun elsewhere.

Once an infusion of cytotoxic drugs has been established, responsibility rests with the nurse to observe the patient and provide continuing physical and emotional support. The point of entry of the needle into the vein should be observed frequently and any comments from the patient about the comfort of the area heeded. Leakage of the drug into the surrounding tissues, known as extravasation, may have disastrous consequences because of its irritant nature.

Any evidence of pain, burning or stinging at the injection site calls for an immediate assessment of the site. The doctor should be called at once and the infusion stopped. A ready-prepared pack for the first aid treatment of extravasation should be brought. The doctor will aspirate with the needle in place as much of the infiltrated drug as possible. Specialist advice should be sought to establish whether an antidote is available. Corticosteroids (to reduce inflammation), antihistamines and analgesics may require to be given. Cold compresses may also be ordered. Thereafter, frequent checking of the site will be required, with careful documenting of progress until resolution occurs. Ideally, drugs liable to cause extravasation should be given through a central line (e.g. Hickman catheter). Cytotoxic drugs that are known to be particularly damaging on extravasation are listed in Box 19.2.

Vomitus, urine and faeces from treated patients may contain unchanged drug or active metabolites. Vomitus from patients who have received an oral dose of a cytotoxic medicine should be considered hazardous for up to 12 h after administration; urine and faeces are potentially hazardous for up to 7 days

---

Box 19.2 Cytotoxic drugs that are particularly damaging on extravasation

- Carmustine
- Dacarbazine
- Dactinomycin
- Daunorubicin
- Doxorubicin
- Epirubicin
- Etoposide
- Idarubicin
- Melphalan
- Mitomycin
- Vinblastine
- Vincristine
- Vindesine
- Vinorelbine

---

following chemotherapy. Disposable utensils should always be used and care taken when placing them in the waste disposal unit to avoid splashing the contents. Skin contact should be avoided by wearing disposable latex gloves, and nurses' uniforms should be protected by a disposable plastic apron. Normal hygiene measures should be employed. Heavily soiled linen of patients receiving cytotoxic drugs should be dealt with as infected linen. It is the responsibility of the nurse in charge of the ward to advise all members of the nursing staff of those patients for whom these precautions must be taken.

PROCEDURE IN THE EVENT OF AN ACCIDENT

SPILLAGE OF A CYTOTOXIC DRUG ON TO INTACT SKIN

If any cytotoxic drug, apart from dacarbazine and melphalan, comes into contact with the skin, the affected area should be flushed with copious amounts of water.

If dacarbazine is spilled on to the skin, it should be washed off immediately with soap and water. In the case of mitomycin, the contaminated skin should be treated with a *fresh* solution of bisodium carbonate 8.4% w/v.

After skin contamination with methotrexate, if transient stinging occurs following washing with water, a bland cream (e.g. aqueous cream BP) should be applied to the affected area.

SPILLAGE OF A CYTOTOXIC DRUG ON TO BROKEN SKIN, INTO EYES OR THROUGH NEEDLE PENETRATION OF THE SKIN

If accidents involve cuts or needle penetration of the skin, the area should be washed with copious amounts of water.

If any cytotoxic drug enters the eye(s), the eye(s) should be irrigated thoroughly with sterile sodium chloride 0.9% solution.

In all such cases, the doctor and person in charge of the ward, department or clinic should be notified. The normal accident-reporting procedure should then be followed and a copy of the accident form sent to the occupational health department.

ORAL ADMINISTRATION

Oral solid dose forms of cytotoxic drugs constitute no risk to the handler if a few simple precautions are taken. If the patient has difficulty swallowing such preparations, advice should be sought from the pharmacy so that an alternative formulation can be provided. In general, tablets should neither be divided nor crushed or capsules opened. All oral dosage forms should be dispensed and administered using a non-touch technique, if necessary wearing disposable gloves. If the outer coating of a tablet or capsule is intact, there will generally be no hazard to the nurse. Disposable spoons and medicine measures should be used. A stainless steel 'triangle' should be used when tablets require to be counted. It should be washed after use. In the event of contamination by free powder or the contents of a capsule, the same principles for dealing with spillage of parenteral drugs apply. To prevent inhalation of powder, it is essential to use a well-fitting face mask. For mopping up spilled powder, a damp disposable towel paper should used. Disposal is by incineration.

MANAGEMENT OF SIDE-EFFECTS

The commonest adverse effects of cytotoxic drugs fall into four main categories:

- bone marrow suppression
- damage to the gastrointestinal mucosa
- damage to the skin and hair
- altered sexuality and fertility.

These effects reflect the areas of the body in which normal cell turnover is greatest. *The severity of side effects will depend on the drug(s) used and the dose given.*

BONE MARROW SUPPRESSION

LOWERED RESISTANCE TO INFECTION

Immunity to infection is provided by the white blood cells. Because of their very rapid rate of turnover, the white blood cells are the ones most readily damaged by cytotoxic drugs. As treatment progresses and the white count falls, the patient's ability to combat infection lessens. Frequent monitoring of the white cell count assists the clinician in deciding whether the patient has sufficient white cells to withstand the next dose of treatment and still combat an infective attack. A white blood count of less than $5 \times 10^9/L$ significantly increases the risk of infection. Care is directed towards minimising the risk of infection. Chemotherapy is likely to be withheld when the leucocyte count is less than $4 \times 10^9/L$.

Decisions sometimes have to be made as to where and how best to nurse in-patients receiving cytotoxic therapy. In the early stages of treating acute leukaemia, for example, when the white count is still at a reasonable level, the patient may be nursed alongside other patients, and indeed this may be important to maintain the patient's morale. As treatment progresses, increasing levels of protection may be necessary. A single room, a laminar air flow unit and protective isolation nursing measures may have to be introduced depending on the white cell count.

Staff caring for an immunosuppressed patient should be free from colds and sore throats, and they must not be involved if they have been in contact with viruses such as measles or chickenpox. Personal hygiene must be of the highest standard, especially hand hygiene. Strict aseptic technique must be employed while carrying out invasive procedures.

Recordings of the patient's temperature and pulse should be taken at least every 4 h. Even a low-grade pyrexia must be reported. Regular inspection of the body for evidence of infection is essential. The commonest sites of local infection are the mouth, axillae, groins and perineum. Infections of lungs, gut and urinary tract produce signs and symptoms with which the nurse should be familiar. Observing, recording, reporting, taking laboratory samples and administering prescribed antibiotics are standard procedures. Fresh blood or a white cell transfusion may be ordered. Nursing care is directed towards keeping the risk of infection to an absolute minimum. An overwhelming infection can have fatal consequences. The dangers of infection cannot be overstated.

In addition to clinical care, a high standard of food hygiene must be observed. Certain foods, (e.g. those containing uncooked eggs, meat or fish) should be totally avoided.

INCREASED RISK OF BLEEDING

Platelets (thrombocytes) are essential for blood clotting. When the platelet level falls below $20 \times 10^9/L$, the risk of spontaneous bleeding is significant. Although the patient's platelet count will be estimated at frequent intervals, it is also important for the nurse to observe for any signs of bleeding. This may range from overt bleeding, such as from an intravenous injection site or menorrhagia, to tiny petechial haemorrhages in the mouth or skin. More sinister is internal bleeding such as a subarachnoid haemorrhage or splenic bleed, which may have fatal consequences. As a safeguard, chemotherapy is withheld when the platelet count falls below $100 \times 10^9/L$.

Efforts must also be made to reduce the risk of bleeding. Injections should be kept to a minimum and restricted to the intravenous route. The risk of bleeding into a large and highly vascular area such as the buttock often makes intramuscular injections unacceptable. Mouthwashes are preferable to the trauma that a toothbrush may place on the gums. An electric razor should be used for shaving to reduce the risk of cuts to the skin. Blood pressure recordings are not taken in thrombocytopenic patients, because the pressure caused by an inflated sphygmomanometer cuff may be enough to cause internal bleeding in the upper arm. Finally, care should be taken when handling and moving such patients, to reduce the likelihood of bruising.

Platelet transfusions are given when the platelet count falls below $10 \times 10^9/L$.

ANAEMIA

When the number of red blood cells or the haemoglobin is reduced, the patient becomes anaemic and will experience breathlessness on exertion, feel the cold and generally lack energy. The reduction in haemoglobin level is gradual, and to an extent this allows the body to adapt. Everyday tasks can still be carried out but require greater effort. Although anaemia is not life-threatening and can be effectively treated with blood transfusions, patients do not feel at their best and may have less of a will to get better. Nursing care is directed towards providing comfort, assistance, reassurance and encouragement. Patients whose haemoglobin has dropped to 8 g/dL are likely to be transfused.

Table 19.4 Cytotoxic drugs known to be emetogenic

Risk of emesis	Example of cytotoxicity
Mild	Etoposide
	Fluorouracil
	Methotrexate
	Vinca alkaloids
Moderate	Cyclophosphamide (intermediate and low doses)
	Doxorubicin
	Methotrexate (high doses)
	Mitoxantrone
High	Cisplatin
	Dacarbazine

DAMAGE TO GASTROINTESTINAL MUCOSA

NAUSEA AND VOMITING

The severity of the symptoms of anorexia, nausea and vomiting are dependent on the drug(s) used, dose, frequency, route and regimen, and patients need to be reassured of this. Not all chemotherapy patients are sick. In some cases, however, vomiting has been so distressing that the patient has refused to accept a subsequent course of treatment. Cytotoxic drugs vary in their potential to cause nausea and vomiting (see Table 19.4). The aim is to try to prevent sickness occurring. Acute symptoms may be reduced in patients with a low risk of emesis by giving, for example, oral prochlorperazine or domperidone in advance. For patients at high risk of emesis, ondansetron and dexamethasone may be given intravenously at the start of treatment.

Care should be taken in positioning the patient in a suitable part of the ward, giving consideration to the comfort of other patients. A supply of disposable sickness basins, towels, paper tissues and disposal bags should be made ready. When appropriate, a container for dentures should be provided. A mouthwash and/or supply of cold water for rinsing the mouth after a bout of sickness should always be available. A call bell must always be to hand. Many patients appreciate the support of a nurse when they are being sick. Privacy is also essential. The patient is alarmed at this time and may be hampered by an intravenous infusion. By placing a hand across the patient's forehead, the nurse can provide a resistance against which to push, reducing the strain on the patient. The nurse can also help to support the sickness basin. Help is also often required to wipe the mouth and dispose of tissues. Sickness basins should be in plentiful supply so that the patient is not faced with a half-filled basin while waiting for the next wave of sickness to come. Used basins should be removed from the bedside immediately and measurements of volume recorded on a fluid balance chart. Repeated vomiting is exhausting for patients and so, whenever possible, they should be given every assistance to try to sleep.

Patients troubled by nausea often find their own ways of minimising the problem. These include, for example, taking small amounts of food and fluid at frequent intervals and listening to relaxation tapes. There is some evidence to suggest that receiving chemotherapy sitting in a chair rather than lying in bed reduces the risk of vomiting. If the patient's condition permits, this is an option that can be offered. Care must be taken to ensure that the chair is comfortable and supportive, that the patient is not allowed to get cold and that the legs are supported if the patient is seated for prolonged periods. Acupressure wristbands have proved a useful non-invasive method of controlling nausea and vomiting in some patients undergoing cytotoxic chemotherapy.

In some cases, past experience of vomiting following chemotherapy can lead to anticipatory nausea. The sight of the hospital, the ward, a particular member of staff, or the arrival of equipment at the bedside can, in themselves, make the patient feel very sick and can even provoke an attack of vomiting. In addition to antiemetic therapy as described, lorazepam may be given to reduce anxiety.

Loss of appetite commonly accompanies treatment with cytotoxic drugs. In the short term, a reduced intake of food does no harm, and so patients who decline a meal should not be badgered about it. Patients should, however, be encouraged to take some nourishment once the acute reaction has passed. To begin with, small amounts of what the patient chooses to take should be given at frequent intervals. Once the intake of very light foods or liquids can be tolerated, the process of increasing the volume and consistency should be a gradual one. Nutritional supplements tend to be rich and strongly flavoured and so are difficult to tolerate in the early stages. They are better reserved for supplementing the diet once it is re-established. Finding foods and liquids that appeal to patients calls for some imagination on the part of the nurse. Involvement of the families is important here in providing patients with their favourite (often homemade) tasty items of food. Flexibility is essential so that patients may eat or drink at any time of the day or night as the fancy takes them. The involvement of the dietitian is of course vital in many cases so that patients' nutritional status can be successfully monitored and maintained.

BREAKDOWN OF ORAL MUCOSA

Very strict attention to oral hygiene is of the utmost importance in patients receiving cancer chemotherapy, especially methotrexate and corticosteroids. Guidance on mouth care should be given to patients at the outset, and they should be encouraged to get into the habit of attending to this themselves whenever this is possible. They should be taught to inspect the mouth regularly and to report any changes without delay, and to rinse the mouth with an effective mouthwash such as chlorhexidine gluconate. When this is not possible, oral hygiene must be carried out by the nurse. Any suspect lesions should be swabbed for culture and sensitivity. Treatment for clinically obvious thrush will be begun before laboratory results are received. Mouth pain may be relieved by using benzydamine hydrochloride oral rinse. Liquids that sting the mouth and hard foods should be avoided. Some patients like to suck crushed ice or lemon and glycerin swabs.

CONSTIPATION

The neurotoxic effect of vinca alkaloids can lead to severe constipation and may result in paralytic ileus. Preventive measures should therefore be taken at the start of treatment. These will include increased fibre in the diet and plenty of fluids.

DIARRHOEA

Fluorouracil and doxorubicin may cause diarrhoea, necessitating the use of codeine phosphate or loperamide and appropriate nursing measures, such as a reduction in dietary fibre and an increase in fluid intake.

DAMAGE TO THE SKIN AND HAIR

EXTRAVASATION

Certain cytotoxic drugs are especially vesicant, and if allowed to leak from the vein into the surrounding tissues can cause burning and necrosis that, in some cases, have resulted in skin grafting and amputation. The nurse plays a vital role in explaining, observing for and reporting this phenomenon. The management of extravasation is described on page 393.

HAIR LOSS

Damage to the hair follicles reduces all hair growth on the body and makes the hair fall out. The term for this is alopecia or epilation. For both men and women,

this is a very distressing side-effect affecting body image, sexuality and self-confidence. Scalp-cooling techniques using gel packs may be used to reduce the concentration of drug in the capillaries of the scalp. The hair should always be groomed gently and, when it is clear that a wig will be required, arrangements if so desired should be made for it to be ordered while the colour, texture and style of the patient's hair are still apparent. The imaginative use of scarves and caps can help the patient through this period. Many patients, however, prefer to have no head covering at all and, particularly when at home, or in hospital where they feel safe, leave the head uncovered, especially when sleeping. The environment should be comfortably warm and free from draughts.

ALTERED SEXUALITY AND FERTILITY

As well as alterations to body image caused by chemotherapy in both male and female patients, there may be a loss of sexual function and ability to reproduce. In the female patient, cytotoxic therapy may cause fibrosis of the ovary, leading to amenorrhoea and sterility. The accompanying fall in oestrogen secretion may produce menopausal symptoms. In the male patient, there may be a total absence of sperm. Impotence and gynaecomastia may alter body image and reduce self-esteem. In both female and male patients, sterility may be temporary or permanent. Although women who have received chemotherapy have subsequently given birth to normal infants, genetic counselling should be given when pregnancy is desired by patients who have previously had chemotherapy, because of the possible effects on the unborn child. For men who have received cancer chemotherapy, 'sperm banking' is a possibility. Suitable contraception is advised in particular situations. If nurses are to help patients to cope with sexual dysfunction caused by treatment, then they need to feel comfortable discussing the subject. When this is not the case, the help of a trained counsellor may be required.

ROLE OF THE NURSE IN CANCER CHEMOTHERAPY

ASSESSMENT OF THE PATIENT

A full nursing assessment should be carried out, because the relationship between the nurse and the chemotherapy patient may last a considerable length of time. Special attention should be paid to patients' understanding of the treatment planned for them, their attitude towards the treatment and their thoughts about the longer term. Measurements of weight and height are taken for use in calculating cytotoxic drug dosages. In patients with acute leukaemia, lymphoma or myeloma, a bone marrow aspiration or trephine biopsy will be carried out at intervals to review progress, and this calls for particular support from the nurse.

With each pulse of treatment and at the start of a new course, there must be a willingness to reassess the patient's condition, checking up on the development of infection or any other new symptoms of note. A review of the patient's psychological condition is equally important.

SUPPORT AND ENCOURAGEMENT

Patients require a careful explanation of their course of chemotherapy, how it is to be given, how it will work and what effects it is likely to have. The challenge for the nurse is to pitch the information at a level the individual patient can cope with. Patients should be gently told that they are to receive powerful drugs that may make them feel less well before they start to get better again. They should be discouraged from comparing themselves with neighbouring patients, as no two patients react in an identical way. Realistic goals should be set in consultation with the patient. For example, the patient may be very anxious to continue working as much as possible throughout the treatment, and this may demand some degree of flexibility on both sides. Patients often need to have information repeated, partly because they have a lot to assimilate and partly because they need the reassurance that treatment is progressing. They need to be reassured that someone will listen to their anxieties. Whenever possible, there should be continuity of nursing staff to ease communication and so that patients can build up a feeling of trust.

Patients spend a lot of time waiting. Most patients accept the fact that they need treatment and just want to get on with it. Waiting for blood results can be tedious. In some cases, the treatment may have to be temporarily stopped because the white count is too low, and this news can be received with disappointment and even anger. The nurse must allow for such reactions and provide the necessary support for both patients and their families.

Chemotherapy patients have a lot to cope with. They may still be coming to terms with their diagnosis at the same time as trying to cope with treatment. They may also be trying to protect their families from the full impact of their condition and the treatment. Although they may be attending as outpatients, they may not be feeling very well. There may be issues that they want to discuss only with their carers in the expectation that they will understand. The ward or clinic becomes something of a haven for them where, for example, hair loss, vomiting and malaise are accepted. Time must be found for the patient who needs to talk. As an active listener, the nurse can gain much valuable information while at the same time helping the patient to offload. Keeping a special record of how patients are feeling about their progress can be extremely helpful to all members of the healthcare team.

SELF-ASSESSMENT QUESTIONS

SECTION A

Outline the information that should be given on a chemotherapy protocol to ensure that safe systems are in place for use of cytotoxic therapy.

SECTION B

1. Which of the following drugs is likely to cause nausea and vomiting?
   a. Dacarbazine
   b. Busulfan
   c. Cisplatin
   d. Cyclophosphamide (high dose)
   e. Doxorubicin
2. Which of the following drugs is likely to cause bone marrow suppression?
   a. Methotrexate
   b. Chlorambucil
   c. Melphalan
   d. Mitomycin
   e. Cytarabine
3. Which of the following drugs is likely to cause alopecia?
   a. Docetaxel
   b. Dactinomycin
   c. Etoposide
   d. Vincristine
   e. Paclitaxel
4. Which of the following drugs is likely to cause cardiotoxicity?
   a. Trastuzumab
   b. Epirubicin
   c. Paclitaxel
   d. Rituximab
   e. Chlorambucil

5. Which of the following drugs is likely to cause pulmonary fibrosis?
   a. Busulfan
   b. Mitomycin
   c. Carmustine
   d. Bleomycin
   e. Chlorambucil
6. Which of the following drugs is likely to cause diarrhoea?
   a. Irinotecan
   b. Fluouracil
   c. Melphalan
   d. Doxorubicin
   e. Methotrexate

SECTION C

1. Which is the odd one out and why?
   a. Domperidone
   b. Cyclizine
   c. Ondansetron
   d. Dexamethasone
   e. Omeprazole
2. Which is the odd one out and why?
   a. Chlorambucil
   b. Melphalan
   c. Interferon alfa
   d. Ciclosporin
   e. Methotrexate
3. Which is the odd one out and why?
   a. Vindesine
   b. Vinblastine
   c. Vigabatrin
   d. Vincristine
   e. Vinorelbine
4. Which is the odd one out and why?
   a. Cisplatin
   b. Methotrexate
   c. Mesna
   d. Cyclophosphamide
   e. Chlorambucil

REFERENCES

British Medical Association and Royal Pharmaceutical Society of Great Britain 2005 British National Formulary. BMJ Publishing Group, London

National Institute for Health and Clinical Excellence (http://www.nice.org.uk)

Scottish Executive 2005 Guidance for the safe use of cytotoxic chemotherapy. Scottish Executive, Edinburgh

FURTHER READING AND RESOURCES

Armstrong AC, Eaton D 2001 Science, medicine and the future: cellular immunotherapy for cancer. British Medical Journal 323:1289–1293

Chung-Faye GA, Kerr DG 2000 Innovative treatment for colon cancer. British Medical Journal 321:1397–1399

Cohen MR, Anderson RW, Attilio RM et al. 1996 Preventing medication errors in cancer chemotherapy. American Journal of Health-System Pharmacy 53:737–746

Curt GA 2001 Fatigue in cancer. British Medical Journal 322:1560

Donovan JL, Frankel SJ 2001 Screening for prostate cancer in the UK. British Medical Journal 323:763–764

Eystein Lønning P 2001 Aromatase inhibitors and inactivators in breast cancer. British Medical Journal 323:880–881

Grampian Medicines Committee 2000 Policies and procedures relating to medicines in Grampian. Grampian Medicines Committee, Aberdeen

Greenwald P 2002 Cancer chemoprevention. British Medical Journal 324:714–718

Grundy M (ed) 2006 Nursing in haematological oncology, 2nd edn. Elsevier, Edinburgh

Health and Safety Executive 2003. Safe handling of cytotoxic drugs M1SC615. HSE Books, Suffolk

Popat S, Smith LE 2006. Breast cancer. Update on Cancer Therapeutics 1:187–210

Royal College of Nursing 2005. Competencies – an integrated competency framework for training programmes in the safe administration of chemotherapy to children and young people. RCN, London

Scottish Intercollegiate Guidelines Network 2005 (updated 2006) Management of breast cancer in women, no. 84. SIGN, Edinburgh

Scottish Intercollegiate Guidelines Network 2005 Management of patients with lung cancer, no. 80. SIGN, Edinburgh

Scottish Intercollegiate Guidelines Network 2006 Management of oesophageal and gastric cancer, no. 87. SIGN, Edinburgh

Sjöström J, Bergh J 2001 How apoptosis is regulated and what goes wrong in cancer. British Medical Journal 322:1538–1539

Walters C 2006 Colorectal cancer: an overview. Pharmaceutical Journal 276:323–326

Xiong GQ, Carr K, Abbruzzese JL 2006 Cytotoxic chemotherapy for pancreatic cancer, advances to date and future directions. Drugs 66:1059–1072

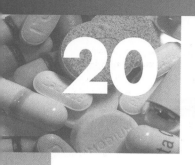

20 Drugs affecting the immune response

CHAPTER CONTENTS

KEY OBJECTIVES

After reading this chapter, you should be able to:

- describe how vaccines elicit an immune response
- discuss the use of vaccines in the UK childhood immunisation programme
- list the use of both normal and specific immunoglobulins
- outline the rationale for the use of antiproliferative immunosuppressants in the treatment of autoimmune disorders
- discuss the nursing care of the immunosuppressed patient.

THE IMMUNE SYSTEM

INTRODUCTION

Every day of our lives, we come into contact with a large variety of micro-organisms such as viruses, bacteria and fungi. Many of these pathogens are capable of causing disease, yet most of the time we do not succumb to infection. Moreover, when we do, the course of disease is usually short-lived. The immune system is the body's defence against potentially harmful substances and micro-organisms.

Specific and non-specific mechanisms take part in the immunological response. The blood and lymphatic systems, bone marrow, thymus gland, liver and spleen interact to make this system effective. The bone marrow is responsible for the production of lymphocytes, which are primed in the thymus gland (T lymphocytes) and possibly the bone marrow itself (B lymphocytes). These immunologically competent cells, together with phagocytes (macrophages), circulate in the blood and lymphatic systems, liver and spleen, ready to react to an invasion by foreign substances (antigens).

In those patients in whom the immune system is defective and immunodeficiency has occurred, there can be a risk of overwhelming and sometimes life-threatening infections. Perhaps the best-known cause of such a condition is infection with the virus HIV, leading to AIDS (see Ch. 15). This virus infects and destroys particular cells of the immune system, without which the patient becomes very susceptible to a variety of bacterial, viral and fungal infections. Immunodeficiencies are also caused by certain rare genetic diseases. Another common immunodeficiency occurs following treatment with drugs that damage the immune system. For example, immunodeficiency is a common side-effect of chemotherapy for cancer, and patients undergoing such treatment become more susceptible to infections. The immune response can

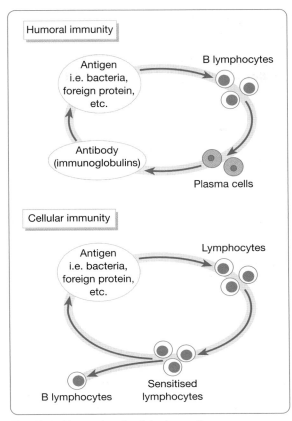

Fig. 20.1 Humoral and cellular immunity.

be used to positive effect with the use of vaccination and is one of the most effective methods of combating infectious disease.

SPECIFIC IMMUNE RESPONSE

When a foreign substance (antigen) enters the body, two different types of immunological response may occur (see Fig. 20.1).

HUMORAL IMMUNE RESPONSE (ANTIBODY-MEDIATED IMMUNITY)

On contact with the antigen, immunologically competent B lymphocytes change into plasma cells (effector cells). These plasma cells are capable of producing specific antibodies, the immunoglobulins. The antibody combines with the antigen (antigen–antibody reaction) and neutralises it, for example by coating bacteria to enhance their destruction by phagocytosis.

Another product of the primary contact of antigen with immunologically competent B lymphocytes is

the memory cells. Memory cells are able to recognise the same antigen on a second contact, which results in a more rapid and sometimes more intense response. Plasma cells are formed much faster, which in turn results in a large amount of antibodies. The capability of the memory cells to recognise specific antigens sometimes years after the primary contact forms the basis of active immunisation against bacteria and their toxins.

CELLULAR IMMUNE RESPONSE (CELL-MEDIATED IMMUNITY)

Depending on the physicochemical properties of the antigen and its way of entry into the body, some antigens cause the production of sensitised lymphocytes, the T lymphocytes, which have antibody-like molecules on their surface (cell-bound antibody). The T lymphocytes are responsible for the specific cell-mediated immune response. On primary contact with the antigen, they proliferate like the B lymphocytes and produce memory cells and effector cells. Unlike B lymphocytes, T lymphocytes produce different types of effector cells that directly take part in the immune reaction:

- cytotoxic effector cells (killer T cells) that can destroy other cells; this reaction to foreign cells is especially important in the rejection of transplanted organs
- T helper cells, which cooperate with the cytotoxic effector cells and also take part in the humoral immune response
- suppressor T cells, which can suppress the function of B lymphocytes and other T lymphocytes.

NON-SPECIFIC IMMUNITY

Apart from the specific immune response, a number of non-specific antimicrobial mechanisms have been recognised. These non-specific factors often operate in conjunction with the specific immune response, which greatly increases the overall effectiveness. These non-specific mechanisms include:

- bactericidal lysozyme, which is present in tears and saliva
- phagocytosis – some leucocytes are able to ingest and kill bacteria
- acute inflammatory response to a foreign substance – release of histamine from sensitised mast cells
- the non-specific antiviral agent interferon, which is a lymphokine produced by T cells in response to viral infections; interferon inhibits the intracellular viral replication (it also acts on the immune system by increasing the cytotoxic activity of T lymphocytes and inhibits the mitosis of tumour cells).

Box 20.1 Common allergens

- House and dust mites
- Grass and tree pollens
- Pet skin flakes or hair
- Fungal or mould spores
- Food (milk, egg, wheat, soya, seafood, fruit and nuts)
- Wasp and bee stings
- Some medicines
- Plants
- Nickel, rubber, preservatives and synthetic resins

Box 20.2 Common symptoms of allergy

- Sneezing
- Wheezing
- Sinus pain
- Runny nose
- Cough
- Nettle rash or hives
- Swelling
- Itchy eyes, ears, lips, throat and palate
- Shortness of breath
- Sickness, vomiting and diarrhoea

ALLERGY

Allergies are very common and affect around one in four people in the UK at some time in their lives. Each year, the numbers increase by 5%, with many more children being affected. Allergies result when the immune system is hypersensitive and over-reactive. The system misidentifies harmless proteins as antigens and then reacts out of proportion to the threat. Any substance that triggers an allergic reaction is called an allergen (Box 20.1). The symptoms may be mildly annoying or a major illness (Box 20.2). Most allergens are not obviously harmful, and have no affect on those individuals who are not allergic. Allergens frequently contain protein, and it is the protein that causes the reaction. Drugs may also cause allergic reactions (e.g. penicillins; see Ch. 10).

Allergy tends to run in families. Someone with an allergic tendency produces far more than the normal amounts of an antibody immunoglobulin E. Allergic individuals also produce more than the normal numbers of mast cells. The mechanism in susceptible individuals involves the production of immunoglobulin E antibody directed against the antigens. Immunoglobulin E binds to the surface of the mast cells and basophils. Subsequent exposure to antigen triggers the release of various substances, predominant among which is histamine. In the worst case scenario, this can result in an anaphylactic reactions (see Ch. 10).

Whenever possible, the most effective way of treating allergies is to avoid all contact with the allergen causing the reaction. Antihistamines treat allergies by blocking the action of the histamine that is released from mast cells (see Ch. 13). Decongestants help to relieve symptoms such as a blocked nose, which is often caused by hay fever, and dust and pet allergies (see Ch. 24). Nasal sprays and eye drops are available; nasal sprays reduce swelling and irritation in the nose, while eye drops relieve sore, itchy eyes. Drugs such as sodium cromoglicate and corticosteroids can be used regularly to stop symptoms developing. These are commonly available as nasal sprays and eye drops.

Another form of treatment is hyposensitisation. This can help those who have a specific allergy (e.g. bee stings). The person is gradually introduced to more and more of the allergen to encourage the body to make antibodies that will stop future reactions. This type of treatment must only be carried out under close supervision from a doctor, because of the risk that it may cause an anaphylactic reaction.

IMMUNISATION

Immunity can be induced, either actively or passively, against a variety of bacterial and viral agents.

ACTIVE IMMUNISATION

The objective of vaccination is to provide protection against certain infections such as diphtheria and tetanus. Active immunity is induced by injection of antigen in the form of inactivated or attenuated live organisms or their products (toxins). This stimulates the production of antibodies and a population of primed cells, which can expand rapidly on renewed contact with the antigen and inactivate the invading organism or its toxins. This means prevention or at least minimisation of the disease. Established disease cannot be treated by this method.

Active immunisation is used for the routine vaccination of babies and children (UK immunisation schedule, Table 20.1), for opportunistic vaccination of previously non-immunised adults (Table 20.2), and for the vaccination of travellers going to specified areas and people at risk from infection through the nature of their work or their lifestyle (Table 20.3).

Table 20.1   UK childhood immunisation schedule

Age at vaccination	Vaccine(s)	Notes
2 months	DTaP/IPV/Hib plus PCV	Pneumococcal vaccine introduced into UK immunisation schedule in 2006.
3 months	DTaP/IPV/Hib plus MenC	–
4 months	DTaP/IPV/Hib plus MenC plus PCV	–
In first year of life	BCG vaccine (for neonates at risk only)	For infants living in areas where the incidence of tuberculosis is greater than 40 per 100 000 *or* with a parent or grandparent born in a country with an incidence of tuberculosis greater than 40 per 100 000.
12 months	Hib/MenC	New combined vaccine introduced into UK schedule in 2006.
13 months	MMR plus PCV	Reviews undertaken on behalf of the Committee on Safety of Medicines and the Medical Research Council have not found any evidence of a link between MMR vaccination and bowel disease or autism.
Before school or nursery entry	DTaP/IPV (low- or standard-dose diphtheria) plus MMR	–
Before leaving school or before employment or further education	Adsorbed diphtheria (low dose), tetanus (DTaP) and IPV	An individual who has received five doses of tetanus vaccine is likely to have lifelong immunity. Individuals aged over 10 years should receive low-dose adsorbed diphtheria.

BCG, bacille Calmette–Guérin; DTaP, diphtheria, tetanus, pertussis (acellular, component); Hib, *Haemophilus* type b conjugate vaccine (adsorbed); IPV, inactivated poliomyelitis vaccine; MenC, meningococcal group C conjugate vaccine; MMR, measles, mumps and rubella vaccine, live; PCV, pneumococcal conjugate vaccine.

Table 20.2   Adult immunisations in those previously unimmunised

Individuals	Vaccine	Notes
Unimmunised women of childbearing age	MMR	Should be tested for rubella antibodies and seronegative women offered rubella immunisation – exclude pregnancy before immunisation.
Any unimmunised adults	DTaP	Three doses at intervals of 4 weeks. Booster dose at least 1 year after primary course and again 5–10 years later. (Booster doses may be required in travellers going to high-risk areas at 10-year intervals.)
At risk individuals	BCG	Contacts of those with active respiratory tuberculosis. Previously unvaccinated new immigrants from countries with a high incidence of tuberculosis, occupational health risk.

BCG, bacille Calmette–Guérin; DTaP, diphtheria, tetanus, pertussis (acellular, component); MMR, measles, mumps and rubella vaccine, live.

Table 20.3 Other vaccines used for specific circumstances

Vaccine	Indications for use
Anthrax vaccine	Individuals who handle infected animals or are exposed to infected animal products. Laboratory staff working with *Bacillus anthracis*.
Botulism antitoxin	Postexposure prophylaxis of botulism.
Cholera vaccine	Travellers to endemic or epidemic cholera areas.
Hepatitis A vaccine	Laboratory staff working with the virus; patients with haemophilia treated with factor VIII or factor IX; travellers to high-risk areas; individuals at risk due to their sexual behaviour; patients with chronic liver disease; staff and residents of homes for those with learning difficulties; sewage workers; parenteral drug abusers; close contacts of confirmed cases of hepatitis A.
Hepatitis B vaccine	Parenteral drug abusers; close contacts of case/carrier; infants born to mothers with hepatitis B; haemophiliacs receiving blood products; chronic renal failure; carers of dialysis patients; healthcare personnel who have direct contact with blood/body fluids; morticians and embalmers; staff and patients of daycare or residential accommodation for learning difficulties; inmates of custodial institutions; travellers to areas of high prevalence at increased risk or staying for long periods; families adopting children from countries with a high prevalence of hepatitis B.
Influenza vaccine	Patients with respiratory disease, chronic heart disease, chronic liver disease, chronic renal disease, diabetes mellitus, immunosuppression (disease or treatment), HIV infection; persons aged over 65 years of age; healthcare workers directly involved in patient care.
Meningococcal A, C, W135, Y vaccine	Travellers going to risk areas (particularly those going to the Haj in Saudia Arabia).
Pneumococcal vaccine	Those aged over 65 years; patients with asplenia or splenic dysfunction, chronic respiratory disease, chronic heart disease, chronic renal disease, chronic liver disease, diabetes mellitus, immune deficiency because of disease; presence of cochlear implant; presence of cerebrospinal fluid shunt.
Rabies vaccine	Laboratory staff who handle rabies vaccines; staff working in quarantine stations; animal handlers and vets likely to be bitten by infected wild animals; bat handlers; travellers going to endemic areas for > 1 month or at increased risk.
Smallpox vaccine	Laboratory workers handling pox viruses (contingency plans for the wider use of vaccine in event of post-eradication era outbreak are being considered).
Tick-borne encephalitis vaccine	Travellers going to those areas of high risk (e.g. forested areas of central and eastern Europe and Scandinavia).
Typhoid	Travellers to countries where sanitation standards may be poor.
Varicella zoster vaccine	Not recommended for routine use. May be used for seronegative individuals who come into close contact with varicella infection or have a high risk of severe varicella infection.
Yellow fever vaccine	Travellers going to endemic areas. Laboratory staff handling the virus or clinical material from patients.

Vaccines are very effective when administered correctly. However, basic personal hygiene remains vitally important, especially for travellers.

TYPES OF VACCINES USED FOR ACTIVE IMMUNISATION

Live attenuated vaccines. Live attenuated vaccines such as those against measles, mumps and rubella (MMR), tuberculosis (bacille Calmette–Guérin, BCG), varicella zoster, smallpox and yellow fever contain strains of attenuated live organisms that, although non-pathogenic, are still capable of producing specific antibodies. Some live vaccines may contain small amounts of agents, such as an antibiotic arising.

There is now overwhelming evidence that MMR does not cause autism. Over the past 7 years, a large number of studies have been published looking at this issue. For the latest evidence, see the Department of Health's website.

Inactivated vaccines. Bacterial and viral vaccines such as pertussis, poliomyelitis and tick-borne encephalitis vaccines contain heat-killed or chemically inactivated organisms. Human diploid cell vaccines such as rabies and hepatitis A vaccines contain organisms cultured on human diploid cells and chemically inactivated. *Haemophilus influenzae* type b (Hib) vaccine, pneumococcal vaccine, influenza vaccine, and hepatitis B vaccine contain immunising components of the organism. Because of their changing nature of the influenza virus, the World Health Organization monitors strains throughout the world. Each year, the World Health Organization makes recommendations about the strains to be included in vaccines for the forthcoming winter. To provide continuing protection, annual immunisation is necessary with vaccine against the currently prevalent strains. Should a new influenza A subtype emerge with epidemic or pandemic potential, a monovalent vaccine against that strain would be considered.

Vaccines such as tetanus and diphtheria vaccine contain bacterial toxins inactivated by formaldehyde to produce a toxoid. Typhoid and meningococcal vaccines are derived from the capsular polysaccharide antigen.

Adsorbed vaccines such as the diphtheria, tetanus, pertussis (acellular, component) vaccine (DTaP) and hepatitis B vaccine are inactivated vaccines adsorbed to an adjuvant such as aluminium phosphate or aluminium hydroxide. The adjuvant releases the antigen slowly and achieves a higher production of antibodies. Combined vaccines such as MMR or DTaP/inactivated poliomyelitis vaccine (IPV)/Hib are available to reduce the number of injections when immunising babies and children.

DURATION OF IMMUNITY

Injection with a vaccine does not provide immediate protection. There is usually an interval of a few days before the first antibodies appear. Inactivated vaccines produce a slow antibody or antitoxin response (primary response). Two injections may be needed to produce this effect. Further injections lead to an accelerated production of antibodies or antitoxins (secondary response) and therefore better protection. If the level of detectable antibody falls, a booster injection may be given to reinforce immunity. Immunity achieved in this way varies from months to years. No vaccine offers 100% immunity, and a small number of individuals get infected despite vaccination. For example 5–10% of children do not respond to the measles component in the first dose of MMR. The risk of measles is reduced by offering an additional dose of vaccine, usually before school entry.

ROUTES OF ADMINISTRATION

Oral vaccines. Most vaccines are administered parenterally. The exception is oral cholera vaccine. It is administered as an oral suspension for dilution with solution of effervescent sodium bicarbonate granules, containing inactivated strains of *Vibrio cholerae* bacteria and recombinant cholera toxin. Live oral polio vaccine is not now part of routine immunisation in the UK and is reserved for outbreak control only.

Vaccines for injection. With the exception of BCG, smallpox and oral cholera, all vaccines should be given by deep subcutaneous or intramuscular injection. The site should be chosen so that the injection avoids major nerves and blood vessels. The preferred sites for intramuscular and subcutaneous immunisation are the anterolateral aspect of the thigh or the deltoid area of the upper arm. The anterolateral aspect of the thigh is the preferred site for infants under 1 year old, because it provides a large muscle mass into which vaccines can be safely injected. If the buttock is used, injection into the upper outer quadrant avoids the risk of sciatic nerve damage. Injection into fatty tissue of the buttock has been shown to reduce the efficacy of hepatitis B and rabies vaccines.

The BCG vaccine must always be given intradermally. The operator should stretch the skin between the thumb and forefinger of one hand, and with the other slowly insert the needle (size 25- or 26-gauge), bevel upwards, for about 2 mm into the superficial layers of the dermis, almost parallel with the surface. A raised, blanched bleb showing the tips of the hair follicles is a sign that the injection has been made correctly. If considerable resistance is not felt, and it is suspected that the needle is too deep, it should be removed and reinstated before more vaccine is given. A bleb of 7-mm diameter is approximately equivalent to 0.1 mL of injection. For BCG, the site of injection is over the insertion of the left deltoid muscle; the tip of the shoulder must be avoided because of increased risk of keloid formations. (It is generally accepted that it is given in the same place for confirmation of previous BCG). For tuberculin sensitivity tests (Mantoux), intradermal injections are given in the middle of the flexor surface of the forearm. This site should not be used for injecting vaccines. Rabies vaccine may be given intradermally if more than one person needs to be immunised or a rapid immunisation is required (e.g. staff caring for a patient with rabies).

CONTRAINDICATIONS

Contraindications apply to the administration of most vaccines. Some of these are outlined below. The current data sheet should always be consulted before the administration of a vaccine. All vaccines are contraindicated in those who have had a confirmed anaphylactic reaction to a previous dose of a vaccine containing the same antigens or another component contained in the vaccine (e.g. neomycin, streptomycin or polymyxin B, which may be present in trace amounts in some vaccines).

In addition, the following individuals should not receive live vaccines.

- Patients with evidence of severe primary immunodeficiency (e.g. severe combined immunodeficiency and other combined immunodeficiency syndromes).
- All patients being treated for malignant disease with immunosuppressive chemotherapy or radiotherapy, and for at least 6 months after stopping treatment.
- All patients who have received a solid organ transplant and are currently on immunosuppressive treatment.
- Patients who have received a bone marrow transplant until at least 12 months after finishing all immunosuppressive treatment, or longer when the patient has developed graft versus host disease. The decision to vaccinate should depend on the type of transplant and immune status of the patient.
- All patients receiving systemic high-dose steroids until at least 3 months after treatment has stopped. This includes children who receive prednisolone, orally or rectally, at a daily dose (or its equivalent) of 2 mg/kg per day for at least 1 week, or 1 mg/kg per day for 1 month. For adults, an equivalent dose is considered to be about 40 mg of prednisolone per day for more than 1 week. There may be individuals on lower doses of steroids who may be immunosuppressed.
- Patients receiving other types of immunosuppressive drugs (e.g. azathioprine, ciclosporin, methotrexate, cyclophosphamide, leflunomide and the newer cytokine inhibitors) alone or in combination with lower doses of steroids. The advice of the doctor should be sought.
- Patients with immunosuppression due to HIV.

There will be very few occasions when deferral of immunisation is required. Minor illnesses without fever or systemic upset are not valid reasons to postpone immunisation. If an individual is acutely unwell, immunisation may be postponed until they have fully recovered. This is to avoid wrongly attributing any new symptom or the progression of symptoms to the vaccine.

Individuals with a confirmed anaphylactic reaction to egg should not receive influenza or yellow fever vaccines. MMR vaccine can be safely given even to most children with a previous history of allergy after ingestion of egg or egg-containing food. For the small number of individuals who have a history of confirmed anaphylactic reaction after any egg-containing food, specialist advice should be sought with a view to immunisation.

There is a theoretical concern that vaccinating pregnant women with live vaccines may infect the fetus. There is no evidence that any live vaccine (including rubella and MMR) causes birth defects, but given the theoretical possibility of fetal infection, live vaccines should generally be delayed until after delivery. Inactivated vaccines cannot cause infection in either the mother or the fetus.

Immunoglobulin may interfere with the immune response to live vaccine viruses, because the immunoglobulin may contain antibodies to measles, varicella and other viruses. Live virus vaccines should therefore be given at least 3 weeks before or 3 months after an injection of immunoglobulin. This does not apply to yellow fever vaccine, because immunoglobulin used in the UK is unlikely to contain high levels of antibody to this virus.

ADVERSE REACTIONS

Adverse reactions to vaccines are usually mild, and severe reactions are very rare. Because vaccines have become safer, the risk associated with immunisation, particularly in children, is very much smaller than the risk of complications of the disease. Most vaccines may produce mild local or systemic reactions such as redness and swelling at the injection site, raised temperature and screaming. Some vaccines such as measles vaccine may cause a mild form of the disease. Parents should be informed about possible adverse effects and advised on fever management after routine immunisation of their children.

Severe site reactions after BCG administration, such as large ulcers, abscesses and keloid formations, are due largely to the wrong immunisation technique (see routes of administration).

Despite the rarity of severe adverse reactions, doctors and nurses always have to be prepared for an anaphylactic reaction after vaccination and must be familiar with the management of anaphylactic shock (see Ch. 9). All anaphylactic reactions should be reported to the Committee on Safety of Medicines using the yellow card scheme.

TUBERCULOSIS: BACILLE CALMETTE–GUÉRIN IMMUNISATION

Vaccination against tuberculosis is discussed in greater detail because of the special tests and immunisation technique involved.

Patterns of tuberculosis in the UK have changed significantly since the BCG programme was first introduced in the 1950s. At that time, 50 000 cases of tuberculosis were reported each year in the UK, with cases occurring across most groups of people in society. Numbers of cases are now approximately 7000 a year. Although they have increased overall since the early 1990s, cases tend to be concentrated in large cities and in specific population groups. As a consequence, in July 2006 the Department of Health announced that routine childhood BCG immunisation programme was to stop. This has been replaced by a policy of identifying and vaccinating those who are most likely to catch the disease.

RECOMMENDATIONS FOR IMMUNISATION

The following groups are recommended for immunisation with BCG provided that successful BCG immunisation has not previously been carried out, the tuberculin test is negative, and there are no other contraindications:

- all infants (aged 0–12 months) living in areas of the UK where the annual incidence of tuberculosis is 40 per 100 000 or greater
- all infants (aged 0–12 months) with a parent or grandparent who was born in a country where the annual incidence of tuberculosis is 40 per 100 000 or greater

- previously unvaccinated children aged 1–5 years with a parent or grandparent who was born in a country where the annual incidence of tuberculosis is 40 per 100 000 or greater; these children can normally be vaccinated without tuberculin testing
- previously unvaccinated, tuberculin-negative children aged from 6 to under 16 years of age with a parent or grandparent who was born in a country where the annual incidence of tuberculosis is 40 per 100 000 or greater
- previously unvaccinated tuberculin-negative contacts of cases of respiratory tuberculosis
- previously unvaccinated, tuberculin-negative new entrants under 16 years of age who were born in or who have lived for a prolonged period (at least 3 months) in a country with an annual tuberculosis incidence of 40 per 100 000 or greater
- high-risk occupational groups (e.g. healthcare staff who will have contact with patients or clinical materials or veterinary staff).

IMMUNISATION REACTION

Normally, a local reaction develops at the injection site within 2–6 weeks; this consists of a small papule increasing in size for a few weeks up to 7 mm in width with scaling, crusting and occasional bruising. Occasionally, a shallow ulcer develops; this should be exposed to the air. The lesion slowly subsides over a period of several months, leaving a small scar.

THE TUBERCULIN TEST

Before BCG immunisation, a tuberculin skin test is carried out; a positive test implies immunity through past infection or immunisation. Test-positive people should therefore not receive BCG. Those with a strongly positive test may have active disease and have to be referred. The Mantoux test is now the only technique for tuberculin testing. It uses purified protein derivative, tuberculin PPD (Statens Serum Institut) and is labelled as 2 TU per 0.1-mL dose (20 units in 1 ml). The higher concentration 10 TU/0.1 mL may be used for a second test if the first test (2 TU per 0.1 mL) is negative (less than approximately 6 mm in diameter) and a retest is considered appropriate for clinical purposes.

The Mantoux test

The solution is injected intradermally, using a 25- or 26-gauge short-bevel needle, on the flexor surface of the forearm at the junction of the upper third with the lower two-thirds. The skin is slightly stretched, and the needle point (held almost parallel with the skin surface, bevel upwards) is inserted into the superficial layer of the dermis. The needle should be visible through the epidermis during insertion. The solution is slowly injected, and a small papule of 8–10 mm in diameter appears and remains for about 10 min. If a papule does not appear, the solution has been injected too deeply. The results should be read 48–72 h later. A positive result (using the Statens Serum Institut PPD) consists of a transverse induration of at least 6 mm diameter; 0–5 mm induration is negative, 6–14 mm is positive, and 15 mm or more is strongly positive.

Factors affecting the tuberculin test

The reaction to tuberculin protein may be suppressed by the following factors:

- glandular fever
- viral infections in general
- live viral vaccines
- Hodgkin's lymphoma
- sarcoidosis
- corticosteroid therapy
- immunosuppressing diseases, including HIV.

Other factors that also affect the consistency of tuberculin testing include patient's age, skin thickness, tuberculin adsorption on to the surface of the syringe and tester/reader variation.

IMMUNISATION OF CHILDREN

The immunisation of babies and children against infectious diseases such as diphtheria, pertussis, tetanus, measles, mumps, rubella and poliomyelitis has greatly reduced infant mortality and permanent physical and mental handicap caused by the illness. The introduction of the Hib vaccine in the 1970s was effective in children over 18 months of age. Pneumococcal immunisation has been introduced into the routine childhood immunisation programme from 2006.

The aim of the vaccination programme is to eliminate these diseases as far as possible from the population. For example, by giving rubella vaccine to young children it is intended to interrupt the circulation of rubella and thereby remove the risk of infection to non-immune pregnant women. Rubella immunisation (using MMR) to non-immune women continues to reduce the considerable risk to unborn babies. To achieve this aim, a high uptake in child vaccinations is required.

RISK GROUPS

The risk groups are HIV-positive persons, children with special conditions, people living in institutions such as old people's homes, occupational risk groups and travellers.

HIV-POSITIVE PATIENTS

HIV-positive patients are at increased risk from infectious diseases. Symptomatic and asymptomatic HIV-positive individuals can receive measles (or MMR), mumps, rubella, polio, whooping cough, diphtheria, tetanus, typhoid, hepatitis A and B, and Hib vaccines, and rabies vaccine as appropriate.

HIV-positive patients should *not* receive BCG or yellow fever vaccines. Travellers intending to visit infected areas where a valid immunisation certificate is required should obtain a letter of exemption from their medical practitioner. Vaccine efficacy may be reduced in HIV-positive individuals, and consideration should be given to the use of normal immunoglobulin after exposure to measles and to varicella zoster immunoglobulin after exposure to chickenpox or herpes zoster.

CHILDREN AND ADULTS WITH SPECIAL CONDITIONS

Some conditions, such as HIV (see above), asthma, chronic lung and congenital heart diseases, Down's syndrome, small-for-dates and prematurity increase the risk from infectious diseases. Children with such conditions should be immunised as a matter of priority. Small for dates and premature babies should be immunised according to the recommended schedule like any other children. Apart from routine immunisations, children and adults at risk should also be immunised against influenza and pneumococcal infections.

Hepatitis B immunisation is recommended for haemophiliacs on regular blood transfusions and patients with renal failure, drug abusers, babies born to hepatitis B carrier mothers and certain occupational groups.

CHILDREN WITH NEUROLOGICAL PROBLEMS

Immunisation of children against whooping cough is recommended when they have established neurological problems such as cerebral palsy. In doubtful cases, advice should be sought from a consultant paediatrician. Children with a personal or family history of febrile convulsions and epilepsy should also receive the pertussis vaccine.

CHILDREN AND ADULTS LIVING IN INSTITUTIONS

Children in residential care are at special risk from measles and should be immunised provided that there are no contraindications. Residents of nursing homes, old people's homes and other long-stay facilities in which rapid spread after introduction of the infection may occur should be immunised against influenza. Hepatitis B immunisation is recommended for staff and clients in residential accommodation, for those with a learning disability, and for inmates of custodial institutions (see Table 20.3).

OCCUPATIONAL RISK GROUPS

Healthcare staff such as doctors and nurses, laboratory staff, veterinary staff, customs officers and prison staff may be at increased risk from infectious diseases such as hepatitis B, tuberculosis and rabies because of the nature of their work; they should be immunised (see Table 20.3).

TRAVELLERS

Travellers to areas where the risk of contracting an infectious disease is especially high, or the nature of travel presents a special risk, or a valid immunisation certificate such as for yellow fever and meningococcal meningitis is required should be immunised. Advice on which immunisation is necessary for which country and on other measures for the prevention of diseases should be obtained from a general medical practitioner or travel clinic well before travelling (see Table 20.3).

Apart from immunisation, the main measure for preventing diseases such as typhoid, cholera and hepatitis A in areas of poor hygiene and sanitation is strict personal, food and drink hygiene. Normal immunoglobulin in now no longer given routinely for protection against hepatitis A, and hepatitis A vaccine is the recommended choice. Immunoglobulin may be indicated in the immunocompromised traveller.

PASSIVE IMMUNISATION

In this method of immunisation, the appropriate antibody or antitoxin against the invading organism or toxin is injected. The antibodies are retrieved from immunised animals (antisera), for example diphtheria antitoxin, which is prepared in horses, or from immunised humans (immunoglobulins). The use of antisera has been widely replaced by the use of human immunoglobulins, because of the serious side effects associated with antisera, such as serum sickness and other allergic-type reactions. Reactions to human immunoglobulins are rare.

TYPES OF HUMAN IMMUNOGLOBULINS

Non-specific polyvalent human immunoglobulin (normal human immunoglobulin) is produced from pooled plasma of a large group of donors, which contains antibodies currently prevalent in the population. Normal human immunoglobulin is used for:

- the protection of immunosuppressed children exposed to measles
- children under 12 months in whom there is a particular reason to avoid measles; immunisation with MMR vaccine should follow after a 3-month interval
- prophylaxis of infections following bone marrow transplantation
- protection of immunocompromised individuals against hepatitis A.

Normal human immunoglobulin is *not* recommended for the protection of previously non-immunised pregnant women exposed to *rubella*. If termination of pregnancy is not acceptable, it may be given to reduce the likelihood of a clinical attack, which may possibly reduce the risk for the fetus. Immunisation with normal human immunoglobulin produces immediate protection that lasts for 4–6 weeks.

Specific immunoglobulins such as tetanus, hepatitis B, cytomegalovirus, rabies and varicella zoster are produced from pooled blood of convalescent patients or recently immunised donors or donors who have a sufficient antibody titre. Specific immunoglobulin is used for postexposure treatment of previously unimmunised patients, usually in combination with the appropriate vaccine. Previously immunised patients need only a booster injection of the appropriate vaccine. Treatment of the established disease with specific immunoglobulins is effective only if a high proliferation of the invading organism, especially viruses, or the bonding of toxins to body structure has not yet taken place. For example, in clinical tetanus a decrease of symptoms is only sometimes possible.

Anti-D (RhO) immunoglobulin is used to prevent a rhesus-negative mother forming antibodies to fetal rhesus-positive cells. It should be injected within 72 h of birth or abortion to protect any subsequent child from haemolytic disease of the newborn.

ADMINISTRATION

Human immunoglobulins are administered intra-muscularly, because of the danger of aggregation and anaphylactic reactions if given intravenously. To produce intravenous preparations, the immunoglobulin has to undergo specific treatment. Intravenous preparations (e.g. tetanus immunoglobulin for intravenous use) is indicated if a large amount of antibody or a quick rise of antibody titre is necessary, as in the case of clinical tetanus. Special formulations of immunoglobulins are also available for intravenous use in replacement therapy, for example, in the treatment of congenital agammaglobulinaemia or idiopathic thrombocytopenic purpura.

STORAGE AND DISPOSAL OF VACCINES

Most vaccines have to be stored and transported under refrigeration at the recommended temperature. This means that a 'cold chain' should be maintained at all times by using insulated cooled containers for the transport of vaccines from one refrigerator to another. The potency of vaccines can be guaranteed only if they have been kept at the recommended temperatures. (Manufacturers' leaflets should be consulted.) For most vaccines, the recommended storage temperature is +2° to +8°. As with all immunological preparations, the cold chain must be maintained during transport and distribution.

Reconstituted vaccines must be used within the recommended period of time, usually between 1–4 h, and safely discarded after an immunisation session. Opened multidose containers of any vaccine have to be discarded after 1 h for non-preservative-containing and 3 h for preservative-containing vaccines. Single-dose containers should be used when possible.

Spillages must be cleared up quickly; gloves should be worn. The spillage should be soaked up with paper towels, taking care to avoid skin puncture from glass or needles. The area should be cleaned according to the local chemical disinfection policy or Control of Substances Hazardous to Health safety data sheets. Gloves, towels, etc. should be sent for incineration. Spillages on skin should be washed with soap and water. If vaccine is splashed in the eyes, they should be washed with sterile sodium chloride solution 0.9% and medical advice sought.

Unused vaccine and spent or partly spent vials should be disposed of by incineration at 1100°C. Local policies for the disposal of vaccine waste should be followed.

CONDITIONS TREATED WITH DRUGS AFFECTING THE IMMUNE SYSTEM

Intervention into this most important defence mechanism is justified only in certain circumstances. Risks and benefits of drug treatment have to be weighed up carefully. Treatment should be initiated only in a specialist unit under the supervision of an experienced physician. Drug treatment is indicated in the following conditions.

ORGAN TRANSPLANTATIONS

The immune system enables the body to distinguish between self and non-self. This causes the rejection of transplanted organs, which are recognised as non-self by the immune system of the recipient. Drugs that act by suppressing the immune response are vitally important in helping to prolong the life of a transplanted organ.

AUTOIMMUNE DISEASES

Sometimes, the body's mechanism for preventing the recognition of self components as antigen is disturbed and the system turns against itself: autoantibodies are produced. All diseases associated with the formation of autoantibodies are called autoimmune diseases. Major examples are:

- systemic lupus erythematosus
- scleroderma
- rheumatoid arthritis
- ulcerative colitis
- myasthenia gravis
- active chronic hepatitis
- chronic glomerulonephritis
- Wegener's granulomatosis.

CANCER

Examples include hairy cell leukaemia, certain lymphomas and solid tumours, and Kaposi's sarcoma associated with AIDS. The treatment of these and other cancers is dealt with in more detail in Chapter 19. It is very important to recognise that treatment with immunosuppressive drugs greatly weakens the patient's defence mechanism. This fact must be taken into account when providing nursing care and planning treatment (e.g. every effort must be made to reduce the risk of infection to a minimum).

MAIN DRUG GROUPS

These drugs may be categorised as *immunosuppressants* and *immunomodulators*.

IMMUNOSUPPRESSANTS

Under this heading, we consider the following:

- antiproliferative immunosuppressants
- corticosteroids

- ciclosporin
- other immunosuppressants.

ANTIPROLIFERATIVE IMMUNOSUPPRESSANTS

Azathioprine, the most commonly used drug in this group, is metabolised to 6-mercaptopurine, which suppresses cell-mediated immune reactions by preventing lymphocyte proliferation and function. Cyclophosphamide and methotrexate may also be used to suppress the immune response.

Azathioprine is used either alone or, more commonly, in combination with corticosteroids and/or other immunosuppressive agents in the management of renal and other organ transplantations and autoimmune diseases (e.g. autoimmune haemolytic anaemia). The therapeutic effect may be evident only after a few weeks and may be corticosteroid-sparing, thereby reducing side-effects associated with high dosage and prolonged use of systemic corticosteroids. Azathioprine is available as both tablets and injection. Whenever possible, oral administration is the preferred route. When the therapeutic effect is evident, doses should be reduced to the lowest effective level and should be maintained indefinitely in transplant patients because of the risk of organ rejection. Elderly patients and patients with renal or hepatic impairment should receive doses at the lower end of the range.

Mycophenolate mofetil has similar actions and uses to azathioprine. Antiproliferative immuno-suppressants are potentially dangerous drugs and have numerous side-effects. Careful monitoring and regular blood counts are required, with dose adjustments if necessary, and patients should be advised about the importance of regular blood counts.

The most important side effects are:
- marrow toxicity, which is dose-related and reversible
- hair loss, usually more significant in transplant patients
- increased susceptibility to viral, fungal and bacterial infections, usually more significant in transplant patients
- increased risk of neoplasia, particularly lymphomas
- gastrointestinal disturbances
- cholestatic hepatotoxicity, which requires an immediate withdrawal of the drug.

CORTICOSTEROIDS (see Ch. 16)

Corticosteroids are powerful immunosuppressants. They suppress the immune function of lymphocytes and interfere with both humoral and cell-mediated immune reactions. They are used to prevent organ transplant rejection, commonly in conjunction with other immunosuppressants. In autoimmune diseases, they are used for their immunosuppressive and anti-inflammatory effects.

CICLOSPORIN

Ciclosporin is a cyclical polypeptide (a complex protein-like substance derived from a soil fungus). It suppresses mainly cell-mediated immune reactions by inhibition of T-lymphocyte proliferation. Ciclosporin is a potent immunosuppressive agent that prolongs the survival of allogeneic transplants involving skin, heart, kidney and other organs. Since the introduction of ciclosporin, the number of successful organ trans-plantations has increased significantly. It is virtually non-myelotoxic and can therefore be used for bone marrow transplantations. It has no cytotoxic actions. Oral ciclosporin is also used for the treatment of severe psoriasis that is unresponsive to other forms of treatment.

Ciclosporin is available as oral (oral solution and capsules) and parenteral preparations. Parenteral therapy is used for initiation of therapy in organ and bone marrow transplantations, usually 1 day before the operation and in the immediate follow-up period. Oral treatment should commence as soon as possible, depending on the patient's condition. If corticosteroids are used at the same time, lower doses are used. Dosage levels are adjusted in the light of blood level determinations. Oral solutions should be mixed with orange juice (or squash) or apple juice to mask the taste (grapefruit juice should not be used and avoided for 1 h before the dose). In order to ensure that the full dose is ingested, the cup or glass should be rinsed.

Side-effects include nephrotoxicity, changes in liver function, gastric disturbances and hypertension (see specialist literature).

OTHER IMMUNOSUPPRESSANTS

These include the calcineurin inhibitors tacrolimus and sirolimus. Monoclonal antibodies basiliximab and daclizumab are also used for prophylaxis of rejection in organ transplantation (see specialist literature). Thalidomide is a potent immunomodulating drug.

INTERFERONS

Type 1 interferons (alfa and beta) are naturally occurring glycoproteins that have complex effects on the immune system and cell function. Type 2 interferons are characterised by gamma interferon. Interferons are available only as injections to be administered subcutaneously, intramuscularly or directly into the lesions of Kaposi's sarcoma.

Interferon alfa is used in the treatment of hairy cell leukaemia, chronic myelogenous leukaemia, AIDS-related Kaposi's sarcoma, hepatitis B and hepatitis C. Interferon alfa is also used as an adjunct in the treatment of malignant melanoma and for the maintenance of remission in myeloma. The most frequently occurring side effects are flu-like symptoms, which can be successfully treated with paracetamol. Interferon alfa also has a suppressive effect on the bone marrow that can lead to leucopenia and thrombocytopenia. Safety has not been established in children, and therefore interferons are usually not recommended for use under the age of 18.

Interferon beta is used in the treatment of relapsing remitting multiple sclerosis. Multiple sclerosis is the commonest demyelinating disease of the nervous system and is the commonest cause of disability in young adults. Multiple sclerosis is thought to be caused by a combination of factors (including viral activity), which leads to an autoimmune destruction of the central nervous system myelin. The mechanisms by which interferon beta produces therapeutic benefits are not well understood but could include the following actions: decrease in proliferation of T cells, restoration of T-suppressor cell function and reduction in the secretion of interferon gamma, which plays a role in the occurrence of spontaneous multiple sclerosis exacerbations. The National Institute for Health and Clinical Excellence (2002) did not recommend the use of interferon therapy in multiple sclerosis. However, a risk-sharing scheme between the manufacturers and the NHS was set up to allow the supply of both interferon beta and glatiramer (another immunomodulating drug) to multiple sclerosis patients.

NURSING THE IMMUNOSUPPRESSED PATIENT

The care of the immunosuppressed patient calls for an understanding, by everyone involved, of the potential dangers of being overwhelmed by infection with little or no resistance to fight it. It falls to the nurse in particular to provide as safe an environment as possible for the patient, and to observe for and act on any signs or symptoms of infection as promptly as possible. There may be an assumption that most infections, with the help of modern medicines, are treatable and that no one is likely to die from infection. In the absence of a functioning immune system, the patient is at very great risk not only from bacterial invasion but also from fungal and viral organisms.

The aspects of care that require special consideration, especially by nurses, may be considered under a number of headings.

Location and method of nursing. Patients who are immunosuppressed require to be isolated from micro-organisms that will harm them. Protection is achieved by using a method of nursing known as protective isolation. The degree of immunosuppression will dictate the degree of protection required. The facilities available will also influence the situation. For some patients, it may be sufficient to nurse them in a single room within the ward. Others will require stricter control of the environment provided by either specially designed units with en suite facilities or a plastic isolator.

Environment. The patient's room should be kept scrupulously clean. Furniture, equipment and the floor should be wiped down daily using a detergent solution. Wherever possible, disposable cloths should be used. Mop heads should be laundered after use. Disposable equipment should be used whenever possible. Otherwise, equipment should be left in the room for the exclusive use of the patient. Flowers should be displayed outside the room, because they or the water they are standing in are potential sources of infection.

Staff and visitors. Those coming into contact with the patient should not pose any risk of passing on infection. Staff suffering from a cold or sore throat or who have any focus of infection (such as an infected finger) should be temporarily employed elsewhere if not absent from duty. Numbers of visitors should be limited, and there should be a restriction on children visiting, because there is an increased likelihood that they will have been in contact with viral infections such as measles or chickenpox that could prove fatal if acquired by the immunosuppressed patient.

Handwashing. Hands are considered to be the prime source of transfer of micro-organisms. They should be thoroughly washed using an antiseptic cleansing solution such as chlorhexidine gluconate solution 20% or alcoholic hand rub before and after all clinical procedures. Procedures such as urinary catheterisation, catheter toilet, wound dressing, venepuncture and endotracheal suction must be carried out using a rigorous aseptic technique.

Food. Cooked food is safer than uncooked food. Fruit and vegetables should always be cooked and salads avoided. Food in tins and sealed packets from reputable firms and within date are considered safe. Bottled water and canned or bottled juices may be used. Tap water should be boiled before using.

Observation. The nurse must be vigilant in observing the development of signs of infection at an early stage. Frequent and thorough inspection of areas likely to be the first focus of infection, such as the mouth, axillae, groins and anal area, should be made. Careful recordings of temperature and pulse should also be made. Any elevation of these vital signs should be reported at once. The development of any other significant features should be noted. For example, a productive cough may signal a chest infection; dysuria, a urinary tract infection; diarrhoea, gastroenteritis. Diagnostic tests such as a chest x-ray and bacteriological examination of appropriate body fluids will be ordered. Good observation, however, is in itself not enough. Careful documenting by each shift of nurses and prompt reporting are also essential.

Finally, it should not be forgotten that isolation can bring with it psychological difficulties, and so nurses must ensure that patients understand the need for such an arrangement and provide as much encouragement as possible.

SELF-ASSESSMENT QUESTIONS

1. Outline the use of immunoglobulins in providing passive immunity.
2. Define active immunity
3. Define passive immunity.
4. Immunosuppressants are of increasing importance in the treatment of life-threatening conditions. What is their purpose?
5. Name four general areas of therapy where immunosuppressant drugs are of high value.
6. Corticosteroids have significant side-effects. Which is potentially the most serious and why?
7. The NHS should provide a full travel vaccination service for the public. Do you agree/disagree? Give reasons for your answer. (No answers provided here).

REFERENCE

National Institute for Health and Clinical Excellence 2002 TA32 beta interferon and glatiramer acetate for the treatment of multiple sclerosis: guidance. NICE, London

FURTHER READING AND RESOURCES

Bong JJ, Lansdown M 2002 Skin cancer in patients on long term immunosuppression. British Medical Journal 324:1344

Department of Health 1996 The green book. Immunisation against infectious diseases. Department of Health, London

Heller T 2001 How safe is MMR vaccine? British Medical Journal 323:838–839

Lee MA 2003 Transplantation: drug aspects of immunosuppression. Hospital Pharmacist 10:201–207

Prasad KR, Lodge JPA 2001 Transplantation of the liver and pancreas. British Medical Journal 322:845–847

Scottish Executive Health Department 2005 Changes to the BCG vaccination programme. Scottish Executive Health Department, Edinburgh

Taylor B, Miller E 2002 Measles, mumps and rubella vaccination and bowel problems or developmental regression in children with autism: population study. British Medical Journal 324:393–396

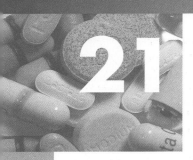

21 Nutrition and blood, fluid and electrolytes

KEY OBJECTIVES

After reading this chapter, you should be able to do the following.

Nutrition:

- identify the type of patients who may benefit from nutritional supplementation
- explain how the basal metabolic index is calculated
- list the foods that may be encouraged before resorting to prescribable supplements
- explain what is meant by enteral tube feeding
- list the indications for parenteral nutrition
- detail the monitoring required during intravenous nutrition
- distinguish between water-soluble and fat-soluble vitamins.

Fluid and electrolytes:

- distinguish between an intracellular compartment, an extracellular space and an intravascular compartment
- identify the main sources of water intake and water loss
- identify how the body is protected from hyperosmolality
- recognise the signs and symptoms of hypokalaemia
- name the main indication for oral rehydration therapy.

Blood:

- name the main constituents of the blood
- state where the blood cells are derived
- state the main functions of the blood cells
- name the clinical features of iron deficiency anaemia
- name the additional features of megaloblastic anaemia
- state the name, dose, frequency of administration and side effects of oral iron
- explain what is meant by pernicious anaemia
- describe the treatment of pernicious anaemia
- describe the role of folic acid in pregnancy.

NUTRITION

INTRODUCTION

People who are ill can greatly benefit from well-managed nutritional support. Team working is the key to the success of this aspect of patient care. Within the nutritional support team, medical, surgical, nursing, dietetic and pharmaceutical skills must be available if patients are to receive high-standard, cost-effective therapy.

Malnutrition occurs in both the community and hospital settings. It occurs when an individual's nutrient intake falls below the metabolic requirements. The early detection of malnutrition is important as, if left untreated, it can severely compromise patient recovery.

The body has only limited reserves of immediately available energy and nitrogen sources. In the absence of adequate food ingestion, energy is derived from stores of glycogen in the liver, from muscle protein, and from fat in adipose tissue. However, glycogen stores are limited and are exhausted within the first 24 h of starvation. Over the next few days, muscle protein is broken down to provide glucose. In more prolonged starvation, fat is used to provide the energy source, and the brain adapts to utilise ketone bodies. When the fat stores have been utilised, accelerated protein breakdown resumes and leads eventually to death.

NUTRITIONAL SUPPORT

The aim of nutritional support is to arrest catabolism due to these losses, to reverse weight loss and to restore the patient to a positive nitrogen balance. This can be accomplished by administering calories, nitrogen (protein), fluid, electrolytes, vitamins and trace elements. The place of nutritional support is well recognised. Advances in the management of severe illness and trauma have meant that more patients survive the initial phase of their illness and require continuing supportive treatment. This involves the administration of appropriate fluids, electrolytes and nutritional requirements.

PROTEIN

If nutrition is deficient, not only does the patient lose weight by the loss of skeletal muscle but also tissue repair and immune mechanisms are significantly inhibited, as these processes require active cell turnover and therefore new protein formation. Amino acids are the building blocks of protein. They can be divided into two groups: essential amino acids and non-essential amino acids. It is necessary that nutrition solutions contain a balanced content of essential amino acids and a broad spectrum of non-essential amino acids.

ENERGY

Energy is provided as carbohydrate or fat.

ELECTROLYTES AND TRACE ELEMENTS

Sufficient quantities of electrolytes and trace elements must be given, not only for maintenance, but also to replace any significant losses. The action of each is summarised below:

- sodium
  — predominant cation in extracellular fluid
  — maintains integrity of cell membrane along with potassium
- potassium
  — major intracellular cation
  — required for transport of glucose across cell membrane
- calcium
  — continuous supply necessary to form and maintain skeleton and to maintain homeostasis in nerve and muscle tissue
- magnesium
  — important factor in many enzyme reactions
- iron
  — required for haemoglobin synthesis
- copper
  — involved in release of iron from liver
- zinc
  — essential for many enzyme reactions
- cobalt
  — essential constituent of vitamin B_{12}
- manganese
  — involved in calcium and phosphorus metabolism
- iodine
  — required in synthesis of thyroid hormones
- fluoride
  — required for maintenance of skeleton
- chromium
  — deficiency leads to glucose intolerance.

VITAMINS

All vitamins can be supplied by parenteral and enteral feeding regimens.

NUTRITIONAL ASSESSMENT

Nutritional support must be designed to suit the particular metabolic and nutritional needs of each individual. Careful assessment of the patient's nutritional state is required before deciding on a treatment plan. This is normally carried out by the dietitian, who will obtain information from a variety of sources, including the patient, relatives, doctor and nursing staff. Close liaison between dietetic, medical and nursing staff is important.

IDENTIFYING THOSE REQUIRING NUTRITIONAL SUPPLEMENTATION

There are many screening tools available to help identify those patients who are at risk of malnutrition. Most of these require the patient's current body mass index (BMI) to be measured and also request that an estimation of the rate of weight loss is determined.

The BMI is calculated as the weight in kilograms over the height in metres squared, i.e.:

$$BMI = \frac{weight\ (kg)}{height\ (m)^2}.$$

$$Percentage\ weight\ loss = \left[\frac{usual\ weight\ (kg)\ -}{\frac{current\ weight\ (kg)}{usual\ weight\ (kg)}}\right] \times 100.$$

Weight categories may be classified in terms of BMI as follows.

- Underweight: < 18 kg/m^2
- Normal: 18–24.9 kg/m^2
- Overweight: 25–29.9 kg/m^2
- Obesity: 30–39.9 kg/m^2
- Extreme obesity: > 40 kg/m^2

Not all patients with a BMI < 18 kg/m^2 are necessarily malnourished. For some healthy individuals, this may be normal. Consideration must also be given to the person's medical condition and evidence of weight loss. Weight loss ≥ 10% of usual body weight is considered significant and requires action. Food and fluid intake are also important and action is required if, over the course of 3 days, patients are:

- leaving more than half of their meals
- unable to eat solid food or having physical feeding problems
- unable to retain or absorb food.

TREATMENT OF MALNUTRITION

It is important to determine the cause of malnutrition because, in many cases, treating the cause can result in improvement in food intake without any major intervention (e.g. poor appetite can be associated with fever, depression and recurrent infection). Treatment of these conditions usually results in improvement in appetite. Patients who have physical disabilities and/or swallowing problems may have their nutritional intake significantly improved by providing modified cutlery and crockery and/or altering the consistency of their food. In cases of acute malabsorption lasting 4 or more days, the cause should be identified and the dehydration corrected by advising adequate fluid intake.

FIRST-LINE ADVICE THAT SHOULD BE GIVEN AT SURGERY OR WARD LEVEL

First-line dietery advice should be tried before any other interventions, unless otherwise directed. Patients should initially be encouraged to:

- eat frequent small meals
- have nourishing between-meal snacks
- use full-fat milk enriched with 4 tablespoons of skimmed milk powder/pint
- add extra cream, sugar and butter to desserts, sauces and breakfast cereals
- use Build Up or Complan as nourishing drinks between meals.

Increasing the energy and protein density of the diet through foods is much more acceptable from the patient's point of view.

PATIENTS WHO MAY BENEFIT FROM NUTRITIONAL SUPPORT THROUGH SUPPLEMENTATION

Dietary supplementation is most appropriately used in patients:

- with malignancy
- before or after major surgery
- with malabsorptive conditions
- with degenerative conditions (e.g. multiple sclerosis, motor neurone disease, Huntington's disease).

It is worth considering nutritional support for those people with:

- pressure sores or leg ulcers
- swallowing difficulties
- dementia
- chronic medical or physical problems.

MONITORING THE PATIENT

Once a patient has been identified as being 'nutritionally compromised', the above first-line advice should be given. It is important that an individual's progress is reviewed to establish the success of first-line treatment. For some patients, modification of their normal diet and possibly the introduction of a non-prescribable product such as Build Up will be sufficient to reverse the nutritional decline. This conservative management of nutritional needs is likely to be supervised by nursing staff either at ward level or in the patient's home. The frequency of review and monitoring will be different in acute and primary care, but it is important to highlight the need for further intervention.

ORAL NUTRITIONAL SUPPLEMENTS (SIP FEEDS)

If the nutritional problem persists, it may be necessary to commence the patient on an appropriate sip feed, the choice depending on patient preference. Referral to the community or hospital dietitian should be considered at this point depending on local protocol.

All patients should be reviewed after being commenced on a sip feed. In primary care, this will usually be after 4 weeks, or sooner if clinically thought necessary. In patients in whom there has been no improvement, referral to the local dietitian should be considered. Most patients usually manage to drink one or two supplements per day in addition to ordinary foods.

In secondary care, this first review may be within 24–48 h. Patients should be reviewed prior to discharge and only be discharged from hospital on a sip feed if it is clinically indicated. At this point, the patient's condition may have resolved, and sip feeding can be stopped or continued for 7 days post discharge.

Once the nutritional problem appears to have resolved, sip feeds and fortified diet should be discontinued and the patient should be encouraged to monitor their weight for 3 months. If problems recur, then the supplements and fortified diet should recommence, and this will become a new episode of care.

TYPES OF SUPPLEMENTS AVAILABLE

Prescribable supplements fall into three main groups.

Sip feeds. This group can be subdivided into complete supplements that contain all the essential nutrients (vitamins, minerals, energy and protein) and incomplete supplements that do not contain a full range of the essential nutrients. The energy content of the supplement varies. Some provide 1 kcal/mL, while others contain 1.5 kcal/mL. Some nutritional supplements have higher fibre content. These products are often based on milk, fruit juice or yoghurt and are available in several flavours. The majority of these products are lactose- and gluten-free and are suitable for patients with malabsorption, diarrhoea and known coeliac disease.

Single-nutrient supplements. These are energy-, protein- or fat-only, depending on the type of supplement, and are available in liquid or powder form.

Box 21.1 Examples of prescribable supplements

Sip feeds
1 kcal/mL
- Enrich
- Clinutren ISO
- Ensure
- Fresubin 1000 Complete

1.25 kcal/mL
- Provide Xtra

1.5 kcal/mL
- Clinutren 1.5
- Enlive Plus
- Enrich Plus
- Ensure Plus
- Fortijuce
- Fortisip

Single-nutrient supplements
- Calogen
- Maxijul
- Maxipro
- Polycal
- Polycose
- Protifar
- Vitapro

Other specialised products
- Calshake
- Elemental 028
- Peptamen
- Scandishake

The energy-only supplements are intended for patients with protein and fluid restrictions.

Other specialised products. A variety of specialised supplements are available, such as semielemental feeds for use with patients who have malabsorption, products such as supplemented puddings for patients with swallowing difficulties, and the less frequently used products specifically for patients with renal disease or liver failure or who are HIV-positive. Dietetic advice is required before patients are commenced on these products.

Examples of prescribable supplements currently on the market are shown in Box 21.1.

Deciding which product to prescribe should be based on patient requirements, taste preference and local policy. Although it is possible to survive on some of the complete supplements in the absence of food, it is generally recommended that supplements are taken in addition to food and should not replace meals or snacks. Supplements used inappropriately can inhibit the patient's ability to resume meeting their nutritional requirements from ordinary food.

WHEN TO REFER TO A DIETITIAN

This will depend on local policy and the nutritional screening tool used. Referral for dietary advice should be considered when:

- the BMI is under 18 kg/m² and there is significant weight loss, i.e. > 10% of usual body weight, and dietary supplements have been prescribed but there is no improvement
- the patient has another medical condition requiring dietary intervention (e.g. diabetes, renal disease, malabsorption)
- the patient's weight and/or intake continue to deteriorate.

The dietitian will complete a full nutritional assessment and recommend specific further treatment for the patient. The dietitian is able to assess the appropriateness of introducing an alternative supplement if there has been an intolerance or palatability problem.

ENTERAL TUBE FEEDING

People who cannot meet their nutritional or fluid requirements and who have a functioning small intestine (e.g. patients with neurological conditions or stroke, who have had head and neck surgery, who have had gut resection or who have other gastrointestinal disease) need to be fed using an alternative method. The most commonly used alternative methods are via a nasogastric, gastrostomy or jejunostomy tube. The decision as to the most suitable method for each individual patient is based on:

- the *length of time* the patient is expected to require feeding by an alternative route; for short-term feeding (e.g. up to 4 weeks), the nasogastric route will be used
- the *functioning of the gastrointestinal tract*; the majority of patients will have a gastrointestinal tract that is fully functional, and long-term feeding will be required – the feeding route used will therefore be gastrostomy.

If the patient's stomach and duodenum need to be temporarily or permanently bypassed, jejunostomy is the required route.

NASOGASTRIC TUBE FEEDING

A fine-bore nasogastric tube is used to facilitate this form of feeding. Because there is a wide range of systems available, it is advisable to seek the advice of the dietitian and nutrition nurse specialist.

The importance of ensuring correct positioning of a nasogastric tube cannot be overemphasised. Confirmation that the tube is not kinked and is in the stomach rather than in the oesophagus or lung must be made before starting a feed, by aspirating the stomach contents and testing with pH-indicating paper.

X-ray confirmation is time-consuming and costly, and so it is now used only for certain categories of patient (e.g. the unconscious) or when neither gastric position nor misplacement has been confirmed by the above test.

In the acutely ill or unconscious patient, it is important to establish that the stomach is emptying. This is an important precaution to take and can prevent potential hazards such as vomiting or gastric reflux, which may lead to aspiration pneumonia. It is also important that the volume of feed given is increased gradually, particularly in patients who have received nothing via their gut for several days, in order to prevent gastrointestinal side-effects.

Regular aspiration of gastric contents is especially important for patients receiving intensive care, for the unconscious and for those on drug therapy that may interfere with absorption. Absorption can be assumed if there is little or no aspirate, abdominal distension or nausea and when bowel sounds are normal. Gastric emptying can be enhanced and gastric reflux minimised by raising the head of the bed while feeding.

A wide range of commercially made preparations are available. For those totally unable to feed in the normal way, it is essential to use nutritionally complete foods, of which there are a number. Nutritional supplements and nutritionally complete foods are classed as borderline substances approved for use in specific clinical conditions such as dysphagia, inflammatory bowel disease, malabsorption states and bowel fistulae. Despite the name given to them, nutritionally complete foods may still not meet the patient's entire needs, and additional vitamins and minerals may be required.

The availability of nutritional preparations, diverse in composition and nutrient ratios, permits the selection of a feed to meet the specific requirements of the patient. Manufactured polymeric feeds generally suit most tube-fed patients. Compared with hospital-made feeds, they are sterile until opened, their composition is known and constant, and they are more convenient. The dietitian will be able to advise on the most appropriate feed to use.

To reduce the risk of bacterial contamination, correct preparation and storage of feeds are necessary. All individually prepared feeds can be stored at room temperature if unopened. The feeds must be clearly labelled to indicate the date and time by which they must be used. To minimise the risk of growth of micro-organisms, hospital-made feeds should be administered within 4–6 h of hanging, and aseptically administered sterile feeds within 12–24 h. Reservoirs and administration sets should be renewed once every 24 h. Bacteriological testing of the feeds should also be carried out as per the local control of infection policy.

TUBE FEED REGIMEN

Nausea and abdominal distension may be induced if the feed is administered too quickly. Continuous administration can minimise this problem, using either gravity drip or pump-assisted feeding. Continuous drip administration also minimises the risk of diarrhoea, which may result from administering bolus feeds, particularly if the feed is hyperosmolar. Pump-assisted feeding will help patients who have some impairment of gastrointestinal function, as the flow rate can be controlled to meet their absorptive capacity, and this is the administration method of choice.

Whatever method of feeding is used, accurate entries should be made on the patient's fluid balance chart and a record kept of the patient's tolerance of the feed. 'Today's feed tolerance will influence tomorrow's feeding regimen'. Doctors and nurses require access to details of the daily regimen, which has been worked out for each patient, including:

- a breakdown of energy, protein, electrolyte values, vitamins and minerals
- the total volume
- instructions regarding the volume of feed to be given per hour and how many hours in a 24-h period the feed is to be administered.

Nurses have a considerable contribution to make to the care of the patient fed by tube. They are involved in:

- assisting in the assessment of the patient's nutritional state
- communicating with dietetic and medical staff
- storing feeds appropriately
- initiating and supervising the feed
- observing the patient (e.g. for respiratory difficulty, tolerance of the feed)

- providing the patient with encouragement
- keeping accurate records.

Diarrhoea in enterally fed patients is not usually caused by the feed. Causes including recent or current drug therapy (e.g. antibiotics) or infection should be ruled out. There are some feeds on the market that are supplemented with soluble fibre, which has been advocated for the treatment of diarrhoea. The soluble fibre provides a substrate for colonic microflora to produce short-chain fatty acids. These fatty acids act in the ascending colon to promote absorption of water and sodium and therefore have a possible role in preventing diarrhoea.

Feeds with fructo-oligosaccharides or prebiotics that are undigested in the small intestine but pass to the colon, where they are fermented, also assist in preventing diarrhoea. Moreover, they selectively promote the growth of bifidobacteria and therefore reduce colonisation by *Escherichia coli* and *Clostridium difficile*. Examples of these feeds are Jevity Plus and Fresubin Isofibre.

ADMINISTRATION OF MEDICINES VIA ENTERAL FEEDING TUBE

Enteral feeding tubes may be used as an alternative route for the administration of medicines. When prescribed by this route, medicines are administered in the form of a solution, suspension or emulsion. If the drug is not normally available in a liquid form, the pharmacist should be consulted for advice and assistance. It may be possible for a liquid form of the drug to be prepared in the pharmacy using a suitable formulation that takes account of the properties of the drug, such as stability in an aqueous form.

Crushing of tablets into the necessary fine powder cannot be achieved satisfactorily on the ward. If tablets are insufficiently powdered, there is a risk of the tube being blocked, with consequent risk of underdosage. It should be borne in mind that some solid dose forms cannot be crushed, even to give a coarse powder. In some cases, the crushing of a tablet may destroy the essential properties of the product.

Apart from using an oral liquid, it may be acceptable to administer the injectable form of the drug via the enteral feeding tube. If this procedure is adopted, clear instruction must be given by the prescriber on the patient's drug prescription sheet. The pharmacist must first be consulted to ensure that the procedure is satisfactory and that there is no suitable alternative. Adding a medicine to a feed is not recommended, as chemical or physical interaction may adversely affect the drug, the feed, or both. An unknown quantity of

---

Box 21.2 Administration of continuous nasogastric feeding using a fine-bore tube

Documentation
- Feed prescription sheet

The medicine
- Feed in feed container

The environment
- Patient seated or in bed; warmth, comfort, privacy (if preferred)

The nurse and the patient
- Patient identified; explanation given to patient

Technique
- Nurse ensures that hands are thoroughly washed before and after feed
- Feeding set connected to feed
- Feed run through to expel air
- Correct position of tube confirmed by:
  — auscultation
  — aspiration of stomach contents (turns pH-indicating paper pink).
- Tube flushed with 20–30 mL of water
- Feeding set connected to tube
- Flow and volume of feed regulated as per feed prescription
- Feed recorded

Hazards
- Aspiration pneumonia

---

the drug may be lost if the food is altered or some is lost due to spillage or leakage from the delivery system.

The standard procedure for checking the position of the tube must be followed before administering medicines via the tube. To administer the medication, the tube is first clamped. The barrel of a suitably sized syringe is then attached. The medicine is poured into it and the clamp released. The medication is allowed to flow in by gravity. The tube is clamped again. Prior to and following the administration of each medication, a volume of water (20–30 mL) should be instilled. This will minimise the risk of tube blockage and ensure that the medicine has passed through the tube and out into the stomach.

ADMINISTRATION OF CONTINUOUS NASOGASTRIC FEEDING USING A FINE-BORE TUBE

For short-term feeding (e.g. up to 4 weeks), a fine-bore nasogastric tube is generally used. This procedure is outlined in Box 21.2.

Throughout the ongoing administration of the feed, the nurse's responsibilities are as follow.

CHECKING THE POSITION OF THE TUBE

Prior to commencing each feed, the position of the tube should be checked.

If the patient is restless or comatose, it is recommended that the tube position be checked more frequently.

If the tube starts to protrude, even as little as 1 cm, it should be removed and a fresh one passed. A partially removed tube must NEVER be pushed back down, as there is a danger of the tube becoming kinked or entering the lungs.

MAINTAINING THE FLOW OF THE FEED

The flow rate should be checked hourly or more frequently as instructed.

- If the rate of flow becomes sluggish, the tube and feeding set should be checked to ensure that they are functioning properly:
  — if the fault is in the tube, it can be flushed through with lukewarm water
  — if the fault is in the administration set, it should be disconnected and replaced.

KEEPING THE TUBE PATENT

Instil 20–30 mL of water through the feeding tube between each feed container change, and before and after each dose of medication, to reduce the risk of occlusion caused by feed or build-up of drug deposits. When the feed is stopped (e.g. X-Ray visit) and on completion of a feed, the tube must be flushed with 20–30 mL of water and plugged or capped. This will trap a column of water in the tube, reducing risk of blockage.

MINIMISING RISK OF INFECTION

The feed container and feeding set should be changed at least once every 24 h.

KEEPING ACCURATE RECORDS

The following records must be maintained:

- feed prescription
- fluid balance chart
- nursing care plan and progress notes.

PROVIDING NURSING CARE AS REQUIRED

- Assisting with the activities of living.
- Special attention to oral hygiene.

REPORTING ABNORMALITIES

The nurse should report any abnormalities.

GASTROSTOMY OR JEJUNOSTOMY TUBE FEEDING

For longer-term feeding, either percutaneous endoscopic gastrostomy or jejunostomy is the preferred option. The overall number of patients who have a gastrostomy has increased. The factors contributing to this increase include developments in healthcare technology, changes in clinical practice and growing numbers of elderly patients.

Non-surgical gastrostomies may be placed radiologically or by endoscopy.

ASSESSMENT FOR GASTROSTOMY FEEDING

All patients require to have their nutritional requirements fully assessed prior to being referred for a gastrostomy procedure. The percutaneous endoscopic gastrostomy tube is normally placed while in secondary care, but the majority of patients then receive their continuing care in the primary care setting in their own home, a nursing home or a community hospital.

TUBE FEEDING SYSTEM

All adults in primary care who have a gastrostomy tube in situ also require the following equipment:

- a feeding pump, with adaptor and battery charger
- supply of giving sets and possibly reservoirs
- pH-indicating paper
- adhesive tape
- 50-mL syringes
- supply of feeding solutions.

PARENTERAL NUTRITION

This method of nutritional support should be used only to prevent or correct malnutrition when no other route for the administration of nutrients is available. The intravenous route is the one referred to in this text. The vein used may be either a peripheral or a central one depending on the likely duration of the therapy.

INDICATIONS

The indications for parenteral nutrition are:

- preoperative – preparation of undernourished patients for surgery, chemotherapy or radiation therapy when the enteral route is not functioning
- postoperative – when complications prevent a return to oral intake (e.g. prolonged postoperative ileus, sepsis or fistulae)
- extensive burns, when nutritional requirements cannot be met enterally

- in some patients with hepatic or renal failure
- when there is impairment of intestinal mobility and/or absorption of nutrients (e.g. chronic gastrointestinal tract disease – Crohn's disease, pancreatitis, short bowel syndrome)
- prolonged coma when the enteral route is not functioning.

INTRAVENOUS NUTRITION SOLUTIONS

Protein is supplied by solutions of crystalline amino acids.

Glucose, which provides 16.8 kJ (4 kcal) per gram, is the best carbohydrate for intravenous use, but glucose solutions of high calorific value are hypertonic and must be infused via a central vein to provide rapid dilution. This minimises the risk of vein thrombosis, which can occur if these hypertonic solutions are infused peripherally. When glucose intolerance occurs, insulin may be required and blood glucose levels should be monitored.

Fat emulsion in the form of a lipid solution of, for example, Intralipid or Ivelip, may also be used as an energy source, providing 37.8 kJ (9 kcal) per gram. Lipid is also used as a source of essential fatty acids and a medium for giving fat-soluble vitamins. Lipid should not be used as the sole caloric source. The fat emulsion is hypotonic and can be infused by peripheral vein. It is incorporated using the 3-L bag, commonly named the 'big bag' system.

Electrolyte levels in intravenous solutions vary according to the individual requirements of the patient. Sodium, potassium, calcium, magnesium and phosphate are added to the nutrient solutions. Sodium acetate, a bicarbonate precursor, is incorporated to regulate the acid–base balance. It is necessary to incorporate trace elements into the intravenous admixture.

All vitamins can be supplied intravenously. Fat-soluble vitamins A, D, E and K are available in commercial preparations. Commercial water-soluble vitamin preparations for addition to intravenous nutrition solutions contain some or all of the following: ascorbic acid, thiamine, riboflavine, niacin, pyridoxine, pantothenic acid, vitamin B_{12} and folic acid.

PREPARATION OF INTRAVENOUS NUTRITION SOLUTIONS

Standard total parenteral nutritional formulations may be acceptable for many patients because of the kidney's ability to maintain homeostasis. No single parenteral regimen would be ideal for all patients because of the wide variety of pathology and differing age groups, or for the same patient throughout. The composition of the solution requires to be determined from day to day by clinical and chemical monitoring. The patient's details are filled in by the prescriber along with the date, day of prescription, duration of prescription, volume of amino acids and glucose solutions, and quantities of electrolytes and other additives.

The advantages of using a system in which the intravenous nutrition is provided in a 3-L bag are:

- the risk of contamination by frequent changes of container and the use of airways and connections is minimised
- it requires changing only once in 24 h and therefore staff time is saved
- amino acids and calorie source are delivered simultaneously, thus spreading the glucose load over 24 h so that the incidence of glycosuria is reduced.

The intravenous admixtures should be prepared in the pharmacy, as pharmaceutical calculations, drug stability, incompatibilities, solubility and sterility are important factors. The ward preparation room is an unsuitable location for aseptic procedures, which are better carried out in the aseptic suite within the pharmacy department.

Amino acids, glucose solutions and lipids are combined in a 3-L pack with additions of vitamins, electrolytes and other small-volume components. Checks are made to ensure compatibility of the components.

INCOMPATIBILITIES

It is essential that potential incompatibilities or the degradation rate of certain additive drugs in the presence of others are taken into consideration. Incompatibilities can usually be avoided or corrected. For example:

- insulin is unstable in the presence of bicarbonate
- insoluble carbonates may form if bicarbonate is added to calcium or magnesium; it is simpler to use a bicarbonate precursor such as sodium acetate
- vitamins are unstable in hypertonic intravenous solutions, especially in the presence of light.

The reaction can be slowed by using a freshly prepared solution and protecting it from bright light. It is essential that the solution be examined prior to setting up and during the infusion, as precipitate may appear after a few hours. Pharmacists are aware that the fat emulsion may 'crack', especially if there are high levels of electrolytes, in particular calcium and magnesium, in the bag. If calcium and phosphate are present above a certain level, a precipitate of calcium phosphate may form, particularly if the solution has been stored in the refrigerator.

Intravenous nutrition and the administration system should not be used as a means of administering drugs. In addition to the risk of contamination, many chemical changes can occur. For example, penicillins are rapidly degraded in amino acid solutions, and tetracyclines form insoluble complexes with calcium and magnesium.

ADMINISTRATION OF INTRAVENOUS NUTRITION

Peripheral intravenous nutrition is suitable for patients requiring up to 7 days' intravenous nutrition. Long-term parenteral nutrition is administered through a central vein, preferably the superior vena cava. In both situations, the line must be inserted following strict skin cleansing and using an aseptic technique.

The care of both the peripheral venous line and the central venous line used with intravenous nutrition should be meticulous. Responsibility for the care of the line is a combined one between medical and trained nursing staff, the overall aim being that no harm should come to the patient. The nurse's role is to explain to patients what is involved and to try to reassure them. It is essential therefore that the nurse is fully conversant with the procedure and associated care.

COMPLICATIONS OF INTRAVENOUS NUTRITION

The major complications associated with intravenous nutrition include:

- complications at line insertion
- sepsis
- line blockage
- air embolism
- phlebitis
- thrombosis
- metabolic complications associated with the nutrients
- mechanical problems
- psychological problems.

It is therefore important that protocols and procedures be designed to minimise the risk of such complications. Key factors in the prevention of complications are:

- meticulous aseptic handwashing
- strict attention to aseptic procedures
- adherence to hospital protocol for care
- staff who are knowledgeable and competent.

CARE OF THE PATIENT RECEIVING INTRAVENOUS NUTRITION

Patients receiving intravenous nutrition should be closely observed for the early detection of complications. Urinalysis should be performed every 4–6 h to note the presence of glucose or ketone bodies. A 24-h urine collection for measurement of urea level is used to estimate the nitrogen balance. The patient should be weighed regularly (e.g. twice weekly). Four-hourly recordings of temperature and pulse are made to detect the development of infection, and the character of the respirations observed to check that there is no embarrassment to the heart or lungs. Accurate recordings of the intake and output of fluid must be kept. Care must be taken to maintain accuracy of fluid recordings, especially on completion of one chart and the commencement of the next (e.g. at midnight). Regular checks should be made to ensure that the prescribed rate of infusion is being maintained and that sufficient volume of feed remains in the infusion pack. A volumetric pump is used so that the nurse is immediately alerted to occlusion of the line or the presence of an air embolus.

Transparent dressings allow for easy visualisation of the insertion site; any evidence of swelling, discoloration or pain should be reported at once.

No medications should be added to any part of the system, nor should it be used for blood sampling or central venous pressure monitoring.

A special cover can be obtained for placing over the bag to protect the feed from strong sunlight. Administration sets made of ultraviolet absorbent material are also available.

The nurse has a vital role not only in minimising the entry of micro-organisms but also in vigilant monitoring of the rate of the infusion. The use of an infusion pump is not a substitute for frequent checking and, if necessary, making minor adjustments to the infusion rate. No attempt should be made to 'catch up' if the infusion is behind time.

The patient receiving nutritional support may be malnourished and/or debilitated to some degree. This patient requires much encouragement. General physical care increases in importance, including skin care, mouth care and exercise within the limitations of the infusion system and/or clinical condition. Bowel activity, which may be reduced, should be carefully noted.

CHANGING THE INFUSION PACK

Accurate identification of the patient is essential. Details on the pack must be compared carefully with the prescription. The infusion solution should be checked to ensure that it is not out of date, that the solution is free from precipitate and that there is no evidence of the bag having been damaged (rendering it unsterile).

Care is needed to connect up the new infusion bag as an aseptic procedure. This can be achieved by thorough handwashing and careful introduction of the administration set into the infusion pack. Utmost care should be taken to avoid perforating the bag. The administration set must be free of air bubbles before setting the rate controller and starting the infusion. A record of the new pack, batch number, and starting time is made and initialled by the nurse(s) involved. The volume of solution that has been administered is recorded on the patient's fluid balance chart.

The method and frequency of changing the administration set and the site dressing are important elements for the nurse to know but are beyond the scope of this book.

INTRAVENOUS NUTRITION AT HOME

An increasing number of patients who have had, for example, small bowel resection with resulting short bowel syndrome, require long-term intravenous nutrition. This may be carried out at home if it is anticipated that more than 3 months' intravenous nutrition will be required. Thorough training is given to the patient and spouse or parent, as appropriate. This will take 2–4 weeks. Nutritional requirements are supplied by the pharmacy in preassembled packs. Other stores or supplies are delivered every 4 weeks. An infusion pump, trolley, refrigerator and intravenous stand can be loaned by commercial companies who specialise in home care delivery systems. The patient's home needs to have suitable facilities for the management of an aseptic infusion system at home (e.g. suitable worktop surface, adequate hand-washing and storage facilities, telephone). If necessary, these requirements should be made available through the occupational therapy and social work departments.

The patient reports to hospital on a regular basis in order that checks can be carried out and, when necessary, the nutritional components altered. The patient must be supplied with a 24-h contact in case there is a need for advice or emergency help. The GP must be made aware of these developments and asked to be involved in shared care with the hospital consultant. Funding and finance are important issues and should be organised prior to the final decision regarding a patient going home on intravenous nutrition.

SUMMARY

Safe intravenous nutrition has been developed by doctors, pharmacists, biochemists, microbiologists, nutrition experts and nurses. The role of the nurse in this form of therapy (whether undertaken in a specialist centre or in the patient's own home) continues to increase. Ideally, a senior nurse with specific responsibility for nutrition patients is appointed. A high standard of nursing care, including assessment of the patient, meticulous levels of hygiene, close observation, accurate recording and prompt reporting is of fundamental importance. When care at this level is assured, the maximum benefit to the patient of this technique, which may be life-saving, is within reach.

VITAMINS

Vitamins are essential substances that are required in daily amounts ranging from micrograms to milligrams for growth, development and maintenance of the body. Many of them are involved in the control of the body's metabolic processes through participation in enzyme reactions. Others have additional roles as structural components of bone and in electrolyte balance. Vitamins are substances that are present in certain foods but that the human body is unable to manufacture.

A good mixed diet provides adequate amounts of vitamins, and some are also formed by bacteria in the colon, so that vitamin supplements are normally unnecessary. Provided a sufficency of vitamins is taken, which should be available in a good mixed diet, there is no advantage to be gained by taking further large doses of the various vitamins unless there is a form of malabsorption. Indeed, further large doses may be harmful. Restricted diets or defective absorption or utilisation of food result in vitamin deficiencies that lead to a number of conditions requiring administration of appropriate vitamins. Other factors leading to vitamin deficiencies include anorexia and vomiting, gastrointestinal disease, liver damage and cancerous conditions. They can also arise in alcoholic patients and in the elderly on poor diets, and also when natural demands for vitamins are increased in fevers, pregnancy, breast-feeding and metabolic disorders.

Vitamins present in food can be divided into two classes: the fat-soluble vitamins (including vitamins A, D, E and K) and the water-soluble vitamins (including vitamins B and C). Table 21.1 outlines the main features of these vitamins.

Table 21.1 Main features of vitamins

Vitamin	Sources	Functions	Results of deficiency	Notes and clinical uses
A	Dairy products (e.g. milk, butter and cream). Also in fish liver oils. Can be formed in the body from carotene, a substance found in carrots, green vegetables and liver.	Formation of rhodopsin, a pigment in some of the light-sensitive cells (rods) in the retina.	Damage to skin and mucous membranes; corneal lesions; night blindness.	Deficiency in UK is rare.
B₁ (thiamine)	Egg, liver, wheatgerm and some vegetables.	Essential for certain stages of carbohydrate metabolism.	–	Deficiency may occur in chronic alcoholism and is best treated by parenteral administration of vitamins B and C. Recommended that use is restricted to essential. Intravenous injection administered slowly (over 10 min). Facilities for treating anaphylaxis should be available. Potentially serious allergic adverse reactions may occur during or shortly after administration.
B₂ (riboflavine)	Same as for vitamin B₁.	Necessary for carbohydrate metabolism.	Ulceration and infection of mucous membranes and skin.	Deficiency occurs only with malnutrition.
Nicotinamide	Animal and vegetable protein. Can be manufactured both by the body itself and by bacteria present in the gut.	–	Pellagra.	Deficiency rare except in general malnutrition.
Pyridoxine	–	Necessary for metabolism of many amino acids.	Peripheral neuropathy, convulsions and anaemia.	Naturally occurring deficiency rare in Britain. An acute deficiency may be induced by treatment with the antituberculous drug, isoniazid, which reacts chemically with pyridoxine, thus neutralising any of the vitamins present in the body. Pyridoxine used to treat deficiency and is used in prophylaxis.

Continued

Table 21.1 Main features of vitamins 'cont ...'

Vitamin	Sources	Functions	Results of deficiency	Notes and clinical uses
B$_{12}$ (hydroxocobalamin)	See page 429.			
C (ascorbic acid)	Fresh fruit and vegetables.	Essential for development of collagen, cartilage and bone, and is concerned in haemoglobin formation and tissue repair.	Scurvy – characterised by subcutaneous haemorrhage.	Scurvy now rare but mild deficiency states may occur during pregnancy and in patients on restricted diets, particularly the elderly.
D (calciferol)	Derived mostly from the diet, especially fish, eggs and liver. Can also be formed in the skin under the influence of sunlight.	To promote the absorption of calcium from the intestine.	Rickets in children, osteomalacia in adults.	Requirements greatest in childhood and during pregnancy and lactation. Deficiency may arise in some ethnic minority groups who have a poor vitamin intake and cover their skin. In most cases, treatment with the natural dietary vitamin (D$_2$ calciferol) is adequate. The hypocalcaemia of hypoparathyroidism requires larger doses.
E (tocopherol)	Wheatgerm, soya bean, lettuce and other green vegetables.	–	In young children with congenital cholestasis, abnormally low concentrations may be associated with neuromuscular abnormalities.	Available synthetically as tocopherols. Little evidence to suggest that oral supplements are essential in adults, even when there is fat malabsorption secondary to cholestasis. Neuromuscular abnormalities caused in children respond only to parenteral vitamin E.
K	Green leafy vegetables. Also produced by bacteria in the intestine.	Essential to assist manufacture, by the liver, of prothrombin and factor VII, needed for coagulation of blood.	Haemorrhage, bruising.	True deficiency rare, as intestinal bacteria synthesise it in sufficient quantity. In newborn, intestinal bacteria are absent, and therefore they are commonly given phytomenadione (vitamin K$_1$) by injection. In adults, deficiency is associated with fat malabsorption from pancreatic disease or obstructive jaundice. Replacement therapy is given in form of menadiol. Oral anticoagulants such as warfarin inhibit the use of vitamin K$_1$, thus preventing manufacture of essential clotting factors. Vitamin K may thus be used as an antidote to warfarin if need be.

BLOOD

INTRODUCTION

Blood consists of a pale yellow fluid called plasma in which red cells, white cells and platelets are suspended. These cellular components all develop in the bone marrow. The blood fulfils a multitude of purposes, the chief functions being the transport of oxygen and nutritional materials to all the cells of the body and the removal of carbon dioxide and waste materials. Oxygen is carried by haemoglobin contained in the red cells, while carbon dioxide is transported partly in the plasma and partly in the red cells.

The main control mechanism ensuring the maintenance of a constant circulating red cell mass is provided by erythropoietin, which is produced by the kidney in response to anoxia and acts on the bone marrow to increase the rate of cell division, cell maturation and haemoglobin synthesis. Abnormality of any of these factors may give rise to anaemia. Excessive blood loss or destruction of blood cells may also lead to anaemia. Anaemia may therefore be defined as a reduction in the normal amount of red cells or haemoglobin, or both. It is said to be present when the haemoglobin concentration is below the normal range for the age and sex of an individual. For adult men, the normal haemoglobin concentration is 130–170 g/L; for women, 120–155 g/L. It is slightly lower in pregnancy.

THE ANAEMIAS

The types of anaemia most often encountered are iron deficiency anaemia and megaloblastic anaemia.

Other conditions of the blood include anaemia associated with chronic renal failure, iron overload, aplastic anaemia and haemolytic anaemia.

IRON DEFICIENCY ANAEMIA

Iron is absorbed as the ferrous salt in the duodenum and upper small intestine. It is carried to the bone marrow for the synthesis of haemoglobin. About 70% of the total body iron is present in erythrocyte haemoglobin. The remainder is stored in the liver, spleen and bone marrow. The absorption of iron is carefully regulated so that just enough is absorbed to make good any deficiency.

Iron is an essential constituent of haemoglobin. When red cells break down, the iron is retained by the body and utilised in the formation of further haemoglobin. In health, the loss of iron from the body is 1–2 mg daily, which is replaced by absorption from a dietary intake of 10–20 mg. Iron is present in red meat, some vegetables, pulses and cereals enriched with iron. The main causes of iron deficiency anaemia are as follows:

- reduced iron stores at birth
- inadequate intake of iron
  — restricted diet
  — malnutrition.
- increased requirements
  — pregnancy
  — breast feeding.
- chronic blood loss
  — profuse menstruation
  — disease of the gastrointestinal tract:
    hiatus hernia
    varices
    haemorrhoids
    ulceration
    colonic carcinoma
    bleeding
  — drug-induced
    aspirin
    non-steroidal anti-inflammatory drugs.
- malabsorption
  — coeliac disease
  — malabsorption syndrome.

CLINICAL FEATURES

The features of iron deficiency anaemia include the general features common to all anaemias (Table 21.2).

The clinical features specific to iron deficiency anaemia include glossitis, angular stomatitis and koilonychia.

ORAL IRON

Iron is usually given orally to correct a deficiency. The following formulations are available:

- ferrous salts in liquid and solid oral dose, including controlled-release preparations
- formulations containing both ferrous sulphate and folic acid for use in pregnancy
- formulations containing vitamins and minerals in addition to ferrous sulphate.

The iron content of commonly used oral iron preparations is given in Table 21.3.

The daily dose of elemental iron should be 100–200 mg. The choice is dependent on efficacy, side effects and cost.

Table 21.2 General features common to all anaemias

Feature	Cause
Fatigue	Lack of oxygen for internal respiration, hence lack of energy
Pallor of mucous membranes and skin	Reduced haemoglobin concentration
Dyspnoea on exertion	Exertion requires more oxygen, therefore more rapid passage through lungs required
Dizziness (fainting)	Reduced oxygen to brain
Feeling of cold	Reduced tissue respiration, therefore reduced production of heat
Palpitations, tachycardia	Compensatory attempt to increase oxygen level in tissues; may lead to cardiac failure
Exacerbation of angina	Angina caused by lack of oxygen to cardiac muscle; reduced oxygen-carrying capacity worsens the angina

Table 21.3 Iron content of oral iron preparations

Iron salt	Amount (mg)	Ferrous iron content (mg)
Ferrous fumarate	200	68
Ferrous gluconate	300	35
Ferrous sulphate	300	60
Ferrous sulphate, dried	200	65

Efficacy. Absorption of a soluble ferrous salt occurs in the upper part of the small intestine where the pH is lower; at higher pH levels, ferrous phosphates form, which are not suitable. The efficacy of an iron preparation depends on how much of its iron content is released in this part of the gastrointestinal tract. Fluids and solid oral dose preparations are preferable to controlled-release preparations, because the latter may release only a proportion of iron in the area where absorption takes place. Some inhibition of iron absorption can occur if it is taken with milk, tea or eggs.

Side-effects. Acceptability by the patient may be influenced by adverse effects. Gastrointestinal disturbances, including nausea, abdominal discomfort, diarrhoea or constipation, may occur. The nausea may be reduced by taking the iron preparation after food. Patients should be advised of the possibility of these side effects and also that iron causes blackening of the stool. Where gastrointestinal disturbances occur with ferrous sulphate, the dose may be reduced or a change to ferrous gluconate or ferrous fumarate may help.

Cost. Controlled-release and liquid preparations are more expensive than simple tablet and capsule forms. Ferrous sulphate 200 mg (65 mg of elemental iron) three times daily provides an effective dose that is relatively inexpensive.

Interactions. Iron salts should not be given with tetracyclines, as the absorption of both drugs is impaired. Antacids and penicillin can also impair the absorption of iron.

Duration of treatment. The haemoglobin concentration should rise by about 100–200 mg/100 mL per day over 3–4 weeks. Treatment of iron deficiency should be continued for 3–4 months after the haemoglobin has returned to normal in order to replace depleted iron stores. Extra encouragement may have to be given to ensure that the patient completes the course of treatment. The underlying cause should have been treated as far as possible.

PARENTERAL IRON THERAPY

When oral iron cannot be tolerated in any form, or there is malabsorption of iron, it may be necessary to give the iron by injection. Iron injections bypass the mechanism that controls the degree of iron absorption, and the dose must be based on the actual iron deficiency as calculated from laboratory test results and the patient's ideal body weight. Iron sorbitol injection is given by *deep* intramuscular injection using the Z-track technique to prevent leakage along the needle track and subsequent staining of the skin (see p. 57). It can also cause severe arrhythmias and anaphylaxis in some patients. As a severe allergic reaction can take place, it is administered to a very limited group of patients, always in hospital and under very close supervision. There is no significant difference in the rate of haemoglobin response to injectable iron compared with oral iron, i.e. a rapid cure of anaemia cannot be effected by use of the injectable route. Iron dextran and iron sucrose injections are also available. Both are given by slow intravenous injection or intravenous infusion.

MEGALOBLASTIC ANAEMIA

Both vitamin B_{12} and folate are necessary for the production of mature red blood cells. Vitamin B_{12} is present largely in meat; folate is found in both animal and plant foods. A deficiency of either will result in megaloblastic anaemia. In the normal person, a factor (the intrinsic factor) is produced by the stomach and is necessary for the absorption of vitamin B_{12} in the intestine. The main causes are as follows.

- Vitamin B_{12} deficiency:
  — malabsorption (due to disease, e.g. Crohn's or resection of the terminal ileum)
  — deficiency of intrinsic factor (as found in pernicious anaemia and after gastrectomy)
  — inactivation of vitamin B_{12} (by abnormal intestinal bacterial flora associated with anatomical abnormality of the small bowel)
  — veganism, when there are low levels of available dietary vitamin B_{12}.
- Folate deficiency:
  — malabsorption (due to disease, e.g. coeliac disease, or resection of the jejunum)
  — increased demands (due to pregnancy and lactation, malignancy, chronic inflammatory diseases, and haemolytic diseases)
  — drugs (e.g. anticonvulsants, including phenytoin and phenobarbital; dihydroxyfolate reductase inhibitors, e.g. methotrexate, trimethoprim, pyrimethamine; H_2-receptor antagonists such as cimetidine or ranitidine, proton pump inhibitors such as omeprazole)
  — inadequate intake of folate (due to dietary deficiency).

PERNICIOUS ANAEMIA

Pernicious anaemia is a particular form of anaemia in which the mature red cells are irregular in shape and size and reduced in number. The cause of pernicious anaemia is an autoimmune gastritis that leads to a deficiency in the production of the so-called intrinsic factor, a protein normally secreted by the stomach and essential for the satisfactory absorption of vitamin B_{12} in the terminal ileum. In addition to the megaloblastic anaemia, the deficiency of vitamin B_{12} leads to degenerative changes in the nervous system that, if untreated, ultimately render the patient immobile.

CLINICAL FEATURES

The megaloblastic anaemias present with the general features common to all anaemias (Table 21.2). In addition, the patient may have a red, raw, ulcerated tongue; a pale lemon-tinted skin (caused by haemolysis as the body recognises the cells as abnormal); and paraesthesia. In very severe cases, ataxia and a spastic weakness of the legs develop – a condition known as subacute combined degeneration of the spinal cord.

The diagnosis of pernicious anaemia is confirmed by the Schilling test, a dual isotope test that confirms malabsorption of vitamin B_{12}. The test involves fasting patients overnight, asking them to empty their bladder in the morning and discarding the urine. Two capsules of short half-life radioactive vitamin B_{12} are given to the patient to swallow with as little water as possible, and hydroxocobalamin 1 mg is given by intramuscular injection. The patient fasts for a further 2 h. A 24-h urine collection is obtained from the time the capsules and injection are given. It is essential that the collection is complete. In health, radioactive vitamin B_{12} would be absorbed into the gut, and excess to requirements (15–40%) would be excreted in the urine. In pernicious anaemia, radioactive vitamin B_{12} is *not* absorbed and therefore passes in the stools instead of the urine (less than 3%).

There are two cobalamins available: hydroxocobalamin, which is highly bound by plasma proteins so that it is excreted slowly and thus its action prolonged, and cyanocobalamin, which is more rapidly excreted.

Hydroxocobalamin is the form of vitamin B_{12} used, as it is retained in the body longer than cyanocobalamin and therefore does not have to be given so frequently. Initial treatment is 0.25–1 mg by intramuscular injection on alternate days for 1–2 weeks, then 250 micrograms weekly until blood counts are within normal range. A course of oral iron may be required to supply the increased number of mature red cells. Thereafter, the maintenance dose is

1 mg every 3 months. Unless it is caused by dietary insufficiency, the lack of vitamin B$_{12}$ in pernicious anaemia is permanent, and therefore replacement therapy must be parenteral and for life. Consequently, education of the patient and relatives is important.

TREATMENT OF OTHER CAUSES OF VITAMIN B$_{12}$ DEFICIENCY

Prophylactic vitamin B$_{12}$ in the form of intramuscular hydroxocobalamin every 3 months should be given after total gastrectomy or total ileal resection and after partial gastrectomy if malabsorption is demonstrated. Prophylactic oral vitamin B$_{12}$ (in the form of cyanocobalamin) at a dose of 50–150 micrograms daily between meals can be given to vegans.

FOLATE DEFICIENCY

Most causes of folate deficiency will yield to a course of treatment comprising 5 mg of folic acid by mouth daily for 4 months. A daily dose of 10 or 15 mg may be necessary when malabsorption occurs. When megaloblastic anaemia is due to dihydroxyfolate reductase inhibitors, the conversion of folic acid to its active metabolites is inhibited. Folic acid will therefore not be effective; folinic acid may be used, 15 mg orally once daily.

Folate deficiency may occur in pregnancy, with the possible development of neural tube defects. Prophylactic folic acid–iron combinations can be given. The level of folic acid in these preparations is insufficient to treat megaloblastic anaemia.

ANAEMIA ASSOCIATED WITH CHRONIC RENAL FAILURE

ERYTHROPOIETIN

Erythropoietin is a hormone manufactured mainly by the kidney that is necessary for erythrocyte formation (Fig. 21.1). If the kidneys fail, the level of erythropoietin in the blood falls, with resulting anaemia. Epoetin is a genetically engineered human erythropoietin.

The commonest use of epoetin is in patients with anaemia of chronic renal failure, especially in patients on regular dialysis, when it has been demonstrated to improve haemoglobin levels and quality of life as well as reducing or abolishing red cell transfusion dependency for these patients. It is also licensed for the treatment of anaemia associated with cancer chemotherapy.

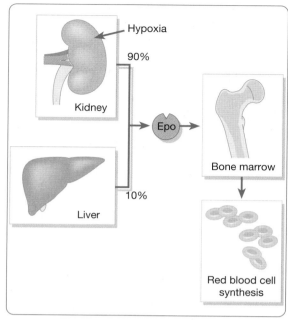

Fig. 21.1 Erythropoietin (Epo) and erythrocyte formation. (From Page CP, Hoffman BF, Curtis M et al. 2006 Integrated pharmacology. Mosby, Edinburgh. With permission of Mosby.)

Prescription would normally be initiated in a specialist hospital clinic setting and continued in primary care in accordance with an agreed form of shared care protocol. The dosage depends on the exact preparation given and is usually administered subcutaneously (most patients can be trained in self-administration). If necessary it can be given intravenously.

Side-effects. There is a dosage-dependent increase in blood pressure, and therefore when hypertension is poorly controlled, blood pressure should be monitored carefully. Common side-effects include flu-like symptoms with fever, myalgia and arthralgia. Darbepoetin is a derivative of epoetin that has a longer half-life and may be administered less frequently than epoetin.

IRON OVERLOAD

Iron overload may occur as a result of repeated blood transfusions to treat haemolytic anaemias. Desferrioxamine is used to reduce the iron level. It is a powerful iron-chelating agent that is given by subcutaneous infusion over 8–12 h, three to seven times a week. The dose should reflect the degree of iron overload. For established iron overload, the dose is usually between 20 and 50 mg/kg daily. Desferrioxamine is also used to treat acute toxicity usually seen in children who have swallowed iron tablets in mistake for sweets. The result of the ingestion of large quantities of iron tablets is severe necrotising gastritis with vomiting, haemorrhage and diarrhoea, followed by circulatory collapse.

Iron excretion induced by desferrioxamine is enhanced by administration of ascorbic acid in a dose of 200 mg daily. It should be given separately from food, as it also enhances iron absorption.

APLASTIC AND HAEMOLYTIC ANAEMIAS

Aplastic or hypoplastic anaemia is an uncommon disease that is caused by depression of the bone marrow. This may affect the formation and development of the red cells, neutrophils or platelets. In 50% of cases, no causative factors can be found; in the others, exposure to certain drugs or chemicals, ionising radiation or viruses may be linked.

Anaemias caused by excessive destruction of red blood cells in the spleen are termed *haemolytic anaemias*. They are due to either breakdown of red blood cells that are defective (congenital haemolytic anaemias) or to the effects of poisons or infection (acquired haemolytic anaemias). It should be noted that haemolytic anaemias are uncommon among the indigenous population in the UK. Among the multi-racial communities in some of the large inner cities, patients with haemolytic anaemia are encountered more frequently. Conditions such as sickle cell anaemia and thalassaemia are associated with a haemolytic process. When possible, the underlying cause should be treated. Splenectomy may be necessary in some cases of haemolytic anaemia.

In either hypoplastic or haemolytic anaemia, red cell transfusions, platelet transfusions and antibiotics may be given as supportive therapy, and bone marrow transplantation may be considered in severe cases if the patient is under 40 and a compatible sibling donor is available.

Corticosteroids have an important part to play in the management of autoimmune haemolytic anaemias. Oral prednisolone is the first-line treatment for autoimmune haemolytic anaemia. This should be prescribed in general practice only after specialist advice and following confirmation of the diagnosis.

There are numerous secondary causes of autoimmune haemolytic anaemia, particularly lymphoproliferative disease, and any suspected case should be referred to a haematologist for investigation and follow-up.

Glucocorticoids quickly slow or stop haemolysis in two-thirds of patients. For severe disease, up to 60 mg of prednisolone can be given daily. Once haemoglobin stabilises, prednisolone may be tapered to 2.5–15 mg daily and continued for 2–3 months before tapering off entirely.

It is advisable to consider cover with H_2 antagonists to reduce gastric side-effects. For patients requiring long periods on steroid therapy, the prophylactic use of bisphosphonates to protect against steroid-induced osteoporosis is indicated.

The appearance of adverse effects is related to the duration of treatment and the dosage used. Gastrointestinal disturbances are common and, at daily doses of 15 mg and over, there is an increased risk of peptic ulceration. Salt and water retention may precipitate heart failure, particularly in the elderly. Steroid-induced hypokalaemia may require potassium supplementation.

With long-term treatment, features of Cushing's syndrome may develop, namely moon face, bruising, hirsutism, impaired glucose tolerance, hypertension, acne, weight gain, osteoporosis and an increased susceptibility to infections. Mental disturbances can occur, including any kind of mood change.

ANAEMIA IN PREGNANCY

Pregnancy increases the daily requirement for iron by approximately 2 mg daily, and a pregnant woman therefore needs 3–4 mg of iron per day. A normal diet contains 10–15 mg of iron.

There is no clear consensus on the use of supplementary iron in pregnancy. Pregnant women who are otherwise healthy do not need routine iron supplements. In women who are at risk of anaemia from previous menorrhagia or poor nutrition, prophylactic iron supplements should be recommended.

Folate supplements are in use for the increased demands of pregnancy. To avoid megaloblastic anaemia in late pregnancy, supplements are advised for those particularly at risk (e.g. those with inadequate diet or for a twin pregnancy).

It has also been shown that administration of folate in the periconceptual period reduces the number of neural tube defects by 75%. For the prevention of a first occurrence of neural tube defects, 400 micrograms of folic acid is recommended daily before conception and then during the first trimester.

DRUGS USED IN NEUTROPENIA

Recombinant human granulocyte-colony stimulating factor stimulates the production of neutrophils and reduces the risks of infection and sepsis in patients by reducing the duration of chemotherapy-induced neutropenia. Human granulocyte colony–stimulating factor (filgrastim and lenograstim) given by subcutaneous or intravenous injection or infusion stimulates the production of neutrophils. These factors are administered daily until the neutrophil count is in normal range or for a maximum number of days depending on which product is being used for which condition.

FLUID AND ELECTROLYTES

GENERAL

Water makes up almost two-thirds of the total body mass (men, 60%; women, 55%). A 70-kg man will therefore contain about 42 L of water and a 70-kg woman nearer 38 L. The reason for this difference between the sexes is that women contain an extra 5% adipose tissue.

Water intake is derived primarily from three sources: ingested water, water contained in food and water produced from the oxidation of carbohydrates, proteins and fats. Water losses occur in the urine and stool as well as evaporation from the skin and respiratory tract.

COMPARTMENTS OR SPACES

The majority of our total body water is held within our cells; this is the intracellular compartment or space (30 L). Bathing the cells and occupying extracellular spaces such as the pleural cavity and joint spaces is a smaller amount of interstitial water (9 L). The intravascular compartment holds the smallest amount of water, at around 3 L (Fig. 21.2).

The interstitial and intravascular compartments make up the extracellular space. Water moves freely between these compartments, but fluids can only be administered into or taken from the intravascular space.

OSMOLALITY

To understand what osmolality is, it is first necessary to understand a few terms.

Solvent. This is a usually liquid substance (such as water) that is capable of dissolving or dispersing one or more substances.

Solute. A solute is a substance (such as carbohydrate or electrolytes) that dissolves in a solvent. So if you put sugar into a cup of water, the sugar would be the solute and the water would be the solvent.

Solution. This is the combination of a solute with a solvent, when the solute has been evenly dissolved in the solvent. An example would be when sugar (the solute) is evenly dissolved in a glass of water (the solvent).

Concentration. A measurement of the amount of a solute compared with the amount of solvent in a solution. As an example, if a high amount of sugar (the solute) were dissolved in a small amount of water (the solvent), the concentration would be high. The concentration would be low if a small amount of sugar was dissolved in a large amount of water.

Semipermeable membrane. A thin layer of tissue that allows some substances in, but not all. For example, the semipermeable membrane may allow a smaller substance in but not a larger one, or it may only allow the solvent (such as water) to pass through but not allow any solutes to pass through. Semipermeable membranes are widespread in the body and surround all cells.

WHAT IS OSMOLALITY?

Osmolality is the concentration of a solution. In other words, it is a measurement of the amount of a solute compared with the amount of solvent in a solution.

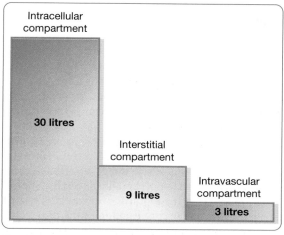

Fig. 21.2 Distribution of water in body compartments.

Table 21.4 Definitions

Term	Definition
Acid–base balance	In health, there is a balance between the carbonic acid (acid) and bicarbonate (base) content of plasma.
Acidosis (metabolic)	Acidosis develops when the plasma level of bicarbonate falls to 15 mmol/L. In severe acidosis, the bicarbonate level may fall below 10 mmol/L.
Alkalosis (metabolic)	Alkalosis develops when the plasma bicarbonate is elevated to 35 mmol/L. The pH of blood also rises.
Anion	Negatively charged ion (e.g. Cl^- or HCO_3^-).
Cation	Positively charged ion (e.g. Na^+ or K^+).
Electrolyte	A chemical substance that dissociates in water to yield ions (charged particles), for example sodium chloride (NaCl) dissociates to yield Na^+ and Cl^-.
Isotonic	The osmotic pressure of plasma is the accepted standard in medicine. An isotonic solution has the same osmotic pressure as plasma. A 0.9% w/v solution of sodium chloride is isotonic with plasma. Solutions with a lower osmotic pressure than plasma are hypotonic. Solutions with a higher osmotic pressure are hypertonic.
Millimole (mmol)	A mole is the molecular weight of a substance expressed in grams. A millimole is 1/1000 of the molecular weight.
Osmolarity	Concentration of solute particles in a given volume of solvent.
Osmosis	When two solutions of different concentration of dissolved solids (solute) are separated by a semipermeable membrane (e.g. cell membrane), water flows to the side of the membrane with the higher concentration of solute. Water flow ceases when the concentrations become equal.
Osmotic pressure	The pressure created by the flow of water due to osmosis.
pH (hydrogen ion concentration)	A measure of the degree of acidity or alkalinity of a solution. A pH below 7 indicates an acidic pH, whereas a pH above 7 indicates an alkaline solution; pH 7.0 is neutral.

PLASMA OSMOLALITY

Plasma osmolality is a function of the ratio of body solute (dissolved substances) to body water. It is regulated by changes in water balance. The distribution of water throughout the body is dictated partly by the size of the compartment available but mainly by tonicity (see Table 21.4 for further definitions). Water balance is adjusted to maintain osmolality at a constant throughout all three compartments (see Fig. 21.3).

Alterations in plasma osmolality of as little as 1–2% are sensed in the hypothalamus. These receptors initiate mechanisms that affect water intake (by thirst) and water excretion (via antidiuretic hormone) to return plasma osmolality to normal.

BODY'S DEFENCE AGAINST HYPEROSMOLALITY

The major defence against hyperosmolality (accumulation of solute in excess of body water) is *increased thirst*. Although the kidney can minimise water losses via the action of antidiuretic hormone, water deficits can be corrected only by increased dietary intake.

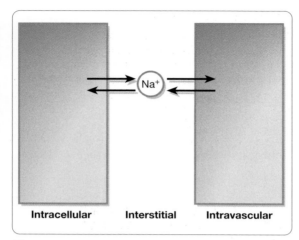

Fig. 21.3   Water balance.

WHEN CAN HYPO-OSMOLALITY RESULT?

Hypo-osmolality can result from excessive body water retention with subsequent dilution of body solutes or from solute loss in excess of water loss (e.g. diarrhoea). Because the kidney excretes large volumes of water daily, persistent water retention resulting in hypo-osmolality occurs only in the presence of decreased renal water excretion. In patients with normal renal function, hypo-osmolality must therefore be due to solute loss in excess of body water loss.

ORAL PREPARATIONS FOR FLUID AND ELECTROLYTE IMBALANCE

Disorders of fluid balance are almost always accompanied by changes in the concentration of plasma sodium, potassium and other electrolytes. Where deficiencies of sodium or potassium occur which are mild to moderate, oral preparations are available to treat these conditions. Where there is an excess of potassium, this may be corrected by administration of an oral preparation.

ORAL POTASSIUM

Normal dietary intake of potassium is more than sufficient to compensate for excretion. Dietary sources include fruit (bananas, oranges, tomatoes, melons and mangos) and vegetables (potatoes).

Lowered potassium levels occur where there is an excessive loss of potassium in the urine or from the gastrointestinal tract. Vomiting, diarrhoea (including through laxative misuse) or colostomies can put patients at risk of potassium depletion. It is important to take a full drug history as long-term administration of drugs such as loop diuretics and thiazides may cause low potassium. This can be avoided by using potassium-sparing diuretics. Corticosteroids can also induce potassium loss. Other causes of low potassium include high aldosterone level (Addison's disease), which promotes potassium excretion, and severe burns resulting in loss of large amounts of potassium through fluid loss.

For patients with mild to moderate hypokalaemia, oral replacement is the method of choice. Effective preparation include soluble tablets (Kloref, Sando-K) or syrup (Kay-Cee-L). However, for some patients a metallic aftertaste or experiencing nausea and vomiting may contribute to non-compliance. Slow release formulations are available, but are less well absorbed. In addition, localised release of high concentrations of potassium which is very irritant can cause intestinal ulceration. They should therefore be swallowed whole with plenty of liquid and avoided last thing at night. Because of these difficulties, slow release potassium tablets should only be used when the liquid preparations cannot be tolerated.

The reference range for plasma potassium is between 3.5 and 5.5 mmol/L. Patients who have mild to moderate hypokalaemia (2.5 – 3.5 mmol/L) may only have minor symptoms. Muscle weakness is the main symptom, but apathy and depression can occur. Symptoms increase with decreasing potassium levels, and arrhythmias, constipation and abdominal discomfort may be experienced. If a patient is being prescribed digoxin, its action is potentiated if low plasma levels are present, leading to increased signs of toxicity such as visual disturbances and arrhythmias.

It is important when taking a drug history to ask the patient if they purchase over-the-counter medicines from their pharmacist or health food products from other sources. An example is where the patient may be purchasing a salt substitute (e.g. LoSalt, Ruthmol). These contain significant amounts of potassium chloride and may cause potassium intoxication in a patient with renal failure.

POTASSIUM REMOVAL

Plasma potassium between 5.5 and 6.5 mmol/L is described as mild hyperkalaemia. A polystyrene sulphate resin should be given. The oral route is preferred (15g 3-4 times daily) because if the rectal route is used (30g in methylcellulose solution), the enema requires to be retained for nine hours (the patient should not have a bowel movement during this time) followed by irrigation to remove the resin. Taken orally, the resin takes at least 24 hours to work and should be stopped as soon as the potassium level reaches 5.0 mmol/L. Laxatives may be required as the resin causes constipation. A sodium resin should not be used when there is hypernatraemia, because the resin liberates sodium as potassium is taken up. Similarly calcium resin must not be used if the patient's calcium levels are already too high.

ORAL SODIUM

In chronic conditions associated with mild or moderate degrees of sodium depletion (e.g. in salt-losing bowel or renal disease), oral supplements of sodium chloride or sodium bicarbonate may be sufficient. In more serious depletion, intravenous administration will be required.

Patients with hyponatraemia may experience nausea, weakness, headache and drowsiness. The degree and nature of the symptoms depend on the level of sodium in the plasma. Concentrations in the region of 120 mmol/L give rise to weakness; at 90–105 mmol/L, neurological signs and symptoms develop.

The dose for prophylaxis of sodium chloride deficiency is four to eight tablets daily with water (in severe depletion, up to a maximum of 20 tablets daily).

ORAL REHYDRATION THERAPY

The oral route is preferred when it is necessary to replace losses of both water and electrolytes lost through diarrhoea. A number of products e.g. Dioralyte, Electrolade, Rapolyte) is available for reconstitution in water. These products contain balanced quantities of sodium and potassium salts, citrate and glucose. The citrate corrects acidosis that occurs as a result of the diarrhoea and also enhances the absorption of sodium. Glucose enhances the absorption of sodium and potassium salts.

The contents of a sachet are poured into a large glass of drinking water (200 ml). This is mixed well and the whole glassful consumed. Once reconstituted, any solution should be used within one hour or within 24 hours if stored in a refrigerator. A basic principle of treatment of diarrhoea is to replace lost fluid and electrolytes and then to maintain sufficient fluid intake to replace fluid loss from stools.

ORAL BICARBONATE

In conditions such as renal tubular acidosis or uraemic acidosis, bicarbonate is administered orally to neutralise the excess acid. Preparations available include sodium bicarbonate capsules (500 mg), sodium bicarbonate tablets (600 mg) and potassium tablets effervescent. The condition requires to be monitored in order that the dose and duration of treatment are tailored to the individual patient's needs.

PARENTERAL PREPARATIONS FOR FLUID AND ELECTROLYTE IMBALANCE

An important way of expressing the strength (concentration) of a medicine is the use of molarity. An understanding of this term will help the nurse particularly in the administration of intravenous fluids. Molarity can be a difficult concept for those who have not had a grounding in chemistry. In order to explain the concept of molarity, it is essential to refer to some basic chemistry:

- each atom has an atomic weight (e.g. sodium, 23; potassium, 39; calcium, 40; and chlorine, 35.4)
- atoms combine to form a molecule, for example sodium (Na) combines with chlorine (Cl) to form sodium chloride (NaCl). Sodium chloride has a molecular weight of 58.4 (the sum of the atomic weights).

MOLE

The term *mole* is defined as follows: one mole of a drug weighs (in grams) the same as the molecular weight of that drug.

For sodium chloride, 1 mole weighs 58.4 g. A molar solution contains 1 mole in 1 L of solvent, i.e. 58.4 g of sodium chloride in 1 L.

Therefore, 1 mmol contains 58.4/1000 g of sodium chloride in 1 L, i.e.

$$\frac{58.4}{1000} \times 1000 \text{ mg in 1 L}$$

$$= 58.4 \text{ mg in 1 L.}$$

One intravenous infusion commonly administered is sodium chloride intravenous infusion 0.9% w/v, which is isotonic with plasma.

The strength is 0.9% w/v of sodium chloride in 100 mL:

Table 21.5 Electrolyte values

Infusion fluid	Na+	K+	mmol/L HCO₃⁻	Cl⁻	Ca²⁺
Normal plasma	142	4.5	26	103	2.5
Intravenous infusions					
Sodium chloride 0.9%	154	–	–	154	–
Compound sodium lactate (Hartmann's)	131	5	29	111	2
Sodium chloride 0.18% and glucose 5%	31	–	–	31	–
Potassium chloride 0.3% and sodium chloride 0.9%	154	40	–	194	–
Sodium bicarbonate 1.26%	150	–	150	–	–
Sodium bicarbonate 8.4%	1000	–	1000	–	–

0.9 g of sodium chloride in 100 mL

= 900 mg of sodium chloride in 100 mL

= 9000 mg of sodium chloride in 1000 mL.

Therefore the number of millimoles is 9000/58.4 mmol/L, i.e. 154 mmol/L.

Solutions of electrolytes are given intravenously to meet normal fluid and electrolyte requirements or to replenish substantial deficits or continuing losses when the patient is nauseated or vomiting and is unable to take adequate amounts by mouth.

In an individual patient, the nature and severity of the electrolyte imbalance must be assessed from the history and the clinical and biochemical examination. Sodium, potassium, chloride, magnesium, phosphate and water depletion can occur singly and in combination, with or without disturbances of acid–base balance (Table 21.5).

INTRAVENOUS SODIUM

For mild to moderate sodium depletion, the oral route is the one of choice. However, where the patient is unable to take supplements orally due to nausea or vomiting and a more severe deficiency exists, an intravenous infusion will be administered. This will also result in the plasma sodium level being increased more rapidly. Intravenous infusion of sodium chloride 0.9% w/v is an isotonic solution and initially 2-3 litres may be given over 2-3 hours, thereafter the infusion rate can be slowed. When the electrolyte levels have been corrected, the infusion rate is set to reflect daily requirements. Compound sodium lactate (Hartmann's solution), in addition to sodium chloride, contains small quantities of sodium lactate, potassium chloride and calcium chloride and is sometimes used instead of injection of sodium chloride 0.9% w/v during surgery. Injection of sodium chloride 0.45% w/v and glucose 2.5% w/v is administered where there is a requirement for both sodium and water.

The administration of sodium intravenously is not without risk. Fluid overload must be avoided. Plasma sodium levels must be monitored, and physical signs such as pulse rate and blood pressure give a good indication of the patient's response to therapy.

INTRAVENOUS GLUCOSE

Injection of glucose 5% w/v is an isotonic solution used largely to replace water deficits where there is no requirement to administer electrolytes. If the patient is unable to take fluid orally, the daily requirement of 1.5 – 2.5 L can be given in this way. Where there is initially a deficit, this volume may have to be doubled. In the treatment of diabetic ketoacidosis, glucose solutions are administered accompanied by a continuing insulin infusion.

INTRAVENOUS POTASSIUM

Intavenous potassium infusions are frequently administered in hospitals, but this procedure can be extremely dangerous if mishandled. It is generally preferred if ready-prepared infusions are available for the nurse to use rather than adding strong potassium chloride solutions (15%) from an ampoule to an infusion. Guidance from The National Patient Safety Agency requires that potassium ampoules are available only in essential clinical areas, due to the dangers posed by mistakes in preparing solutions which may result in toxic hyperkalaemia. Any addition of potassium chloride to infusion fluids must be carefully calculated and checked, and particular attention paid to ensure thorough mixing.

Rates above 20 mmol/h should only be used in critical care areas because of potential cardiac effects. Fast replacement may be required before emergency surgery because low potassium levels make inhaled anaesthetics more likely to cause arrhythmias. Potassium-containing intravenous infusions are best managed using infusion pumps with adequate controls. Careful monitoring of the plasma potassium level is required to determine when this has returned to normal and also to avoid the risk of hyperkalaemia developing.

BICARBONATE

Sodium bicarbonate is used to control severe metabolic acidosis (as in renal failure). Because this condition is usually accompanied by sodium depletion, this is first corrected by the administration of sodium chloride 0.9%, provided that the kidneys are not primarily affected and the degree of acidosis is not so severe as to impair renal function. In these circumstances, 0.9% infusion of sodium chloride alone is usually effective, as it restores the ability of the kidneys to generate bicarbonate.

A total volume of up to 6 L (4 L of sodium chloride 0.9% and 2 L of sodium bicarbonate 1.26%) may be necessary in the adult. In severe shock, due for example to cardiac arrest, metabolic acidosis may develop without sodium depletion. In these circumstances, sodium bicarbonate is best given in small volumes of hypertonic solution, such as 50 mL of 8.4% solution intravenously; plasma pH should be monitored.

MINERALS

CALCIUM SUPPLEMENTS

Calcium is found in the bones and teeth in combination with phosphate to give strength and rigidity. More than 99% is combined with phosphorus and concentrated in the skeletal system, with only a small proportion present in the plasma (extracellular fluid). Calcium is important in blood coagulation processes, neuromuscular functions and cardiac activity. Intake is mainly dietary (especially dairy products), and excretion is mainly in the faeces. Small amounts are excreted in the urine. Vitamin D and gastric pH influence the absorption of calcium. Regulation of calcium metabolism is by parathyroid hormone, vitamin D and calcitonin.

Calcium supplements are usually required only when dietary calcium intake is deficient. This dietary requirement varies with age and is relatively greater in childhood, pregnancy and lactation due to an increased demand, and in old age due to impaired absorption. In osteoporosis, a calcium intake that is double the recommended amount reduces the rate of bone loss.

PHOSPHATE

Phosphate occurs mainly in the intracellular fluid and in combination with calcium is a constituent of bones and teeth. Phosphate also helps to maintain acid–base balance by providing a buffer system. Phosphates are important in a number of metabolic processes, especially carbohydrate metabolism. Phospholipids are important structural components of cell membranes. Phosphate regulation is linked closely with calcium metabolism. Parathyroid hormone liberates phosphate, and vitamin D probably enhances renal excretion of phosphate. Phosphate is widely present in foodstuffs, especially milk and other dairy products. Excretion is via the urine and faeces.

FLUORIDE

Systemic fluoride supplements can play an important role in reduction of the incidence and extent of dental caries. However, it should be considered as one component in a number of measures including reducing sugar intake and regular brushing of teeth. Indeed, the topical action of fluoride on enamel through use of a suitable toothpaste may be more important than the systemic effect.

Daily administration of fluoride tablets or drops is a suitable means of supplementation where the fluoride content of drinking water is less than 700 micrograms per litre.

SELF-ASSESSMENT QUESTIONS

SECTION A

1. What are the benefits of five fruit and vegetables a day?

2. What are our main sources of energy?
3. What foodstuff is rich in potassium?
4. What does BMI stand for, what purpose does it serve and how is it calculated?
5. What is a sip feed?
6. What are the dangers of enteral feeding?
7. By what means is the correct location of a fine-bore nasogastric tube established?
8. What precautions require to be taken when preparing a parenteral feed?
9. What observations or recordings should be made throughout the administration of a parenteral feed?
10. What problems may arise when putting medicines down an enteral tube?

SECTION B

The following agree to meet up for a meal after being in hospital. The menu is shown in Figure 21.4. What would you advise each of them to have and to avoid, and why?

- Charlie has type 1 diabetes.
- Lou had a deep vein thrombosis and is taking warfarin.
- Dorothy has osteoporosis and is taking risedronate.
- Alfred has a duodenal ulcer and is on triple therapy.
- Reg suffers from depression and is taking phenelzine.

SECTION C

1. What features are common to all anaemias?
2. What is the commonest type of anaemia?
3. Name the hormone produced in the kidney in response to anoxia.
4. Which of the blood cells is necessary for fighting infection?
5. Name the test used to diagnose pernicious anaemia.
6. What is the treatment for pernicious anaemia?
7. Name a deficiency in pregnancy that can cause neural tube defects.
8. What does G-CSF stand for?
9. What drug is used to treat iron overload?
10. How should intramuscular iron be administered?
11. What foodstuff may inhibit absorption of iron?
12. Name the factor whose deficiency can lead to pernicious anaemia.

SECTION D

1. On average, how much fluid does a person consume in 24 h?
2. On average, how much urine does a person pass in 24 h?

Menu

Lentil soup with a wholemeal, crusty roll
Smoked mackeral paté
Melon cocktail

Roast beef and Yorkshire pudding
Fried haddock
Spaghetti bolognese
Steak and kidney pie
Chicken curry

Boiled potatoes
Roast potatoes
French fries
Boiled rice

Carrots
Broccoli
Peas
Parsnips
Green salad

Sticky toffee pudding with cream
Lemon cheesecake with cream
Apple pie and custard
Ice cream – various flavours
Fresh fruit salad
Cheese board: Stilton, Camembert, mature cheddar

Drinks menu

White wine
Red wine
Fresh orange juice
Grapefruit juice
Tomato juice
Cranberry juice
Tea or coffee

Fig. 21.4   Sample menu.

3. How much saliva does a person produce in 24 h?
4. How much blood does the body contain?
5. What are the main sources of fluid in the body?
6. Name four types of diuretic.
7. Distinguish between haemodialysis and peritoneal dialysis.
8. Define electrolyte.
9. Define hypokalaemia.
10. Define hypernatraemia.

FURTHER READING AND RESOURCES

[Anonymous] 2006 Primary vitamin D deficiency in adults. Drug and Therapeutics Bulletin 44:25–29

Cannaby A-M, Evans L, Freeman A 2002 Nursing care of patients with nasogastric tubes. British Journal of Nursing 11:366–372

Manning E 2002 Management of vitamin and mineral deficiencies. Prescriber 13:43–64

Murphy A, Scott A 2000 Artificial nutritional support: what are the options? Hospital Pharmacist 7:146–153

Ruxton C 2004 Fruit and vegetables and their impact on disease. Nutrition in Practice 5:1–4

Thomson EC, Naysmith MR, Lindsay A 2000 Managing drug therapy in patients receiving enteral and parenteral nutrition. Hospital Pharmacist 7:153–163

Ward N 2005 Clinical nutrition: physiology and treatment of intestinal failure. Hospital Pharmacist 12:9–12

Wechalekar A, Smith A 2005 Diagnosis and treatment of anaemia in primary care. Prescriber 16:43–60

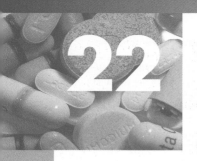

22 Drug treatment of musculoskeletal and joint diseases

CHAPTER CONTENTS

KEY OBJECTIVES

After reading this chapter, you should be able to:

- outline the anatomy and physiology of the synovial joint
- discuss the principles of treatment of rheumatoid arthritis and the main groups of medicines used
- discuss the rationale for the differences in treatment strategies between rheumatoid arthritis and osteoarthritis
- outline the main side-effects of non-steroidal anti-inflammatory drugs (NSAIDs)
- list the groups of patients most at risk from the side effects of NSAIDs
- outline the monitoring requirements for the disease-modifying antirheumatic drugs
- identify non-pharmacological methods that can ameliorate the symptoms of rheumatoid arthritis
- discuss the role of corticosteroids in the treatment of rheumatoid diseases
- name three drugs that can precipitate the onset of gout
- outline the pharmacological treatment options in acute gout.

INTRODUCTION

The term *musculoskeletal and joint diseases* includes conditions that affect the bones, joints, and ligaments, such as the various forms of arthritis, connective tissue diseases, osteoporosis, gout, soft-tissue rheumatism and back pain. These conditions can be a source of pain that affect widespread parts of the body or only defined local areas. It is estimated that more than 7 million adults in the UK, 15% of the population, have long-term health problems due to arthritis and related conditions. An even greater number, 9 million people, visit their GP each year with arthritis or related problems. The commonest condition, osteoarthritis, is increasing in prevalence as the population ages. At least 4.4 million people in the UK have radiographic evidence of moderate to severe osteoarthritis in their hands. The incidence rates of rheumatoid arthritis appear to be remaining steady, affecting approximately 0.8% of the UK population, having fallen during the 1970s and 1980s. As well as rheumatoid arthritis and osteoarthritis, there are more than 200 different types of arthritis and related conditions. Many of these occur relatively infrequently, but some such as ankylosing spondylitis, systemic lupus erythematosus, juvenile idiopathic arthritis and gout, affect significant numbers of people.

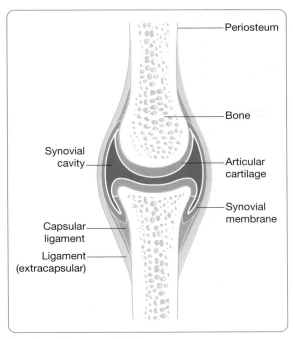

Fig. 22.1   The synovial joint.

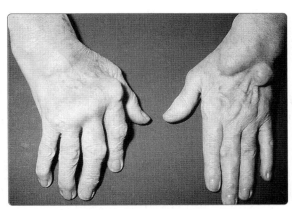

Fig. 22.2   Rheumatoid arthritis in the hands. (From Huckstep RL Sherry E 1994 Color guide – orthopaedics and trauma. Churchill Livingstone, Edinburgh. With permission of Elsevier.)

ANATOMY AND PHYSIOLOGY

Movement of the bony framework results from the contraction of muscles at the joints. Although some joints (e.g. vertebral joints) have only slight movement caused by compression of cartilage, the majority of joints in the body (e.g. the hip joint) are freely movable as the result of the contraction of muscles surrounding them and are known as synovial joints (Fig. 22.1).

A synovial joint has a surrounding fibrous sleeve, the capsular ligament, which joins the bones together, so protecting the joint without hindering movement. The articular cartilage is a smooth surface on the parts of the bones in contact to allow free articulation of the joint. The synovial membrane secretes a thick fluid, known as synovial fluid; which lubricates the joint and holds the bones in close proximity to one another, providing nourishment for the structures within the joint cavity. As well as lining the capsule, the synovial membrane covers the bony surfaces within the joint not covered by articular cartilage. Many joints have ligaments continuous with the capsule that provide further stability. Muscles or muscle tendons stretch across the joint, and movement of bones occurs when these muscles contract and shorten or relax and lengthen. The joint structures and the muscles involved are supplied by both nerves and blood vessels. Synovial joints are predominant in the limbs, where mobility is important.

RHEUMATOID ARTHRITIS

CLINICAL FEATURES OF RHEUMATOID ARTHRITIS

Rheumatoid arthritis affects approximately 0.81% of the population and is more common in women than in men (ratio 2.7:1). There are around 12 000 new cases of rheumatoid arthritis in the UK each year. It is a chronic inflammatory autoimmune disease affecting the synovial membrane. It occurs at a ratio of 1:9:12 in the young to middle-aged to elderly populations. In affected joints, the synovium becomes thickened; the amount of synovial fluid increases and the ligaments and tissues around the joint become inflamed, causing a build-up of pressure within the joint. The joint hurts because nerve endings are irritated by the chemicals produced by the inflammation and the capsule is stretched by the swelling in the joint. Granulation tissue forms on the articular cartilages of the affected joints. In time, this may erode not only the cartilages but also bone and even ligaments and tendons in the area. As the disease progresses, there is additional and cumulative damage to the joints, leading to increasing deformity, pain and loss of function (Fig. 22.2). The course of rheumatoid arthritis is variable and unpredictable, but for a significant number of patients it is a severe disease resulting in persistent pain and stiffness, progressive joint destruction, functional decline and premature mortality. Typical clinical features of rheumatoid arthritis include:

- joint pain, swelling and tenderness
- stiffness following inactivity (often worse in the morning)
- systemic flu-like symptoms
- synovitis
- extra-articular features.

Ankylosing spondylitis is another autoimmune inflammatory arthritic disease in which the sacroiliac and vertebral joints become ossified.

PRINCIPLES OF TREATMENT OF RHEUMATOID ARTHRITIS

Curative treatment, although highly desirable, has yet to be achieved. At present, the goals of management in rheumatoid arthritis are to relieve pain, stiffness and swelling; to prevent disease progression and deformities; to improve morbidity and function of joints; and as far as possible to maintain the patient's normal lifestyle.

Drug treatment is only one element of the overall management that should also involve a combination of interventions, including exercise, physiotherapy, occupational therapy, education, emotional support and rest. The management plan should be individualised based on considerations such as joint function, degree of disease activity and the patient's age, gender, occupation and response to previous therapy.

DRUG TREATMENT OF RHEUMATOID ARTHRITIS

SIMPLE ANALGESIA

Analgesics are used early in the treatment of rheumatoid arthritis and are often an adjunct to non-steroidal anti-inflammatory drugs (NSAIDs) and disease-modifying anti-rheumatic drugs (DMARDs). Paracetamol, codeine and combination medications containing paracetamol are effective in reducing pain in rheumatoid arthritis. Combination analgesic preparations reduce the scope for effective titration of the individual component in the management of pain. Simple analgesics should be used in place of NSAIDs if possible, and DMARDs should be introduced early to suppress disease activity.

NON-STEROIDAL ANTI-INFLAMMATORY DRUGS

Mode of action

Non-steroidal anti-inflammatory drugs are effective in providing symptomatic relief of pain and stiffness but do not influence the progression of rheumatoid arthritis. NSAIDs have anti-inflammatory, analgesic and antipyretic properties.

It is believed that NSAIDs produce their anti-inflammatory effect by inhibition of prostaglandin synthesis. There are over 20 different naturally occurring prostaglandins, which are widely distributed throughout the body because they are synthesised by virtually every tissue. Prostaglandins are formed in the body by the enzymatic oxygenation of arachidonic acid and linoleic acid, the key enzyme involved being cyclo-oxygenase (COX). Prostaglandins are very potent chemicals with a broad range of activities, which include:

- inhibition of gastric acid secretion
- bronchial relaxation
- vasodilator and hypotensive activity, including control of blood flow through the renal medulla
- mediation of some aspects of inflammation.

In rheumatoid arthritis, it appears that control over the balanced production of prostaglandins is, to some extent, lost, and this results in excessive production of prostaglandins involved in inflammation. Administration of NSAIDs blocks the action of the enzyme COX, which effectively reduces the synthesis of prostaglandins. The therapeutic outcome is a reduction in pain, tenderness, swelling and temperature in the affected joints; decreased stiffness; and increased joint movement. COX is present in different forms; COX-1 is present in the stomach and produces prostaglandins that protect the gastric mucosa, and COX-2 is present only at sites of inflammation.

CHOICE OF NSAID

Patient response to NSAIDs is highly variable, and therapeutic trials with several NSAIDs may be necessary to determine the best agent. It is estimated that 60% of patients will respond to any one NSAID. The drug should be changed after 1 week if there has been no response and an analgesic effect is the desired outcome, or after 3 weeks if an anti-inflammatory effect is desired. Approximately 10% of patients will not find any NSAID beneficial. As a general principle, NSAIDs should be prescribed initially at the lowest recommended dose and only one NSAID should be prescribed at any one time.

There are over 20 NSAIDs available, and these vary in half-life, dose, potency and side-effect frequency. They are also available in a variety of dosage forms, such as modified-release oral preparations, suppositories, injections and topical preparations. Ibuprofen is the most commonly used first-line agent, as it combines good efficacy with fewer side effects than other NSAIDs, but its anti-inflammatory properties are weaker. Many patients with rheumatoid arthritis find ibuprofen relatively ineffective even on maximal doses of 600 mg three times a day. Naproxen is a good choice, as it combines good efficacy with a low incidence of side-effects (but more than ibuprofen) when taken at a dose of 500 mg twice daily. Diclofenac has actions and side-effects similar to those of naproxen. Fenoprofen is as effective as naproxen, and flurbiprofen may be slightly more effective. Both are associated with slightly greater gastrointestinal side-effects than ibuprofen. Fenbufen may have a lower risk of gastrointestinal bleeding but has a high risk of rashes, especially in seronegative rheumatoid arthritis, in psoriatic arthritis and in women.

CYCLO-OXYGENASE (COX)-2

Standard NSAIDs act by direct inhibition of both COX-1 and COX-2 via blockade of the COX enzyme site. The subsequent inhibition of prostaglandins reduces inflammation but also has collateral effects on platelet aggregation, renal homeostasis and gastric mucosal integrity. In an effort to reduce the side effects of NSAIDs, particularly gastrointestinal side effects, agents have been developed that selectively block COX-2 with minimal effect on COX-1.

There are four COX-2 selective agents available: etodolac, meloxicam, etoricoxib and celecoxib. Etodolac and meloxicam inhibit COX-2 up to 50 times more than COX-1, and newer agents celecoxib and etoricoxib are even more COX-2 selective. Celecoxib and etoricoxib are thought to inhibit COX-2, whereas meloxicam and etodolac are thought to have high COX-2 selectivity rather than complete inhibition. COX-2 selective agents are recommended only for use in patients who are at particularly high risk of developing gastroduodenal ulcer, perforation or bleeding, but they are not recommended for routine use.

Side-effects of NSAIDs

Toxicity is a major factor, and side-effects are related to dose and duration of therapy. Common side-effects are gastrointestinal toxicity (there is a linear increase in risk with age), fluid retention and hypertension. Other less common but potentially serious side-effects are renal disease and hypersensitivity (including asthma). Uncommon and not usually serious side-effects are headaches, dizziness, tinnitus, rash (particularly with fenbufen) and abnormal liver function tests (particularly with diclofenac).

The use of NSAIDs is associated with gastrointestinal toxicity (see Ch. 11). The following side-effects occur to a varying extent with all preparations and all routes of administration:

- dyspepsia
- gastric erosions
- peptic ulceration
- small bowel inflammation and bleeding
- perforation
- haematemesis or melaena
- occult gastrointestinal blood loss and anaemia.

The annual relative risk of mortality attributed to NSAID-related gastrointestinal adverse effects is four times that for those not using NSAIDs. The rate of NSAID-related serious gastrointestinal complications requiring hospitalisation has decreased in recent years. The reason for this is likely to be multifactorial. Intensive education programmes have alerted physicians and patients to the use of newer, less toxic NSAIDs and non-NSAID analgesics in populations at high risk. There has also been a much wider use of gastroprotective therapy such as proton pump inhibitors, prostaglandin analogues and H_2-receptor antagonists. Of these, proton pump inhibitors are the most effective and most commonly used. Although selective inhibitors of COX-2 are associated with a lower risk of serious upper gastrointestinal side-effects (they can still cause dyspepsia) than non-selective NSAIDs, concerns have emerged concerning their cardiovascular safety. In December 2004, the Committee on Safety of Medicines (CSM) issued advice that any patient receiving a COX-2 selective inhibitor who has ischaemic heart disease or cerebrovascular disease should be switched to alternative treatment as soon as possible. Celecoxib and etoricoxib are contraindicated in ischaemic heart disease, cerebrovascular disease, peripheral arterial disease and moderate to severe congestive heart failure. There is no justification for prescribing a COX-2 selective agent in combination with gastroprotective agents.

Risk factors for NSAID-associated gastroduodenal ulcers include a previous history of ulcer, higher doses of NSAIDs, combination use of NSAIDs, concomitant use with oral corticosteroids and comorbidity. Cigarette smoking and significant alcohol consumption possibly may also increase the risk. It is important to note that the use of an enteric-coated, parenteral or rectal NSAID preparation is *not* protective. The systemic effects of NSAIDs are the predominant cause of damage.

NSAID (both COX-2 selective and non-selective) use is also associated with renal disease. Prostaglandins regulate and maintain intrarenal perfusion, particularly under conditions in which renal blood flow may be reduced (e.g. dehydration or blood loss, cardiac failure, chronic renal failure, diuretic use or hypertension). By inhibiting prostaglandin synthesis under these conditions, NSAIDs may further impair intrarenal blood flow, contributing to renal impairment (or overt renal failure), hyperkalaemia, oedema and hypertension. These problems are particularly likely in the elderly.

Following reports of severe cystitis, the Committee on Safety of Medicines (CSM) has recommended that tiaprofenic acid should not be given to patients with urinary tract disorders and should be stopped if urinary symptoms develop.

The CSM has also warned that worsening of asthma can be related to the ingestion of NSAIDs, either prescribed or purchased over the counter.

Strategies to minimise the risk of NSAID toxicity are summarised in Box 22.1.

ASPIRIN AND SALICYLATES

Aspirin, as an anti-inflammatory analgesic, largely takes second place to NSAIDs. The required dose of aspirin for active inflammatory joint disease is at least 3.6 g daily. Gastrointestinal side-effects such as nausea, dyspepsia and gastrointestinal bleeding may occur with any dosage, but anti-inflammatory doses are associated with a much higher incidence of side-effects. Owing to an association with Reye's syndrome, aspirin-containing preparations should not be given to children under 16 years unless specifically indicated (e.g. for juvenile arthritis).

DISEASE-MODIFYING ANTI-RHEUMATIC DRUGS

Rheumatoid arthritis should be treated as early as possible with DMARDs to control symptoms and delay disease progression. All patients with persistent inflammatory joint disease of greater than 6–8 weeks' duration and already receiving simple analgesics and NSAIDs should be considered for referral for specialist rheumatology opinion and DMARD therapy, preferably within 12 weeks. Early and sustained treatment with DMARDs slows erosive joint destruction and improves long-term disease outcome. They may also improve extra-articular symptoms such as vasculitis.

Mode of action of DMARDs

The precise mechanism of action of these drugs is unclear. All the DMARDs inhibit the release, or reduce the activity, of inflammatory cytokines. Activated T lymphocytes appear to be particularly important in this process, and it is known that methotrexate and ciclosporin both inhibit T cells. They do not produce an immediate effect but require 4–6 months of treatment to produce full benefit.

Use of DMARDS

Early DMARD therapy in rheumatoid arthritis is important to maintain function and reduce later disability. DMARD therapy should be sustained in inflammatory disease in order to maintain disease suppression. DMARD choice should take into account patient preference and existing comorbidity (see Table 22.1 for DMARD profiles). Patients should be counselled about the benefits and risks of specific DMARDs and should be provided with additional written information. Clear advice about monitoring of specific DMARDs should be available to the patient, GP and practice nurse. Good liaison between primary and secondary care is essential. Rheumatology nurse specialists have an important role in this aspect of care.

Sulfasalazine, methotrexate, intramuscular gold and penicillamine have a comparable clinical effect on disease activity, but the first two are the current DMARDs of choice because of their more favourable efficacy, toxicity profiles and relatively speedier onset of action. Hydroxychloroquine and auranofin (oral gold) are relatively weak DMARDs with a slower onset of action. Successive DMARDs are required for most patients in the medium to long term.

TUMOUR NECROSIS FACTOR BLOCKADE

The DMARDs often produce only delayed, inadequate or temporary responses or troublesome unwanted effects. Drugs that block the effects of tumour necrosis factor (TNF) offer a novel approach. TNF is a product

Table 22.1 Profiles of disease-modifying antirheumatic drugs

Drug	Dose	Non life-threatening side-effects	Potentially life-threatening side-effects	Monitoring requirements
Azathioprine	1–2.5 mg/kg per day (maximum 3 mg/kg)	Nausea, vomiting, hair loss	Neutropenia, thrombocytopenia, hypersensitivity reactions, liver impairment, pancreatitis	FBC, U&E, LFT at baseline then FBC and LFT weekly for first 4 weeks or until maintenance achieved, then monthly thereafter
Auranofin	6 mg/day increasing to 9 mg/day if no response	Diarrhoea, rash, pruritus	Thrombocytopenia, agranulocytosis, leucopenia and neutropenia, anaphylactic reactions hepatotoxicity, pulmonary fibrosis	FBC, U&E, urinalysis, LFT at baseline then FBC, platelets, U&E, urinalysis fortnightly for 3 months, then monthly; annual chest X-ray
Ciclosporin	2.5 mg/kg per day increasing to a maximum of 4 mg/kg per day	Paraesthesia, tremor, fatigue, hypertrichosis, gingival hypertrophy	Hypertension, renal and hepatic dysfunction, hyperlipidaemia, hyperuricaemia, hyperkalaemia, hypomagnesaemia, pancreatitis	Blood pressure, U&E, urinalysis, FBC, lipids at baseline then U&E, LFT, FBC fortnightly for first 3 months, then monthly thereafter; lipids every 6 months and blood pressure at each monitoring visit
Hydroxychloroquine	200–400 mg/day	Gastrointestinal disturbance, headache, skin rash, hair loss	Retinal damage, thrombocytopenia, agranulocytosis, electrocardiogram changes, cardiomyopathy	Renal function tests and LFT before treatment; visual acuity test every year
Leflunomide	100 mg/day for 3 days then maintenance dose of 10–20 mg/day	Anorexia, weight loss, nausea, vomiting, alopecia, headache, dizziness	Leucopenia, thrombocytopenia, anaphylactic reaction, hypertension, hepatitis, liver failure, birth defects when taken during pregnancy	FBC, U&E, platelets and LFT, blood pressure before treatment then every 2 weeks for 6 months, then every 8 weeks; blood pressure monthly for first 6 months then 8-weekly thereafter; effective contraception required during therapy and for 2 years after discontinuation
Methotrexate	7.5–20 mg ONCE a week	Nausea, anorexia, rash, abdominal discomfort, diarrhoea, alopecia, headache, drowsiness	Leucopenia, thrombocytopenia, pulmonary toxicity, hepatotoxicity	FBC, renal function tests and LFT, urinalysis, chest X-ray at baseline, then FBC, U&E and LFT weekly until 6 weeks after last dose increase, then monthly thereafter

Continued

Table 22.1 Profiles of disease-modifying antirheumatic drugs 'cont ...'

Drug	Dose	Non life-threatening side-effects	Potentially life-threatening side-effects	Monitoring requirements
Penicillamine	125–250 mg/day initial dose increasing to 500–750 mg/day maintenance taken before food (maximum 1.5 g/day)	Nausea, taste disturbance, rash	Proteinuria associated with nephritis, thrombocytopenia, leucopenia	FBC, platelets, renal function, urinalysis before treatment then every 1–2 weeks until dose is stable, then monthly thereafter
Sodium aurothiomalate	10-mg test dose to exclude hypersensitivity, then 50 mg weekly until evidence of remission, then dose interval increased to 4-weekly; discontinue if no response seen after total of 1 g has been given	Rash, pruritus	Thrombocytopenia, agranulocytosis, leucopenia and neutropenia, anaphylactic reactions, hepatotoxicity, pulmonary fibrosis	FBC, urinalysis, U&E; LFT at baseline; FBC, platelets, U&E prior to each injection
Sulfasalazine	500 mg/day increasing by 500 mg/week up to maintenance dose of 2–3 g/day in divided doses	Nausea, diarrhoea, rash, coloured urine, headache, staining of soft contact lenses, photosensitivity, abnormal LFT, reversible oligospermia	Leucopenia, neutropenia, thrombocytopenia, hepatitis, hypersensitivity reactions	FBC, platelets; LFT at baseline then monthly for first 6 months then every 3 months for the next 6 months; if results have been stable, then 6-monthly

FBC, full blood count; LFT, liver function tests; U&E, urea and electrolytes.

of macrophages that acts on the immune system to induce the production of powerful proinflammatory mediators. Etanercept (twice-weekly subcutaneous injections), adalimumab (weekly or fortnightly subcutaneous injection) and infliximab (intravenous infusion repeated 2 weeks and 6 weeks after initial infusion, then repeated every 8 weeks) are selective immunosuppressants that inhibit the activity of TNF. They are used for the treatment of highly active rheumatoid arthritis in adults who have failed to respond to at least two standard DMARDs, including methotrexate. Etanercept, adalimumab and infliximab should be used under specialist supervision and withdrawn if there is no response after 3 months. Infliximab must be given concomitantly with methotrexate. Adalimumab should be used in combination with methotrexate, but it may be given alone if methotrexate is inappropriate. Anakinra is currently not recommended for routine treatment of rheumatoid arthrits except as part of a long-term clinical trial.

Adalimumab, etanercept and infliximab have been associated with infections, sometimes severe, that include tuberculosis and septicaemia. They can also cause nausea, abdominal pain, heart failure, hypersensitivity reactions, fever, headache, depression, lupus erythematosus-like syndrome, pruritus and blood disorders.

CORTICOSTEROIDS

Systemic corticosteroids have long been used in the management of rheumatoid arthritis and were the first drugs to result in reversibility of the disease. However, their place in therapy is still controversial.

Corticosteroids suppress cytokines and produce a rapid improvement in signs and symptoms of the disease. They have a potent anti-inflammatory effect. Unfortunately, the side-effects associated with long-term, high-dose therapy (e.g. osteoporosis, diabetes mellitus, hypertension and peptic ulceration) have severely limited the long-term role of corticosteroids in rheumatoid arthritis.

Place of corticosteroids in therapy

Oral prednisolone can be used to provide temporary relief until a DMARD becomes effective or in patients with aggressive disease whose pain cannot be adequately controlled with a combination of DMARDs (step-up or step-down approach). Once commenced, systemic corticosteroids can be difficult to withdraw, as the disease tends to flare with dose reductions.

In order to minimise side-effects, a daily maintenance dose of 7.5 mg of prednisolone, or less, given as a single dose in the morning, should be used.

Oral corticosteroids are not recommended for routine use, as there is no sustained clinical or functional benefit and there is a high risk of toxicity with long-term use. The lowest possible dose of corticosteroid should be used for the shortest possible time. Oral corticosteroids should be withdrawn slowly to avoid rebound flare of symptoms. Patients should be warned of the risks of corticosteroids at the outset and issued with a steroid warning card. They should be monitored closely for side-effects such as diabetes, cataract and infection. There should be adequate prophylaxis and treatment of osteoporosis in patients taking oral corticosteroids.

Intra-articular corticosteroid administration can effectively relieve pain, increase mobility and reduce deformity in one or more joints. Examples of drugs that are given via this route are methylprednisolone acetate and triamcinolone acetonide. The duration of response to intra-articular steroids is variable. The dose used is dependent on the joint size. Methylprednisolone acetate 40 mg or up to 40 mg of triamcinolone acetonide are suitable for use in large joints (e.g. knees).

Intra-articular injections can be used for rapid and sometimes sustained symptomatic relief in target joints. Intra-articular injections to any one joint should not be given more than three times in 1 year. When intra-articular injections are being administered:

- a sterile technique should be used
- patients should be advised to seek help if the joint fails to settle after injection.

THE ROLE OF THE MULTIDISCIPLINARY TEAM

There are many general measures that can be used to help patients with rheumatoid arthritis. The nurse has a key role to play in providing education to patients. Provision of information on the disease and its therapies gives patients a realistic outlook and allows them to be involved in therapeutic decisions. Education also emphasises the role of patients in controlling their own disease.

Because much of the pain and stiffness associated with rheumatoid arthritis comes from periarticular tissues, such as muscle and tendons, physiotherapists can advise on exercises and mobilisation techniques that can be tailored to the needs and capabilities of individual patients. Use of hydrotherapy may also help to improve mobility and general fitness as well as maintaining muscle bulk around the joints.

Occupational therapists can provide appliances and devices to help patients with the activities of daily living. These include, for example, grab rails and adaptors for keys and taps. In addition to educating patients on their drug therapy, pharmacists can provide a range of devices that may assist compliance, such as the Dosett tray and wing caps on tablet bottles.

The role of the dietitian is also important. Some trials have suggested a consistent but modest benefit from the inclusion of fish oil, fish supplements or evening primrose oil in the diet. Various elimination diets have also been proposed. A diet that involves avoiding red meat, dairy products, fruit, herbs, additives and preservatives is popular with patients. Perhaps most important is weight management; impaired mobility may lead to an increase in weight, which in turn may increase the workload on affected joints.

Joint replacement has been one of the greatest advances in the management of rheumatoid arthritis. Other surgical procedures that are beneficial include tendon transfers (manipulation to reduce deformity) and synovectomy (removal of the synovial membrane, which is often undertaken in patients with rheumatoid arthritis of the knee). Function may be greatly improved after tendon transfer, particularly in the hand. Although used less frequently, synovectomy can usefully debulk a synovial mass, resulting in reduced pain.

OSTEOARTHRITIS

CLINICAL FEATURES OF OSTEOARTHRITIS

Osteoarthritis is a degenerative non-inflammatory disease. Articular cartilage gradually becomes thinner, because its replacement does not keep pace with its removal. Bone, formed at the margin of the articular cartilage, enlarges and may deform the affected joints and interfere with movement. Involvement of the knee, hip or other joints may become a major disability requiring surgical replacement.

DRUG TREATMENT OF OSTEOARTHRITIS

SIMPLE ANALGESICS

Pain is the main reason why patients with osteoarthritis seek help from healthcare professionals. However, drug treatment is an adjunct and not a substitute for other types of treatment. As osteoarthritis has only a minor inflammatory component, paracetamol is now accepted as first-line therapy in uncomplicated osteoarthritis. It can be taken in a regular full dosage (up to 4 g daily) or on an as-required basis.

The effect of compound analgesics, which are commonly prescribed for osteoarthritis, is often disappointing, as many contain subtherapeutic doses of opioids. However, preparations with a full dose of the opioid component often cause unwanted side-effects, such as constipation, especially in elderly patients. Analgesics such as co-codamol and co-dydramol are generally thought to be no more effective than paracetamol alone and are probably best avoided, as they may be more hazardous in overdose.

ORAL NSAIDS

Osteoarthritis is primarily a non-inflammatory disease, although NSAIDs are frequently prescribed. NSAIDs should be reserved for patients whose symptoms are not controlled by other means or to manage acute exacerbations that are associated with inflammation.

Individual choice should be based on relative safety, patient acceptability and cost. Ibuprofen therefore should be used first line, because of its good safety profile and low cost. The usefulness of NSAIDs is limited by their side-effects. These can be a particular problem in the elderly or in those with poor renal function. If it is absolutely essential to use an NSAID in an elderly patient or in a patient with a previous history of peptic ulceration, the concurrent administration of an H_2 antagonist, misoprostol, or a proton pump inhibitor must always be considered.

In patients with renal insufficiency, NSAIDs should be avoided whenever possible or used in very low doses if the benefits are expected to outweigh the risks. In such cases, serum creatinine, urea and electrolytes must be monitored regularly.

TOPICAL NSAIDS AND RUBEFACIENTS

Rubefacients act by counterirritation, and the pain is relieved by any method that produces irritation of the skin. They usually contain a combination of ingredients such as camphor or methylsalicylate. Capsaicin can also be used topically for the symptomatic treatment of osteoarthritis.

A wide range of topical NSAIDs is available in a variety of formulations, such as gels, foams, creams, ointments and sprays. These products are promoted on the basis that they diffuse rapidly and directly into joints. This is claimed to result in high local and low plasma concentrations of the drug and theoretically gives a lower risk of systemic side-effects than oral NSAIDs. However, there is still the risk of a hypersensitivity reaction.

THE ROLE OF THE MULTIDISCIPLINARY TEAM

As for rheumatoid arthritis, patients who are overweight should be encouraged to lose weight so as to reduce stress on their joints and to increase their mobility. This strategy is particularly beneficial in patients with osteoarthritis of the knee.

Physiotherapists contribute significantly to management by advising on exercises tailored to the patient's needs, which can help to preserve the function of the joint as well as protect it from further damage. Physiotherapy can also help patients regain muscle strength around weakened joints, improve the range of movement of affected joints and enhance general well-being. It is vital that patients are given a clear explanation of the nature of their disease, methods of management and likely prognosis as soon as osteoarthritis is diagnosed. This will help them to come to terms with the disease, understand how it will affect their life and how they can work with healthcare professionals to manage their condition. Providing social contact and access to telephone helplines allows patients to discuss their disease (with other patients, therapists and support groups) and share experiences, which can also effectively improve symptoms.

GOUT

CLINICAL FEATURES OF GOUT

Gout is characterised by higher than normal levels of uric acid in the blood because of either overproduction or defective excretion by the kidneys. Uric acid is a waste product of the breakdown of cell nuclei and is produced in excess when there is large-scale cell destruction (e.g. following trauma, malignancy, treatment with cytotoxic drugs and starvation). The excess uric acid forms sodium urate crystals that are deposited in joints and tendons (Fig. 22.3). Acute inflammation is due to substances released by phagocytes that have ingested the crystals.

Acute gout often presents as a hot, red, swollen, exquisitely painful and tender joint. This may be associated with fever, leucocytosis (raised number of leucocytes) and raised erythrocyte sedimentation rate. Lower limbs are most commonly affected, including the metatarsophalangeal joints (at the base of the toe), ankles and knees, but the wrist and small joints of the hand can also be affected. Ninety per cent of initial attacks are monoarticular, and most resolve spontaneously within a few days. Symptom-free intervals occur between attacks, but subsequent attacks tend to be more severe, longer in duration and often involve additional joints.

Chronic tophaceous gout can develop after several years of acute attacks, with progressive damage to cartilage, periarticular bony erosions evident on X-rays and deposition of tophi leading to disability. Tophi are amorphous deposits of uric acid and can appear either in association with acute gouty attacks or in a more chronic form. Tophi can develop in cartilage, synovium, bursae or tendon sheaths and are commoner in previously damaged joints.

There is an increasing tendency for the development of tophaceous gout in the elderly, particularly women on diuretics. The onset may be insidious, without acute attacks, and there may be confusion with osteoarthritis, as it often affects the distal interphalangeal joints.

DRUGS CAUSING HYPERURICAEMIA AND GOUT

Certain drugs can precipitate an attack of gout:

- thiazide and loop diuretics can precipitate an attack of gout by inhibiting the tubular secretion of uric acid
- aspirin in low doses inhibits the tubular secretion of uric acid
- cytotoxic drugs causing a high rate of cell kill may increase purine production, with a consequent increase in the production of uric acid, which may result in an acute attack of gout.

DRUG TREATMENT OF GOUT

The therapeutic approach to gout entails two phases; first, the elimination of pain and joint inflammation,

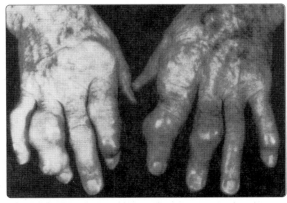

Fig. 22.3   Gout in the hands. (From Andreoli TE, Carpenter CCJ, Griggs RC et al. (eds) 2004 Cecil essentials of medicine. Grune & Stratton, New York. With permission of Elsevier Inc.)

and second, the reduction of blood uric acid levels to normal and the resorption of tophaceous deposits.

Management of acute gout

Acute attacks of gout are usually treated with NSAIDs such as diclofenac, indometacin, ketoprofen, naproxen, piroxicam or sulindac. A beneficial effect can be observed within hours of ingesting an NSAID, but an attack may take several days to resolve completely. Severe pain intensity may warrant concurrent use of analgesics such as paracetamol or codeine.

Colchicine is probably as effective as NSAIDs. Its therapeutic effect is due to immobilising polymorphonuclear leucocytes arriving at the acutely inflamed joint so that they enter the joint in fewer numbers, resulting in less phagocytosis of urate crystals and release of lysosomal enzymes into the joint. One milligram of colchicine is given initially, followed by 500 micrograms every 2–3 h until relief of pain is obtained, or vomiting or diarrhoea occurs, or until a total dose of 6 mg has been reached. The course should not be repeated within 3 days.

Most common side-effects are nausea, vomiting and abdominal pain. The use of colchicine is limited by the development of toxicity at higher doses, but it is of value in patients with heart failure because, unlike NSAIDs, it does not induce fluid retention. Moreover, it can be given to patients receiving anticoagulants.

Long-term control of gout

Patients who are obese should be encouraged to lose weight, and those who overindulge in alcohol should be encouraged to consider the risks. This is on the basis that there is a good correlation between the level of uric acid and body weight and also excessive alcohol intake, because alcohol stimulates purine synthesis in the liver, which breaks down to form uric acid. Long-term management and prophylaxis of gout can be achieved in two ways:

- blocking the production of uric acid by the administration of a xanthine-oxidase inhibitor such as allopurinol
- increasing the excretion of uric acid by the administration of a uricosuric drug such as sulfinpyrazone or probenecid (the latter now only available in the UK on a named-patient basis).

Frequent recurrence of acute attacks of gout may call for the initiation of long-term ('interval') treatment. For long-term control of gout, the formation of uric acid from purines may be reduced with the xanthine-oxidase inhibitor allopurinol, or the uricosuric drug sulfinpyrazone may be used to increase the excretion of

uric acid in the urine. Treatment should be continued indefinitely to prevent further attacks of gout by correcting the hyperuricaemia. These drugs should never be started during an acute attack. The initiation of treatment may precipitate an acute attack, and therefore colchicine or an anti-inflammatory analgesic should be used as a prophylactic and continued for at least 1 month after the hyperuricaemia has been corrected (usually about 3 months of prophylaxis). However, if an acute attack develops during treatment, the treatment should continue at the same dosage and the acute attack should be treated in its own right.

Allopurinol is a well-tolerated drug that is widely used. It is especially useful in patients with renal impairment or urate stones when uricosuric drugs cannot be used; it is *not* indicated for the treatment of asymptomatic hyperuricaemia. It is usually given once daily, because the active metabolite of allopurinol has a long half-life. Maintenance doses range from 100 mg/day in mild conditions to 900 mg/day in severe conditions, but doses over 300 mg daily should be divided. It may occasionally cause rashes.

Sulfinpyrazone can be used instead of allopurinol or in conjunction with it in cases that are resistant to treatment. It is initiated at doses of 100–200 mg/day given with food or milk, increasing over 2–3 weeks to 600 mg/day. This is continued until serum uric acid levels are normal, then the dose is reduced to a maintenance dose of 200–300 mg/day. It can cause gastrointestinal disturbances and occasionally allergic skin rashes, and rarely acute renal failure, hepatitis and blood disorders.

MYASTHENIA GRAVIS

CLINICAL FEATURES OF MYASTHENIA GRAVIS

Neuromuscular transmission depends on the release of acetylcholine from the nerve terminal. This is followed by an interaction between the neurotransmitter acetylcholine and receptor sites on the postsynaptic membrane. This results in an action potential being triggered, leading to muscle contraction.

Myasthenia gravis is an acquired autoimmune disorder involving the production of antibodies to the acetylcholine receptors at the neuromuscular junction. Acetylcholine is therefore blocked at nerve endings, and this leads to muscle weakness affecting more commonly the external ocular muscles, causing ptosis and diplopia; the bulbar muscles, causing dysphagia; or indistinct speech and occasionally aphasia. Neck and shoulder muscles may also be affected such that patients have difficulty holding up the head and raising the arms. Limb muscles may be affected and movement restricted. These symptoms may be exacerbated by emotional disturbances, strenuous exercise and pregnancy. The condition has a remitting and relapsing course. In the UK, the prevalence is around one in every 10 000 people. Between the onset ages of 15 and 40, about 75% of patients are female, but between the ages of 50 and 75, about 60% are male.

TEST FOR MYASTHENIA GRAVIS

Acetylcholine is broken down by the enzyme acetylcholinesterase. If acetylcholinesterase is inhibited, the concentration of acetylcholine at the motor end plate rises and its action is potentiated. Inhibition of acetylcholinesterase results in an increase in the concentration of acetylcholine at the neuromuscular junction, thus overcoming the reduction in functioning receptors. Edrophonium chloride is an acetylcholinesterase inhibitor (anticholinesterase) with a very short duration of action and is used to test for the presence of myasthenia gravis when antibody assays are not available or the titre is normal. In patients with muscle weakness when fatigued, a raised serum titre of antibody to acetylcholine receptors (present in about 85% of cases) establishes a firm diagnosis. For more immediate diagnosis and in seronegative tests, an intravenous edrophonium chloride test can be done.

A test dose of edrophonium chloride 2 mg intravenously is given, followed 30–60 s later (if no adverse drug reaction has occurred) by 8 mg. A positive response, defined as improvement in strength (e.g. recovery of ptosis, increased limb strength or increased vital capacity) will occur within 20–30 s of injection and subside after about 3 min.

Muscarinic side effects of anticholinesterases include increased sweating, salivary and gastric secretion, increased gastrointestinal and uterine motility, and bradycardia. Adverse effects such as severe bradycardia and cholinergic crisis leading to respiratory arrest occur occasionally. Severe cholinergic reactions can be countered by injection of atropine sulphate, which should always be available. It is recommended that resuscitation equipment is also available and to premedicate with atropine sulphate 600 micrograms intravenously. Edrophonium chloride can also be used to determine over- or undertreatment. In patients overtreated with anticholinesterases, administration will have no effect or it will intensify symptoms. In contrast, undertreated patients will show a transient improvement in muscle power.

DRUG TREATMENT OF MYASTHENIA GRAVIS

Anticholinesterases are first-line treatment for myasthenia gravis and provide symptomatic relief. They are of greatest benefit in patients with mild symptoms, often completely correcting weakness in those cases and improving the strength of those moderately affected. Neostigmine can be given orally or by subcutaneous or intramuscular injection and has a maximum duration of action of 4 h. It has pronounced muscarinic effects (including increased salivation and colic) and may need to be given up to every 2 h. Pyridostigmine is fewer powerful and has a slower onset of action but a longer duration of action than neostigmine. It also has fewer muscarinic side-effects and is therefore the treatment of choice. The usual starting dose of pyridostigmine is 30–60 mg every 4–6 h. The maximum daily dose is 720 mg. Distigmine has the longest action, but the danger of a cholinergic crisis caused by an accumulation of the drug is greater than with shorter-acting drugs.

Adverse effects of these drugs (colic, diarrhoea) can usually be controlled by propantheline 15 mg three times a day and 30 mg at night. Excessive dosages should be avoided, because they may impair neuromuscular transmission and precipitate cholinergic crisis. This is due to flooding the neuromuscular junction with acetylcholine, resulting in continual stimulation of postsynaptic acetylcholine receptors. The membrane is not allowed to repolarise, and this results in a depolarising block. In patients taking a high dosage of an anticholinesterase, cholinergic toxicity can be distinguished from myasthenic crisis by the presence of hypersalivation, lacrimation, increased sweating, vomiting and miosis.

Anticholinesterases are used as first-line therapy, but when they fail to control symptoms completely corticosteroids and a second-line immunosuppressant such as azathioprine may be used. Plasmapheresis or infusion of intravenous immunoglobulin may induce temporary remission in case of severe relapse.

SKELETAL MUSCLE RELAXANTS

Patients with various disorders of the musculoskeletal system and of the central nervous system, for example multiple sclerosis, may suffer from muscle spasm. This spasm may produce pain and deformity. Treatment with drugs is generally only moderately effective. The drugs used in the treatment of muscle spasticity are diazepam, baclofen, dantrolene and tizanidine.

Diazepam has some antispasmodic effect, but sedation can be a problem, particularly on higher doses. Baclofen acts at the spinal level similarly to diazepam. Adverse effects such as sedation and hypotonia can be limiting. Dantrolene acts directly on skeletal muscle. It is used in severe spasticity, multiple sclerosis, spinal cord injury and stroke. Dosage should be increased slowly, but if no benefit has been obtained after about 6 weeks the drug should be withdrawn. Drowsiness may be a problem if the patient has to drive or operate machinery. Tizanidine is an α_2-adrenoceptor agonist indicated for spasticity associated with multiple sclerosis or spinal cord injury.

SELF-ASSESSMENT QUESTIONS

1. Miss D. is in her late twenties and has just been diagnosed with early rheumatoid arthritis. She has no other medical problems. She has symptoms that include joint pain and early morning stiffness, but as yet she has no joint deformities. Her erythrocyte sedimentation rate and C-reactive protein are both raised. Suggest what medication may be appropriate and what monitoring requirements may be needed.

2. Which of the following is the appropriate way to start sodium aurothiomalate?
   a. 10mg test dose followed by 50mg injection weekly.
   b. Give 50mg injection once a month until stable.
   c. Give test dose of auranofin (oral gold) first
   d. 50mg IM every 2 weeks.

3. List some of the activities of prostaglandin.

FURTHER READING AND RESOURCES

[Anonymous] 2001 Etanercept and infliximab for rheumatoid arthritis. Drug and Therapeutics Bulletin 39:49–52

Akil M, Amos RS 1995 Rheumatoid arthritis: clinical features and diagnosis. British Medical Journal 310:587–590

Alldred A 2005 Gout: pharmacological management. Hospital Pharmacist 12:395–400

Arthritis Research Campaign 2002 Arthritis: the big picture. Online. Available: http://www.arc.org.uk/about_arth/bigpic.htm

Bakr M, Waller DG 2005 COX-2 inhibitors and the cardiovascular system: is there a class effect? British Journal of Cardiology 12:387–391

Harris A 1996 Management of myasthenia gravis. Pharmacy in Practice 6:350–351

Johnstone A 2005 Gout: the disease and non-drug treatment. Hospital Pharmacist 12:391–394

National Institute for Clinical Excellence 2001 Guidance on the use of cyclo-oxygenase (COX) II selective inhibitors, celecoxib, rofecoxib, meloxicam and etodolac for osteoarthritis and rheumatoid arthritis. Technology appraisal guidance no. 27. NICE, London

Parkinson S, Alldred A 2002 Drug regimens for rheumatoid arthritis. Hospital Pharmacist 9:11–15

Scottish Intercollegiate Guidelines Network 2000 Management of early rheumatoid arthritis. SIGN guideline no. 48. SIGN, Edinburgh

Simpson C, Franks C, Morrison C et al. 2005 The patient's journey: rheumatoid arthritis. British Medical Journal 331:887–889

Starey N 2001 NSAIDs in the treatment of osteoarthritis. Evidence Based Medicine in Practice 3–9

Drug treatment of eye conditions

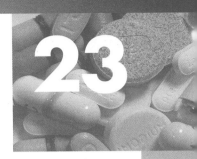

CHAPTER CONTENTS

KEY OBJECTIVES

After reading this chapter, you should be able to:

- demonstrate a working knowledge of the structures of the eye
- give one example of an antibiotic, an antiviral, a local anaesthetic, and a preparation used to treat tear deficiency
- define glaucoma, blepharospasm and cataract
- explain what mydriatics and cycloplegics are and what they are used for
- describe the procedures for instilling drops/applying ointment to the eye
- list the precautions that must be taken when treating eye conditions.

INTRODUCTION

The benefits of healthy eyesight are enjoyed by most people in the developed world. However, the impact on eye health of the ageing process and modern lifestyles present many challenges to all those involved both in research and the delivery of eye care. In the developing world, the problems of meeting the urgent need to improve eye health are massive and sadly still not always being met.

Conditions presented in UK ophthalmology departments and in general practice range from conjunctivitis (which has a variety of causes), eye trauma and tear deficiency to sight-threatening glaucoma, cataract and degenerative eye diseases. Some of these conditions are amenable to topical or systemic medication and/or surgery. The treatment of chronic degenerative eye conditions presents special problems.

Although the eye has built-in protective mechanisms, great care is needed to avoid microbial contamination and to maintain the stability and potency of topical eye preparations both in use and in storage. It is imperative to avoid cross-infection in all settings in which eye care is provided. The need to reduce the risk of infection when an eye injury is being investigated is critical, as it is in surgery.

Cataracts are a common cause of loss of useful sight in older people. Surgical procedures are widely and successfully carried out to correct this condition. Although no pharmacological treatment is available for cataracts, topical pre- and postoperative medication play a vital part.

There is a need to be aware that eyes can be significantly damaged or irritation caused by systemic drug treatment given for unrelated conditions, by improper care of contact lenses and by excipients such as preservatives contained in eye drops.

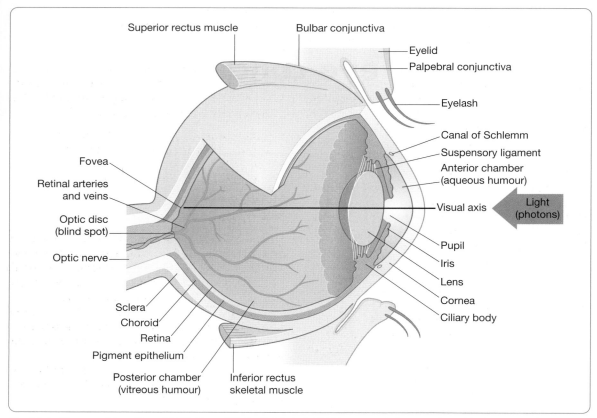

Fig. 23.1   The eye. (From Page CP, Hoffman BF, Curtis M et al. 2006 Integrated pharmacology. Mosby, Edinburgh. With permission of Mosby.)

Many patients will need topical medication in the longer term. Such patients should be given support and guidance in using eye drops safely and effectively. Compliance aids can bring significant benefit to patients in the community, saving nursing time and achieving a better outcome for patients (see p. 469).

For some serious eye conditions (which may be hereditary), treatment options are limited. In particular, age-related macular degeneration can be treated with photodynamic therapy. As with all eye conditions, the aim is to minimise loss of useful vision and to protect or improve the vision the patient currently enjoys using all possible means.

As people are increasingly being encouraged to be more proactive in managing their own health, the need to value and protect healthy eyes cannot be overstated. A diet rich in antioxidants, regular eye checks and the use of eye protection will greatly benefit the individual and the NHS.

Nurses are increasingly carrying out ophthalmology procedures exclusively performed in the past by an ophthalmologist. Routine testing prior to examination by an ophthalmologist is part of the role of the nurse working in the outpatient department. Pre- and postcataract removal assessment, preparation and aftercare are the responsibility of nurses specialising in ophthalmic nursing. Eye care in general will continue to be an essential component of the total care of those unable to do this for themselves. A clear understanding of the subject is therefore of relevance to those working in any branch of nursing, be it in the patient's home or in hospital.

ANATOMY AND PHYSIOLOGY

The eye is a spherical organ situated in the orbital cavity, whose bony walls and fat help to protect it from damage. The visible part of the eye is only a proportion of the whole, so that the eye is best considered in vertical cross-section viewed from the side (see Fig. 23.1).

The walls are in three layers. The outermost layer is a fibrous coat consisting of the sclera (the white of the eye) covering all but the anterior part of the eye, which is transparent and known as the cornea.

In the middle is a vascular layer that, like the sclera, covers the posterior five-sixths of the eye and is known as the choroid. The anterior sixth comprises the ciliary body, an essential part of the process of accommodation of the eye, and the iris, the pigmented muscular structure that gives the eye its colour and serves, through autonomic nervous stimulation, to control the amount of light entering the eye.

In the centre of the eye is the eyeball, which consists of an anterior and a posterior segment separated by the lens. The anterior segment is in turn made up of an anterior chamber and a posterior chamber separated by the iris. Both chambers contain a transparent fluid, known as aqueous humour, secreted by the ciliary glands. Aqueous humour circulates from the posterior chamber through the pupil into the anterior chamber and back to the general circulation via the trabecular meshwork and then the canal of Schlemm. In health, the intraocular pressure (IOP) of fluid remains fairly constant. The remaining larger posterior segment of the eyeball is known as the vitreous body and is filled with a transparent, jelly-like substance that, along with the aqueous fluid, helps keep the shape of the eye.

The eye is protected by accessory organs, which include the eyebrows, eyelids and eyelashes and the lacrimal apparatus.

The lacrimal apparatus (see Fig. 23.2) is essential for the flow of tears. Tears are composed of water, salts and a bactericidal enzyme, lysozyme. Added to this fluid are oily secretions from the meibomian glands. These combined fluids serve to protect the eye in several ways:

- moistens the eye, keeping out debris and micro-organisms
- the constant washing of the fluid over the cornea, through blinking, removes grit
- the lysozyme helps to prevent microbial infection
- the oily nature of the fluid helps to keep the conjunctiva from drying up.

The tear film has remarkable properties; flower-like crystal patterns up to 50 millionths of a metre across are thought to provide protection to the eye when we blink (Petrov 2006).

COMMON EYE CONDITIONS

- Red eye (including glaucomas)
- Eyelid disorders
- Lacrimal disorders
- Drug-induced ocular disorders

RED EYE

Patients often present with a red eye. This rather obvious sign should be fully investigated to ensure that any very serious condition (e.g. glaucoma) does not go undetected. Causes of red eye include:

- conjunctivitis – bacterial, viral, allergic, chemical
- corneal ulceration due to microbial infection
- episcleritis and scleritis
- acute closed-angle glaucoma (ACAG)
- foreign body in the eye.

EYELID DISORDERS

Lumps. It is important to ensure that any lumps on the eyelid are carefully investigated to exclude serious conditions such as basal cell carcinoma. Commonly presenting conditions are chalazion (meibomian cyst) and stye, a local infection of a lash follicle.

Drooping of the eyelid (ptosis). This condition may indicate the presence of a serious disease such as myasthenia gravis or a condition that may arise due to the ageing process.

Children who present with a drooping eyelid must be very fully investigated by a specialist, as this may indicate a serious condition.

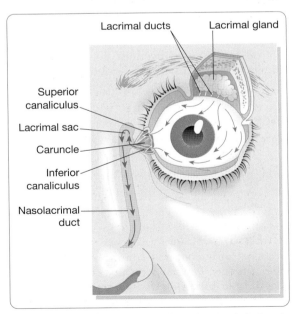

Fig. 23.2 The lacrimal apparatus. (From Waugh A, Grant A 2001 Ross and Wilson anatomy and physiology in health and illness, 9th edn. Churchill Livingstone, Edinburgh. With permission of Elsevier.)

Patients with thyroid disease sometimes develop proptosis that may require surgery. If fulminant disease threatens a patient's vision, high doses of corticosteroids, or emergency radiotherapy, may save the patient's sight.

Facial palsy may cause symptoms of ocular exposure. Exposure keratitis may result, and this can lead to blindness. The use of lubricants in reversible cases will protect the eye in the short term. Surgery is indicated in some cases. A gold weight may be implanted in the upper eyelid to facilitate closure.

INFLAMMATORY EYELID DISORDERS

These include the following.

Blepharitis. This is a chronic condition in which the patient complains of sore eyelids. Styes often accompany blepharitis, and the lid margins are inflamed and crusted. The condition may be present in patients suffering from an inflammatory skin disease such as eczema.

Acute inflammatory conditions of the eyelids must be taken as indicating a potentially serious condition that could result in loss of sight or the spread of a life-threatening infection.

Orbital cellulitis. This may result from the spread of infection from sinuses. Urgent specialist treatment is required in such cases.

Allergy. Allergic reactions can occur as a result of contact with a wide range of allergenic materials from plant or animal sources. Cosmetics may also cause allergic reactions.

Viral infections. Infections due to the herpes simplex or herpes zoster virus can result in a vesicular rash on the eyelid.

LACRIMAL DISORDERS

EXCESSIVE TEAR PRODUCTION

Some patients may experience a watering eye owing to blockage of the lacrimal sac or nasolacrimal duct. Surgery may be indicated to resolve this problem.

DRY EYE SYNDROME

This is a fairly common condition, especially in older patients. Patients with this condition suffer considerable discomfort that is due to a deficiency of either aqueous humour or the mucin component of the tear film. It is often associated with rheumatoid arthritis (Sjögren's syndrome) and autoimmune diseases such as pemphigoid. Certain drugs may be a cause of dry eye syndrome, e.g. clomethiazole.

DRUG-INDUCED OCULAR DISORDERS

Between 1964 and 2004, 4.3% of reported adverse drug reactions involved ocular disorders (Cox 2006). The drugs involved include corticosteroids (topical and systemic), which may cause steroid glaucoma and cataract, and anticholinergics, which may cause dry eye and raised IOP.

EYE INJURIES

Eye injuries can result from a number of causes, notably foreign bodies, blunt injury or chemical damage. Injuries arising from the use of metal tools on wood, glass, stone or metal can result in penetrating injuries to the eye. Chemical damage to the eye must be treated with copious amounts of a suitable irrigating fluid (Dunne et al. 1991) such as sterile sodium chloride 0.9% solution or sterile water. In emergency situations, freshly drawn tap water may have to be used. Eye injuries due to chemicals of alkaline reaction, such as lime, need to be treated very urgently, because alkalis have a penetrating action on ocular tissue, causing iritis and cataract formation.

PRE- AND POSTOPERATIVE TREATMENT

Local eye treatment, both pre- and postsurgery, will depend on the condition being treated and the surgical procedures used. The main agents used are summarised in Table 23.1. Single-use containers must be used to reduce the likelihood of infection. If these are not available, a container should be reserved for the specific use of a named patient. It should be noted that many eye drop formulations contain preservatives and other adjuncts. These may cause sensitivity reactions.

MEDICAL CONDITIONS AND THE EYE

Many serious medical conditions have ocular symp-toms. Examination of the eye may lead to the diagnosis of a serious general condition (e.g. diabetes mellitus, rheumatoid disease or hypertension). Systemic treat-ment is indicated in these conditions, the details of which are given in relevant chapters.

Table 23.1 Drugs used in association with ophthalmic surgery

Drug	Presentation	Uses and notes
Acetylcholine	1% irrigation	Surgical procedures that require rapid and complete miosis.
Apraclonidine	0.5% eye drops 1% eye drops	Short-term treatment of chronic glaucoma. Control of intraocular pressure postoperative situations.
Diclofenac sodium	0.1% eye drops (single-dose units)	Inhibition of intraoperative miosis during surgery for cataract. Also has anti-inflammatory and pain-relieving properties.
Fluorescein sodium	1 or 2% single-dose containers	For the detection of lesions and foreign bodies. Single-use containers are essential to reduce the risk of infection.
Flurbiprofen sodium	0.03% eye drops in polyvinyl alcohol 1.4%	Similar uses to diclofenac sodium. Reduction of inflammation postoperatively.
Ketorolac trometamol	0.5% eye drops	As for flurbiprofen sodium.
Rose bengal	1% eye drops (single-use containers)	Similar use to fluorescein but more expensive. A local anaesthetic is required to prevent stinging.
Sodium chloride	As a 0.9% solution or as a component of balanced salt solution (British National Formulary)	For irrigation during surgery.

GLAUCOMA

Glaucoma is the commonest cause of blindness in the world. It is characterised by a raised IOP, which leads to cupping and degeneration of the optic disc, impairment of optic nerve head function and nerve fibre-type visual field loss. If the condition is untreated, defects in the field of vision enlarge, leading to visual loss. Normal IOP is 16 ± 3 mmHg. A pressure of 21 mmHg (measured by tonometer) or higher may represent a pathological condition and requires treatment. High IOP causes compression of the microcirculation of the optic disc, resulting in ischaemia, the extent of which will depend on the IOP and vascularity/blood supply of the optic disc. Some eyes can withstand an IOP of 30 mmHg or more without damage, owing to the presence of a good blood supply to the optic disc. In other eyes, a pressure of less than 21 mmHg can cause visual impairment. IOP is maintained as a result of balance between inflow and outflow of aqueous humour, which is secreted constantly by the ciliary body. The aqueous humour circulates around the lens before passing through the pupil into the anterior chamber. Aqueous humour leaves the eye through the angle of this chamber by filtering through the trabecular meshwork, and is returned to the general circulation via the canal of Schlemm. In addition to raised IOP, other risk factors for developing glaucoma include age, race and family history. These factors must all be taken into account when diagnosing the condition.

An increased IOP can result from an increased production of aqueous humour or from impaired drainage (Fig. 23.3). In clinical practice, most cases of glaucoma arise from poor drainage of the aqueous humour from the anterior chamber. This is believed to result from a progressive degenerative process in the trabecular meshwork and the endothelium of the canal of Schlemm.

TYPES OF GLAUCOMA

Glaucomas can be divided into two main categories, namely primary open-angle glaucoma (POAG) and primary angle-closure glaucoma (PACG).

PRIMARY OPEN-ANGLE GLAUCOMA

This is the most common form. Patients may not notice the gradual visual loss taking place, presenting only when serious damage has occurred. Hereditary factors are involved, and diabetics and very short-sighted people are especially at risk of developing this condition. Prevalence increases in the over-80 age group to 10%. Screening is advisable in certain situations (e.g. in older people and children of

Table 23.2 Treatment of primary open-angle glaucoma with beta-blockers

Drug	Form and dose	Actions and indications	Contraindications, side-effects and nursing points
Betaxolol	Drops 0.5%, twice daily; also available as a suspension	These drugs reduce the secretion of aqueous humour by blocking beta adrenoceptors in the iris and ciliary body and are used in the treatment of chronic open-angle glaucoma. Long-term treatment is indicated with these drugs so as to achieve prolonged reduction of intraocular pressure.	History of cardiovascular disease, asthma. Systemic absorption can occur, causing beta-blockade. Patient should be encouraged to shut the eyes for several minutes, or the punctum should be occluded. These eye drops may cause bronchospasm and cough due to systemic absorption. This may be of particular concern in older patients. Betaxolol is the only selective β_1-blocker but may still cause problems in susceptible patients.
Carteolol	Drops 1 and 2%, twice daily		
Levobunolol	Drops 0.5% once or twice daily		
Metipranolol	Drops 0.1% twice daily		
Timolol	Drops 0.25 and 0.5% twice daily; also available as a 0.25% gel-forming solution for a longer action, daily		

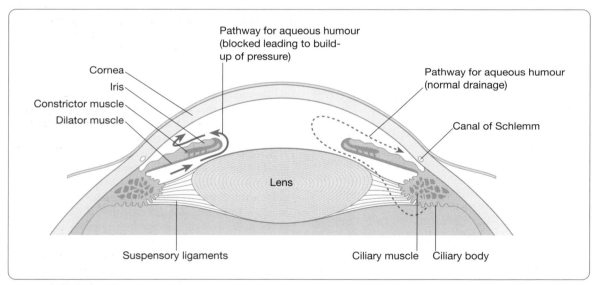

Fig. 23.3 The anterior chamber of the eye, showing the normal pathway for secretion and drainage of the aqueous humour and blocking of circulation.

affected patients). Treatment of POAG is summarised in Tables 23.2–23.4. Latanoprost (and other prostaglandin analogues) is used to treat POAG as a once-daily eye drop. This costly product is reserved for use in patients in whom first-line treatments are inappropriate. The drug acts by increasing uveoscleral outflow. Patients should be monitored for changes in eye pigmentation.

Brimonidine, a selective second-generation α_2-adrenoceptor agonist, reduces IOP by reducing aqueous humour production and enhancing uveo-scleral outflow. Because this drug has no clinically significant effect on the heart or lungs, it may be a suitable alternative to beta blockers.

Carbonic anhydrase inhibitors act on the form of the enzyme found in the ciliary epithelium, reducing the production of aqueous humour.

PRIMARY ANGLE-CLOSURE GLAUCOMA

In this condition, the affected eye is hard, red and painful and the presentation is acute. The distinction between open-angle glaucoma and closure-angle

Table 23.3 Treatment of primary open-angle glaucoma with parasympathomimetics and sympathomimetics

Drug	Form and dose	Actions and indications	Contraindications, side-effects and nursing points
Parasympathomimetics (miotics)			
Carbachol	Drops 3%, up to four times daily	Now seldom used. Acts in a manner similar to that of pilocarpine.	History of cardiovascular disease. Systemic absorption can occur. Sweating, colic, bronchospasm and hypersalivation can occur (see also p. 142).
Pilocarpine	Drops 0.5–4%, three to six times daily; also available as an ophthalmic gel 4%	Opens up the trabecular meshwork resulting in improved drainage/outflow.	Pilocarpine should not be used if there is retinal disease. Dangers of absorption (see above).
Sympathomimetics (mydriatics)			
Adrenaline (epinephrine)	Drops 0.5 or 1%, once or twice daily	Indicated in the treatment of open-angle glaucoma; causes increase in outflow of aqueous humour and dilates the pupil.	Not used for the treatment of PACG Cardiovascular problems due to systemic absorption. Stinging and redness of the eye.
Brimonidine	Drops 0.2%	Used to treat primary open-angle glaucoma in patients for whom beta-blockers are contraindicated or as an adjunct treatment to beta blockers.	A selective α_2-adrenoceptor stimulant. Use with caution in patients with cardiac disorders.
Dipivefrine	Drops 0.1%, twice daily	A prodrug that is converted into the active drug (adrenaline) in the eye.	As for adrenaline but may be less of a problem owing to the prodrug action.

Table 23.4 Treatment of glaucomas with carbonic anhydrase inhibitors

Drug	Form and dose	Actions and indications	Contraindications, side effects and nursing points
Acetazolamide	250-mg tablets or sustained-release capsules 0.25–1 g daily individual doses (injection also available).	Acetazolamide inhibits carbonic anhydrase. This enzyme regulates bicarbonate production. Bicarbonate anions balance sodium cations involved in aqueous humour secretions. Mainly used in the treatment of PACG to reduce intraocular pressure prior to surgery.	Acetazolamide may induce a mild acidosis. It is contraindicated in idiopathic renal hyperchloraemic acidosis. The drug is also contraindicated in conditions associated with electrolyte level disturbances (e.g. Addison's disease). Careful monitoring of fluid and electrolyte state is required in long-term therapy. Periodic blood cell counts are advisable. Patients should be advised to report any unusual skin rashes. The appearance of significant side effects should be reported at once. It may be necessary to terminate treatment. Not recommended for long-term use.

Continued

Table 23.4 Treatment of glaucomas with carbonic anhydrase inhibitors 'cont'd...'

Drug	Form and dose	Actions and indications	Contraindications, side-effects and nursing points
Brinzolamide	Eye drops 10 mg/mL two to three times daily	Used alone or with beta-blockers in raised intraocular pressure and open-angle glaucoma.	Local irritation, taste disturbance and significant systemic effects (see specialist literature).
Dorzolamide	2% drops applied three times daily if used alone; in combination with timolol 0.5%, twice-daily applications required	Reduces intraocular pressure in primary open-angle glaucoma. A topical carbonic anhydrase inhibitor. Treatment of primary open-angle glaucoma when beta-blockers alone are inadequate.	Severe renal impairment, hyperchloraemic acidosis, pregnancy and breast feeding.

glaucoma is made on the basis of the appearance of the anterior chamber angle on ocular examination. In this form of glaucoma, drainage of the aqueous humour is blocked by the iris. IOP builds up very quickly, vision becomes blurred and there is headache, sickness and ocular pain. Older and long-sighted people are more at risk than younger people of developing this condition.

Primary open-angle glaucoma and PACG are separate entities that require different management. PACG requires urgent intervention. Initially, IOP is reduced medically, followed by surgery to prevent recurrence. In both cases, the aim of treatment is to reduce IOP and maintain the reduction. Common glaucomatous conditions are compared and summarised in Table 23.5.

SECONDARY GLAUCOMAS

These conditions result from developmental abnormalities and acquired defects. A detailed discussion of these conditions is beyond the scope of this text. The developmental abnormalities that can result in glaucoma include inborn errors of metabolism and certain skeletal, cardiovascular and ocular changes that occur in conditions such as Marfan's syndrome. Acquired defects that may result in glaucoma include ocular inflammatory conditions, degenerative conditions, tumours, trauma and postoperative complications. Drug treatment, especially local application of potent corticosteroids (betamethasone and dexamethasone), can cause glaucoma of the chronic open-angle type. Any drug that dilates the pupil may result in PACG. Patients with narrow angles only are at risk of developing

this dangerous condition. Both local and systemic drugs can cause PACG in susceptible patients. Atropine (antimuscarinic drug) and phenylephrine (sympathomimetic) are potential causes of PACG. Systemically administered drugs that have an antimuscarinic (parasympathetic blocking) action or side-effects can precipitate closed-angle glaucoma. The main groups of drugs that can cause problems (especially in older people) are:

- antidepressant drugs of the tricyclic group (e.g. amitriptyline)
- anti-Parkinson's disease drugs (e.g. trihexyphenidyl [benzhexol])
- atropine-like drugs (antimuscarinics)
- pseudoephedrine, which may be present in cough medicines or decongestant preparations.

TREATMENT OF INFECTIONS OF THE EYE

Many infections of the eye are amenable to treatment with topical antimicrobial agents. Whenever possible, the drugs used are those that are not used to treat systemic infections, so as to reduce the risk of resistance developing. In severe infections, it may be necessary to use supporting systemic therapy. Tables 23.6 and 23.8 provide summaries of the main topical anti-infective agents. Acanthamoeba keratitis may arise from poor contact lens hygiene. Treatment requires intensive therapy managed by a specialist. Fungal infection of the cornea can be very difficult to manage. Referral to a specialist centre is required.

Table 23.5 Primary glaucomas: a comparison

Primary open-angle glaucoma or chronic simple glaucoma (POAG)	Acute closed-angle glaucoma or primary angle-closure glaucoma (PACG)
• In this condition, the angle of the anterior chamber is open	• In this condition, the angle of the anterior chamber is closed
• Incidence rises with age, onset insidious	• Incidence rises with age
• Equally common in both sexes	• Female:male ratio 4:1
• More common in Afro-Caribbean population than in white people	• Acute rise in IOP to 70–80 mmHg; hard, painful red eye
• Predisposing factors include high myopia asymmetric IOP and non-ocular diseases such as diabetes mellitus and hypothyroidism	• Peripheral iris obstructs angle of anterior chamber (structurally predisposed eyes are when anterior chamber is narrow)
• Caused by obstruction to the outflow of aqueous humour through the trabecular meshwork	• Causes include mature cataract, dilatation of pupil by dim light or drugs
• IOP rises above the normal range of 10–21 mmHg	• Symptoms include pain, blurred vision, nausea and vomiting
• Raised IOP damages retinal nerve cells (anoxia caused by compression of blood vessels)	• Emergency treatment of this condition is essential
• Loss of visual field results	
Treatment	
Drugs are used that cause reduction of formation of aqueous humour or increase outflow of aqueous humour	Medical reduction of IOP followed by iridectomy
• Drugs reducing aqueous humour formation: beta-blockers, carbonic anhydrase inhibitors and selective adrenergic agonists	• Acetazolamide (IV) used perioperatively (side effects and dosage levels require careful monitoring and preclude the use of this drug for chronic management except as a last resort); mannitol by IV infusion may also be used to reduce IOP
• Drugs increasing outflow: parasympathomimetics and prostaglandins	• Parasympathomimetics may be used after IOP has been lowered
• Sympathomimetics have a dual action (see Table 23.8)	• A beta-blocker may be preferred, because the miotic effect of pilocarpine may result in the formation of posterior synechiae
• Latanoprost (or bimatoprost) (prostaglandin analogues) may be used when other drugs are inappropriate; this drug may cause changes in eye coloration – monitoring is essential	• Because the other eye is at risk of developing primary angle-closure glaucoma, appropriate topical medication will be required (pilocarpine or a beta-blocker; see Tables 23.7 and 23.8)
The aims of treatment should be a 20–30% reduction of IOP at which damage occurred	

IOP, intraocular pressure.

Table 23.6 Anti-infective drugs: antibacterials[a]

Drug	Form and dose	Actions and indications	Contraindications, side-effects and nursing points
Chloramphenicol	Eye drops 0.5%, two drops every 3 h or more frequently; eye ointment 1%	Used for both treatment and prevention of bacterial infections (e.g. conjunctivitis). Eye ointment useful for application at night (long action). Valuable to prevent secondary bacterial infection in viral conjunctivitis.	As with all eye drops, there is a possibility of transient stinging on application. The risk of aplastic anaemia from absorption on long-term use is not well founded.
Ciprofloxacin	Eye drops 0.3%	Antibacterial in corneal ulceration.	Must be used intensively throughout the day and night (see British National Formulary for details). May cause localised itching and burning, and bitter taste due to systemic absorption.
Framycetin with gramicidin and dexamethasone	Drops containing framycetin 0.5% gramicidin 0.005% dexamethasone 0.05%	Bacterial infections (e.g. conjunctivitis).	Most antibacterial agents are applied several times daily depending on clinical need. All locally applied anti-infective agents have the potential to cause sensitivity reactions. Antibacterial agents combined with corticosteroids should not be applied when viral infections are present – or suspected – because local defence mechanisms will be compromised.
Gentamicin	Drops 0.3%	Bacterial infections; a broad-spectrum agent.	Has poor ocular penetration and potential toxicity. These problems limit its use.

[a]Other antibacterial eye preparations available include gentamicin (ointment), levofloxacin (drops) and polymyxin in various combinations. Propamidine is a non-antibiotic preparation used in the treatment of acanthamoeba keratitis (see the British National Formulary for details).

Table 23.7 Anti-infective drugs: antifungals

Drug	Form	Indications	Notes
Natamycin	Drops 5%	Fungal keratitis	Applied every 30 – 60 min for 72 h
Amphotericin	Drops 0.15%	Fungal keratitis	Prepared aseptically from injection

The treatment of fungal infections of the eye is highly specialised and requires skilled diagnosis and treatment. The preparations used are not available from normal commercial sources. (see British National Formulary)

Table 23.8 Anti-infective drugs: antivirals

Drug	Form and dose	Actions and indications	Contraindications, side-effects and nursing points
Aciclovir	Eye ointment 3%, five times daily	Herpes simplex infections and herpes simplex keratitis.	Treatment must be continued 3 days after healing.
Ganciclovir	Slow-release ocular implant, inserted surgically	To treat sight-threatening cytomegalovirus retinitis in AIDS patients. Topical treatment does not replace systemic therapy.	–

LOCAL ANAESTHETICS

Local anaesthetics (see Table 23.9 and p. 285) are applied to the eye to relieve pain following injury or to reduce discomfort prior to ophthalmological procedures. Hypersensitivity may occur, and stinging on application may be a problem.

TREATMENT OF TEAR DEFICIENCY

Tear deficiency (see Table 23.10) produces a very troublesome 'dry eye' condition leading to sore, uncomfortable, 'gritty' eyes. The condition can be alleviated by the regular use of water-based lubricant eye drops or by simple eye ointment for use at night.

TREATMENT OF INFLAMMATORY EYE CONDITIONS

The local application of corticosteroids to the eye is potentially hazardous (see p. 456). The anti-inflammatory action is, however, very valuable. Local application of corticosteroids in cases of undiagnosed infection (e.g. herpes simplex viral infection) can lead to a rapid worsening of the condition, which may even cause the loss of an eye. Anti-inflammatory drugs are detailed in Table 23.11.

MYDRIATICS AND CYCLOPLEGICS

These drugs (antimuscarinics and sympathomimetics; see Table 23.12) dilate the pupil and paralyse ciliary muscles. The main uses of these drugs are pre- and postoperatively and in diagnostic procedures (e.g.

refraction). The pain due to certain eye injuries (e.g. corneal abrasion) can be relieved by the application of homatropine eye drops. Adverse effects are briefly described in Table 23.12. Many eye drops contain very toxic drugs and should be safely stored when not in use.

BLEPHAROSPASM

Botulinum A toxin, produced by the bacterium *Clostridium botulinum* type A, is one of the most powerful neurotoxins known. It can be fatal in severe untreated cases of botulinum food poisoning. The toxin paralyses muscles by blocking the release of acetylcholine from the presynaptic neurones. The effect is irreversible and remains until new nerve end plates form.

A standardised preparation suitable for medicinal use of the toxin (botulinum A toxin–haemagglutinin complex) is licensed for the treatment of blepharospasm and hemifacial spasm. The potency of the product is expressed in units. The toxin's muscle-weakening action is exploited therapeutically in some dystonias (involuntary muscle spasms), the injection being indicated for blepharospasm and hemifacial spasm. Sufferers typically have uncontrollable blinking spasms in both eyes, symptoms usually starting insidiously in the 50–70 age group. Spasms become more frequent and severe, with both eyes clamping shut, resulting in many patients effectively being blind. Botulinum A toxin injection (120 units per affected eye) reduces the intensity of the spasm in 2–5 days. Further injections (into the medial and lateral orbicularis oculi of the lower lid) are required every 8 weeks. There is no evidence that repeat treatment leads to resistance. However, there are adverse effects: blurred vision,

Table 23.9 Local anaesthetics

Drug	Form and dose	Actions and indications	Contraindications, side-effects and nursing points
Lidocaine (lignocaine)	Drops 4% with fluorescein 0.25%	Local anaesthetic with staining agent to help in the diagnosis of ocular lesions. The dye (fluorescein) is taken up by the damaged tissue.	–
Oxybuprocaine	Drops 0.4%	Local anaesthetic.	–
Proxymetacaine	Drops 0.5%	Local anaesthetic.	Causes less stinging than other agents and is useful for children.
Tetracaine (amethocaine)	Drops 0.5 and 1%	Local anaesthetic.	Local sensitivity reaction to the drug or preservative used in the eye drops may occur.

Table 23.10 Preparations for tear deficiency

Drug	Form and dose	Actions and indications	Contraindications, side-effects and nursing points
Acetylcysteine and hypromellose	Drops 5%/0.35%; apply four times daily	This product provides lubrication, and the acetylcysteine has a mucolytic action that is useful when accumulations of mucus occur.	As with other eye conditions, appropriate eye hygiene must be carried out to reduce discomfort from crusting on the eyelid margins.
Carbomers	See BNF		
Hypromellose	Drops 0.3%, used hourly if necessary (a range of products are available)	Lubricant in tear deficiency.	Frequent applications needed. In-patients may prefer self-administration of these drops when this can be arranged. The choice of a particular preparation will be determined by acceptability to the patient.
Paraffins	Liquid or with yellow soft paraffin	Lubricant in recurrent corneal epithelial erosion.	Cause visual disturbance. Best used before sleep.
Polyvinyl alcohol	Drops 1.4%	Lubricant in tear deficiency.	Mucomimetic action. May provide a longer period of relief from symptoms than is provided by hypromellose.
Povidone	Drops 5%	Lubricant in tear deficiency.	–

Table 23.11 Anti-inflammatory drugs[a]

Drug	Form and dose	Actions and indications	Contraindications, side-effects and nursing points
Corticosteroids			
Betamethasone (other topical corticosteroids are available; see British National Formulary)	0.1% every 1–2 h for acute phase; reduce frequency and use eye ointment 0.1% at night	Indicated for the short-term treatment of inflammatory conditions such as uveitis and scleritis. Also used postoperatively to reduce inflammation.	Expert supervision of topical corticosteroid therapy is required, because the dangers from topical therapy are significant. Steroid glaucoma may result and undiagnosed herpes simplex infection may be aggravated, leading to loss of vision or even of the eye. As in other conditions, therapy with corticosteroids can produce great benefits for patients, but the dangers and side-effects must be guarded against by all concerned with the patient's care.
Other anti-inflammatory drugs			
Antazoline	Drops: antazoline 0.5% with xylometazoline 0.05%; apply four times daily	Allergic conjunctivitis.	To be avoided in patients with cardiac disease, hypertension, etc. because of possible systemic absorption. Avoid in PACG.
Nedocromil sodium	Drops 2%; apply four times daily	Allergic conjunctivitis and vernal keratoconjunctivitis.	Transient burning and stinging.

[a]Other products are available for the treatment of seasonal allergic conjunctivitis (e.g. azelastine and related drugs; see the British National Formulary for details).

Table 23.12 Mydriatics and cycloplegics (antimuscarinics)

Drug	Form and dose	Actions and indications	Contraindications, side-effects and nursing points
Atropine	1% eye drops and eye ointment	Long-acting (7 days) antimuscarinic. Dilates pupil and paralyses ciliary muscle.	As with other eye drops, there are risks of systemic absorption resulting in dry mouth etc. Patients at extremes of age are more likely to suffer side-effects than are other patients. Mydriatics may precipitate PACG.
Cyclopentolate	Eye drops 0.5 and 1%	Used for producing cycloplegia for refraction in young children. Effect lasts for up to 24 h. Also used for relieving pain from pupillary spasm in eye injuries.	Contraindications similar to those of other drugs in this class.
Homatropine	Eye drops 1%	Similar to cyclopentolate.	–
Tropicamide	Eye drops 0.5 and 1%	Similar to cyclopentolate. Very short-acting mydriatic (3 h).	–

local pain, swelling, ptosis, dry eye and photophobia. In view of the nature of the side-effects, it is vitally important to counsel the patient before the treatment is administered.

Botulinum B toxin is used in specialist centres to treat spasmodic torticollis (cervical dystonia).

ADMINISTRATION OF EYE PREPARATIONS

The eye is a delicate and vital structure that protects itself in several ways. The immediacy of the blink reflex is evidence of the protective response made to the slightest threat to the eye. An ophthalmic procedure, be it the application of eye drops or of ointment, is approached against this background. Despite the fact that many patients may tolerate more painful procedures with equanimity, procedures involving the eye can cause particular anxiety. Ophthalmic treatment calls for a manner that conveys confidence to patients, helping to ensure that they are relaxed before, during and after the procedure. As with all procedures, a clear explanation is given to patients to gain their cooperation.

Risks of infection must be guarded against by washing the hands with a suitable antiseptic cleansing solution before and after each procedure. If there is a discharge from the eye or evidence of old ointment, it may be necessary to swab the eye first. A damaged eye is particularly susceptible to infection so, whenever possible, a single-use presentation (e.g. of an eye drop) is used. This is especially important when a suspected corneal abrasion is being examined using fluorescein. Where single-dose units are not available, or when larger volumes are required, a separate multidose container should be used for each patient. Care must be taken not to contaminate the dropper or nozzle of eye preparations. Patients who have undergone surgery as an outpatient and have evidence of a recent ocular infection should be given a fresh supply of eye drops after the operation, a separate bottle being supplied for each eye if both require treatment.

When applying eye medication, the standard procedures for administering and recording medicines are followed. All containers should be labelled with the patient's name and the date of opening. The label on the eye preparation should be compared with the prescription. The special points to note are:

- the name of the medication and the strength (usually expressed as a percentage)
- the amount

- which eye is to be treated, if not both
- the time
- the frequency of administration
- that the preparation is in date.

As with other forms of medication, eye drops may be administered once only (including preoperatively) or on a regular basis. Intensive treatment may also be indicated such as in the case of an infection. In order to convey all the necessary information, a specially designed prescription sheet is required (Fig. 23.4). This should enable prescriptions to be written for non-standard intervals, regular intervals and on a once-only basis.

In order that the medication is administered safely and effectively, it is important to position the patient suitably. The head requires to be tilted back and maintained in a steady position so that the risk of damaging the eye by contact with the equipment in use is minimised. To achieve this, the patient should be lying or else sitting, in which case the head should be supported by a pillow or the back of the chair. When possible, the nurse should work from the affected side so as to be close to the working area and in greater control of the procedure.

As always, safety aspects should be considered. Good lighting is essential for carrying out procedures on delicate structures such as the eye. Light should be from above and behind the nurse. With photophobic patients, consideration must be given to light reaching them, otherwise they may be unable to open their eyes. Movements of the hand should be gentle and controlled. Gloves are not worn, as the disposable type are seldom close-fitting and therefore in danger of causing damage if they are allowed to touch the sensitive corneal surface of the eye. In all cases, the nurse must be alert to any sign of adverse reaction to a drug used locally in the eye. This may take the form of a worsening of inflammation or spread of inflammation to surrounding skin.

In the event of the wrong preparation having been administered or the wrong eye being treated, the doctor must be notified *at once* so that any corrective action may be ordered without delay.

TEACHING PATIENTS TO ADMINISTER EYE MEDICATIONS

Nurses play an important role in teaching patients to master the technique of self-administration of eye medications. Compliance and independence will be more readily achieved when the patient is provided with motivation and encouragement.

When teaching a patient to administer an eye medication, the special points to emphasise are:

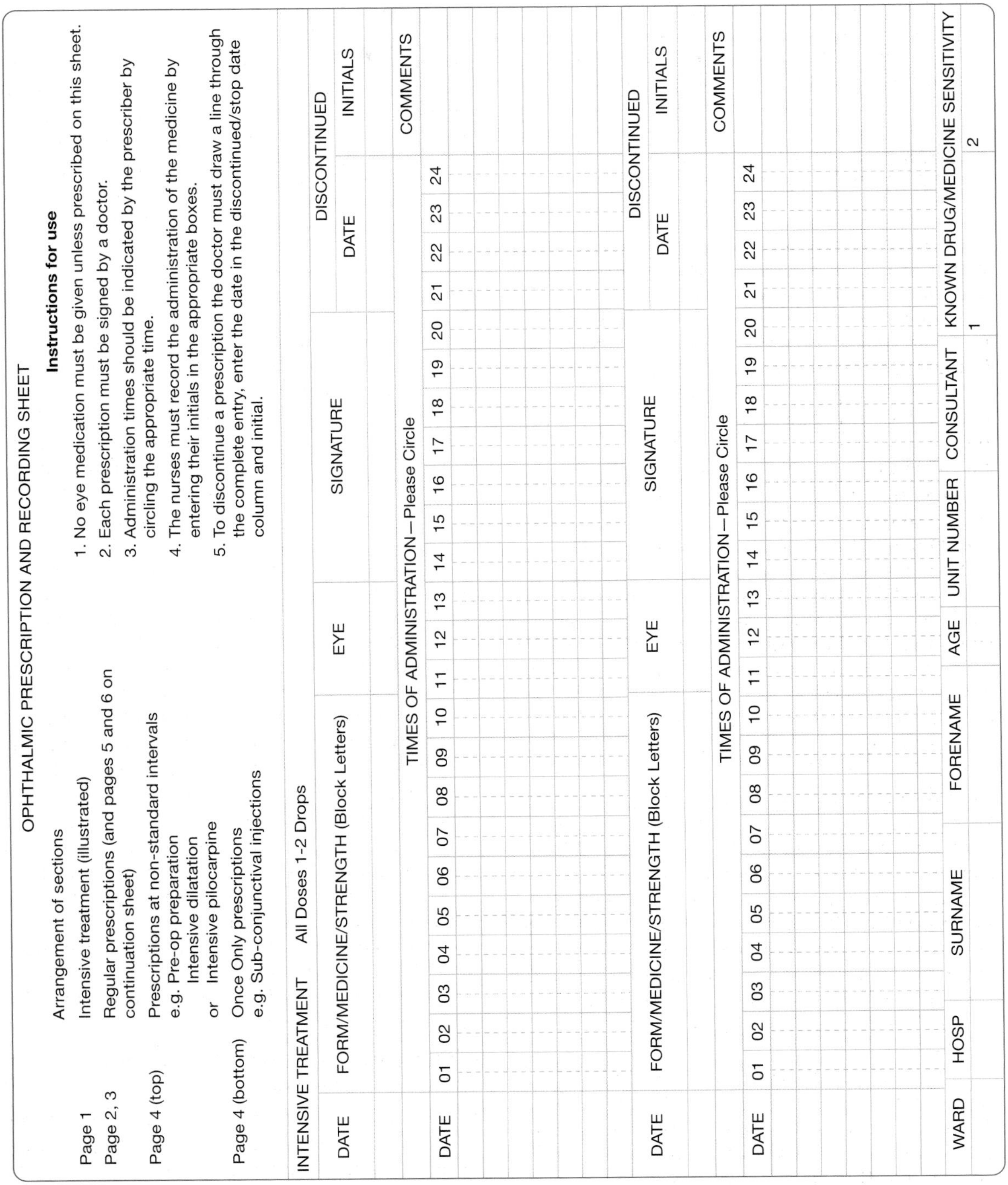

OPHTHALMIC PRESCRIPTION AND RECORDING SHEET

Instructions for use

Arrangement of sections

Page 1 Intensive treatment (illustrated)

Page 2, 3 Regular prescriptions (and pages 5 and 6 on continuation sheet)

Page 4 (top) Prescriptions at non-standard intervals
e.g. Pre-op preparation
Intensive dilatation
or Intensive pilocarpine

Page 4 (bottom) Once Only prescriptions
e.g. Sub-conjunctival injections

1. No eye medication must be given unless prescribed on this sheet.
2. Each prescription must be signed by a doctor.
3. Administration times should be indicated by the prescriber by circling the appropriate time.
4. The nurses must record the administration of the medicine by entering their initials in the appropriate boxes.
5. To discontinue a prescription the doctor must draw a line through the complete entry, enter the date in the discontinued/stop date column and initial.

INTENSIVE TREATMENT All Doses 1-2 Drops

DATE	FORM/MEDICINE/STRENGTH (Block Letters)	EYE	SIGNATURE	DISCONTINUED DATE	DISCONTINUED INITIALS

TIMES OF ADMINISTRATION — Please Circle

DATE	01	02	03	04	05	06	07	08	09	10	11	12	13	14	15	16	17	18	19	20	21	22	23	24	COMMENTS

DATE	FORM/MEDICINE/STRENGTH (Block Letters)	EYE	SIGNATURE	DISCONTINUED DATE	DISCONTINUED INITIALS

TIMES OF ADMINISTRATION — Please Circle

DATE	01	02	03	04	05	06	07	08	09	10	11	12	13	14	15	16	17	18	19	20	21	22	23	24	COMMENTS

WARD	HOSP	SURNAME	FORENAME	AGE	UNIT NUMBER	CONSULTANT	KNOWN DRUG/MEDICINE SENSITIVITY
							1 2

Fig. 23.4 Ophthalmic prescription and recording sheet.

- the need to wash the hands thoroughly first
- the need to avoid contamination
- the importance of using only the prescribed medications.

Because of the systemic toxicity of many ophthalmic drugs, it is especially important that all eye preparations are kept out of the reach and sight of children. Similarly, safe disposal of any remainder when treatment is discontinued, or the container changed, is essential.

Patients may be helped to select for themselves a suitable position in which to administer the medi-cation. To instil eye drops, some patients find that lying flat and feeling for the lower lid is a successful method with gravity assisting. This may be inconvenient or impossible for others, and they may prefer to work in front of an up-standing mirror, although coordination of the hand and eye may take time to master by this method. Self-application of an eye ointment and removal or insertion of a contact lens or artificial eye are best performed in front of a mirror.

COMPLIANCE AIDS

A number of patients experience problems using eye drops, owing to difficulty in aiming the drops and squeezing the plastic bottle (Winfield et al. 1991). Aids to the instillation of eye drops are available that assist patients to use their eye drops in accordance with the prescriber's directions. The type of aid needed will depend on the patient's particular needs. If the patient has difficulty in aiming the bottle, an Easidrop or Autodrop should be considered. These devices are designed to help the patient to position the dropper to expel a drop. Squeezing the bottle can be a particular problem for older patients, whose grip strength may be reduced. For patients who have difficulty in both aiming and squeezing the bottle, the Opticare device or Opticare-Arthro (Figs 23.5A & B) may be useful. Whichever device is selected, the patient should be given guidance and instruction in its use. In some circumstances, it may be appropriate for the patient to use the selected device in the ward for a period prior to discharge so as to help ensure continuity of treatment. The use of a compliance aid often helps the patient gain benefit from the treatment and at the same time achieve greater independence. There is also potential to achieve better use of resources if the number of visits by a district nurse to instil eye drops can be reduced.

EYE DROPS

Eye drops are sterile aqueous solutions or suspensions, presented in multiple application dropper bottles that may be of glass fitted with a glass dropper. A more usual presentation is a flexible plastic container with an orifice through which drops are expelled with pressure of the fingers. Although eye drops in multiple application containers contain preservatives, there is always a risk of contamination in use. A multiple application container should be used for not more than 4 weeks in the community and 1 week in hospital wards, after which the original container should be rejected and if necessary a new container started. In each case, the multiple-application pack is for the use of an individual patient. In some formulations, a shorter 'life' may be indicated on the label.

Single-application containers should always be used in surgical procedures, because of the increased risk of infection. Solutions presented in this way do not contain preservatives, and so a new single-use unit should be used for each application. Both single-

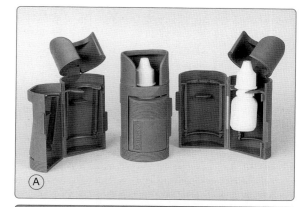

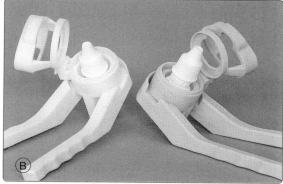

Fig. 23.5 **(A)** Opticare device and **(B)** Opticare-Arthro for arthritic patients.

application and multiple-application packs should have tamper-evident closures and packaging.

The question of the number of drops that can be instilled into the eye requires clarification. One drop from an eye dropper is 50 microlitres (μL) and will overload the average conjunctival sac, which has a capacity of 25 μL (Lessar and Fiscella 1985). To overcome this, when more than one drop of the same preparation is to be instilled (or another preparation used) an interval of 5–10 min should elapse before instilling the second drop. This may present difficulties in ophthalmology units, where a considerable number of patients may be receiving several different forms of drops in succession.

If there is a high rate of tear secretion, aqueous solutions will be quickly diluted or eliminated from the eye into the nasolacrimal duct, thus becoming unavailable for ophthalmic absorption but available for systemic absorption. This may result in systemic side effects (e.g. dry mouth with atropine). Some practitioners recommend pressure over the punctum after administration as a means of restricting tear flow into the duct.

The frequency of instillation of drops varies and will depend on, for example, the degree of infection or inflammation. In the treatment of acute glaucoma, a very intensive regimen of instillation is followed initially, which is then gradually reduced in frequency to hourly, continuing until the IOP is controlled and the pupil pinpoint.

Every effort is made to avoid causing irritation to the eye. Drops used straight from the refrigerator cause discomfort for the patient. If eye drops have been refrigerated, sufficient time should be allowed for the drops to attain room temperature before use. A drop instilled from a height greater than 2.5 cm directly on to the cornea will cause stinging. Any irritation caused by faulty technique will result in increased tear secretion with consequent loss of therapeutic benefit owing to a dilution effect. In addition, the patient will often react by squeezing the lids in an accentuated blink reflex, expelling the solution between the lids or down the nasolacrimal duct.

If, after the instillation of drops, the patient complains of irritation of the skin or a feeling of heat and tightness, an allergic reaction should be suspected and the doctor informed.

INSTILLATION OF EYE DROPS

When the eyes are sticky, this procedure (see Fig. 23.6) is preceded by bathing the eyes using sterile sodium chloride 0.9% solution. Drops should be instilled just inside the lower eyelid on the upper rim of the

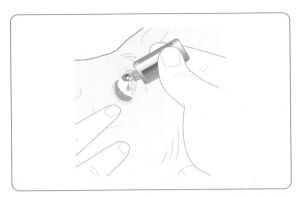

Fig. 23.6   Instillation of eye drops.

inferior fornix, as the conjunctiva in this area is less sensitive than that overlying the cornea. The drops will run into the pocket of the lower fornix, which allows some delay before they drain into the nasolacrimal duct (Box 23.1).

EYE OINTMENTS

In addition to the more commonly used eye drops, many ophthalmic drugs are available as eye ointments (see Fig. 23.7). Eye ointments are essentially dispersions of the active ingredient in a sterile bland base, such as soft paraffin, polyethylene glycol or a specially formulated gel. Useful properties of eye ointments include:

- duration of action longer than that of eye drops
- reduction in systemic absorption (useful in young children)
- an emollient soothing action
- ease of application
- long shelf-life.

Eye ointments soften crusts, thus preventing adherence of eyelids and eyelashes when the patient is asleep. However, there may be some interference with vision owing to the smearing of the cornea with the ointment base (Box 23.2).

RODDING

This procedure is done to prevent formation of adhesions between the eyelid and the eyeball, which can arise as the result of chemical burns of the conjunctiva. In the first few days after injury, the procedure is likely to be uncomfortable and a local anaesthetic such as tetracaine (amethocaine) 0.5% eye drops is instilled in advance. Sterile petroleum jelly is used to lubricate the rod in most cases, although sometimes an antibiotic ointment may be prescribed. By passing the rod under the upper eyelid then moving it from side to side,

Box 23.1 Administration of eye drops

Documentation
- Prescription and recording sheet

The medicine
- Eye drops in accordance with prescription and at room temperature
- Eye drops in date

The environment
- Well-lit location with no through traffic

The nurse and the patient (general)
- Identification of patient and comparison with prescription
- Cooperation and relaxation of patient achieved by careful explanation and gentle approach
- Patient discouraged from rubbing eye and reassurance given that blurring of vision is normal and will soon pass
- General comfort of patient on completion of procedure

The nurse and patient (specific)
- Encouragement to open eye and look upwards

Technique (general)
- Patient's head supported and nurse working from patient's affected side
- Hand hygiene before and after each treatment

Technique (specific)
- Eversion of lower eyelid
- Adequate warning to patient prior to actual instillation
- Instillation from correct height
- Extreme care to avoid touching any part of the eye
- Immediate replacement of cap if multiple-application bottle in use
- Excess medication mopped from cheek

Hazards
- Physical trauma
- Infection
- Systemic absorption

Special features
- Self-medication with or without compliance aid

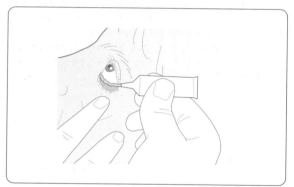

Fig. 23.7 Administration of eye ointment.

Box 23.2 Administration of eye ointment (see Fig. 23.7)

Documentation
- As for instillation of eye drops

The medicine
- Eye ointment in accordance with prescription

The environment
- As for eye drops

The nurse and the patient (general)
- As for eye drops

The nurse and the patient (specific)
- Patient encouraged to close eyes for approximately 1 min after application of ointment

Technique (general)
- As for eye drops

Technique (specific)
- Nozzle held 2.5 cm above patient; ointment squeezed along lower lid from inner canthus outwards

Hazards
- Physical trauma
- Infection

exerting slight pressure outwards, any adhesions are broken down and a film of grease is left between the two surfaces.

CLEANSING THE EYE

The eye may be cleansed by bathing and irrigating.

EYE BATHING

This procedure (Box 23.3) may be used to soothe the eye(s) and to remove crusts from the eyelid(s).

Box 23.3 Eye bathing

Documentation
- Nursing care plan

The medicine
- Sterile 0.9% sodium chloride solution

The environment
- As for instillation of eye drops
- Tray or trolley cleaned, pack and solution prepared as for surgical dressing

The nurse and the patient
- As for eye drops

Technique (general)
- As for eye drops

Technique (specific)
- Uninflamed, uninfected or operated eye bathed first
- Upper lid bathed with patient looking down; lower lid with patient looking up
- Sterile technique
- Each eye swabbed from inner canthus out to prevent infection of the punctum, the lacrimal apparatus or the other eye
- Each swab used once and discarded
- Dry wool never used, as it may leave wisps attached to the eyelashes; swabs always well rung out

Hazards
- Physical trauma
- Infection

IRRIGATION OF THE EYE

In an acute emergency, clean water may be used for the removal of irritant chemicals (Box 23.4). When it is carried out in an accident and emergency department or occupational health centre, the volume and nature of the irrigation solution and the equipment used will depend on the agent that has caused the injury. Sterile sodium chloride 0.9% solution is usually used.

CARE OF AN ARTIFICIAL EYE

Patients who have had enucleation of an eye performed and have been fitted with a temporary shell or prosthesis should have the prosthesis removed twice a day, or according to the surgeon's preference, to allow it and the socket to be cleaned with sterile sodium chloride 0.9% solution. The prospect of this activity calls for some degree of fortitude, but the nurse's mind will quickly be concentrated on the technique involved and on the great need to provide the patient with encouragement.

At first, patients are likely to be understandably tense and frightened that the procedure will be painful. They should be warned that they will feel the presence of something in the socket, but that there will be no pain. About 3–4 days following the operation, the prosthesis is replaced with an artificial eye.

In due course, patients may be taught to carry out eye toilet. When the socket is completely healed, patients will be able to rinse the artificial eye under running water and come to no harm.

Box 23.4 Irrigation of the eye

Documentation
- Dependent on condition being treated: nursing care plan or standard prescribing and recording sheet

The medicine
- Sterile sodium chloride 0.9% solution (sachet, plastic bag or prefilled disposable undine) or special irrigation solution
- As prescribed at body temperature

The environment
- As for eye bathing

The nurse and the patient
- As for eye drops

Technique (general)
- As for eye drops

Technique (specific)
- Sterile technique

- Patient holding receiver firmly against appropriate cheek with head tilted slightly towards receiver
- Patient allowed to become accustomed to temperature of solution by pouring a little over cheek first
- Eyelids held apart using thumb and forefinger
- Solution directed in steady stream over eyeball from inner canthus outwards
- Patient asked to move eyeball up, down and from side to side so that entire eye is cleansed
- Eyelids and cheek left dry
- Eyepad applied if instructed

Hazards
- Physical trauma
- Infection

When a patient with an artificial eye requires to have the eye stored for any length of time, for example during surgery, it should be placed in a container of sodium chloride 0.9% solution so that it does not dry out and become rough.

CONTACT LENSES

Because of the increased use of contact lenses and the very discreet nature of many of them, nurses must make a conscious effort to ask patients whether they wear contact lenses or to observe whether lenses are in use. This should be done on the patient's admission to hospital. Lenses should be removed for safekeeping before any general anaesthetic. They should also be removed prior to any eye procedure to prevent irritation and so as not to be spoiled, unless medical advice has been given to the contrary. Great care must be taken in storing them, because they are easily damaged and are both costly and inconvenient to replace. They are normally kept in a specially supplied contact lens case, although in an emergency a suitable alternative such as a universal container may have to be found. The container should be labelled with the patient's name, ward and unit number and stored in a safe place.

Handling of lenses should be kept to a minimum, and they should not be allowed to dry out because of the danger of cracking. Lens solution is normally brought into hospital by the patient, but if this is not available sterile sodium chloride 0.9% solution serves just as well. Contact lens hygiene is vitally important in preventing the development of acanthamoeba keratitis, which can damage eyesight. Disposable contact lenses are also available.

To remove a lens, the hands should be washed, rinsed and dried, leaving no trace of soap that could be conveyed to the lens and irritate the eye. The patient is asked to tilt the head back, as recommended for any eye procedure, and to look up. Using the index finger, the lens is gently slid downwards on to the bulbar conjunctiva and then lifted off the conjunctiva with the thumb and index finger. The utmost care is required not to drop a lens, as it may then be very difficult to find.

DRUGS AND CONTACT LENSES

Consideration needs to be given to contact lenses and the concurrent administration of medicines. Some patients find that inserting contact lenses is painful, and so they may be prescribed local anaesthetic eye drops to instil in advance. It is now well recognised that soft, hydrogel lenses can absorb drugs and preservatives in certain preparations instilled into the eye, leading to toxic reactions. Coloured eye drops such as rose bengal will stain soft contact lenses permanently. Rifampicin, used in the treatment of tuberculosis, and sulfasalazine colour body secretions, including the tears, an orange-red, leading to pigmentation of the contact lens. In certain conditions, however, the water absorption property of the lens can be used to advantage; a soft hydrophilic lens may be inserted to avoid repeated instillation of drugs such as pilocarpine in the treatment of glaucoma. Unless medically contraindicated, soft lenses are better removed during the period that the patient is receiving treatment. Hard lenses are not affected in this way.

Adverse effects from many drugs taken systemically can occur. A number of drugs (e.g. antihistamines, antimuscarinics, phenothiazines, some beta blockers, diuretics and tricyclic antidepressants) cause a reduction in tear secretion, causing blurred vision. Oral contraceptives may also cause ocular complications.

Drugs that reduce blinking, such as anxiolytics, hypnotics, antihistamines and muscle relaxants, can affect contact lens wear. Drugs that increase tear secretion include ephedrine and hydralazine, and they too can cause eye problems in those who wear contact lenses. Contact lens wearers may also experience ophthalmic discomfort in association with taking drugs such as isotretinoin, primidone and aspirin.

SELF-ASSESSMENT QUESTIONS

1. What do the following terms mean?
   a. Mydriatic
   b. Cycloplegic
   c. Parasympathomimetic
   d. Sympathomimetic
2. Match the following drugs to their mode of action.

Aciclovir	Diagnostic stain
Sodium chloride	Artificial tears
Oxybuprocaine	Mydriatic
Fluorescein	Antifungal
Betamethasone	Anti-inflammatory
Chloramphenicol	Irrigation
Timolol	Antiviral
Tropicamide	Local anaesthetic
Ketoconazole	Antibacterial
Hypromellose	Reduces intraocular pressure

3. What are tears composed of?
4. What purpose do they serve?
5. How may infection be minimised in a patient receiving eye drops?

6. For how many days may a multidose eye drop container be used by an individual patient?

7. How would you care for an unconscious patient's contact lenses?

8. Why is it vital to identify and treat glaucoma promptly?

REFERENCES

Cox A 2006 Prevention and management of drug-induced ocular disorders. Prescriber June:39–42

Dunne A et al. 1991 Eye irrigation: practice procedures and problems. Hospital Pharmacy Practice 1:219–226

Lessar TS, Fiscella RG 1985 Antimicrobial drug delivery to the eye. Drug Intelligence and Clinical Pharmacy 19:642–654

Petrov PG 2006 Crystal tears. British Journal of Ophthalmology 90:139

Winfield AJ, Williams A, Jessiman D et al. 1991 Assisting patients with their eyedrops: 1. Identifying the problems. British Journal of Pharmaceutical Practice 13:10–14

FURTHER READING AND RESOURCES

[Anonymous] 2001 New guidance on the use of eye preparations [editorial]. Pharmaceutical Journal 267:307

Dunne A, Winfield AJ, Williams A et al. 1991 Eye irrigation: practice, procedures and problems. Hospital Pharmacy Practice October:1–4

Elton M 2005 Conjunctivitis and chloramphenicol. Pharmaceutical Journal 274:725–728

Fraser S, Bunce C, Wormald R et al. 2001 Deprivational late presentation of glaucoma: case-control study. British Medical Journal 322:639–643

Fraser S, Manvinkar S 2005 Glaucoma: the pathophysiology and diagnosis. Hospital Pharmacist 12:251–254

Haylor V, Jones J 2007 Use of preserved eye preparations – is the Society's guidance still relevant? Pharmaceutical Journal 278:186

Husband H, Worsley A 2005 Glaucoma: pharmacological treatment. Hospital Pharmacist 12:255–260

Newport A, Lockwood B 2005 Use of nutraceuticals for eye health. Pharmaceutical Journal 275:261–264

Royal College of Ophthalmologists 2001 Guidelines for the management of ocular hypertension and primary open-angle glaucoma. RCO, London

Williams A, Winfield AJ 1990 Topical medication for eye patients. Nursing Times 86:42–43

Winfield AJ, Jessiman D, Williams A 1990 A study of the causes of non-compliance by patients prescribed eye drops. British Journal of Ophthalmology 74:477–480

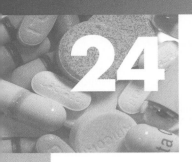

24 Drug treatment of ear, nose and oropharynx

KEY OBJECTIVES

After reading this chapter, you should be able to:

- describe the presentation of acute otitis media and discuss treatment options
- describe how to administer ear drops
- discuss the treatment of fungal infections of the oropharynx
- explain the importance of oral hygiene as part of patient care
- describe how to administer nasal drops.

INTRODUCTION

Disorders of the ear, nose and oropharynx vary greatly in their implications for patients. Unless effectively treated, these conditions can at best cause a great deal of misery for patients and at worst may be life-threatening. Underlying causes of the patient's condition must be identified and dealt with, if necessary by a combination of local and systemic therapy and surgery. Some local preparations may be helpful but over-reliance should not be placed on these. Simple remedies should always be considered. The nurse's role in providing effective aural, nasal and oral care is pivotal. Self-care is to be encouraged through teaching.

DRUG TREATMENT OF DISORDERS OF THE EAR

ANATOMY AND PHYSIOLOGY

There are three main parts to the ear (Fig. 24.1):

- outer ear – pinna (auricle) and external auditory canal
- middle ear – tympanic membrane and ossicles
- inner ear – cochlea and vestibular labyrinth.

Sound waves reaching the pinna are channelled through the external auditory canal to the tympanic membrane (eardrum), which vibrates in response. These vibrations are transmitted through the ossicles to the cochlea, which converts them into impulses for transmission by the auditory nerve to the brain. The middle ear connects to the throat via the eustachian tube.

COMMON CONDITIONS

Each part of the ear may be affected by disease. The outer ear may be affected by skin conditions such as eczema, dermatitis and furuncles (boils), with itching and pain as the presenting symptoms. Inflammation of the external auditory canal/pinna is known as *otitis externa*. Wax (cerumen), secreted by cells in the external auditory canal, may cause some loss of hearing when production is excessive. The ciliated epithelial cells that line the middle ear secrete mucus. *Otitis media*

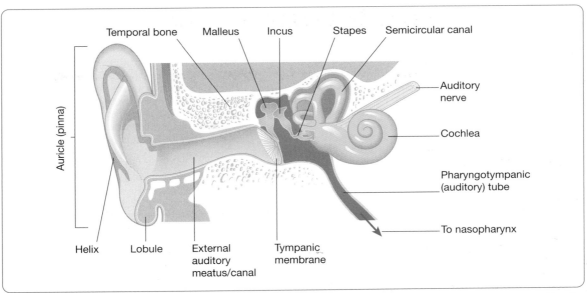

Temporal bone   Malleus   Incus   Stapes   Semicircular canal

Auditory nerve

Cochlea

Pharyngotympanic (auditory) tube

To nasopharynx

Auricle (pinna)

Helix   Lobule   External auditory meatus/canal   Tympanic membrane

Fig. 24.1   The ear. (From Waugh A, Grant A 2001 Ross and Wilson anatomy and physiology in health and illness, 9th edn. Churchill Livingstone, Edinburgh. With permission of Elsevier.)

with effusion ('glue ear') is a condition in which the middle ear becomes congested with mucus. When the mucosa becomes infected, resulting in pus formation, the resulting painful condition is known as acute otitis media. Occasionally, pressure build-up will cause the tympanic membrane to rupture; this results in pressure release and subsidence of pain. Repeated episodes of infection with recurrent discharge of pus may lead to persistent rupturing of the tympanic membrane and the condition known as chronic otitis media. Conditions affecting the inner ear are dealt with in Chapter 14. In the investigation of all significant ear problems, suitable hearing tests should be carried out. In addition, it is vitally important to exclude serious underlying conditions.

The main features and treatment of otitis externa and the various forms of otitis media are outlined in Table 24.1.

TREATMENT OF OTITIS EXTERNA

A furuncle is an infected hair follicle, usually caused by *Staphylococcus aureus*. This can be very painful, especially when the pinna is moved. Applying a hot flannel to the infected ear and the use of simple analgesics may be sufficient, but oral antibiotics may be necessary if symptoms are very severe.

In acute otitis externa, the ear appears red, swollen or scaly and it is important to exclude underlying otitis media before treatment is started. Acetic acid

ear drops act as both antifungal and antibacterial agent in the external ear canal; they can be purchased over the counter for mild otitis media and are less likely to cause superinfection. Aluminium acetate ear drops have astringent properties and may be used to reduce inflammation. Topical corticosteroids such as betamethasone or prednisolone can also be used if infection is not present. When infection is suspected, a topical anti-infective agent that is not used systemically can be used (e.g. neomycin or clioquinol).

TREATMENT OF OTITIS MEDIA

Acute otitis media often follows an upper respiratory tract infection and can be viral or bacterial. Most, 75% (Scottish Intercollegiate Guidelines Network 2003), acute otitis media occurs in children under 10 years of age. Otitis media with effusion, or glue ear, is a chronic inflammation of the middle ear accompanied by accumulation of fluid. It occurs in 10% of children and in 90% of children with cleft palates. Untreated or resistant glue can lead to some forms of chronic otitis media. Key elements of treatment of all forms of otitis media are aural toilet, exclusion of complicating factors and the need to ensure that an acute condition does not become chronic. Most uncomplicated cases resolve without the need for antibacterial treatment, and use of simple analgesia such as paracetamol is effective. The Committee on Safety of Medicines has stated that treatment with a topical aminoglycoside

Table 24.1 Treatment of common forms of otitis

Condition	Main features	Treatment
Otitis externa	Inflammation of meatal skin, associated with infection and/or eczema. Itching and pain without hearing loss. Predisposing factors include loss of self-cleaning epithelium. Overenthusiastic cleaning of the ears (e.g. cotton buds, syringing) may be a contributing factor.	Exclude chronic otitis media before initiating treatment. Aural toilet, astringent ear drops (e.g. aluminium acetate, antimicrobial agents) may be indicated depending on swab/culture. If eczematous condition is present, topical steroids may be required.
Otitis media	Hearing impairment, earache – due to inflammation or infection.	See otitis media with effusion, acute otitis media, chronic otitis media
Otitis media with effusion	Hearing impairment, earache. As with acute otitis media, worse in water.	Observation, pain relief and antibiotics, simple analgesics for pain in acute conditions. Surgery required in order to achieve resolution of the condition.
Acute otitis media	Earache, discharge, hearing impairment, tympanic membrane inflamed, fever, lymphadenopathy. Occurs from first year of life onwards. Referral for specialist advice is needed in cases of acute pain or neurological involvement.	Local treatment with antibiotic ear drops is of no value. The aim is to avoid progression to chronic otitis media. Oral antimicrobial agents are widely used. A pragmatic approach is adopted, choice of antibiotic depending on pathogen present. Oral amoxicillin is the first choice. Antibiotic resistance is a growing problem. Prophylactic antibiotics may be needed if acute otitis media is recurrent.
Chronic otitis media	History of childhood ear problems, recurrent discharge, hearing problems. If neurological symptoms occur (e.g. vertigo), urgent referral to specialist. The condition occurs in approximately 5% of the adult UK population. It should be noted that there are linkages between the above conditions.	Aural toilet to remove debris (e.g. keratin and necrotic bone). Antibiotic treatment, depending on sensitivity of organisms.

antibiotic is contraindicated in those patients with a perforated tympanic membrane. However, some specialists do use these cautiously in the presence of perforation in patients with otitis media when other measures have failed. The risk of ototoxicity arising from the infected pus is greater than the risk of side effects from the antibiotic.

Although antibiotics are widely used to treat acute otitis media, the role of these agents has been questioned. The evidence to show that any improved outcome is achieved with antibiotic therapy is sparse. Infecting organisms are commonly *Streptococcus pneumoniae*, *Haemophilus influenzae*, staphylococci and streptococci. In children without systemic symptoms,

oral amoxicillin or erythromycin may be started if there is no improvement within 72 h, or earlier if deterioration occurs. Treatment is usually only for 5 days.

REMOVAL OF EARWAX

Earwax is a combination of cerumen, sebum, dead cells, sweat, hair and dust. In most circumstances, it is not necessary to clean the ear canals. However, sometimes earwax can build up and impede the passage of sound. It is sometimes possible to loosen small amounts of earwax using wax-softening drops alone. Syringing with warm water using an ear syringe or an electronic pulsed water unit (Box 24.1) is carried

---

Box 24.1 Syringing the ear

The medicine
- Tap water at body temperature (38°C)

The environment
- Usually GP's clinic or surgery by practice or district nurse

The nurse and the patient
- Hand hygiene before and after procedure
- Patient given clear explanation of what is involved
- Patient informed that there may be some discomfort
- Privacy, warmth, comfort
- Patient seated in upright chair with towel over appropriate shoulder
- Patient asked to hold receiver against neck just below ear to be treated

Technique
- Syringe filled with water or pulsed water unit primed and air expelled
- Pinna pulled up and back
- Fluid directed along roof of auditory canal without undue force but at a steady rate
- Content of returned fluid observed
- Procedure repeated until all wax removed
- Meatus inspected periodically using otoscope to check that wax has been removed and ear has not been damaged
- Patient understanding checked, as hearing may be affected
- External auditory meatus gently but thoroughly mopped dry

Hazards
- Infection of the middle ear, resulting from rupture of the tympanic membrane
- Otitis externa

ADMINISTRATION OF EAR PREPARATIONS

As always, the standard procedure for prescribing and recording medications must be followed. Hands should be washed before and after each procedure, and each patient should have a separate medicine container. When checking preparations against the prescription, special note should be made of the strength of the medication and, for example, the number of drops to be instilled and whether both ears are to be treated. Explanation of the procedure is important in order to gain the patient's cooperation so that the medication is allowed to take maximum effect with minimal discomfort. Correct positioning of the patient helps to minimise discomfort and ensure penetration of the medication to the part where it is intended to take effect. Before instilling drops, instructions may be given by the doctor to mop the ear canal using a cotton-tipped applicator for better penetration of the medication. Ear drops are solutions or suspensions of active ingredients in water, propylene glycol or other suitable vehicle. Ear drops should be used in the temperature range between room and body temperature. If ear drops are instilled from a bottle recently stored in a refrigerator, they may cause a mild vertigo.

Patients may be helped to feel more secure throughout the procedure if they are given an absorbent tissue to hold. For patients receiving ear drops who are unable to maintain the required position, a wisp of cotton wool may be *gently* placed in the ear canal to ensure that the drops remain in contact with the epithelium. The prescribed volume of ear drops may range from two to four drops. Glass droppers are rarely used, but if one is used it is important to check the top of the dropper each time to ensure that it is not chipped or cracked. Most ear drops come in plastic bottles with an integrated dropper attached. Box 24.2 details the step by step process for instillation of ear drops.

Ear ointments have properties similar to those of ointments in general. Some eye ointments may also be prescribed for ear conditions. The customary way of introducing an ointment into the ear is to insert ribbon gauze that has been impregnated with the ointment. The wick is left in for 24 h. Oral analgesics may be required prior to removal of the wick each day.

out to remove plugs of wax that block the ear causing discomfort and deafness, or when closer inspection of the eardrum is required. Syringing is preceded for several days by a course of wax-softening drops such as olive or almond oil (care must be taken for those with nut allergy) or sodium bicarbonate ear drops. Some proprietary preparations contain an organic solvent that may cause sensitisation and should be used only when oil or sodium bicarbonate ear drops have failed. Because of the potential danger of perforating the tympanic membrane, the ear is examined by a doctor

Box 24.2 Instillation of ear drops

Documentation
- Standard prescribing and recording sheet

The medicine
- Prescribed ear drops
- Separate bottle for each patient
- At room temperature, at least

The nurse and the patient
- Patient identified
- Patient given explanation
- Patient assisted as necessary into position either sitting with head tilted to one side *or* lying on side with ear to be treated uppermost
- Patient's clothing protected
- Patient made comfortable

Technique
- If instructed, external auditory meatus gently mopped with cotton-tipped applicator
- Hand hygiene before and after actual instillation of drops
- Bottle shaken if it contains a suspension and required amount drawn into dropper (if ear drops come with separate dropper)
- Cartilaginous part of pinna gently pulled up and back (for a child, down and back)
- Drops instilled in external canal without allowing dropper or top of bottle to come into contact with ear
- Gentle massage applied over tragus to help work in drops
- Patient encouraged to maintain position for several minutes to allow drops to reach eardrum
- Cotton wool ball lightly placed in external meatus if necessary
- Excess medication wiped away

DRUG TREATMENT OF DISORDERS OF THE NOSE

ANATOMY AND PHYSIOLOGY

The nasal passages are lined by a highly vascular mucous membrane covered with ciliated epithelium that warms and moistens the entering air and traps a certain amount of dust. When the mucous membrane is congested or inflamed, there is considerable resistance to inflow and breathing through the nose is correspondingly difficult. The nose and nasal sinuses produce a litre of mucus in 24 h, and much of it passes into the stomach via the nasopharynx (Fig. 24.2).

NASAL ADMINISTRATION OF DRUGS

Many low molecular weight, non-polar drugs in solution are able to penetrate the nasal epithelium with ease. Some molecules demonstrate 100% bio-availability compared with intravenous administration. Large molecules experience increasing difficulty with absorption, a characteristic that is similar to that found in the gastrointestinal tract. There are a number of nasally delivered, systemically acting drugs on the market in different therapeutic categories, including desmopressin and nicotine, with a growing number of products in the pipeline. There are many reasons for this change, including improved patient compliance (elimination of needles), avoidance of first-pass metabolism and rapid onset of action.

COMMON CONDITIONS AND THEIR TREATMENT

NASAL ALLERGY

Examples of nasal allergy include hay fever and allergic rhinitis. Sodium cromoglicate inhibits the release of chemical mediators such as histamine from mast cells. It is these mediators that, when released in response to exposure to an allergen, cause an allergic reaction. Sodium cromoglicate is used prophylactically, and treatment should be commenced several weeks before the hay fever season commences and continued on a regular basis.

In severe rhinitis, administration of a corticosteroid such as beclometasone or budesonide (in a spray form) directly into the nose decreases inflammation and oedema of the nasal mucosa. Corticosteroids (as a spray) should not be administered in the presence of nasal infection. The possibility of systemic absorption of corticosteroids must always be considered. Systemic corticosteroids may be required in short courses for severe conditions. Oral antihistamines may also be required (see Ch. 13). Azelastine and levocabastine are antihistamines available for use as a nasal spray. In cases in which there are severe associated symptoms (e.g. allergic conjunctivitis), supplementary medication may be required.

NASAL CONGESTION

Congestion occurs in vasomotor rhinitis, nasal polyps and the common cold. Sodium chloride 0.9% solution, given either as nasal drops or nasal spray, may relieve nasal congestion by helping to liquefy mucous secretions. Symptoms of nasal congestion associated with vasomotor rhinitis can be relieved in the short term by decongestant drops or sprays. These are

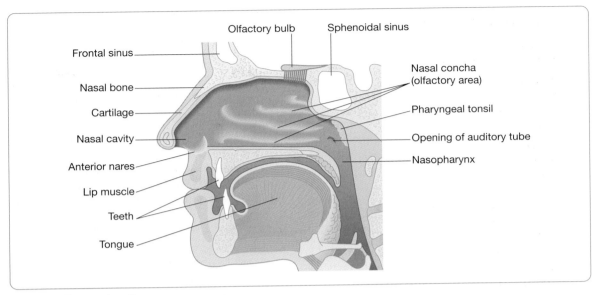

Fig. 24.2 The nasal cavity.

sympathomimetic drugs that cause vasoconstriction of the mucosal blood vessels and provide relief of congestion. The most significant adverse reaction is rebound nasal congestion if treatment is prolonged. They should be used for no more than 5–7 days to avoid rebound congestion. Ephedrine nasal drops are the safest preparation and can give relief for several hours. Xylometazoline (nasal drops or spray) is much longer acting than ephedrine but more likely to cause rebound nasal congestion. Ipratropium nasal spray (an antimuscarinic agent) is used to treat watery rhinorrhoea.

SINUSITIS

Acute sinusitis frequently follows a viral upper respiratory tract infection. It is caused by inadequate ventilation and drainage in the paranasal sinuses. Bacterial infection may develop if the sinuses are blocked with mucus. Facial pain and headache are common and may be associated with nasal congestion and postnasal drip. An antibiotic (e.g. amoxicillin, doxycycline, erythromycin) and a topical decongestant spray are valuable. Steam inhalations and analgesics will provide symptomatic relief.

NASAL INFECTION

Local antibiotics have little place in the treatment of nasal infections, but a cream containing chlorhexidine 0.1% and neomycin sulphate 0.5% is applied locally in the treatment of staphylococcal infections and prophy-

laxis against nasal carriage of staphylococci. Recolonisation frequently occurs. Intranasal chlorhexidine has been reported to cause anaphylactic circulatory arrest when applied to mucous membranes. In cases in which a reaction is possible, careful history taking is essential. If in doubt, chlorhexidine must be avoided in susceptible patients (Chisholm et al. 1997).

A nasal ointment containing mupirocin is available for hospital use in the eradication of nasal carriage of methicillin-resistant *Staphylococcus aureus*.

EPISTAXIS (NOSEBLEED)

Epistaxis may result from a variety of causes, including disordered clotting mechanisms. Persistent epistaxis requires full investigation. Packing, surgery and/or cautery may be required in some instances.

Nasal packs may be used to control severe epistaxis and as a rule are inserted by the doctor. Patients understandably are often very alarmed by the blood loss and require a nurse to stay with, and reassure, them. The insertion of a pack into the nasal cavity is done with the patient sitting up with clothing suitably protected. Using a suitable size of nasal speculum, the doctor, with the aid of forceps, inserts sterile half-inch (1 cm) ribbon gauze that has been impregnated with bismuth iodoform paraffin paste. Alternatively, a Brighton catheter or a Foley catheter may be inserted into the nose and inflated to stop the bleeding. Patients appreciate a mouthwash after a nosebleed and may get rid of clots from the back of the throat by gargling.

It is often advisable to administer an oral analgesic prior to removal of a nasal pack that, with drying, becomes painful to remove. To begin with, only half of the packing should be gently pulled out to see what happens. If there is no bleeding, the remainder can be removed, but if the first stage has caused bleeding the remainder of the pack should be left in place and a further attempt made later.

ADMINISTRATION OF NOSE PREPARATIONS

The principles of administering nasal preparations are similar to those identified for the administration of ear preparations, as described previously in this chapter. Nasal preparations usually take the form of nasal drops. Box 24.3 details the procedure involved in the instillation of nasal drops. Care should be taken when patients have a history of epistaxis. Nasal drops should be allowed to reach room temperature prior to instillation if previously stored in the refrigerator. Instead of instilling drops, medications may be sprayed into the patient's nose in powder form using a nasal insufflator. A nasal spray is also available that

is inserted into the anterior nares. The container is squeezed two or three times to instil the medication. The effect, however, is very transient because the cilia lining the nasal cavities remove the drug in about 20 min. The nasal mucosa is utilised as a route for the administration of certain medications; nasally administered insulin has recently been formulated. The position of the patient is important in ensuring that nasal drops reach the appropriate area (Fig. 24.3).

DRUG TREATMENT OF OROPHARYNGEAL DISORDERS

ANATOMY AND PHYSIOLOGY

The oropharynx consists of the oral cavity within which there are the gums, teeth, hard palate, soft palate and uvula, tonsils and tongue. The oral cavity is lined throughout with mucous membrane containing small mucus-secreting glands. Three pairs of salivary glands, namely parotid, submandibular and sublingual, also pour their secretions into the mouth. These combined secretions make up saliva, which contains water, mucus, mineral salts and salivary amylase. Approximately 1.5 L of saliva flow through the mouth in 24 h; its purpose is to lubricate the oral cavity, initiate the digestion of starches and assist with chewing, swallowing and speaking. The output of saliva is increased by the sight of food, eating and drinking, brushing the teeth, and movement of the jaws.

The lining of a healthy mouth is moist and pink. The teeth are free from caries, the papillae on the tongue are visible and the lips intact. There is no discomfort or odour.

COMMON CONDITIONS AND THEIR TREATMENT

Careful assessment and investigation of all oral lesions is essential, because the lesion may be an indication of the presence of a serious underlying medical condition. Patients with long-standing oral lesions that do not respond to standard treatments should be investigated using microbiological, biochemical, haematological and immunological tests. Biopsy may be required in order to eliminate malignant disease.

There are many causes of oral ulceration; infection, trauma, blood disorder, gastrointestinal disease, nutritional deficiency and drug therapy causing immunodeficiency such as cancer chemotherapy all predispose to a breakdown of the oral mucosa. Treatment of the underlying condition should resolve

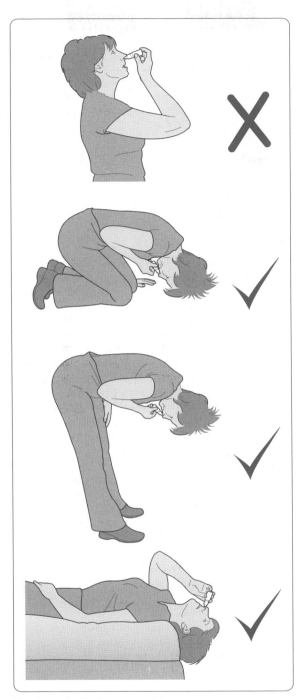

Fig. 24.3 Instillation of nasal drops.

the oral problem. Aphthous ulcers are very painful, non-specific mouth ulcerations that are difficult to treat. Good oral hygiene is an essential part of the treatment of all oral lesions.

SORE THROAT

Sore throat caused by bacteria or (more usually) viruses is a common condition. It is often very difficult to identify the cause. Unless the sore throat is associated with respiratory distress (when hospital admission is called for), simple management methods are appropriate. Salt water gargles, paracetamol or a soothing lozenge may be helpful. Compound analgesics and non-steroidal anti-inflammatory drugs are not recommended. Oral rinses containing an anti-inflammatory drug (benzydamine) may be worthwhile. The cause(s) of recurrent sore throat should be investigated in detail. Failure of previous therapy may be a cause (owing to inadequate therapy and/or non-compliance). Antibiotic therapy (phenoxymethylpenicillin 500 mg four times daily for 10 days) may be required if the presence of β-haemolytic *Streptococcus* is confirmed, if there is a history of valvular disease, if there is marked systemic upset or peritonsillar cellulitis or if the patient is at increased risk of acute infection (e.g. immunosuppressed). The use of antibiotics to prevent the complications of streptococcal pharyngitis (rheumatic fever or acute glomerular nephritis) is not supported by the evidence (Scottish Intercollegiate Guidelines Network 1999). Surgery (tonsillectomy) is normally carried out only following assessment of the patient (against defined criteria) over a 6-month period. Long-term treatment with certain drugs (see p. 150) may be a cause of a persistent sore throat. This cause should always be eliminated by careful investigations, including the patient's detailed drug history.

ACUTE TONSILLITIS

The condition presents with sore throat, often with pain on swallowing, pyrexia and upper respiratory infection, possibly associated with otalgia. Children are most commonly affected. Difficulties may arise in determining whether the infecting organism is bacterial or viral. On examination, the tonsils are engorged with or without purulent discharge, with localised lymph node enlargement. Treatment is designed to alleviate symptoms. Antibiotic therapy should not be delayed until the results of a swab have been obtained. Oral phenoxymethypenicillin (or erythromycin in persons with penicillin hypersensitivity) is the first line of treatment. Ampicillin should be avoided, because in cases of glandular fever an erythematous rash will develop. If first-line antibiotics fail, a cephalosporin or co-amoxiclav may be required. Increased fluid intake, analgesia or a suitable oral rinse will be helpful. Glandular fever (infectious mononucleosis) is associated with very swollen tonsils often covered with

Table 24.2 Some drugs used for the treatment of aphthous ulcers

Drug	Notes
Benzydamine hydrochloride	Used as a mouthwash or solution spray to relieve pain and inflammation.
Hydrocortisone lozenges (2.5 mg)	Held in the mouth as near as possible to the ulcer to reduce inflammation.
Doxycycline	May be of benefit in the form of a mouthwash.
Carmellose sodium	May relieve some discomfort arising from ulceration by protecting the ulcer site.
Triamcinolone dental paste	A specially formulated paste designed to adhere to mucous membranes. Contains a potent corticosteroid. Care should be taken to treat any concomitant infection that may be present.
Choline salicylate dental gel	May provide some analgesic action, but excessive use can irritate the mucosa and itself cause ulcers.

a dirty yellow membrane. Management of glandular fever is directed towards alleviating symptoms. Antipyretics and analgesics will be needed.

ORAL ULCERATION, INFLAMMATION AND SUPERFICIAL INFECTIONS

Ulceration of the oral mucosa may be caused by many factors (e.g. trauma, carcinoma), and it is important to establish a diagnosis in each case, as specific management is required. Aphthous ulcers are difficult to treat because of the problem of maintaining an adequate concentration of drug in contact with the lesions. Table 24.2 gives some drugs that may be prescribed. Mild oral lesions are treated with a salicylate-containing gel, but this is not suitable for prolonged use in children owing to the possibility of absorption of salicylate leading to adverse reactions. Doxycycline mouthwash has been used for severe recurrent aphthous ulceration. Although it may reduce the duration and severity of ulcers, it can cause oral candidiasis and a burning-like sensation of the pharynx. The contents of a doxycycline 100-mg capsule are dispersed in water and rinsed around the mouth four times a day.

Simple warm saline mouthwashes may relieve the pain of traumatic ulceration. Secondary bacterial infection may occur with any ulceration and can increase discomfort and delay healing. Hexetidine solution 0.1% w/v has antibacterial and antiprotozoal activity. It is used in the treatment of gingivitis and pharyngitis and for oral hygiene generally. The

solution (15 mL) should normally be used undiluted, although some patients may find the taste rather unpleasant. It should be used two to three times daily. Chlorhexidine or povidone–iodine mouthwashes may also be beneficial and accelerate healing of recurrent apthous ulcers.

Hydrogen peroxide solution 6% (20 vols) is an oxidising agent that, when in contact with organic matter, effervesces, releasing oxygen; this has some mechanical cleansing action. This solution is particularly useful in dealing with anaerobic organisms that cause acute gingivitis or when the tongue is so heavily furred that other solutions are rendered ineffective. To minimise the likelihood of local irritation, 15 mL is diluted with a cartonful of warm water. The mouth should be rinsed for 2–3 min two to three times per day.

Fungal infections

Fungal infections of the mouth, principally candidiasis (thrush), are especially likely to arise in patients who are debilitated or immunosuppressed. The commonest groups affected are the very young, the elderly and those receiving a course of broad-spectrum antibiotic, cytotoxic medication, or intensive chemotherapy for AIDS.

Nystatin (suspension or pastilles) is commonly used to treat oral candidiasis. The medication should be retained in the mouth for as long as possible to ensure maximum effect. Patients will need to be given guidance on the best way to use the particular product and the need to avoid eating or drinking for a short time after treatment.

Amphotericin, in the form of suspension (or lozenges), is an alternative antifungal agent, especially when the infecting organism is resistant to nystatin. Miconazole is an antifungal agent with a wide spectrum of activity against pathogenic fungi and some Gram-positive bacteria. An oral gel is available containing 125 mg in 5 mL. The gel is retained in the mouth in contact with the lesion for as long as possible.

When candidal infection has been diagnosed, the care of a patient's dentures becomes a particularly important part of oral hygiene. First, the dentures should be removed and left to dry for 8 h. They should then be immersed in sodium hypochlorite or chlorhexidine gluconate 0.2% (if denture made of chrome cobalt) overnight and rinsed well before being reused. This should be repeated twice weekly. If possible, the patient should stop using the dentures for 2 weeks. Miconazole, either in the form of an oral gel or a denture lacquer, may be prescribed for application to the surface of the denture as part of the overall care and treatment of oral candidiasis.

Viral infections

Viral infections of the mouth include herpetic stomatitis. Vesicles form in the mouth, and these break down to give ulcers. The use of chlorhexidine mouthwash will control plaque accumulation and help to control secondary infection. In severe herpetic stomatitis, a systemic antiviral such as aciclovir, valaciclovir or famciclovir is required. Aciclovir is available over the counter for the treatment of cold sores. Treatment also includes a soft diet with good fluid intake. Good oral hygiene is essential. Supplementary treatment with antibiotics, antifungal agents and analgesics may be required. Herpes infection of the mouth may also respond to rinsing the mouth with doxycycline.

TONGUE LESIONS

Black hairy tongue and furred tongue are treated with a combination of oral hygiene and appropriate therapy when a specific underlying condition can be identified.

Oral leukoplakia is caused by the Epstein–Barr virus and presents as white plaques on the tongue. Biopsy of the mucous membrane reveals precancerous changes. It can occur in smokers and when there has been long-standing infection such as chronic candidiasis and tertiary syphilis. It can also occur in AIDS patients. Treatment of the underlying cause generally resolves the condition.

OTHER ORAL LESIONS

These are:

- blisters due to pemphigus vulgaris
- benign mucous membrane pemphigoid
- oral manifestations of lichen planus
- erythema multiforme (may be caused by a drug reaction)
- angina bullosa haemorrhagica.

Treatment of the above conditions involves oral hygiene, topical corticosteroids, local antiseptics and analgesics, and in the case of erythema multiforme a course of oral/systemic corticosteroids may be required.

- Gingivitis may arise because of poor oral hygiene but may present as acute necrotising ulcerative gingivitis that requires antimicrobial therapy (metronidazole).
- Squamous cell papilloma: these benign lesions are caused by the human papillomavirus. Treatment is surgical excision to prevent recurrence.

MALIGNANT DISEASE

Oral cancer is rare, but suspicious presentations (long-standing ulceration or white patches) should be referred for specialist investigation and treatment.

PREPARATIONS USED IN GENERAL CARE OF THE MOUTH

The preparation selected for use will depend on local guidelines as contained in a nursing formulary or laid down in some other way, although it cannot be overemphasised that the frequency and standard of mouth care are every bit as important as the individual mouthwash solutions used. The properties of two commonly used preparations are described below.

Mouthwash solution tablets can be used. One tablet dissolved in 125 mL (one paper carton) of water yields an aromatic, pleasant-tasting alkaline solution containing thymol, which has mild antimicrobial and deodorant properties.

Compound thymol glycerin, when diluted with three times its volume of water, yields a solution with similar properties to that produced by dissolving a mouthwash solution tablet. Both solutions are used to freshen the mouth and for mechanical cleansing. Most patients with a sore mouth appreciate the soothing properties of warm mouthwashes. However, some patients, especially if they are pyrexial, welcome the refreshing effect of a cold mouthwash.

Care must be taken to avoid microbial contamination of thymol mouthwashes by rejecting any unused solution on completion of the procedure. Thymol, in the concentrations normally present in mouthwash solutions, is only a very weak antimicrobial agent. If solutions become contaminated, bacterial growth can occur, with consequent risk of infection, especially in immunosuppressed patients.

ORAL HYGIENE

More and more people are retaining their teeth into old age and require to care for them. In many cases, the need to carry out oral hygiene in one form or another to rid the mouth of debris is part of everyday living. When illness presents, the need for oral hygiene is much greater. For example, with anorexia, vomiting, constipation, pyrexia, dehydration and fatigue, the tongue and the teeth become dry and coated, and if left uncared for result in a foul taste, bad smell and the development of oral sepsis.

When fluid intake has to be restricted, the mouth quickly becomes dry, as it does when a patient is mouth breathing or receiving continuous oxygen therapy. Patients who are immunosuppressed, as the result of a disease such as leukaemia or treatment such as radiation or cytotoxic drugs, are prone to mouth infections. The cells of the oral mucosa and salivary glands divide at a moderately rapid rate. Anticancer treatments aimed at rapidly replicating malignant cells are unfortunately not sufficiently selective, and so the mouth is often adversely affected. Diuretics, psychotropics and insulin, as well as sympathomimetic and parasympathomimetic agents, all alter salivary function. Antibiotics may encourage opportunistic bacteria to flourish in the mouth by reducing the resident flora. The many situations regarded as high risk for developing some form of discomfort of the mouth are evidence of how important this procedure is for nurses.

Some patients can be left to attend to this aspect of their care; some simply need to be prompted or given encouragement. Other patients are capable of carrying out the procedure for themselves but may need assistance in gathering together the necessary equipment. Many patients are wholly dependent on the nurse to meet every need. The purpose is to remove and prevent the build-up of plaque, to stimulate the flow of saliva and to reduce the risk of complications such as candidal infection and parotitis. The three direct methods employed are:

- brushing the teeth with toothpaste and water
- rinsing the mouth with mouthwash solution
- swabbing the mouth (Box 24.4).

Whenever possible, patients should be encouraged to brush their teeth in the usual way or have their teeth brushed for them. Patients with a reduced platelet count whose gums are very liable to bleed are nevertheless also encouraged to use a toothbrush, although it must be a soft one. Alternatively, an electric toothbrush may be used because the brushes rotate and are less traumatic than a conventional toothbrush.

Mouthwashes are easier for patients to manage when they feel weak and unwell. Swabbing with a swabbed finger, although not a pleasant procedure

---

Box 24.4 Swabbing the mouth

The medicine
- Mouthwash solution tablets
- Soft paraffin

The environment
- Privacy, warmth, comfort

The nurse and the patient
- Patient given explanation, if appropriate, of what is involved
- Patient assisted, if necessary, into position that allows ease of access

The technique
- Nurse ensures that hands are socially clean before and after procedure
- Patient's dentures removed if appropriate
- Mouth examined using spatula and torch to identify area requiring greatest attention (e.g. tongue)
- Solution prepared
- Excess solution squeezed from each swab before use
- Oral cavity gently and systematically wiped from inside using mouthwash solution
- Each swab used for one wipe only and then discarded
- Mouth reinspected
- Soft paraffin applied sparingly to lips if indicated
- Dentures thoroughly brushed before being replaced
- Discarded material carefully disposed of
- Patient made comfortable
- Observations noted on nursing records

Hazards
- Infected mouth
- Spread of infection to other patients
- Inhalation of swab or solution by unconscious patient

for the patient, is essential for those who are acutely ill, unconscious or in the terminal stages of illness. This approach needs to be gentle yet effective. The airway of the unconscious or semiconscious patient must be protected at all times. Because of the danger of inhalation, any excess of the solution used for cleaning the mouth should be wrung out of the swab before use. Very ill patients will require to have the mouth cleaned at least every 2 h. Whichever method is applied, the aims of oral care are the same, i.e. to cleanse and moisten the mucosa.

There are further ways of helping to keep the mouth of conscious patients clean and moist. Apart from encouraging and facilitating nasal breathing, imaginative ideas of suitable food and drinks, if permitted, may be put into practice. Flavoured ice lollies, chips of ice, boiled sweets or chewing gum may help. Fruit juices, especially those containing lemon, stimulate the flow of saliva and are cleansing and refreshing but may cause the mouth or lips to sting if the mucosa is irritated or broken.

In summary, the role of the nurse in oral hygiene is:

- to assess the state of the patient's mouth
- to select the appropriate method of oral hygiene for the patient
- to estimate the amount of assistance the patient requires with the procedure
- to assist the patient with oral hygiene as required
- to observe, report and record details of the condition of the patient's mouth
- to teach aspects of oral hygiene to patients and relatives.

Special measures taken to keep a patient's mouth clean and comfortable are generally required only for as long as the patient is acutely ill. As the patient's general state of health improves, there is usually a corresponding improvement in the condition of the mouth.

CARE OF THE MOUTH IN SPECIAL SITUATIONS

REDUCED SALIVARY FLOW

Dry mouth (xerostomia) can cause considerable discomfort. It may result from a reduction in salivary flow such as occurs with:

- certain drugs (e.g. antispasmodics and tricyclic antidepressants or drugs having antimuscarinic side effects)
- radiotherapy to the head and neck
- infection of a salivary gland

- inflammation of the mouth or throat
- dental or oral surgery.

Local and systemic treatments are available. Artificial saliva products containing electrolytes and gelling agents at neutral pH are available as a spray, lozenge or pastille.

Pilocarpine (a muscarinic drug) is administered as a tablet (5 mg) in cases of salivary gland malfunction following radiotherapy for head and neck cancers. The contraindications and side effects are very significant, as would be expected from a potent muscarinic drug (see p. 145).

In general, lozenges, sprays, etc. have little proven therapeutic benefit but do offer some comfort when required. Boiled sweets or chewing gum (preferably low sugar) may be just as helpful.

LOWERED RESISTANCE TO INFECTION

In situations in which patients are receiving chemotherapy or radiotherapy, or are immunosuppressed for any other reason, chlorhexidine gluconate 0.2% may be used prophylactically in the form of a mouthwash. The solution (10 mL, four or five times per day) should be held in the mouth for 1 min before being expelled. In view of possible incompatibility, 30 min should be allowed to elapse before using toothpaste. The patient should be warned that the solution may cause brown staining of the teeth. On completion of treatment, staining can be removed by a dentist. Stained fillings may have to be replaced.

POST TONSILLECTOMY

Mouthwashes are administered after tonsillectomy to remove blood clots from the throat. Using the mouthwash as a gargle may help to clear the throat by mechanical action. The solutions used in this situation are intended to:

- detach blood clots and debris (hydrogen peroxide solution)
- ease pain using local analgesic (benzydamine hydrochloride solution)
- treat or prevent infection (povidone–iodine solution)
- cleanse and refresh (thymol mouthwash solution).

POSTRADIATION INFLAMMATION OF THE THROAT

Patients receiving radiotherapy to the head and neck or the chest can suffer from an extremely sore throat. This may be soothed without aggravating the existing reaction by using sodium bicarbonate solution or povidone–iodine solution as a mouthwash or gargle.

SELF-ASSESSMENT QUESTIONS

1. Outline some of the issues involved in mouth care in patients undergoing chemotherapy and what the patient can do to minimise problems.
2. What is the main danger of syringing an ear?
3. At what temperature should ear and nose drops be administered?
4. On what occasions is care of the mouth especially important?
5. How would you recognise oral thrush?
6. What is the treatment for oral thrush?
7. Name a drug that can damage gingival tissue causing hyperplasia.
8. When is it especially important to ensure good oral hygiene in patients receiving drug therapy for osteoporosis?
9. What are the dangers of using a muscarinic drug (pilocarpine) for the treatment for xerostomia?
10. Name a drug that can be administered by the nasal route to produce a systemic effect.
11. Is the routine use of corticosteroid nasal sprays to be cautioned against? If so, why?
12. Is the nose a 'safe haven' for potentially dangerous pathogens? If so, how is this dealt with to reduce the risk of infection?

REFERENCES

Chisholm DG, Calder I, Peterson D et al. 1997 Drug points: intranasal chlorhexidine resulting in anaphylactic circulatory arrest. British Medical Journal 315:785

Scottish Intercollegiate Guidelines Network 1999 Management of sore throat and indications for tonsillectomy. Publication no. 34. SIGN, Edinburgh

Scottish Intercollegiate Guidelines Network 2003 Diagnosis and management of childhood otitis media in primary care. Publication no. 66. SIGN, Edinburgh

FURTHER READING AND RESOURCES

Allen S 2006 Outer and middle ear problems. Pharmaceutical Journal 276:83–86

Heals D 1993 A key to wellbeing: oral hygiene in patients with advanced cancer. Professional Nurse 8:391–398

Howarth H 1977 Mouth care procedures for the very ill. Nursing Times 73:354–355

Ludman H 1988 ABC of ear, nose and throat. British Medical Association, London

Peate I 1993 Nurse-administered oral hygiene in the hospitalised patient. British Journal of Nursing 2:459–462

Torrance C 1990 Oral hygiene. Surgical Nurse 3:16–20

Drug treatment of skin disorders

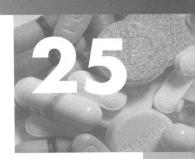

25

KEY OBJECTIVES

After reading this chapter, you should be able to:

- describe the layers of the skin
- describe the role played by the accessory organs of the skin
- describe the clinical features of eczema
- list the types of preparations used in eczema
- describe the clinical features of psoriasis
- list the treatments available for psoriasis
- distinguish between a cream and an ointment
- list the precautions that should be taken when administering topical corticosteroids
- outline the management of infestation by pediculi
- describe how you would ease the distress caused by pruritus
- discuss the psychosocial effects of a chronic skin condition
- describe the process of wound healing
- identify the components of wound assessment
- list the groups of patients at greatest risk of developing pressure ulcers
- give examples of a wound-cleansing agent and a desloughing agent
- state the one essential action that can reduce the incidence of wound infection.

INTRODUCTION

As the skin is the largest organ of the body, it follows that all skin diseases require prompt, expert management and the use of preventive strategies whenever possible, including public health campaigns. Skin diseases affect 20–33% of the population (All Party Parliamentary Group on Skin 1997) at any one time, but the perception that skin diseases are not

487

important sadly may still be encountered. Specialist services are under great pressure, and it is essential that, both from the patient's point of view and NHS costs, primary care services are able to offer a range of effective treatments. Skin diseases range from those conditions that resolve with time and the use of suitable treatment regimens (medication and physical methods) to those that may prove fatal (melanoma). In some cases, skin diseases cause discomfort and embarrassment. Patients can be scarred emotionally as well as physically by some conditions, notably acne vulgaris. Treatment regimens may be time-consuming and inconvenient for patients and carers. However, more cosmetically acceptable topical products have eased some of the burden.

Unlike such conditions as hypertension and certain metabolic disorders, it is very difficult to measure the severity of skin diseases. Patients' perceptions of their condition may not always equate to the nurse's assessment. People with chronic skin diseases may have to run the gamut of suggestions of well-meaning relatives and friends, including avoiding the temptation to use unproven, unorthodox treatments. Many remedies for common skin conditions are available over the counter. These may be useful, especially when used with the guidance of suitably trained nurses and other health professionals. Some skin diseases that have a genetic component continue to present major challenges for clinicians and researchers.

Improved training for all those involved in skin care services will greatly benefit both the patient and the NHS, as will the recognition that skin diseases can be a major cause of suffering and morbidity.

ANATOMY AND PHYSIOLOGY

The skin provides a waterproof surface, retains essential fluids, acts as a barrier against infections and is a major controller of body temperature, the heat of the body being regulated by the blood vessels and sweating. It protects underlying organs from physical, chemical and other injuries. The nerve endings in the skin serve as a relay between external influences and internal organs. The skin acts as an organ of expression, betraying the innermost feelings – anxiety by sweating, anger by a red flush and fear by pallor. It is an important store for water, containing 18–20% of the total water content of the body, which is distributed mainly in the dermis. This percentage decreases with age.

For practical purposes, the skin can be considered in three layers (Fig. 25.1):

- epidermis
- dermis
- accessory organs (e.g. sweat glands, sebaceous glands, nails and hair follicles).

EPIDERMIS

The outermost layer of the skin is the epidermis. The epidermis itself has five layers. From the inside out, they are:

- the stratum basale, where active columnar cells (keratinocytes) divide
- the stratum spinosum, which consists of several layers of irregularly shaped cells
- the stratum granulosum, where granules are visible in the cells' cytoplasm
- the stratum lucidum, a layer of living cells that contains a translucent compound from which keratin is formed; this layer is only present in the palms of the hands and soles of the feet
- the stratum corneum, a horny layer of thin, flat, non-nucleated cells that have become keratinised, i.e. when the protoplasm has been replaced by keratin, a protein that toughens the epidermis and renders it waterproof; the surface of the skin is composed of dead cells that are constantly being rubbed off.

Within the epidermis, a continuous synchronised process takes place in which the cells of the stratum corneum that flake off are replaced at the same rate by new cells generated in the stratum basale. The process repeats itself as the new cells migrate through the epidermal layers, gradually changing in shape and size and in turn reaching the surface, where they are shed.

Specialised cells, known as melanocytes, are to be found in the basal layer. They are responsible for the production of melanin, a protective pigment released following exposure to sunlight.

DERMIS

The dermis is thicker than the epidermis and consists of two layers of fibrous connective tissue (collagen) that support the epidermis and give it its elasticity. The papillary layer lies next to the epidermis and, as its name implies, is made up of papillae – tiny projections containing capillaries that nourish the epidermis and nerve endings responsible for the reflex action in response to painful stimuli. The reticular layer consists of a thick mesh of collagen fibres that make the skin strong and flexible. Blood vessels, nerves and fatty tissue are also present, and it is throughout

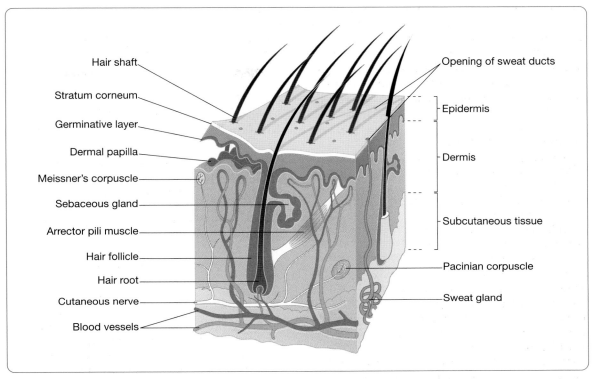

Fig. 25.1 Skin structure.

this layer that the sweat glands, sebaceous glands and hair follicles are located.

ACCESSORY ORGANS

SWEAT GLANDS

Millions of tiny sweat glands are located in the dermis all over the body. There are two types of sweat gland.

Exocrine glands are the commoner type and are mostly concentrated in the palms, soles and forehead. They become active when the body temperature rises through exercise, a hot environment or emotional stress. They promote cooling by evaporation of their secretion on the skin's surface.

Apocrine glands are found in the axillary, anal, genital and mammary areas of the body. Sweat is produced by these glands under the influence of the sympathetic nervous system when emotionally stressed.

SEBACEOUS GLANDS

Sebaceous glands are situated in the dermis. Their function is to produce sebum, an oil containing fatty acids, cholesterol and substances toxic to bacteria.

Sebum is discharged through the sebaceous duct into the hair follicle, moving along the shaft of the hair to the skin surface, keeping both the skin and the hair soft. The glands are located all over the body, except the palms and soles, in close association with body hair.

NAILS

The nails are keratinised epidermal cells that have a horny texture and serve to protect the fingers and toes. A nail consists of:

- a body, which is the exposed part – it is an extension of the germinative area of the epidermis and is composed of a greatly thickened stratum lucidum; the area beneath the nail body is highly vascular
- the lunula (moon-shaped), under which are the epithelial cells
- the cuticle, a fold at the base and sides of the nail
- the nail root, whose cells dictate the rate of nail growth.

HAIR

A hair behaves in a similar way to a nail, in that it is formed by a group of cells at its base that multiply and push forwards to the surface of the skin, where it is ultimately shed or removed. The base of each hair, referred to as the bulb, is situated in the dermis. A pointed projection of the dermis protruding into the hair bulb is known as the papilla. The papilla nourishes the cells of the hair follicle housing the hair root. The root is the part beneath the surface of the skin; the shaft is the visible part. By the time the hair follicle reaches the surface, its cells have become hard and keratinised.

COMMON CONDITIONS AND THEIR TREATMENT

ECZEMA

Eczema is recognised by a characteristic inflammatory reaction in the skin caused by a number of factors, internal, external or a combination of these. Internal (constitutional) factors are thought to underlie a number of different types of endogenous eczema. Filaggrin (filament-aggregating protein) is an important protein in the formulation of the outer (protective) layer of the skin. There is evidence to suggest that mutations of the filaggrin gene are involved in eczema and the related condition asthma (Smith 2006). For those forms of eczema associated with external factors (exogenous), the term *dermatitis* still tends to be used. Lawton's classification of eczema (Hughes and Van Onselen 2001) is given in Box 25.1.

Eczema may be further subdivided into acute, subacute and chronic forms. When there is an acute reaction, the clinical features include erythema and small vesicles that break down causing weeping, oedema and scaling. In subacute eczema, features of both acute and chronic eczema are in evidence. The skin is red and thickened as the result of inflammation and scratching to relieve the associated itch. Many patients are very troubled by itching. The scratching is often followed by serious local damage, leading to lichen simplex, a leathery patch in an accessible area of the patient's skin. In chronic eczema, the same features are present, although they are less pronounced, but there is more thickening and scaling. Pigmentation may be increased.

ENDOGENOUS ECZEMA

Atopic eczema

This form of eczema commonly arises in infancy. There is a hereditary tendency to develop immediate allergic reactions with inflammation, intense itch and excoriation, especially on the face and skin creases. It is strongly linked with a history (personal or close family) of other atopic diseases such as asthma and hay fever.

EXOGENOUS ECZEMA

Contact dermatitis

This form of skin disease is associated with exposure to an irritant or an allergen. Contact irritant dermatitis is more common than the allergic form. Contact with highly toxic substances such as acids may result in an acute irritant dermatitis. Repeat exposure to certain less toxic substances such as detergents may also lead to an irritant dermatitis, although it may take longer to appear. Contact irritant dermatitis is more prevalent among people in certain occupations, such as hairdressing and nursing. The hands are most commonly affected. On first exposure to an offending allergen, susceptible individuals are unaware of an immune response developing. It is only on subsequent exposure to the allergen that there is an eczematous reaction at the point of contact. Contact allergic dermatitis arises in susceptible individuals who have a hypersensitivity to certain materials (e.g. rubber), metals (e.g. nickel) and perfumes (e.g. in soap).

TREATMENT

Eczema and dermatitis are treated similarly, but it is especially important in cases of dermatitis to avoid or remove the causative agent (e.g. cosmetic, household cleaner). Treatment with bland emollients is often helpful (allowing patient choice). Creams for direct application are easy to use and provide welcome relief from itching. Emollient bath additives are useful in many cases of dry skin. The use of

---

Box 25.1 Classification of eczema

Exogenous
- Contact irritant
- Contact allergic
- Photosensitive

Endogenous
- Atopic eczema
- Seborrhoeic
- Discoid
- Gravitational
- Pompholyx

Unclassified
- Asteatotic
- Lichen simplex
- Juvenile plantar dermatosis

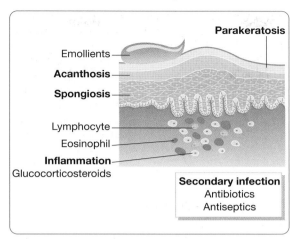

Fig. 25.2 Sites of drug action in eczema. (From Page CP, Hoffman BF, Curtis M et al. 2006 Integrated pharmacology. Mosby, Edinburgh. With permission of Mosby.)

topical corticosteroids, starting with a mild product then moving to a moderate product depending on response, provides symptom control. Overuse of corticosteroids must be avoided due to the dangers of absorption leading to systemic side effects (see p. 341). Alternating emollients with corticosteroids may be a useful strategy.

Coal tar preparations have a limited place in the treatment of chronic atopic eczema. Poor acceptance by the patient and possible long-term side effects have curtailed their use. Ichthammol has properties similar to those of coal tar but is milder in action. Ichthammol has antipruritic properties that may be useful in chronic eczema.

In situations in which allergy and/or infection are present, oral antihistamines or antibiotics will be required. The use of gamolenic acid in atopic eczema is not based on firm evidence of therapeutic benefit. Seborrhoeic eczema of the scalp is treated by shampoos containing coal tar or selenium, or a specially formulated corticosteroid scalp preparation in the form of a mousse. The preferred treatment is a shampoo containing ketoconazole, an antifungal agent. Figure 25.2 shows the sites of action of various treatments. Table 25.1 outlines the use of immunosuppressant drugs in both eczema and psoriasis.

PSORIASIS

Psoriasis is a chronic skin disorder characterised by circumscribed red plaques covered by thick, dry, silvery adherent scales that make the skin itchy and unsightly.

It occurs when there is an excessive production of epidermal cells and the shedding of old skin cells remains normal, resulting in the characteristic lesions of psoriasis. It may occur at any age and can appear in any area of the body, although lesions more frequently arise on bony prominences such as the elbows, knees and sacral area. The scalp is another common site. There are numerous types of psoriasis whose names reflect such aspects as the appearance of the skin, the location of the plaques, the presence of papules or pustules, whether it is of an acute or chronic form, and whether it is localised or generalised. The cause of this condition is not known, but genetic factors and trigger factors such as stress and certain drugs (non-steroidal anti-inflammatory drugs and angiotensin-converting enzyme inhibitors) may be involved. Fig 25.3 shows the sites of drug action in psoriasis.

TREATMENT

Topical and oral therapies are available, many of which require specialist advice. For mild conditions, an emollient may be useful to minimise scaling. This will seldom provide adequate relief but can be helpful when plaque thickness has been reduced by other therapies. Salicylic acid (2% ointment) has keratolytic properties. Care should be taken with products containing high concentrations of salicylic acid to control the amounts applied in order to avoid absorption leading to systemic toxicity.

Coal tar preparations have anti-inflammatory and antiscaling properties. Choice of product will depend on the site of the plaques and the preference of the patient. Dithranol is a more potent agent than coal tar. The use of dithranol requires expert management by prescriber, nurse and patient. Dithranol acts by combining with deoxyribonucleic acid, resulting in the inhibition of nucleoprotein synthesis and so diminishing cellular proliferation. Short-contact applications of 1 h are effective, the strength of dithranol depending on the patient's condition within a range of 0.15–2%, often incorporated in Lassar's paste. Dithranol can cause severe skin irritation and, for this reason, it must be used strictly in accordance with the prescription. It must be applied only to psoriatic plaques (protecting surrounding skin), commencing with a low concentration and gradually increasing this to an optimum concentration that produces a therapeutic effect without irritation. Dithranol stains skin purple-brown, but this fades in 2–3 weeks. It is essential for nurses to wear gloves and avoid all contact, especially with the eyes, when applying dithranol preparations. Hands should be thoroughly washed after use.

Table 25.1 Immunosuppressant drugs used in the treatment of skin diseases

Drug	Indications	Dose, route and notes	Mode of action, toxicity and side-effects[a]
Azathioprine	Severe refractory eczema	See specialist literature. As with all drugs in this class, monitoring for toxicity throughout treatment is essential.	Interferes with purine synthesis and is cytotoxic; metabolised to mercaptopurine, which inhibits DNA synthesis. Depresses bone marrow. May cause nausea and skin eruptions and is mildly toxic to the liver. Vomiting.
Ciclosporin	Severe psoriasis, severe eczema	See specialist literature.	Immunosuppressant. Decreases proliferation of T cells. Reduces function of effector T cells and reduces T-cell-dependent B-cell responses. Causes nephrotoxicity and has other side effects.
Hydroxycarbamide	Severe psoriasis	See specialist literature.	Inhibits ribonucleotide reductase. Causes bone marrow depression.
Methotrexate	Severe psoriasis	Dose (10–25 mg weekly) adjusted in accordance with severity of condition and haematological or biochemical response.	Folate antagonist. Causes depression of bone marrow and damage to the gut. Since the dose is <u>weekly</u> great care is needed managing this therapy.
Mycophenolate mofetil	Severe refractory eczema	See specialist literature.	Restrains proliferation of both T and B lymphocytes. Reduces production of cytotoxic T cells.

If the above treatments and photochemotherapy are ineffective or poorly tolerated, the following may be used.

Drug	Indications	Dose, route and notes	Mode of action, toxicity and side-effects[a]
Efalizumab	Severe chronic plaque psoriasis	By SC injection 700 micrograms/kg then 1 mg/kg weekly.	Works by binding to CD2 on memory effector T lymphocytes, inhibiting their activation in plaques.
Etanercept, infliximab	Licensed for psoriatic arthritis not previously treated with methotrexate	See specialist literature and NICE guidance	Tumour necrosis factor-α inhibitors/anticytokines. Use with caution if there is predisposition to infection.
Pimecrolimus	Acute treatment of mild to moderate atopic eczema not controlled by maximal topical corticosteroids	Cream 1%. Avoid contact with eyes and mucous membrane.	This drug is a calcineurin inhibitor. It reduces inflammation by a number of complex mechanisms (see specialist literature).
Tacrolimus	Moderate to severe atopic eczema not controlled by maximal topical corticosteroid therapy	Topical application of 0.1 or 0.03% ointment twice daily for 2 weeks depending on response. Avoid excessive exposure to sunlight. As with pimecrolimus, this product may be useful when there is a particular risk from corticosteroid absorption.	As pimecrolimus.

[a]See also Chapters 19 and 20.

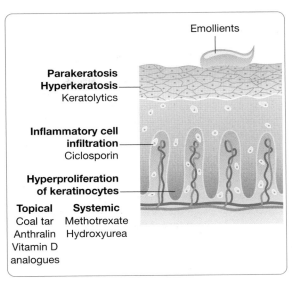

Emollients

Parakeratosis
Hyperkeratosis
Keratolytics

Inflammatory cell
infiltration
Ciclosporin

Hyperproliferation
of keratinocytes

Topical	Systemic
Coal tar	Methotrexate
Anthralin	Hydroxyurea
Vitamin D	
analogues	

Fig. 25.3 Sites of action of various treatments for psoriasis. (From Page CP, Hoffman BF, Curtis M et al. 2006 Integrated pharmacology. Mosby, Edinburgh. With permission of Mosby.)

A range of strengths of dithranol is available in cream formulations, which are easier to apply than stiff pastes. Contact time will depend on the strength of active ingredient (e.g. 0.1% overnight contact, 1–2% maximum of 1 h). A novel dermal delivery system for dithranol presents dithranol (1 or 3%) in a special cream. The dithranol is incorporated in a protective 'sandwich' that maintains the chemical stability of dithranol. Contact time is 30 min for the 3% cream when used on the scalp under medical supervision.

Topical corticosteroid creams have a limited place in the treatment of plaque psoriasis. Skin atrophy can result and render the condition intractable to treatment. A mild or moderate corticosteroid may be used in the flexures. Potent corticosteroids may be used on the scalp in the short term.

Calcipotriol (a derivative of vitamin D) is used topically for mild to moderate plaque psoriasis. A scalp preparation is available. Unlike dithranol, it is easy to use and is non-staining (van der Vleuten 2001). Calcitriol and tacalcitol are used for similar conditions. These products should be used only in accordance with clearly defined 'dosage' regimens, i.e. quantity and frequency of application.

For more severe psoriasis not responding to topical treatments, oral treatments may be required.

Acitretin (a vitamin A derivative) is an oral retinoid. This should be prescribed only by or under the supervision of a consultant dermatologist; 25–30 mg is administered daily for 2–4 weeks, then adjusted according to response. This will usually be in the range of 25–50 mg daily for a further 6–8 weeks; however, a higher dose and longer treatment time may be needed. Side effects include dryness and cracking of the lips, pruritus and nosebleeds. Acitretin is teratogenic, and contraceptive measures in women who may become pregnant should be commenced at least 1 month before treatment initiation and continued for at least 2 years following cessation of the drug. Tazarotene is a retinoid available as a gel formulation for the treatment of mild to moderate plaque psoriasis affecting up to 10% of skin area.

TREATMENT OF SKIN DISEASES WITH IMMUNOSUPPRESSANTS

Immunosuppressants are used in the treatment of certain skin diseases that are unresponsive to other forms of treatment (see Table 25.1). In view of potentially serious side effects (see Ch. 20), the use of these drugs is restricted to specialist units.

Oral treatment of severe resistant psoriasis with ciclosporin may be used under close specialist supervision. Side effects and contraindications may be severe. Dosage is initially 2.5 mg/kg daily in two divided doses, gradually increasing to 5 mg/kg per day. Treatment is discontinued if no improvement is seen in 6 weeks.

Methotrexate is used in severe, resistant cases of psoriasis under hospital supervision. It is a folic acid antagonist that inhibits cellular proliferation. In view of the toxicity of this drug, it is very important to monitor the patient's response and to adjust the dose accordingly.

PHOTOCHEMOTHERAPY

Photochemotherapy involves the use of an oral photosensitising agent (a psoralen, P) and exposure to ultraviolet A light (UVA). The treatment, known as PUVA, is used for both initial treatment and maintenance therapy of most forms of psoriasis. Long-term dangers of this form of therapy are not yet confirmed, but there are theoretical risks of neoplastic skin diseases.

Appropriate treatment of psoriasis improves the appearance of the skin. However, because drugs cannot cure the underlying cause of the disorder, psoriasis tends to recur.

Psoriasis in all its forms can have a very damaging psychological impact on patients. Full support,

> **Box 25.2** Summary of main treatment options for psoriasis
>
> **Topical**
> - Keratolytics
> - Coal tar
> - Dithranol
> - Steroids
> - Vitamin D analogues
> - Phototherapy: ultraviolet B
>
> **Systemic**
> - Psoralens and ultraviolet A (PUVA)
> - Retinoids
> - Methotrexate
> - Ciclosporin

counselling and advice are essential, as is compliance by the patient.

The main treatments of psoriasis are summarised in Table 25.1 and Box 25.2.

ACNE

Acne vulgaris is a common condition affecting mainly adolescents, but it can occur later in life. It is caused by excess production of sebum by the sebaceous glands, leading to a blockage of hair follicles by skin debris and hardened sebum. Acne normally affects the skin on the face and neck and less frequently the back and chest.

Acne may be classified as follows.
- Mild:
  — papules (inflamed spots)
  — pustules (raised, pus-filled spots with a white centre)
  — comedones (blackheads, which are dark owing to the effect of oxygen on sebum).
- Moderate: more extensive papules and pustules with possible scarring
- Severe: many papules and pustules with significant scarring.

TREATMENT

Treatments available include topical and systemic (oral) preparations. Topical products are intended to remove follicular plugs and reduce skin bacterial flora. Benzoyl peroxide alone or in combination with an antimicrobial agent is widely used. Such products have both a keratolytic and an antimicrobial action. Irritation of the skin commonly occurs but will normally subside. Azelaic acid (25% cream) has similar actions to benzoyl peroxide. Gels containing nicotinamide (4%) have an anti-inflammatory effect that may be valuable in mild to moderate inflammatory acne.

Tretinoin reduces sebum production. When applied to the skin, it produces an erythematous reaction, and skin peeling may occur after application for several days. Topical preparations of erythromycin, tetracycline or clindamycin are useful in patients with mild to moderately severe acne. A combination product of an antibiotic and a retinoid is available for topical use. Topical corticosteroids should not be used for acne.

Topical retinoids (forms of vitamin A) have anti-comedogenic properties, both locally and systemically. Creams and gels of both tretinoin and isotretinoin are available. Redness of the skin and peeling may occur, which should settle in time. Contact with mucous membranes and eyes must be avoided. Both topical and oral retinoids are contraindicated in pregnancy and eczema. Adalpene is a retinoid-like drug used topically.

If acne is severe, a course of oral tetracycline or erythromycin may be prescribed: 250 mg three times daily before meals for 1–4 weeks then reduced to twice daily until improvement occurs. Several months' treatment or even longer may be required. If resistance to tetracycline antibiotics or erythromycin occurs, trimethoprim (see p. 303) may be useful but should be initiated only by a specialist. Female patients must stop tetracycline if they become pregnant, because this drug is deposited in developing teeth and bones of the fetus. If the treatments described above are unsuccessful, isotretinoin, an oral drug, may be prescribed. This has an action that is similar, but more powerful, to that of tretinoin. It is a hospital-only preparation and should be prescribed only by or under the supervision of a hospital consultant. Side effects include dry lips, nosebleeds and some loss of hair. Isotretinoin is teratogenic and must not be given to pregnant women. Contraceptive measures in women who may become pregnant must be effective and must last for 1 month after completion of treatment. Broad-spectrum antibiotic treatment can compromise the effectiveness of combined oral contraceptives. This is thought to be due to the effect of the antibiotic on the gut flora, which is responsible for recycling ethinylestradiol from the large bowel. Suitable guidance must be given to patients using oral contraception.

Hormone therapy (co-cyprindiol) has an anti-androgenic effect. The drug reduces sebum secretion when given daily (one tablet) starting on Day 1 of the menstrual cycle. Figure 25.4 shows the sites of action of the drugs used. The side-effects are as for COCs.

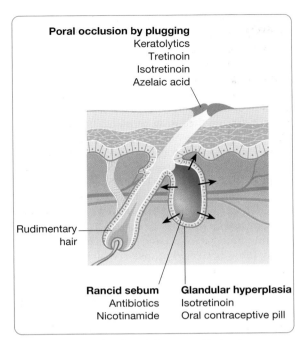

Fig. 25.4 Sites of action of drugs used to treat acne. (From Page CP, Hoffman BF, Curtis M et al. 2006 Integrated pharmacology. Mosby, Edinburgh. With permission of Mosby.)

Poral occlusion by plugging
Keratolytics
Tretinoin
Isotretinoin
Azelaic acid

Rudimentary hair

Rancid sebum
Antibiotics
Nicotinamide

Glandular hyperplasia
Isotretinoin
Oral contraceptive pill

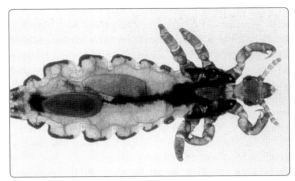

Fig. 25.5 Head louse. (From Paller AS, Mancini AJ 2005 Hurwitz clinical pediatric dermatology. Saunders, Edinburgh. With permission of Elsevier Inc.)

ROSACEA

Rosacea is a form of acne but, unlike acne vulgaris, it is not comedonal. As with acne vulgaris, the condition, characterised by facial flushing, causes considerable distress to those affected. The condition can develop if not treated, leading to persistent facial erythema and inflammatory episodes with swelling, pustules and papules.

The causes of this disorder are poorly understood, but ultraviolet light, extremes of temperature and certain foods and drink are thought to act as triggers. Emotional stress can exacerbate the condition.

TREATMENT

Antibiotic treatment is used to reduce inflammation. In mild cases, topical metronidazole (cream) is commonly used. For more severe rosacea, an oral antibiotic such as oxytetracycline (500 mg twice daily) or tetracycline (500 mg twice daily) may be added. When these drugs are contraindicated, as in renal impairment, doxycycline (100 mg daily) may be used instead. In severe cases, minocycline (100 mg daily) may be further added. When there is resistance to antibiotics or there are persistent clinical features,

oral tretinoin may be prescribed. Laser therapy may be required for the treatment of telangiectasia.

As well as complying with the prescribed treatment, patients can assist by avoiding or reducing their intake of spicy foods, chocolate, hot drinks, alcohol, etc. A non-irritant sunscreen should be used to prevent a worsening of the condition. Redness may be effectively disguised with the assistance of a camouflage cream.

URTICARIA (HIVES OR NETTLE RASH)

This condition is characterised by the appearance of itchy weals on the skin. The causes of acute urticaria include hypersensitivity reactions due to insect bites, stings, foodstuffs and some drugs (see p. 152). Chronic urticaria has no obvious cause (idiopathic). Angioedema may occur with urticaria or as a separate condition. In this condition, the swellings are deeper and may last for up to 48 h. Some drugs, notably angiotensin-converting enzyme inhibitors, may cause serious life-threatening angioedema (see p. 150). Detailed investigations are required that include tests for allergies, blood tests and tests for thyroid function. Treatment includes topical agents (moderately potent corticosteroids) and/or oral antihistamines (see p. 153). Acute cases (which may involve airway obstruction) require adrenaline (epinephrine) subcutaneously.

PEDICULOSIS

Contrary to popular belief, head lice (*Pediculus humanus capitis*; Fig. 25.5) are not confined to dirty long hair. In fact, they flourish on both clean and dirty hair (both short and long) and are passed from person to person when one head is in prolonged contact with another. They are not caused by bad hygiene. Often, adults will be involved in the passing on of the infestation. The head louse would appear to have a preference for the blood of children. The reason for this is not understood. As boys get older, they are much less susceptible to infestation than are girls. Mixing at home, at school or while playing increases the risk to all children. There is never a single case of head lice.

Lice are born, live and die on the host, leaving the head only to transfer to a similar environment. They spend their time feeding off the scalp and reproducing. The eggs laid are glued to the base of a strand of hair and are well camouflaged, as they change in colour to match the skin. Once the eggs incubate, each hatches to produce a louse that, left untreated, will eventually sap the host's strength and leave the person generally unwell. The empty shells remain firmly glued as the hair continues to grow, and they change to a pure white colour, distracting attention from any new live eggs that are always laid at the base of a hair. It is the white shell left behind that is called a nit.

TREATMENT

It is essential that the correct diagnosis is reached by a healthcare professional before treatment is begun. A living, moving louse must be found to confirm the diagnosis. Detection of live lice is by wet combing, which involves intensive combing for at least 30 min over the whole scalp at 4-day intervals for a minimum of 2 weeks using a plastic detection comb and hair conditioner. The most successful formulations for treating lice are lotions and liquids that stay on the head long enough to kill eggs as well as lice. Lotions, being of an alcohol base, are unsuitable for young children or those with asthma or eczema, in which case liquids must suffice. Shampoos are too diluted to be effective.

In order to prevent resistance developing, a mosaic approach is currently recommended whereby if, out of three possible treatment options, the first one fails, treatment moves to the second option and so on to the third (Aston et al. 1998). The insecticides available are malathion (liquid and lotion), permethrin (cream), phenothrin (liquid, alcoholic lotion and mousse), and carbaryl (liquid and lotion). Malathion is an organophosphate that should not be used more than once a week and for not more than 3 consecutive weeks. Carbaryl is considered a potential human carcinogen and is therefore a prescription-only medicine. Whichever course of treatment is selected, two applications of insecticide should be made 7 days apart. The head should be thoroughly checked

2–3 days after the final application, using a plastic detection comb.

When applying a lotion or liquid to the head, it is important to use enough of it (at least 50 mL per application; more if the hair is thick). It should also be remembered that it is the scalp that has to be treated rather than the hair. The hair should be parted while it is still dry and the lotion sprinkled into the parting until the whole scalp has been moistened, taking care to avoid contact with the eyes. The scalp is massaged gently, paying particular attention to the back of the head and to the areas behind the ears. The hair may then be combed and should be allowed to dry naturally. The application is removed 12 h later using ordinary shampoo.

If one member of a family is affected, the whole family must be treated to make certain that they are all free from infestation. Classmates should be treated similarly. Mothers should be advised to make a regular check on their children's heads and to encourage combing of the hair, especially at bedtime.

Nurses in the community, at school and in hospital should exercise diplomacy when dealing with affected patients or explaining the condition to a child's parents. While not wanting to create offence or embarrassment, the nurse, as a health educator, must ensure that this particular problem is not allowed to go unchecked.

SCABIES

Sarcoptes scabiei is the mite responsible for the parasitic infection scabies. The mite burrows into the outer layers of the skin, especially of the flexures, where, after fertilisation, the female lays its eggs. An intensely pruritic rash caused by an allergy to the mite's excretions develops 2–6 weeks after initial infection, along with a widespread rash. Scabies is a contagious disease most commonly seen in children, teenagers and those living in institutions.

TREATMENT

The diagnosis of scabies is confirmed by identification of the mite with the naked eye or with the assistance of a magnifying glass, or by sending skin scrapings for laboratory analysis.

Treatment involves the application of a scabicide to cool, dry skin. Permethrin 5% cream or malathion 0.5% aqueous solution may be used. The treatment should be applied to the whole body from the neck down and left on the skin for 8–12 h (permethrin) and 12 h (malathion). The webs of fingers and toes should receive special attention. Where treatment has failed, the head should also be treated. Permethrin and malathion should be applied twice, 1 week apart. The infected patient (with or without symptoms), all members of the patient's household and anyone who has had skin to skin contact within the last 2 months should be treated at the same time.

PRURITUS

Pruritus or itching is considered to be due to the stimulation of the subepidermal nerve plexuses by proteolytic enzymes that are released from the epidermis as a result of either primary irritation or allergic sensitisation reactions.

Pruritus may be localised or generalised. Itching in localised parts of the body is often the result of local causes. Itching around the anus may be the result of threadworm infestation in children or from haemorrhoids. Genital pruritus in women (pruritus vulvae) may be caused by vaginal infections such as *Trichomonas vaginalis* or, in older women, by hormone deficiency. It may be the result of a skin condition or a systemic disorder. Itching is a common symptom of many skin disorders, including:

- eczema
- psoriasis
- lichen planus
- urticaria
- body lice
- scabies
- fungal infection.

It can also be an important feature of systemic disorders, such as:

- blood disorders (e.g. haemachromatosis, polycythaemia, lymphomas)
- endocrine disorders (e.g. diabetes)
- liver disease (e.g. obstructive jaundice)
- renal disease (e.g. chronic renal failure).

Drug hypersensitivity may also cause severe itching.

TREATMENT

Although scratching may provide temporary relief, it often exacerbates the condition by increasing inflammation. Assessment of the patient with pruritus involves first establishing the underlying cause so that appropriate therapy can be initiated. When local applications are to be used for symptomatic relief, the patient's history must be checked for previous allergy and the skin inspected for signs of excessive dryness, cracking, weeping or broken areas. The patient must be given instruction on the correct method of application and advice to refrain from scratching or rubbing – which damages the epidermis and creates a vicious circle of lesion, more scratching and further damage.

A number of types of medication are used for the relief of skin irritation. Itching from dry skin is often soothed by a simple emollient. For mild itching arising from sunburn, urticaria or insect bites, a cooling lotion such as calamine, with the possible addition of menthol, may be helpful. The menthol, however, may give rise to hypersensitivity reactions in some patients. Crotamiton (10%) in a cream or lotion form may be useful in some cases of pruritus. Doxepin is available as a cream (5%) for use in pruritus of eczema. Because of the possibility of systemic side effects, the cream should be applied thinly, not exceeding 3 g per application. Oral antihistamines should be used in allergic rashes. Chlorphenamine (chlorpheniramine) is an inexpensive antihistamine that is short acting and mildly sedating. When the irritation prevents sleep, a sedating antihistamine (e.g. promethazine) taken at night promotes sleep as well as relieving itching. The sedating oral antihistamine alimemazine may be useful in some cases of urticaria and pruritus.

Topical antihistamines are on sale to the public, but these are generally not recommended due to the likelihood of localised skin reactions. Such products may be useful for short-term therapy (up to 3 days).

The risk of using preparations for pruritus other than simple emollient and soothing preparations is that prolonged or heavy use may cause skin irritation, resulting in aggravation of the itching. Because itching can be a symptom of many underlying conditions, treatment should be reviewed after a week.

PRE-MALIGNANT AND MALIGNANT CONDITIONS

Such conditions may be treated by the carefully controlled application of a cream containing 5% w/v fluorouracil.

SKIN PREPARATIONS

Diseases of the skin are treated by both topical (local) and systemic therapy. A wide range of products are now available, ranging from relatively simple emollients to sophisticated formulations containing potent drugs.

EMOLLIENTS AND BARRIER PREPARATIONS

Emollients are used when a moisturising type of product is likely to be beneficial. They soothe and hydrate the skin and are indicated for dry scaling disorders. Frequent application is required, because their effects are short-lived. They are useful in various dermatological conditions, such as dry eczematous disorders and, to a lesser extent, psoriasis. A wide range of emollient preparations is available. The choice of product will depend on consideration of the patient's condition, the patient's preference and clinical experience.

Both aqueous cream and emulsifying ointment have emollient properties, and either may be used for handwashing or in the bath as a soap substitute to prevent the drying effect of soap on the skin. Several proprietary emulsions are available for use in the bath as 'all over' emollients. Patients should be warned that the bath will be slippery.

Emollients are available for use in conditions such as ichthyosis, traumatic dermatitis, dry eczema, certain types of psoriasis and also when movement of a joint is impaired by dryness or cracking of the overlying skin. Aqueous cream, which contains emulsifying ointment 30% in water, is a light emollient. White soft paraffin (white petroleum jelly); emulsifying ointment that contains emulsifying wax 30%, white soft paraffin 50% and liquid paraffin 20%; and liquid and white soft paraffin ointment (50/50) are more greasy. E45 cream contains light liquid paraffin 12.6% and white soft paraffin 14.5% as well as hypoallergenic lanolin. Lanolin may cause sensitisation in some patients. This should be suspected if an eczematous reaction occurs at the site of application.

Barrier creams are used to provide protection against repeated hydration and irritation, which can result in napkin rash, intertrigo, pressure sores and problems in areas surrounding stomata. Zinc and castor oil ointment is an effective emollient and barrier preparation with mild astringent properties. However, there is no substitute for diligent nursing care. Rashes may clear when left exposed to the air, and an emollient may be helpful. Barrier creams often contain water-repellent substances such as dimeticone or other silicones, but it is doubtful whether these water-repellent creams are any more effective than traditional compound zinc ointments.

Emollients have tended to be undervalued and underused in general care and wound management. Brown and Butcher (2005) have identified that healthcare practitioners need guidance and advice on emollient therapy to improve their care delivery.

TOPICAL CORTICOSTEROIDS

Topical corticosteroids are used for the treatment of a wide variety of inflammatory conditions of the skin other than those due to an infection. Corticosteroids suppress various factors causing inflammation, but

---

> **Box 25.3** Topical corticosteroids grouped according to potency
>
> **Mild**
> - Hydrocortisone 1%
>
> **Moderately potent**
> - Alclometasone dipropionate 0.05%
> - Clobetasone butyrate 0.05%
>
> **Potent**
> - Beclometasone dipropionate 0.025%
> - Betamethasone 0.1%
> - Diflucortolone valerate 0.1%
> - Fluocinolone acetonide 0.025%
> - Hydrocortisone butyrate 0.1%
>
> **Very potent**
> - Clobetasol propionate 0.05%
> - Halcinonide 0.1%

---

they are not curative because the underlying cause of the inflammation is not affected. When treatment is discontinued, the condition may recur. Despite their disadvantages, corticosteroids remain a cornerstone of the treatment of many skin diseases. It will be noted that there are many different corticosteroid compounds available for topical use. The different chemical compounds used are chosen for therapeutic properties that are influenced by the chemical structure of the compound.

The choice of a topical corticosteroid must be made with care. In most cases, a mild corticosteroid is used at the start of treatment. The rule of thumb is to use the minimum amount of the lowest potency corticosteroid. If a patient ceases to respond to a particular corticosteroid, another of similar potency may be tried before resorting to a more potent corticosteroid. Topical corticosteroid preparations are categorised into four groups according to potency (Box 25.3). A number of the products listed in Box 25.3 are available in a formulation that includes an antimicrobial agent (e.g. neomycin).

Adequate use of emollients may reduce the need for corticosteroid creams. When large areas are to be covered by corticosteroid preparations, the nurse or patient should wear gloves and the preparation should be applied sparingly. Application of excessive quantities of external corticosteroid preparations can result in undesirable local and systemic side-effects. The more potent the preparation, the more care is required, as absorption through the skin can cause pituitary adrenal suppression. The body's immune system is suppressed, thus increasing the risk of infection. Absorption is greatest from areas of thin skin and raw surfaces, and the effect is increased by occlusion. Very potent corticosteroids should be used only for short periods. Local side-effects of topical corticosteroids include:

- thinning of the skin, sometimes resulting in stretch marks, which may be permanent
- fine blood vessels under the skin surface possibly becoming prominent and resulting in a red rash if the vessels become damaged (telangiectasia); because the skin on the face is especially vulnerable to such damage, topical steroids are not usually prescribed for use on the face
- increased hair growth
- a possible temporary reduction in pigmentation at the site of application
- acne at the site of application in some patients
- delayed wound healing.

Some proprietary topical corticosteroid preparations contain antibiotics or other antibacterial agents. These may be prescribed when infection complicates the underlying condition. It should be noted that preparations containing hydrocortisone (up to 1%) are available over the counter for the treatment of dermatitis, insect bite reactions and mild to moderate eczema. Pharmacists provide advice on the use of these products to ensure appropriate use.

TOPICAL ANTIMICROBIALS

Antibacterial, antifungal and antiviral preparations are used for skin infections that are not too deeply seated and are therefore amenable to local therapy. Topical antimicrobial therapy should be carefully managed and avoided if at all possible, owing to local sensitisation reactions. The problem of bacterial resistance is of major concern, and it follows that the antimicrobial agents used topically should ideally not be the same as those agents used systemically. Table 25.2 summarises the main drugs used together with indications and precautions.

DISINFECTANTS (BIOCIDES)

Disinfectants have little or no place in wound management procedures (see p. 509) and in the preparation of skin prior to surgery. Alcoholic solutions (70% v/v) alone, or containing chlorhexidine 0.5% w/v, are often used for such purposes. Chlorhexidine combined with a cleansing agent may be used if the patient's skin is contaminated.

Single-use sachets and sterile disposable equipment should be used whenever possible to reduce the risk of cross-infection when performing a dressing. Hand preparation prior to surgical procedures is carried out using a detergent–chlorhexidine (a quaternary ammonium compound) combination and a suitably thorough technique. Alcoholic chlorhexidine solution may be useful as a hand rub after washing, but this will not achieve decontamination of unwashed skin. A handwash containing povidone–iodine is an alternative to chlorhexidine, but iodine may cause sensitisation in some individuals. All health authorities have an infection control policy. See page 294 for the management of methicillin-resistant *Staphylococcus aureus* (MRSA).

Mupirocin should be used only to treat MRSA, otherwise fusidic acid may be used to treat acute impetigo (a highly contagious infection of the skin, usually starting as facial erythema and progressing to pustules and crusts).

Hard surfaces may be treated with ethyl or isopropyl alcohol (70% v/v) in a suitable form (spray or swab). Glutaraldehyde solution has a place in the disinfection of surgical equipment that cannot be heat-treated. However, special precautions must be taken to avoid contamination of the environment with fumes of the product. Phenolic compounds are seldom used today.

SUNSCREENS

Sunlight is composed of a spectrum of wavelengths of electromagnetic radiation. Of these, ultraviolet radiation can be particularly harmful to the skin. The medium wavelengths (290–320 nm, ultraviolet B) cause sunburn and longer-term changes that may lead to skin cancer and ageing. People vary widely in their sensitivity to ultraviolet radiation. Fair-skinned people have least tolerance and burn easily, whereas people with darker skin can withstand exposure for longer periods without noticeable harm. In addition, ultraviolet radiation may be harmful in certain diseases (e.g. lupus erythematosus and rosacea). Certain drugs such as chlorpromazine, demeclocycline and amiodarone can increase the skin's sensitivity to sunlight, and in all these cases protection will be required even for short periods of exposure.

Sunscreens contain substances such as ethylhexyl *p*-methoxycinnamate, titanium dioxide, zinc oxide, avobenzone and aminobenzoic acid, which absorb ultraviolet B (medium-wavelength solar ultraviolet radiation) and, in this way, provide protection. A range of sunscreens is available, graded according to the degree of protection: the sun protection factor (SPF). This figure indicates the amount of ultraviolet radiation that will be absorbed; the higher the SPF, the

Table 25.2 Topical antimicrobial agents

Drug or product	Indications	Notes, side-effects and precautions
Antibacterial agents		
Mupirocin 2% cream and ointment	Gram-positive infections	Unrelated to any other antibiotics. Not suitable for pseudomonal infection. Not to be used for longer than 10 days to reduce risk of resistance developing. Avoid use in hospitals.
Neomycin 0.5% cream (often in combination with other antibiotics)	Bacterial infections	Not to be used to treat large areas, as it may be absorbed and cause ototoxicity. Not used systemically. Care in patients at extremes of age and in renal impairment.
Silver sulfadiazine 1% cream	Prophylaxis and treatment of burns	Compound of silver and a sulphonamide. Contraindicated in pregnancy and breast-feeding. Itching, rashes and argyria have been reported.
Antifungal agents		
A wide range of drugs is available. Some examples are: • benzoic acid compound ointment • clotrimazole • econazole • ketoconazole • miconazole • terbinafine • tioconazole	Fungal skin infections	Valuable antifungal drugs but may cause local irritation, allergic reactions and stinging. These drugs are available as creams, gels, ointments, dusting powders and shampoos. Choice of product will depend on nature and site of the infection. A nail laquer containing amorolfine is available for the treatment of onychomycosis.
Antiviral preparations		
Aciclovir (5%) and penciclovir (1%) available as creams	Labial and genital herpes simplex infections; systemic therapy needed for more deep-seated infections	Apply five times daily at first sign of attack. Penciclovir is applied every 2 h during waking hours for 4 days.
Formaldehyde Glutaraldehyde Podophyllum resin Podophyllotoxin (the active component of the resin)	Plantar warts Persistent warts Genital warts	All these drugs are potent agents that must be prescribed and used with great care so as to avoid adverse reactions in both patients and healthcare staff. Salicylic acid (a keratolytic) may be combined with podophyllum resin for the treatment of plantar warts.

greater the degree of protection. For skin protection in dermatological conditions, an SPF of 15 or more is required. An SPF of 15 should allow a person to remain 15 min longer in the sun without burning. However, this is only a guide. For maximum benefit, the sunscreens must be applied frequently. They are applied before sunbathing to prevent erythema. People with fair skin should start with a sunscreen with a higher SPF. As the skin tans, a lower SPF may suffice. Prolonged exposure of skin to strong sunlight increases the long-term risk of skin cancer, due to the damaging effects of both ultraviolet B and ultraviolet A (long-wavelength [320–400 nm] solar ultraviolet radiation). The only really safe approach is to wear appropriate clothing, because sunscreens do not prevent long-term damage that may be caused by ultraviolet A. Some products are available that provide protection against ultraviolet A and B.

Photodamaged skin may be treated with diclofenac gel for up to 90 days. Tretinoin cream (0.05%) may also be used but may take 3–4 months to achieve benefit.

SHAMPOOS

Dandruff (*pityriasis capitis*) is the condition in which the accumulation of dead cells on the scalp results in flaky scaling. Regular washing with a mild shampoo several times a week may be sufficient to keep the scalp free of dandruff. However, many people find that a medicated shampoo is required. Shampoos containing tar extracts may be useful, as they soften the dead scales and make them easier to remove. Shampoos containing pyrithione zinc reduce the formation of dandruff by slowing the growth of skin scales and have the advantage of not having to be prescribed. The use of selenium sulphide–containing shampoos is no more beneficial than non-medicated shampoos. When dandruff is severe and unresponsive to these treatments, ketoconazole shampoo, alone or in conjunction with weak corticosteroid gels or lotions applied to the scalp, may be helpful.

ANTIPERSPIRANTS

Hyperhidrosis (overproduction of sweat) may be a localised or a more generalised problem. A generalised problem condition can be treated with an antimuscarinic, but side effects (see p. 145) may limit the use of this form of treatment. Localised hyperhidrosis may respond to treatment with a paint containing 20% w/v aluminium chloride in alcohol. The paint is applied overnight to the area affected following careful cleaning and drying. In very resistant cases, surgery may be required to remove areas of maximum sweat production. Botulinum A toxin (see p. 465) by local injection may be useful in intractable cases.

PROBLEMS ASSOCIATED WITH SKIN PREPARATIONS

Table 25.3 indicates some of the potential problems of using certain dermatological preparations. The list should not be regarded as fully comprehensive, but it does identify the major problem areas likely to be encountered by nurses.

TOPICAL THERAPY IN SKIN DISORDERS

THE COMFORT OF THE PATIENT

Treatment of the skin, whether carried out at the bedside or in a treatment room, calls for consideration of a number of factors. First and foremost, privacy must be provided and maintained, and every effort must be made to ensure that the dignity of the patient is preserved. The room should be adequately ventilated but free of draughts.

When caring for patients with a disorder of the skin, the nurse should ensure that the environment is conducive to good communication. Here, an individualised approach to the patient is of paramount importance. The treatment of patients with an apparently similar condition should play no part. Only in a one-to-one situation can there be a satisfactory exchange of views leading to better understanding. The chances of patients maintaining compliance with the treatment prescribed and achieving concordance will be greatly increased if they are helped by the nurse to understand the rationale behind it.

Irrespective of the treatment being followed, all patients with skin conditions need to be cared for with sensitivity. Feelings of shame, disgust and fear have for long troubled patients with skin diseases, often forcing them to hide from the gaze of others. To some extent, this situation has been perpetuated by the attitude of health professionals towards these patients. Sadly, staff may make patients with skin conditions feel unclean by isolating them unnecessarily in single rooms and adopting overprotective measures while treating them. In time, the patient may respond with antisocial behaviour that, in turn, may affect the attitudes of others until what can only be described as a 'leper complex' develops. Unless it is absolutely necessary to do otherwise, these patients should be shown the same consideration afforded to all other patients. Trust and confidence need to be restored by adopting an open and optimistic outlook. This in itself has a beneficial 'therapeutic' effect.

The possibility that a skin disorder has been caused by an underlying systemic condition should not be overlooked (Table 25.4).

ASSESSMENT

There is no substitute for identifying the cause of the problem and tackling it at source. Because two people suffering from the same condition will rarely present in an identical way, it is essential that a thorough assessment is made by examination and questioning. Both visual (often using a hand lens) and tactile examination will be required. Temperature, tension and sensitivity of the skin may be ascertained by careful touching of the affected part(s) using a disposable plastic glove as appropriate. When it is suspected that a skin condition is due to a reaction to an irritant or allergen, systematic questioning may

Table 25.3   Problems associated with some dermatological preparations

Problem	Ingredient causing problem	Methods of risk reduction and precautions
Absorption: systemic	Azelaic acid, corticosteroids (especially potent agents), neomycin, salicylic acid, terbinafine	Avoid contact by using disposable gloves or applicator if available. Wash hands after use (nurse and patient). Occlusive dressings increase absorption – use only when and as prescribed. Discontinue breast-feeding owing to risks.
Eye irritancy	Aluminium chloride, benzoyl peroxide, carbaryl, dithranol, podophyllum resin, sulphur	Never use on face. Patient should be warned not to rub eyes when (or after) using product. Wash hands after use.
Flammable products	Alcohol (especially in high concentrations), collodions, ether	Should never be used near naked flame, electric heaters or other ignition sources.
Granuloma	Talc in dusting powders	Avoid contact with broken skin and body cavities.
Infection	Many dermatological preparations, especially those containing a high percentage of water and/or prepared by dilution of a proprietary product; preservative system may be inadequate	All dermatological products should be used with care to avoid contamination and cross-infection. Observe expiry dates and conditions of storage. Single-use packs should be used for preservative-free products. Particular care is needed when large areas of broken skin are involved.
Irritancy of respiratory tract	Dusting powders, pressurised aerosol	Take care to avoid inhalation, especially in sensitive subjects.
Photosensitivity	Antihistamines, coal tar, tretinoin	Patient should be warned to avoid exposure to strong sunlight.
Sensitisation reactions	Antihistamines, local anaesthetics, neomycin	Be alert to this possibility. Use of product may have to be discontinued.
Skin and fair hair	Clioquinol, coal tar products, dithranol	Patient should be warned in advance about possible discoloration of skin and/or hair.
Skin irritancy	Dithranol, formaldehyde, malathion, podophyllum resin, sulphur, tioconazole	Should be applied only to those areas to be treated. Normal skin may be protected by a bland agent (e.g. soft paraffin). Confine application to lesions.
Staining of personal linen and the patient's bath	Coal tar products, dithranol, potassium permanganate	Patient should be warned in advance.

help to identify the cause, as will carefully managed patch testing.

TREATMENT SELECTION

Selection of a product by either doctor or nurse requires care, because the choice is extremely wide; the British National Formulary (BNF) alone contains several hundred different topical applications. In addition, specially formulated products can be prescribed for patients whose needs cannot be met by an 'off the shelf' formulation. In this case, the range of products available is as wide as the prescriber's imagination.

Many skin conditions require the attention of a consultant dermatologist (or other clinician) who will prescribe the treatment. Products containing antibiotics, corticosteroids or other potent drugs come administration and recording of such products should be in accordance with established policies and procedures for medicines management.

Special prescription sheets are required for the prescribing of topical preparations in hospital, as it is necessary to incorporate a greater amount of information than the standard in-patient prescription sheet allows. The prescription should include the following.

- Date of the prescription.
- Name of the preparation; a specially made-up formula may consist of several different substances that should be listed.
- Formulation and its strength; when necessary, details such as aqueous or oily should be given, and it is better, when possible, to describe the strength as a percentage – ratios (e.g. 1:9) can be misleading.
- Quantity to be applied; this may be difficult to quantify. 'Sparingly', 'liberally', '1 cm' or 'a worm' are expressions that may be used. The most commonly used instruction given is 'as sparingly as possible'.
- Site(s) for application; these should be described specifically (e.g. 'all active areas', 'wherever the skin is dry'). Vague expressions such as 'all over' should be avoided.
- Dressings and bandages to be used; the size of each should be appropriate to the size of the patient's lesion.
- Number of times of administration; this should span a 24-h period and should be divided evenly throughout the patient's waking day.
- Prescriber's signature.

Prescribing systemic therapy for dermatological conditions is carried out in the same way as all other systemic prescribing.

FORMULATION OF TOPICAL PREPARATIONS

Several different pharmaceutical preparations (ointments, lotions, etc.) are available, each of which has distinctive physical characteristics quite apart from the nature of the active ingredient. In some instances, products are used solely for their physical properties (e.g. emollients, barrier preparations and sunscreens). Although a detailed discussion of formulation aspects is outside the scope of this book, certain important principles are emphasised below, because they have practical implications for the nurse. Typically, a pharmaceutical product intended for topical application will have some, or all, of the following components.

Table 25.4 Skin manifestations of systemic diseases

Systemic disease	Skin manifestation(s)
Chronic obstructive airways disease	Dusky hue or bright pink
Chronic renal failure	Yellow-brown, uraemic frost
Congestive cardiac failure	Cyanosed, oedematous
Diabetic coma	Dry, smelling of acetone
Hypertension	May be highly coloured
Hypoglycaemia	Profusely sweating
Iron deficiency anaemia	Pale
Myxoedema	Dry, coarse
Obstructive jaundice	Deep yellow, itching
Pernicious anaemia	Pale lemon-tinted
Thyrotoxicosis	Warm, moist
Viral diseases of childhood	Characteristic rashes, itching

into this category, because the use of these agents is accompanied by certain risks. Symptoms may be masked by the use of corticosteroids, and the use of certain antibiotics is associated with sensitisation reactions.

Those who have been trained to prescribe from an extended Nurse Prescribers' Formulary (see p. 88) will be able to prescribe a range of treatments for minor ailments of the skin (e.g. acne; atopic dermatitis; contact dermatitis; chronic skin ulcers) and injuries (e.g. abrasions, bites – animal and human, burns and scalds, and minor lacerations).

PRESCRIBING OF TOPICAL PREPARATIONS

Topical preparations that contain a specific drug should be regarded in exactly the same way as any other medicine. It follows therefore that prescribing,

ACTIVE INGREDIENT(S)

The concentration of the active ingredient(s) will normally be expressed as a percentage weight in weight (e.g. 1% w/w hydrocortisone cream).

VEHICLE

The overall characteristics of the product will depend on the vehicle chosen. The vehicle may be aqueous, non-aqueous, liquid or semi-solid depending on the properties required and nature of the active ingredient. Penetration of the active ingredient into the skin is influenced by the properties of the vehicle and nature of the condition being treated. The make-up of the vehicle used in proprietary preparations varies greatly. In order to help trace the source of a local reaction to a product, it may be necessary to seek information on all the components of the product in order that the source of the problem can be identified. In some situations, it may be necessary to prescribe a product by proprietary name to ensure consistency of product.

ANTIMICROBIAL PRESERVATIVE AGENT

The risk of microbial contamination of topical products, especially those containing a high proportion of water, during their use is significant, and so it is essential, unless the product is a single-use pack, to include an antimicrobial agent. Chlorocresol and the hydroxybenzoates are commonly used. These preservatives may cause sensitisation in some patients.

EMULSIFYING OR SUSPENDING AGENT

These are required to give a product physical stability; for example, an emulsifying agent stabilises oil-in-water preparations, and a suspending agent is necessary when insoluble powders of high density are included in a liquid preparation.

OTHER ADDITIVES (EXCIPIENTS)

A buffering agent may be included to give a preparation with a pH approximating that of normal skin. Various stabilisers, antioxidants and fragrances may be added. One or more of these chemicals may cause sensitisation in some patients. Patch testing may be used to identify an allergy to an excipient that must be avoided when prescribing.

TOPICAL PREPARATIONS AND THEIR USE

The terms *cream*, *ointment*, *lotion*, etc. are precise but may not always be used correctly. Care should be taken to determine the actual properties of the product, which may not always be reflected by the name.

CREAMS

Creams are normally oil-in-water emulsions that, because water is the continuous phase, are easily removed, even from hairy areas, by normal cleansing procedures. The evaporation of the water present in the cream produces a useful cooling effect. Drainage from a lesion is facilitated, because creams absorb exudates. Drugs normally incorporated into creams include corticosteroids, antibacterials and antifungal agents. Good penetration of the active ingredient into the skin is achieved and may be enhanced because of the presence of a surfactant (emulsifying agent) in the cream. Creams also have a softening effect on thickened tissues.

Although creams normally contain an antimicrobial preservative, they should be used with great care to avoid microbial contamination, because the antimicrobial agents available for incorporation into creams have a limited spectrum of activity. The antimicrobial agent (and/or active ingredient) may cause skin sensitivity in some patients. Creams are more cosmetically acceptable than ointments, especially when applied to the face, as they disappear when rubbed into the skin.

OINTMENTS

It is very important to distinguish between ointments and creams, because the formulations have different properties. Ointments are normally greasy anhydrous preparations that do not mix with water and therefore should not be applied to exuding lesions. They are occlusive and encourage hydration. Ointments are more difficult than creams to remove from the skin. Soft paraffins are widely used in ointment bases, incorporating liquid paraffin to achieve the required consistency. Ointments soften crusts but are generally not suitable for application to hairy areas. They are particularly useful for application to dry scaly areas.

Being non-aqueous, antimicrobial agents are only occasionally required to be included in ointments, and so there may be less risk of sensitisation from this source than with creams. However, lanolin (wool fat) and derivatives are sometimes included in ointments and may cause contact sensitivity.

OTHER PREPARATIONS

Products are also available that combine the properties of both ointments and creams. Such formulations are described as ambiphilic. The formulation is a stable emulsion system with a uniform distribution of fat and water.

Application of creams and ointments. Ointments and creams generally have different properties, and the indications for their use relate to these. The most important aspect, however, is to use a preparation that is acceptable to the patient. Creams and ointments are best applied in the same way as make-up. Small dots of the product are placed at suitable intervals over the area to be treated. Using the tip of the index finger and/or second finger for small areas (fingertip unit) and the palm of the hand for larger areas, the cream should be spread evenly as far as it will go within the area to be treated. Dressings may be required to cover areas to which creams and ointments have been applied.

PASTES

These preparations are essentially similar to ointments but contain a high proportion of powders, have a very stiff consistency and will adhere to lesions at body temperature. Pastes also have protective properties. Lassar's paste, for example, contains 24% w/w zinc oxide and 24% w/w starch with 50% white soft paraffin and 2% salicylic acid.

Application of pastes. Pastes should be applied only to specific lesions (e.g. in psoriasis) and not to the surrounding skin. When a paste contains a highly active ingredient (e.g. dithranol), it will be necessary to protect the skin adjacent to the lesion with a bland product such as yellow soft paraffin. If the paste is soft enough (temperature will obviously influence the consistency of the product), it may be applied with the finger(s) of a gloved hand. Pastes that cannot be applied in this way may be applied with a wooden spatula. Pastes will seldom require to be covered with a dressing, except when it is necessary to protect the patient's linen from staining by the active ingredient. They are not popular with patients, as they are messy and difficult to apply.

Paste bandages

A range of bandages are available that are impregnated with a zinc oxide paste combined with coal tar, calamine or ichthammol. Paste bandages are used for the treatment of conditions such as eczema, leg ulcers and chronic dermatitis.

DUSTING POWDERS

Dusting powders are of two main types: medicated and non-medicated. All dusting powders have a basis of starch (absorbent) and talc (lubricant). Non-medicated powders are used in general nursing care to reduce friction and absorb moisture between folds of skin. The skin should be clean and well dried before each application. Excessive use should be avoided, because 'caking' in folds of skin may result, causing local irritation or trauma.

Medicated powders have a limited place in the active treatment of skin diseases, because it is generally not possible to achieve a satisfactory concentration of active ingredient at the site of the lesion for any length of time. Dusting powders containing suitable active ingredients are mainly used in prophylaxis (e.g. the prevention of athlete's foot or the prevention of neonatal staphylococcal cross-infection). Dusting powders containing antibiotics are occasionally used in the treatment of superficial bacterial infections such as impetigo, when the powder will tend to stick to the lesions.

LOTIONS

Lotions are normally simple formulations containing active ingredients in an aqueous solution or suspension. Occasionally oily lotions are used, but such preparations have properties very different from those of a lotion with an aqueous base, because they are water-in-oil emulsions. Lotions with an aqueous base are used in weeping eruptions, when they cool and dry the skin by evaporation. In very acute conditions, lotions are used to relieve superficial inflammation and assist in the removal of crusts. When even the presence of fine solid particles cannot be tolerated by the patient, lotions that are simple solutions are used until the most acute phase of the condition has passed. Then lotions containing powders in suspension can be used. The cooling properties of a lotion may be enhanced by the addition of alcohol to the vehicle, but this may cause stinging. Excessive cooling due to the use of lotions must be avoided, especially in the elderly.

Lotions may be useful for the application of a drug to a hairy area of the body where the use of a greasy ointment or stiff paste would be inappropriate or impracticable. In very acute conditions, lotions may be applied as wet dressings using lint or other closely woven fabric. As with all dressings, care should be taken on removal to avoid damaging the epithelium. Any dressings that have dried out should be thoroughly wetted with the lotion before being carefully removed. Lotions may also be applied to small lesions using cotton wool, or to larger areas using a suitable flat brush.

PAINTS

Paints are solutions of the active drug in a suitable solvent, such as water, alcohol or a mixture of solvents, depending on the nature of the active ingredient. Application to the skin is normally by means of a brush.

PRESSURISED AEROSOLS

Pressurised aerosols are widely available for the application of drugs to the skin in conditions such as superficial bacterial infections. Protective applications can also be applied in this way. It is important to use the product in accordance with the manufacturer's recommendations, and to ensure safe disposal of the empty canister. Pressurised aerosols are convenient to use and confer the advantages of a non-touch technique, but they are relatively expensive.

SKIN-CLEANSING PROCEDURES

SKIN CLEANSING

Before applying a topical preparation, the skin should be clean. To prevent accumulation, previous applications to the skin should be removed. This is especially important when drugs such as corticosteroids are involved. In order to remove creams, paints, powders or lotions, the patient or the site should be bathed using simple soaps and warm water; perfumed toilet soap should be avoided. Pastes, ointments and certain paints are best removed with cotton wool soaked in liquid paraffin or olive oil.

BATHING

With increasing changes in the skin towards dryness after about the age of 35, the tendency should be towards a reduction in the frequency in bathing. Soaking in a hot bath makes the skin dry owing to loss of natural oils and causes epidermal cells to shrink on drying. Any itching of the skin is increased. Showering may be more appropriate. A conscious effort should be made to adjust routine and not to overwash patients, particularly elderly people and those patients whose skin is noticeably dry. Nurses are well placed to make an assessment of the patient's skin and decide on the care required.

Patients with skin conditions should be advised to resist the temptation to use any cosmetic bath additives. Detergents or antiseptics may cause the patient further problems and should be avoided. To occlude the skin and thus prevent drying by evaporation, liquid paraffin or olive oil may be used. An emollient such as emulsifying ointment may be added to the bath water. This also acts as a mild occlusive and helps to retain moisture in the skin. An oily bath is obviously exceedingly dangerous, and therefore it is vitally important that the patient is forewarned of the risk of slipping. The nurse should make a careful judgement as to whether the patient can be safely left to get out of the bath unaided. In any case, the bath should be emptied before the patient climbs out. A secure bath mat and grab rails should be made available. After using an emollient, the bath needs careful cleaning. It should be filled full with hot water and have a suitable detergent added, having first ensured that there are no patients in the vicinity who may mistakenly think that the bath has been filled for their use. The bath is then allowed to empty and, as it does so, the water should be agitated and the sides cleaned to remove all traces of the emollient.

SCALP TREATMENT

Shampoos may be used for cleaning or for treatment purposes. Triethanolamine lauryl sulphate 40% forms the basis of many shampoos. It has no additives and is the least irritant. It is therefore useful as a simple cleansing agent for the scalp.

Psoriasis of the scalp may be treated by first descaling using a keratolytic overnight for up to a week. Topical corticosteroids are used when the scalp is inflamed. In the long term, analogues of vitamin D may be used.

Precautions have to be taken to protect the eyes and face from contact with shampoos used as treatment. The patient should be warned to keep the eyes closed throughout the procedure. With gloved hands, two applications are made – the first, a thorough wash to cleanse the scalp, the second, active treatment. Between applications and at the finish, the shampoo should be rinsed out of the hair. The hair is dried with a hairdryer as soon as possible. Some scalp applications (and other dermatological products) are flammable, and when using such products patients should be warned not to dry the hair near a naked flame or take other precautions.

APPLICATION OF TOPICAL PREPARATIONS (Box 25.4)

If the condition is acute, then the frequency of the treatment and the strength of the active ingredient(s) may be increased – rather than increasing the amount applied. It is only the active ingredient(s) in contact with the affected skin that is going to aid healing – not the layers on top. 'A little can do a lot of good, a lot can do a lot of harm' is a maxim worth remembering.

PATIENTS' RESPONSE TO TREATMENT

In-patients undergoing treatment for a skin condition should be given the opportunity to express how they feel their condition is responding, and the comments should be recorded in the patient's progress report. The opportunity will often arise during a treatment session. It is not sufficient for nurses to express their view of progress being made. Whatever the nurse

Box 25.4 Application of topical preparations

Documentation
- Special prescription sheet for topical medicines

The medicine
- Creams, ointments, pastes, dusting powders, lotions
- Paints as prescribed

The environment
- Such as to ensure privacy
- Adequately ventilated but free of draughts

The nurse and the patient
- Patient identified
- Explanation given to patient
- Willingness of nurse to listen to what patient wants to say
- Patient given realistic encouragement

Technique
- Hand hygiene before and after administration
- Polythene gloves worn by nurse
- Preparations applied gently and sparingly
- Dressing kept to minimum size necessary

Hazards
- Irritation of the skin
- Infection from contaminated containers

observes about patients or their skin, it is important to record what patients say – even if it is simply that they are feeling better or worse.

PATIENT COMPLIANCE

Skin conditions are frequently of a chronic or recurring nature, which often necessitates teaching patients and/or relatives how to continue treatment. Advice given may include appropriate skin cleansing and the method of application, as well as any special precautions such as skin protection and protection of personal linen. Teaching should be realistic and helpful if a reasonable degree of compliance is to be ensured. There would be little point in asking a patient to apply a tar preparation before going out in the evening, because of its antisocial effect. To most patients, a large unsightly dressing would be equally unacceptable. For the application of an ointment, some disabled patients may find a long-handled ointment applicator of assistance in reaching inaccessible parts of the body. When there is a degree of difficulty in applying skin preparations, in the absence of a capable family member it is essential to arrange for the treatment to be carried out by the district nurse.

SAFETY AND STORAGE

In hospitals, topical applications must be kept in a locked cupboard set aside for external preparations, careful attention being paid to expiry dates. To prevent cross-infection, patients should be supplied with individually dispensed skin applications. When this is not possible, a quantity of the preparation should be removed from its container with a spatula. If more of the preparation is required, a new spatula should be used. Because rolling up a collapsible tube to expel the contents may obliterate the label, it is preferable to squeeze the tube progressively along its entire length.

HAZARDS

Nurses should be aware of the potential hazards inherent in treating skin conditions. Moreover, they should take the opportunity given to them to set a good example to the patient when carrying out treatments. The precautions to be taken are as follows:

- Skin preparations should be applied strictly in accordance with the prescription.
- Polythene gloves should be worn when applying any preparation to the skin (unless a spatula or brush is being used) so that the nurse does not risk absorbing the active ingredients.
- Creams may support bacterial growth and should therefore be used with care to avoid microbial contamination. All creams will bear an expiry date after which the preparation should not be used.

Particular care should be taken when applying topical corticosteroids

Topical corticosteroids. Although these products are very effective, the risks of inappropriate use are very significant (see p. 499). Application must always be in accordance with the prescription. Nurses applying topical corticosteroids should take precautions to prevent contamination of the product and the possibility of absorption of the active ingredient. Patients will need guidance on the amounts to be used. The fingertip unit (Long et al. 1998) is a useful method of providing guidance to patients (see BNF).

TISSUE VIABILITY AND WOUND MANAGEMENT

A detailed discussion of this topic is beyond the scope of this text. In view of the importance to the nurse of wound management, however, the basic principles are outlined below.

Box 25.5 Classification of wounds

- Acute wounds (heal by primary intention):
  - surgical wounds
  - wounds resulting from trauma
  - burns (including chemical and electrical) – may behave like chronic wounds.

  It should be noted that all acute wounds have the potential to become chronic due to infection or other factors, but they generally heal over a short period of time.
- Chronic wounds (heal by secondary intention):
  - leg ulcer – open lesion between the knee and the ankle joint that remains unhealed for at least 4 weeks (Scottish Intercollegiate Guidelines Network 1998)
  - pressure ulcer
  - wound arising from medical condition (e.g. diabetes).

  Chronic wounds are associated with a number of risk factors:
- poor circulation (failure of valves in veins)
- immobility (may be due to disease)
- smoking
- obesity
- diabetes (sensorily deprived)
- older people
- inadequate nutrition
- medication (e.g. vasoconstrictors).

Table 25.5 Stages in the healing process

Stage	Notes
Haemostasis	This is the first and vital stage. The damaged vessel 'attracts' platelets, which aggregate, producing more platelets and factors influencing the clotting mechanism.
Inflammation	This is a normal response and is essential for wound healing to take place. This phase lasts for a few days in acute wounds, but in chronic wounds it may last for a much longer period. The inflammatory process can be observed by the nurse and is characterised by redness, swelling, heat and pain. Inflammation is a complex physiological process.
Proliferative phase	The release of growth factors stimulates the formation of new blood vessels, which deliver vital oxygen and nutrients to the tissues. Granulation tissue is built up. This tissue is bright red and is moist.
Maturation	This process may take a considerable time (many months) to complete. During the process, strengthening of the wound occurs, changes in the vascular network will occur and paler scar tissue will develop.

TYPES OF WOUND

The nurse is likely to encounter different types of wound, each of which requires the application of appropriate management techniques if a good outcome is to be achieved for the patient. Two broad classifications can be considered, namely acute wounds and chronic wounds. Acute wounds include incised wounds resulting from surgery or trauma, and chronic wounds include leg ulcers and pressure ulcers (see Box 25.5). Within each class of wound, distinctive physiological processes take place that need to be understood if healing is to be achieved.

THE HEALING PROCESS

Great advances have been made in the understanding of this vital process, the stage of which should be considered against the background of the physiology and functions of intact skin. Many factors influence wound healing, but it should be recognised that not all wounds can be successfully healed. The aim in such situations is to give the patient the best possible quality of life. Table 25.5 summarises the stages in the healing process.

ASSESSMENT OF THE WOUND

A full assessment must be carried out before any treatment is applied (Box 25.6). Any worthwhile assessment must be carried out on a continuing basis. Different systems have been developed (Fletcher 2003), but it is important to ensure consistency of approach from each practitioner. This may not always be easy to achieve in practice. The wound-healing continuum (Kingsley et al. 2004) has been advocated as a means of achieving consistency. This approach

Box 25.6 Wound assessment

Wound assessment should include the following.

- Location of wound
- Cause of wound, relevant illnesses, nutritional status
- Form:
  - superficial break
  - sinus
  - cavity.
- Aetiology:
  - venous or arterial leg ulcer
  - pressure sore[a]
  - dehisced wound
  - diabetic foot ulcer
  - burns.
- Tissue type:
  - granulating
  - epithelialising
  - sloughy
  - necrotic
  - clinically infected.
- Size:
  - length
  - width
  - depth
  - area.
- Exudate:
  - low
  - medium
  - heavy.
- Pain assessment
- General skin condition

[a]Calculate pressure sore risk assessment score (National Prescribing Centre 1999).

Table 25.6 Colour and wound assessment

Colour of tissue during healing	Tissue type and discussion
Black	Indicates eschar or necrosis. Eschar (dead/dry tissue) must be removed to facilitate a moist environment.
Black/yellow Yellow Yellow/red	This is slough tissue that cannot be removed by irrigation. Slough is adherent, fibrous tissue derived from protein, fibrin and fibrinogen. Slough provides an ideal culture medium for the growth of bacteria and must be removed if normal healing is to be achieved.
Red moist tissue	At this stage, new blood vessels are developing and granulation tissue is being formed. This is normally a good sign.
Red/pink Pink	Re-epithelialisation will now be taking place, leading to healing.

is based on the colour of the wound, which is a reasonable indicator of the type of tissue present in the wound (Table 25.6).

In addition to the visual assessment of the wound, a full patient history must be taken and all the other relevant factors taken into account (e.g. patient lifestyle). Any key risk factors identified must be addressed, such as incontinence. Careful note must be taken of any exudates and the condition of the surrounding tissue. The wound should be measured and a photograph taken. In order to establish whether the ulcer is arterial or venous (and hence needing a totally different approach to treatment), measurement of the ankle brachial pressure ratio index using handheld Doppler is essential in assessing chronic leg ulcers (Scottish Intercollegiate Guidelines Network 1998).

TREATMENTS

Having assessed the wound and carried out any necessary investigations, treatment can be initiated. Many factors must be taken into account, but an outline of a possible treatment plan is given in Table 25.7. The acronym TIME (Sibbald *et al* 2003) is a useful concept: T, tissue; I, infection; M, moisture balance; E, epidermal advancement.

WOUND-DRESSING SELECTION

Great progress has been made in the development of wound dressings. Simple fabric-based 'passive' dressings have largely been replaced by dressings designed to interact with the wound to promote healing. The BNF lists the properties of an ideal dressing, but it is explained that the selection of a dressing should keep the wound moist but avoid maceration. The wound should be kept free from infection and excessive slough. Foreign matter (fibres and chemicals) should not be liberated into the wound, and an optimum temperature should be maintained. Frequent changes should be avoided and an optimum pH value and patient comfort maintained. Manufacturers' instructions should be

Table 25.7 Treatment objectives

Objective	Treatment and notes
Debridement	An essential first step, which may be carried out surgically (in some cases under operating theatre conditions) or by facilitating natural breakdown of the eschar by adding moisture by means of suitable dressing. A dressing may be needed to remove some of the moisture present but avoiding drying out of the wound. Maggot larvae are used to rapidly liquefy dead tissue. It should be noted that anti-infective agents are seldom required, but if these are indicated sensitivity tests should be carried out.
Facilitation of granulation and epithelialisation	The red/pink stages of the wound indicate the need for the maintenance of an environment that encourages the development of new blood vessels and epithelial growth. An adequate moist environment must be maintained and the very fragile (one cell thick layer) protected from trauma.

followed. Table 25.8 outlines the range of dressings available (BNF classification).

WOUND INFECTION

The presence of bacteria in chronic wounds can influence the clinical outcome. It is essential to establish the bioburden (Browne et al. 2001) of the wound and initiate treatment, depending on the severity of the infection (local or systemic; see Ch. 15). Prevention is better than treatment, and every effort must be made to avoid infection from whatever source.

LOCAL MEDICAMENTS

Local antimicrobial therapy has a limited place in wound management. Silver compounds and medical-grade honey are used in various forms (e.g. in gels, tulles or alginate dressings).

OTHER FORMS OF WOUND MANAGEMENT

Vacuum systems are used to aid the closure of major wounds.

Magnetic therapy is a very old treatment that has made a recent comeback (Jackson 2006). It is used in the treatment of leg ulcers and it is claimed that it could revolutionise their management. The magnet-containing device is designed to be wrapped round the leg and worn for 24 h. It is said to work by promoting part of the tissue-healing mechanism, increasing proliferation of connective tissue cells and improving blood circulation (Wang 2006).

SELF-ASSESSMENT QUESTIONS

1. Distinguish between:
   a. eczema and psoriasis
   b. a cream and an ointment
   c. acne and acne rosacea
   d. a hydrogel and a hydrocolloid dressing.
2. Describe:
   a. the side-effects of topical corticosteroids
   b. five local causes of pruritus and five systemic
   c. two antibacterial, two antifungal and two antiviral skin preparations
   d. the precautions that should be taken when applying topical preparations.
3. What:
   a. are the key factors to consider when assessing a wound?
   b. type of dressing would you use for a sloughy wound?
   c. are *Pityiarisis capitis* and *Sarcoptes scabiei*?
   d. does SPF stand for and why is it important?
   e. does PUVA stand for and what is it used for?
   f. are the drawbacks in using dithranol in the treatment of psoriasis?
   g. drug normally associated with the treatment of cancer may be used to treat psoriasis?
4. A mother with two children aged $3\frac{1}{2}$ and $1\frac{1}{2}$ years is making repeated requests for what seems excessive amounts of betamethasone cream. She suffers from mild eczema. What would you do?

Table 25.8   Classification of dressings

Type	Notes and uses
Alginates	Variety of products available. Absorbent: used on moderately or highly exudating wounds. Not suitable for eschar or dry wounds. Wide range available, from low to high absorbency.
Foam	May be useful in hypergranulating wounds. Donate moisture to wounds to facilitate natural (autolytic) debridement. Some absorptive properties.
Hydrogel	To be avoided in presence of infection. Can be shaped to wound.
Hydrocolloid	Used to facilitate rehydration and autolytic debridement of dry sloughy or necrotic wounds. Promote granulation.
Vapour-permeable films and membranes	Allow passage of water vapour and oxygen but are a barrier to water and micro-organisms. Suitable for mildly exuding wounds. Provide moist environment. Comfortable for the patient. May be used as a secondary dressing over alginates or gels. Useful to protect fragile skin from minor damage.
Low-adherence dressing and wound contact materials	Used in combination under secondary absorbent dressings. Products available include: • tulle dressings – fibres impregnated with soft paraffin to prevent fibres sticking to the wound • medicated tulle dressings containing chlorhexidine • povidone–iodine fabric – impregnated fabric with a polyethylene glycol basis. Can be removed by irrigation. Iodine has a wide (but short-lived) antibacterial action but may be absorbed systemically. Perforated film absorbent dressings are suitable for wounds with mild to moderate exudates. Not suitable for leg ulcers or wounds producing viscous exudates.
Odour absorbent	Some infected wounds are malodorous and require this type of dressing. Charcoal (activated) is the absorbent, sometimes in combination with other agents (e.g. silver).
Surgical absorbents	Cotton wool, lint gauze and non-woven fabrics are used as secondary absorbent layers for heavily exuding wounds. Major disadvantages such as adherence, shedding of fibres and dehydration properties preclude use directly on wound surfaces.
Support bandages or compression bandages	Many types are available (see British National Formulary).
Medicated bandages	Zinc paste-impregnated bandages are used for the treatment of leg ulcers. They can be left undisturbed for up to 4 weeks. Coal tar or ichthammol may be incorporated for use in chronic eczema (see p. 506).
Barrier film surgical adhesive tapes	Used to protect vulnerable, sore, damaged skin around wounds. Available for application as a spray or foam (see British National Formulary). These are used to retain dressings. Synthetic adhesives have been developed to reduce allergic reactions.

REFERENCES

All Party Parliamentary Group on Skin 1997 An investigation into the adequacy of service provision and treatments for patients with skin diseases in the UK. All Party Parliamentary Group on Skin, London

Aston R, Duggal H et al. 1998 Head lice: a report for consultants in communicable disease control (CCDCs). Public Health Medicine Environmental Group Executive Committee, London

Brown A, Butcher M 2005 A guide to emollient therapy. Nursing Standard 19:68, 70, 72

Browne P, Dow G, Sibbald RG 2001 Infected wounds: definitions and controversies. In: Falanga V (ed.) Cutaneous wound healing. Martin Dunitz, London

Fletcher J 2003 The benefits of applying wound bed preparation into practice. Journal of Wound Care 12:347–349

Hughes E, Van Onselen J (eds) 2001 Dermatology nursing: a practical guide. Churchill Livingstone, Edinburgh

Jackson W 2006 The resurgence of magnetic therapy. Pharmaceutical Journal 276:480–481

Kingsley A, White R, Gray D 2004 The wound infection continuum: a revised perspective. Applied Wound Management Supplement Wounds-UK, Aberdeen, pp. 13–18

Long CC, Mills CM, Finlay AY 1998 A practical guide to topical therapy in children. British Journal of Dermatology 138:293–296

National Prescribing Centre 1999 Modern wound management dressings. Prescribing Nurse Bulletin 1:6

Scottish Intercollegiate Guidelines Network 1998 The care of patients with chronic leg ulcers. SIGN, Edinburgh

Sibbald J et al. 2003 Preparing the wound bed: focus on infection and inflammation. Ostomy Wound Management 49:23–51

Smith FJ 2006 Filament-aggregating protein. National Genetics 38:337–342

van der Vleuten CJM 2001 Management of scalp psoriasis: guidelines for corticosteroid use in combination treatment. Drugs 61:1593–1598

Wang L-N 2006 Leg ulcers and the first magnetic device on the NHS. In: Jackson W (ed.) The resurgence of magnetic therapy. Pharmaceutical Journal 276:480–481

FURTHER READING AND RESOURCES

Barneston RS, Rogers M 2002 Childhood atopic eczema. British Medical Journal 324:1376–1379

Bellingham C 2001 Proper use of topical corticosteroids. Pharmaceutical Journal 267:377

Berth-Jones J, Tan E, Maibach HI 2004 Eczema and contact dermatitis. Health Press, Oxford

Connolly M 2005 Current treatment options for head lice and scabies. Prescriber May:31–46

Cunliffe B 2001 Acne. Pharmaceutical Journal 267:749–752

Harding KG, Morris HL, Patel GK 2002 Healing chronic wounds. British Medical Journal 324:160–163

Hart J 2002 Inflammation 1: its role in the healing of acute wounds. Journal of Wound Care 11:205–206

Kelly CJG, Ogilvie A 2001 Raised cortisol excretion rate in urine and contamination by topical steroids. British Medical Journal 322:594

Maillard J-Y 2005 Biocides: health care applications. Pharmaceutical Journal 275:639–642

National Prescribing Centre 1999 Using topical corticosteroids in general practice. MeReC Bulletin 10:21–24

Naumann N, Lowe NJ 2001 Botulinum toxin type A in the treatment of bilateral primary axillary hyperhydrosis: randomised, parallel group, double blind, placebo controlled trial. British Medical Journal 323:596–598

Tredget EB, Demare J, Chandran G 2005 Transforming growth factor-beta and its effect on re-epithelialisation. Wound Repair and Regeneration 13:61–67

Williams H 2002 New treatments for atopic dermatitis. British Medical Journal 324:1533–1534

Palliative care

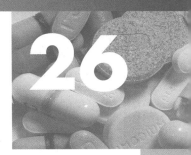

26

KEY OBJECTIVES

After reading this chapter, you should be able to:

- identify the essential components of palliative care
- state what should be included in the assessment of pain
- describe what is meant by the pain-relief ladder
- explain how the dose of morphine for breakthrough pain is calculated
- discuss the common side effects of morphine
- discuss the advantages and disadvantages of morphine
- define adjuvant therapy
- discuss the place of syringe drivers in palliative care
- name the common symptoms other than pain experienced by the dying patient
- describe what is meant by a 'good death'.

INTRODUCTION

When there is advanced disease with no curative treatment, emphasis must be placed on the palliation of symptoms so as to allow the best possible quality of life for patients and their families (World Health Organization 1990).

Specialist palliative care is available as day hospice care, in-patient hospice care and home care teams often known as Macmillan teams. The gold standards framework for community palliative care provides a framework to improve the organisation and quality of care for patients and their families in the community during their last year of life (NHS Education for Scotland [Pharmacy] 2006). The preferred place of care is another concept that contributes to quality of life and of death and can form the basis of care planning (NHS Education for Scotland [Pharmacy] 2006).

Palliative care requires multidisciplinary effort. Its essential components are:

- assessment of the symptoms and needs of the patient
- controlling pain and other distressing symptoms
- helping patients and families cope with the emotional upset and practical problems that arise
- helping people to deal with spiritual questions
- helping people live as actively as possible despite illness
- supporting families and friends in their bereavement.

In palliative care, dying is considered to be a normal process. It is neither hastened nor postponed. Relief from pain and other distressing symptoms is of prime importance. Physical, psychological, social and spiritual aspects of care are integrated to allow the patient to live as actively as possible. Support for the family is provided during the patient's illness and in bereavement.

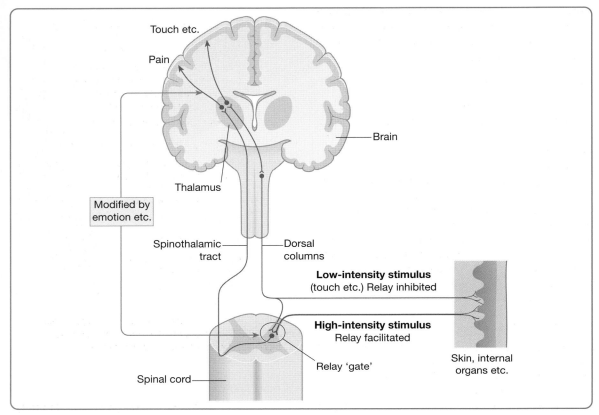

Fig. 26.1 Pathways involved in the perception of pain. (From Greenstein B, Gould D 2004 Trounce's clinical pharmacology for nurses. Churchill Livingstone, Edinburgh. With permission of Elsevier Ltd.)

PAIN

When tissue is damaged, pain may be felt at the site. Damage to nerve endings in skin or internal organs sends impulses to the brain, which interprets these impulses as pain (Fig. 26.1). Medicines that relieve pain may act at different sites along the nerve pathways; for example, local anaesthetics inhibit conduction in nerves carrying impulses from the painful area, and opioid analgesics act on the central nervous system, reducing the sensation of pain.

The body produces its own chemicals, endorphins, which relieve pain (Hughes et al. 1975). When the body feels pain, it is a warning that something is wrong, an injury has been incurred or the body is unwell. The body has its own means of making the pain more bearable. When severe pain is experienced, the body releases endorphins. They act at μ receptors in the central nervous system. Opioid drugs also act at these sites, resulting in analgesia.

PAIN IN PALLIATIVE CARE

Although palliative care comprises several different but complementary elements, the effective relief of pain is perhaps the major challenge facing clinical staff. Multiple pains are often reported by patients with advanced malignant disease. In addition to having pain, the patient may feel depressed and demoralised. Sleep may be prevented. The pain may 'spill over' and affect the patient's family and friends. Just as the presentation of pain can vary, so too can the causes of pain and the sites involved. The treatment chosen will be greatly influenced by the nature of the pain.

As with any treatment programme, it is important to take a careful history and to recognise that the patient will have the expectation of becoming pain-free without reduction in mental alertness. The patient's previous experience may result in fear due to the expectation of pain. Tensions may result that can greatly increase the patient's pain and associated problems. Opportunity should be given to talk over worries and fears. A basic principle is to seek to anticipate crises and avoid having to resort to injections if at all possible.

ASSESSMENT OF PAIN

The basis of successful palliative care is assessment. At an appropriate time and without tiring the patient, details of how the illness began and how the patient and family have coped with it should be established.

Assisting the patient in the completion of some form of pain assessment tool can help to identify the location of the pain, when it arises and its exact nature. The effect of medication or any other activity that helps, as well as those things that make the pain worse, can be recorded. The severity and the nature of the pain can vary, and so it is essential that these are continually reviewed and, when necessary, modifications made to the treatment regimen.

PAIN THRESHOLD

The pain threshold is variable. It changes with external and internal influences (e.g. low self-esteem is linked with a low pain threshold). The following can help to raise the pain threshold and make it much more bearable: symptom control, good quality sleep, a feeling of security and support, treatment of anxiety and depression, helpful explanation, relaxation (perhaps through diversional activities) and the resolution of emotional conflicts.

TREATMENT OF PAIN

The management of pain in malignant disease and palliative care is underpinned by the World Health Organization's pain-relief ladder (World Health Organization 1990; Fig. 26.2). The steps of the ladder represent the severity of the pain and the level of drug therapy required. Analgesics should be given regularly 'by the clock' rather than on an 'as required' basis. The choice of therapy thus depends on the severity of the pain (Table 26.1). Mild pain is treated with a *non-opioid* analgesic drug such as paracetamol or a non-steroidal anti-inflammatory drug that, if given regularly, will often make the use of opioids unnecessary. If pain persists or worsens after the maximum recommended dosage has been reached, these may be changed to a *weak opioid* such as dihydrocodeine or codeine.

In many cases, strong opioids such as morphine or diamorphine may be anticipated and in these cases step 2 of the ladder is missed. There is no advantage

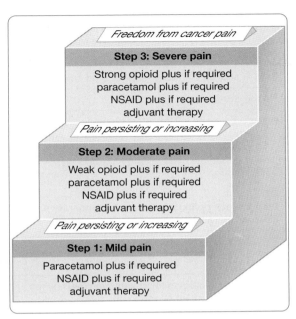

Fig. 26.2 The World Health Organization's pain-relief ladder. NSAID, non-steroidal anti-inflammatory drug. (Courtesy of the World Health Organization.)

in changing to a different weak opioid or combining two together; the patient should be changed to a strong opioid analgesic.

Pain relief should be:
- by the clock
- by the mouth
- by the ladder.

TREATMENT WITH STRONG OPIOIDS

There is no maximum dose.

The overall aim of treatment is to keep the patient pain-free and alert. This is achieved by *regular* administration of the selected dose. Extensive experience has shown that strong opioids are the most valuable drugs in achieving pain relief for many cancer patients with severe pain. Morphine is the strong opioid of choice. The determination of the starting dose will depend on the patient's previous history of analgesic use and on renal function, as outlined in Table 26.2.

Treatment should be commenced with an immediate-release preparation (e.g. Oramorph or Sevredol) at a dose of 10 mg regularly every 4 h plus as-required morphine for breakthrough pain. To calculate the dose for breakthrough pain, divide the total daily dose by 6, and this should be administered as required (consider using a lower dose, 5 mg, if the patient is

Table 26.1 Products used in pain relief

Drug	Dose
Step 1: non-opioid analgesics for mild pain	
Paracetamol	500 mg–1 g orally 4–6-hourly (maximum daily dose 4 g).
Non-steroidal anti-inflammatory drugs[a]	
Ibuprofen	400 mg 8-hourly with or after food.
Diclofenac	75–150 mg daily in two to three divided doses with or after food.
Naproxen	500 mg–1 g daily in one or two divided doses with or after food.
Step 2: weak opioid analgesics for moderate pain (plus, when required, non-opioid adjustment)	
Dihydrocodeine	30–60 mg 4–6-hourly (maximum 240 mg daily).
Codeine	30–60 mg 4 h (maximum 240 mg daily).
Step 3: strong opioids for severe pain (plus, when required, non-opioid or adjuvant)	
Morphine	Strong opioid of choice.
Diamorphine	Very soluble and therefore useful by the parenteral route. It is given subcutaneously (by injection or by syringe driver), intramuscularly and by slow IV injection.
Fentanyl	Initial dose '25' patch or calculated when previous strong opioid has been used. Replaced after 72 h. Apply to non-irritated, non-hairy area in torso or upper arm and rotate site.
Hydromorphone	1.3 mg 4-hourly, increased if necessary according to severity of pain.
Oxycodone	Initially 5 mg every 4–6 h, increased if necessary according to severity of pain, usual maximum 400 mg daily.

[a]Non-steroidal anti-inflammatory drugs are useful for musculoskeletal inflammatory-type pains. They are contraindicated if there is active peptic ulceration or thrombocytopenia. Caution is required in asthma and in cardiac and renal impairment.

frail or elderly or has renal impairment). Pain should be titrated successfully with 4-hourly oral morphine before the patient is changed to a controlled-release preparation. After 24 h, controlled-release morphine suspension may be used in patients who have difficulty in swallowing controlled-release tablets.

To calculate the controlled-release dose, add the total morphine dose taken in the previous 24 h, i.e. regular doses plus as-required doses.

Convert to a modified-release morphine preparation, for example:

MST (12-hourly = twice-daily administration)

MXL (24-hourly = once-daily administration).

The last 4-hourly morphine dose should be given with the first dose of controlled-release morphine.

An immediate-release preparation should be prescribed as required for breakthrough pain. Regular review is essential. Daily increments of 25–50% are reasonable. If the dose is escalating more quickly, then reassess whether the pain is opioid-responsive and whether addition of an adjuvant would be useful.

Table 26.2 Determination of initial morphine and diamorphine dose

Patient's analgesic history	Dose of morphine equivalent	Dose of diamorphine by infusion
Previously controlled on non-opioid (e.g. 1 g paracetamol four times daily)	5 mg of morphine 4-hourly*	10 mg of diamorphine over 24 h
Previously controlled on weak opioid (e.g. dihydrocodeine 60 mg 6-hourly)	10 mg of morphine 4-hourly	20 mg of diamorphine over 24 h
Poor renal function (glomerular filtration rate less than 50 mL/min; potential problem with the elderly)	Doses given (see above*) should be reduced by 50%	
Poor hepatic function	Severe hepatic failure has an effect on morphine metabolism and there may be a need to reduce the dose of morphine	

CASE STUDY

A 56-year-old woman has metastatic colorectal cancer. Despite regular paracetamol and dihydrocodeine, her pain remains poorly controlled.

INITIATING TREATMENT

Discontinue dihydrocodeine. The appropriate starting dose of morphine is 10 mg. This is prescribed as:

10 mg of Oramorph to be given 4-hourly as required.

AFTER 24 H

She has used three doses of Oramorph with benefit, i.e.:

total daily morphine requirement = 3 × 10 mg

= 30 mg.

This can now be converted to modified-release morphine, for example MST Continus 15 mg twice daily (or MXL 30 mg once daily).

The new breakthrough dose is calculated as total daily dose divided by 6, i.e. 5 mg of Oramorph as required.

REVIEW

When next seen, she says that she has needed to use her breakthrough medication six times most days to control her pain, i.e.:

total daily morphine requirement = regular + as required

= (2 × 15 mg) + (6 × 5 mg)

= 60 mg.

The new modified-release morphine dose is MST Continus 30 mg twice daily (or MXL 60 mg once daily).

The new breakthrough dose is 60 mg divided by 6, i.e. 10 mg of Oramorph as required.

PRESCRIBING POINTS FOR OPIOID ANALGESICS

The equivalent single doses of strong analgesics are shown in Table 26.3. Opioid analgesics share many side effects, most commonly nausea, vomiting, constipation and drowsiness. Nausea and sedation usually resolve after 2–3 days. Laxatives should be started as soon as opioids are prescribed. There is no benefit in combining opioid analgesics. Side-effects are not reduced, and assessment of response may be obscured. Oral morphine is available as a solution, suspension, tablets and capsules.

Table 26.3 Equivalent single doses of strong analgesics

Opioid analgesic	Dose (mg)
Morphine salts (oral)	10
Diamorphine hydrochloride (IM)	3
Hydromorphone hydrochloride	1.3
Oxycodone (oral)	5

Table 26.4   Non-oral routes for opioids

Route	Notes
Intravenous or intramuscular	Suitable when relief of pain can be achieved by 4-hourly injections. Greater frequency than this is not acceptable. Diamorphine is more soluble than morphine, and the dose can be given in a smaller volume of water. Diamorphine can be combined with certain drugs (e.g. levomepromazine [methotrimeprazine]).
Rectal	Morphine can be given rectally in doses similar to oral doses. The rectal route may not be acceptable to some patients.
Intrathecal	Combination of low-dose strong opioid and bupivacaine can be given intrathecally. This treatment is suitable for ambulant patients, but spinal catheter care requires special skills.
Transdermal	Fentanyl is available as skin patches only when patient has chronic stable pain and is unable to take morphine. Transdermal systems are expensive and have a slow onset of action. Careful conversion from oral morphine is necessary to achieve equivalent dose.

PATIENT ISSUES

Patients (and healthcare professionals) may have anxieties about morphine. Some of the commonly held beliefs include:

- addiction
- tolerance
- euphoria
- respiratory depression.

These do not occur for the following reasons.

- People are able to stop taking morphine if other interventions successfully reduce pain (e.g. nerve block). Morphine needs to be increased in response to advancing disease process, not because of tolerance.
- Tolerance to strong opioids is not usually a practical problem. Used regularly as an analgesic, it does not directly affect mood, but mood may be improved because of pain relief.
- A therapeutic dose of morphine – when pain is controlled but the patient is not drowsy – does not cause respiratory depression.
- Opioid-induced drowsiness usually diminishes after the first few doses.
- Naloxone (injection) is an opioid antagonist used for the reversal of opioid-induced respiratory depression.

ADMINISTRATION

Whenever possible, the oral route should be used, because it allows the patient to maintain some degree of analgesia control and is preferable to the pain caused by injections into an often emaciated patient. Nausea, vomiting or dysphagia may make it impossible, however, to administer opioids by mouth, and/or the patient may be too weak or drowsy to cope safely with this method. A summary of non-oral routes of administration of opioids is given in Table 26.4. If patients are changed to alternative routes of administration, it is important that they are returned to oral therapy as soon as this is possible. The oral route is the route of choice and when possible should be used.

ADJUVANT DRUG THERAPY

Opioid drugs are, in some patients, ineffective in dealing with particular types of pain, and more specific treatment may be required. These include bone pain, neuropathic pain, muscle spasm, colic and headache. Commonly used adjuvant drugs are listed in Table 26.5. Neuropathic pain is generally managed with a tricyclic antidepressant and certain antiepileptic drugs.

A variety of other forms of therapy are used to relieve pain, promote relaxation and enhance well-being in the terminally ill patient. Treatment that may be used to complement drug therapy includes transcutaneous electrical nerve stimulation, nerve block, progressive muscle relaxation and body massage.

TRANSDERMAL ROUTE

Transdermal preparations of fentanyl may be used when the patient has been stabilised but is unable to take oral morphine. The analgesic levels of fentanyl can be expected 6–12 h after initial application of the patch. It is therefore important to cover this period of time with alternative analgesia until the fentanyl dose builds up (see Table 26.6).

Table 26.5 Adjuvant drugs

Drug	Indication(s)	Dose
Amitriptyline	Neuropathic pain	Initial dose 10 mg at night, increased to 75 mg. Stop if no response.
Clonazepam	Neuropathic pain	0.5–1.5 mg at night.
Gabapentin	Neuropathic pain	Initial dose 300 mg, increased according to response to 1.8 g daily in divided doses.
Dexamethasone	Neuropathic pain, raised intracranial pressure, headache	Trial of a steroid is an appropriate first step. 4–8 mg, 8 a.m. and noon.
Diazepam	Muscle spasm	2–5 mg three times daily (short-term use only).
Hyoscine butylbromide	Visceral colic	20 mg SC bolus, 60 mg SC infusion over 24 h.

Table 26.6 24-h doses of morphine equivalent to fentanyl patches

Morphine (mg daily)	Fentanyl[a]
90	'25' patch
180	'50' patch
270	'75' patch
360	'100' patch

[a]'12' patch, 12 micrograms/h, is available for titrating upwards.

PARENTERAL ADMINISTRATION

When there is no choice but to give a strong opioid parenterally, the subcutaneous route is preferred because it is the least painful method. Diamorphine is very often chosen in preference to morphine, because a very small quantity of diluent is required to reconstitute the powder formulation. The use of an ambulatory pump allows continuous subcutaneous infusion treatment to be delivered and a steady concentration of analgesia to be achieved without the need for repeated injections.

USE OF SYRINGE DRIVERS IN PALLIATIVE CARE

Analgesics in palliative medicine with or without accompanying agents such as antiemetics, sedatives or antimuscarinics are commonly administered by the subcutaneous, epidural or intrathecal route using a syringe driver set at a fixed rate normally measured in mm/h (see Fig. 26.3). This method of administration is indicated when the patient has difficulty in swallowing, is vomiting, has an intestinal obstruction or has diarrhoea affecting absorption. It may be used when the patient is semi-conscious or unconscious.

Ambulant patients are not restricted, because the device is lightweight and may be carried and concealed in a holster. It is especially useful in palliative care, as it reduces the need for repeated injections and provides a steady-state concentration of drug in the plasma.

Care must be taken to observe for and respond to any signs of inflammation at the infusion site, which would be painful and interfere with absorption of the medication.

When setting up a syringe driver, the same care is needed as with the administration of any medication. The drug(s) should be drawn up in a small amount of diluent as prescribed, using a 20-mL syringe. When irritation may be a problem (e.g. with cyclizine), greater dilution using a 30-mL syringe will help reduce this. Water for injections is normally used, as there is less likelihood of precipitation, although a few drugs (e.g. ketamine, ketorolac, octreotide) must be diluted with sodium chloride 0.9% solution. Using the appropriate diluent is important in reducing the risk of incompatibility and inflammation at the chosen site. Further diluent is drawn up, measured against a ruler with a millimetre scale from the first line on the syringe to the rubber bung of the plunger, attached to the giving set and then used to prime the tubing. This should use approximately 2–4 mm of

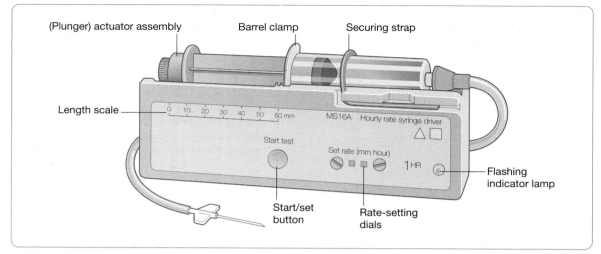

Fig. 26.3 Graseby Medical MS 16A hourly rate syringe driver. (From Mallett J, Dougherty L (eds) 2000 Manual of clinical nursing procedures. Blackwell, Oxford. With permission of Blackwell.)

solution and means that the first syringe will finish in 22–23 h. Details of the contents of the syringe should be entered on the additive label, which is then attached to the syringe (and not the driver). Great care must be taken to place the syringe safely in the driver, with the actuator release button moved into place. The rate should be carefully checked.

The needle is inserted at an angle of 45° into the anterior aspect of the upper arm or thigh or into the anterior chest or abdominal wall. While the infusion is in progress, 4-hourly assessment of the patient's pain should be carried out. At the same time, the infusion site should be checked for signs of inflammation or leakage and the syringe and tubing checked for cloudiness of contents. Checks should also be made and recorded of the rate setting and the length of fluid remaining. The number of millimetres of content should tally with the length expected. Unless there are problems, the site may last for up to 1 week.

As with all infusion devices, care must be taken to handle the equipment carefully. It should not be allowed to get wet, and the progress of the plunger must not be impeded in any way. The driver may be encased in a plastic bag while the patient is bathing or showering.

PREPARATIONS GIVEN VIA SYRINGE DRIVER

Diamorphine is the opioid of choice for subcutaneous injection (see p. 59) and, if required for more than 24 h, for subcutaneous infusion also, as it is more soluble than morphine. If the patient has been receiving oral morphine, the equivalent subcutaneous

Table 26.7 Converting oral morphine to subcutaneous diamorphine

Oral morphine	SC diamorphine equivalent[a]
IR 30 mg 4-hourly	10 mg 4-hourly
CR 60 mg 12-hourly	40 mg in 24 h
CR 60 mg 12-hourly plus IR 20 mg × 3 for breakthrough pain	60 mg in 24 h

CR, controlled release; IR, immediate release.
[a]SC diamorphine is three times more potent than oral morphine.

dose of diamorphine is calculated as one-third of the oral morphine dose (see Table 26.7).

It is important to prevent breakthrough pain when changing from oral to subcutaneous analgesia, and it is recommended that EITHER:

• the subcutaneous infusion is started more than 2 h before the previous oral dose wears off

OR

• a loading dose equivalent to the patient's 4-hourly oral dose is given subcutaneously as the syringe driver is started.

Only certain drugs may be mixed with diamorphine, and only in certain combinations. Mixtures of diamorphine and various other drugs have been administered in day-to-day practice in response to patient needs, although extensive stability data are generally lacking. Nevertheless, experience has shown that few, if any, problems arise if attention is paid to the following.

- Drug combinations should be used within 24 h of admixture.
- Visual inspection of the mixture to detect signs of cloudiness or precipitation, particularly when higher doses of diamorphine are used.
- When several drugs are going to be administered to a patient, and there is doubt as to whether they are compatible in the required dosage, the use of two syringes should be considered.

The following are compatible duos:

- diamorphine/levomepromazine
- diamorphine/haloperidol
- diamorphine/metoclopramide
- diamorphine/cyclizine
- diamorphine/midazolam
- diamorphine/clonazepam
- diamorphine/hyoscine hydrobromide
- diamorphine/hyoscine butylbromide.

Compatible trios

The following information is only a guideline. As concentration increases, the risk of precipitation increases.

- Diamorphine/metoclopramide/midazolam.
- Diamorphine/cyclizine/hyoscine hydrobromide.
- Diamorphine/levomepromazine/hyoscine hydrobromide.

Dexamethasone may give rise to solution difficulties in mixtures, and it is preferable to give subcutaneously twice daily.

Table 26.8 provides suggested doses of drugs to be used in syringe drivers. The procedure involved in the use of syringe drivers is listed in Box 26.1.

SYMPTOMS OTHER THAN PAIN

While pain relief is the cornerstone of care in terminal illness, it is important not to neglect other symptoms that may trouble the patient. Indeed, the alleviation of symptoms such as anxiety and depression can raise the pain threshold, enabling the amount of analgesia to be reduced.

NAUSEA AND VOMITING

Nausea is a distressing symptom at any time, whether or not the patient vomits. In turn, it leads to loss of appetite and loss of weight. Nausea and vomiting are common in patients with advanced malignancy and in the last weeks of life.

There are many causes of nausea and vomiting in terminally ill patients. The choice of antiemetic should be made on the basis of cause and the site of action of specific drugs. Opioids may cause nausea and vomiting in one-third of patients, although this often resolves within 7 days. Alternative strategies may be more appropriate than drug therapy.

Table 26.8 Suggested doses of drugs to be used in syringe drivers[a]

Drug name	Doses often used in practice for palliative care
Cyclizine	150 mg/24 h: antiemetic
Dexamethasone	4–16 mg/24 h: corticosteroid
Diamorphine	No dose limit Maximum concentration: • when used alone, 200 mg/mL • if mixed with other drugs, 150–200 mg/mL opioid analgesic
Haloperidol	2.5–10 mg/24 hours: antiemetic 5–15 mg/24 h: tranquilliser
Hyoscine butylbromide	60–120 mg/24 h: antispasmodic
Hyoscine hydrobromide	0.6–2.4 mg/24 h: antiemetic, antisecretory
Levomepromazine	5–25 mg/24 h: antiemetic 12.5–200 mg/24 h: tranquilliser
Metoclopramide	30–100 mg/24 h: antiemetic
Midazolam	20–100 mg/24 h: sedative
Octreotide	300–600 micrograms/24 h: reducing intestinal secretions in intestinal obstruction and in small bowel fistulae

[a]It is important to remember that the above are only guidelines and that the prescriber is responsible for checking that each medication prescribed is appropriate, not contraindicated, and in the correct dose.

- Constipation-induced nausea and vomiting should always be excluded.
- Psychological factors such as stress and anxiety are potential causes of nausea and vomiting. In such cases, consideration should be given to counselling, explanation of the condition and use of anxiolytics.

Box 26.1 Procedure involved in the use of syringe drivers

- As much care is required in reading the prescription and the details on the label as when preparing to administer any other medicine.
- The amount of diluent is dependent on the number and volume of drugs to be given.
- The size of syringe is 5, 10, 20 or 30 mL.
- Syringe drivers are available that may be set at:
  — *either* millimetres per hour (for rapid infusions)
  — *or* millimetres per 24 h (for palliative care).
- It should be emphasised that these settings express the *distance* travelled by the plunger within a span of time, and not the volume of the drug.
- For convenience, the volume of drug(s) and diluent should be made up to 48 mm.
- To set the rate:
  — measure the distance the plunger has to travel from the first line on the syringe to the black rubber bung of the plunger
  — dial this amount on the syringe driver
  — fill the connecting tubing (the first will run through 1–2 h early, but subsequent syringes will run on time)
  — insert battery into driver
  — press start/test or booster button once.

  Check within the first half hour that the plunger is proceeding as intended.

(After Regnard et al. 2004.)

- Small, more frequent meals can help alleviate vomiting due to 'squashed stomach' syndrome.
- Many people find cooking smells alone can cause nausea, and so it can be helpful to have meals that can be heated quickly in a microwave. Some people find that eating cold food causes less nausea.
- Distraction and relaxation techniques may be helpful.

In any patient, more than one cause of nausea and vomiting may be present. Up to one-third of patients require more than one antiemetic to control their symptoms. The commonest mistake is to use the oral route for antiemetics when nausea is established or vomiting is present.

Drugs used to alleviate nausea and vomiting are listed in Table 26.9.

ANOREXIA

Often, no reason can be found for loss of appetite in terminal illness. If an underlying cause can be found, it should be treated. Causes range from anxiety and depression, nausea and a dry mouth, ill-fitting dentures and oral thrush to drug treatment, chemotherapy or radiotherapy and hypercalcaemia. Meals should be small and light, consist of what patients fancy and be served when they ask for something to eat. Some patients may like and benefit from an aperitif in the form of sherry, whisky or brandy. There may be a place for the use of appropriate nutritional adjuncts on the advice of the dietitian. Relatives understandably are disappointed and distressed when the patient has no interest in food, and so they may need encouragement of a different sort at this time. Options for drug therapy include dexamethasone (2–4 mg oral daily), prednisolone (15–30 mg oral daily) or metoclopramide (10–20 mg oral daily before meals).

Table 26.9   Drugs that alleviate symptoms of nausea and vomiting

Drug	Indication	Dose
Metoclopramide	Vomiting associated with gastritis, functional bowel obstruction	10 mg three times daily
Haloperidol	Vomiting caused by hypercalcaemia, renal failure	1.5 mg once or twice daily
Cyclizine	Nausea and vomiting due to mechanical obstruction, raised intracranial pressure, motion sickness	50 mg up to three times daily
Levomepromazine	Used if first-line antiemetics are inadequate	6–25 mg daily

CONSTIPATION

Difficulty in moving the bowels is common in cases of advanced cancer and is a major cause of anxiety and discomfort. The aim is prevention, and it is good nursing practice to ask, assess, document and review regularly. As always, it is essential to carry out a thorough assessment before embarking on treatment. This may include a rectal examination to establish whether the rectum is full. Note should be taken of any faecal smearing suggestive of overflow. Faecal impaction can lead to many other problems, including urinary retention, overflow, restlessness, confusion and falls, each one leading to the next. Evidence of intestinal obstruction should be reported at once and any measures to relieve constipation withheld until the patient has been examined by a doctor.

Drug treatment is the commonest cause of constipation, especially when opioids such as morphine or codeine-containing substances are being used. In terminal illness, laxatives should be started along with opioid treatment, or for anyone receiving antimuscarinics. As the opioids are increased, so too should be the dose of laxative.

The choice of laxative and dose should be tailored to each patient's needs. Most patients will benefit from a faecal softener with a peristaltic stimulant (e.g. co-danthramer), or docusate with senna can be used.

DIARRHOEA

Before treating diarrhoea, it is important first to exclude the most common causes, namely excessive use of laxatives, impaction with overflow and diet. Profuse watery diarrhoea can leave the patient dehydrated and exhausted. A high intake of fluid is essential, and the patient will need as much rest and assistance as required. Loperamide has an antimotility effect. The dose is 4 mg taken initially then 2 mg oral after each loose stool, up to 16 mg daily. If a patient is already taking morphine, there is little point in adding codeine.

DYSPHAGIA

Patients may have difficulty in swallowing, because it is painful to do so (e.g. in oesophageal thrush) or because there is a partial obstruction (e.g. in oesophageal spasm or carcinoma), in which case food will be regurgitated. Mealtimes are no longer enjoyable, and yet the patient may still have a desire to eat. Weight may be lost quickly and the patient starts to feel weak. An appropriate consistency of food should be used and referral made to the dietitian. Dexamethasone 8 mg daily for several days may decrease oedema and maintain the oesophageal lumen.

HICCUP

Terminally ill patients sometimes develop persistent hiccup caused by gastric distension, which is exhausting. It interferes with eating, speaking and sleep and may be a source of disturbance for others. Hiccup may respond to simple measures initially, such as 20 mL of peppermint water or one or two heaped teaspoons of granulated sugar.

Hiccup due to gastric distension may respond to a preparation containing an antacid and an antiflatulent, e.g. Altacite Plus, Asilone, Maalox Plus. The management of intractable hiccup includes:

- metoclopramide 10 mg 6–8-hourly plus antacid
- chlorpromazine 10–25 mg 6–8-hourly (this is sedating, and so patients should be counselled accordingly)
- nifedipine 10–20 mg 12-hourly
- baclofen 5–10 mg 12-hourly (can be increased slowly – watch for side effects)
- high-dose dexamethasone 16 mg daily if cerebral irritation.

If all else fails, midazolam by subcutaneous infusion may be required.

ORAL COMPLICATIONS

Problems in or around the mouth are often a great source of discomfort to the dying patient. There may be problems in keeping the mouth clean, and frequent attention is important. The mouth may be dry and make for difficulty in speaking and eating. Some drugs, notably morphine sulphate and antimuscarinics such as hyoscine, may make the mouth feel dry (White et al. 1989). Bacterial, viral or fungal infections of the mouth may cause severe pain and difficulty in swallowing. Ulceration may occur. Halitosis may be a source of embarrassment to the patient and/or family (see also p. 485).

Simple non-specific, prophylactic measures of mouth care should always be employed to prevent or relieve such distressing problems. These include:

- regular mouthwashes (chlorhexidine gluconate mouthwash 0.2%: 10 mL twice daily)
- 50:50 mixture of dry cider and tonic or soda water can be very useful and palatable!
- pineapple juice
- sucking crushed ice
- frequent sips of iced water
- benzydamine (Difflam) oral rinse (may be beneficial if the mouth is painful).

RESPIRATORY SYMPTOMS

DYSPNOEA

As with all other symptoms in terminal illness, any underlying cause should be treated if possible. For example, if there is evidence of airways reversibility bronchodilators may be used. Otherwise, opioids are used to control dyspnoea.

Breathlessness at rest may be relieved by regular oral morphine in carefully titrated doses starting at 5 mg every 4 h. The morphine reduces the sensitivity of central chemoreceptors to rises in the concentration of carbon dioxide and also reduces respiratory drive and eases the sensation of dyspnoea.

If the patient is already receiving morphine, the morphine dose should be increased by 20–30%. There may be a place for using anxiolytics in some patients. Sublingual lorazepam 0.5–1 mg is used for shortness of breath. Diazepam 5–10 mg daily may be helpful for dyspnoea associated with anxiety. A corticosteroid such as dexamethasone 4–8 mg daily may also be helpful if there is bronchospasm or partial obstruction. Five millilitres of nebulised 0.9% sodium chloride solution aids expectoration of thickened secretions.

Positioning patients in bed with the help of suitably placed pillows or nursing them comfortably in an upright chair instead of in bed creates a challenge for the nurse. Methods of promoting relaxation should be provided. Loose clothing and an open window or a fan may assist. Fluids and oral care may have to be increased to relieve dryness of the mouth caused by mouth breathing and oxygen therapy.

INTRACTABLE COUGH

Like hiccup, a persistent cough can be painful and distressing, leaving the patient exhausted and others disturbed. Simple linctuses may be tried, as well as moist inhalations. Oral morphine hydrochloride solution may be needed and is given initially as 5 mg every 4 h. In patients already receiving morphine for pain control, the morphine dose should be increased by 20–30%.

EXCESSIVE RESPIRATORY SECRETION ('DEATH RATTLE')

Accumulation of secretions in the pharynx, trachea and bronchi, colloquially referred to as 'death rattle', is generally seen only in patients who are too weak to expectorate. The noise is distressing for family members and other patients, but the patient will not be aware. An explanation to the relatives will help reduce their anxieties and concerns. Repositioning the patient and occasional, gentle suctioning will provide some relief.

Excessive respiratory secretion may be reduced by subcutaneous injection of hyoscine hydrobromide 400–600 micrograms every 4–8 h. Alternatively, glycopyrronium may be given by subcutaneous or intramuscular injection in a dose of 200 micrograms every 4 h.

SKIN CONDITIONS

PRURITUS

Itching of the skin is a troublesome feature of terminal illness and can be the source of irritability and disturbed sleep. Especially problematic is itching due to obstructive jaundice, which may be extremely persistent and difficult to manage in some patients and yet mysteriously vanish in others. Drug reactions may be present (associated rash, recent introduction of opioid, etc.), and so medication review is necessary. Dry skin is a common cause of pruritus in advanced cancer and often responds to simple measures, i.e.:

- using emollients (e.g. aqueous cream)
- using soap substitutes when bathing
- avoiding overheating
- discouraging scratching
- patting the skin dry with a towel rather than rubbing.

The drug treatment of pruritus may include anti-histamines but should always be used in conjunction with good skin care.

SWEATING

Underlying causes such as anxiety, menopausal flushing, infection and thyrotoxicosis should be excluded. Hot drinks and hot baths should be avoided. The patient may be tepid sponged if unable to take a cool shower. Clothes and bedding should be made of cotton and changed as soon as they are damp. Patients may appreciate having their hair washed or at least dried. The use of a single room may allow the environmental temperature to be controlled without upsetting other patients. A bedside fan may offer some relief if carefully positioned. Care must be taken to prevent chilling the patient. Cold drinks and oral hygiene are important. An antimuscarinic such as propantheline 15–30 mg 8–12-hourly may be helpful.

CENTRAL NERVOUS SYSTEM SYMPTOMS

INSOMNIA

It is important to assess the situation fully and to establish what 'difficulty in sleeping' means to the individual patient. Any obvious causes should be treated. Patients should be discouraged from taking naps during the day and should stick to their normal bedtime. Various methods of relaxation may be utilised. Stimulant drugs should be used only in the early part of the day. A milky drink free from caffeine may help before going to bed. As well as a quiet, comfortable environment, peace of mind is essential. A short-acting benzodiazepine such as temazepam will help the patient to fall asleep.

ANXIETY

Listening is of paramount importance. The patient will need reassurance about worries and fears and the meaning of symptoms. Drug treatment takes second place to identifying and dealing with the underlying cause of the patient's anxiety. Antipsychotics such as haloperidol and chlorpromazine may be used in low doses for severe anxiety. They have a moderately sedative action. Diazepam 2.5–5 mg 8-hourly is the drug of choice if a regular anxiolytic is required, because of its long half-life. Lorazepam 0.5–1 mg sublingually may be used in severe acute anxiety.

CONFUSION

When it can be identified, the underlying cause should be treated. There are many possible reasons why a patient may be confused, including hypoxia, cerebral metastases, infection, hypercalcaemia, uraemia and constipation. Confusion may also be drug-induced or result from withdrawal from a drug.

A quiet, well-lit room should be provided and care delivered in a calm, reassuring manner. Staff should introduce themselves and explain any procedure before commencement. Relatives will also require understanding care.

Restlessness and confusion may require treatment with haloperidol 1–3 mg by mouth every 8 h. Chlorpromazine 25–50 mg by mouth every 8 h is an alternative but causes more sedation. Levomepromazine (methotrimeprazine) is also used occasionally for restlessness.

DEPRESSION

It is important to recognise that the patient may become clinically depressed at this time. Emotional support and encouragement will be needed. Antidepressant therapy generally takes about 3 weeks to take effect (see Table 26.10 for doses). Many patients respond to this type of treatment, although not all.

ASCITES

The development of peritoneal metastases from primary tumours of the bronchus or breast results in the distressing accumulation of fluid in the peritoneal cavity known as ascites. A slow reduction in the ascites may be achieved with the administration of spironolactone 200–400 mg daily by mouth. Furosemide 40–80 mg daily by mouth may be added if spironolactone alone is not giving the desired effect. Once the effect is achieved, the loop diuretic should be reduced or stopped.

Table 26.10 Doses of antidepressant therapy

Drug	Dose and frequency
Amitriptyline	75–150 mg oral at night
Sertraline	50–200 mg oral daily
Mirtazapine	15–45 mg oral daily
Venlafaxine	75–150 mg oral daily

SELF-ASSESSMENT QUESTIONS

1. Name a corticosteroid used to relieve intracranial pressure.
2. Name a tricyclic antidepressant used to treat neuropathic pain.
3. Name two drugs used to control excessive respiratory secretions.
4. Give two advantages to the transdermal route for administering pain relief.
5. Give two indications for the use of antacids in palliative care.
6. Morphine is preferred to methadone for the relief of intractable pain. Why?
7. Which two drugs may cause a dry mouth?
8. To which class of drugs do these drugs belong?
9. Antiemetics used in palliative care may have side effects. Name an antiemetic and its side-effects.
10. Give three reasons for the choice of the parenteral route in palliative care.
11. By what route is fentanyl administered?
12. Give one example of the following:
    a. a non-opioid
    b. a weak opioid
    c. a strong opioid (long-acting)
13. Give two examples of adjuvant drug therapy used in palliative care.
14. What do you understand by the term *palliative care*?

15. Using the British National Formulary, identify the most appropriate drugs for treating the following symptoms:
    - diarrhoea
    - anxiety
    - anorexia
    - constipation
    - dry mouth
    - pruritus
    - sweating
    - hiccup
    - dysphagia
    - dyspnoea
    - confusion
    - mouth problems
    - insomnia
    - depression
    - intractable cough
    - ascites.

REFERENCES

Hughes J, Smith TW, Kosterlitz HW et al. 1975 Identification of two related pentapeptides from the brain with potent opiate agonist activity. Nature 258:577–579

NHS Education for Scotland (Pharmacy) 2006 Pharmaceutical care of people requiring palliative care. NES, Edinburgh

Regnard C, Kindlen, Alport S 2004 Procedures in palliative care: 1. Setting up a syringe driver. Worksheet. Coleman Education Centre, St Oswald's Hospice, Newcastle-upon-Tyne

White ID, Hoskin PJ, Hanks GW et al. 1989 Morphine and dryness of the mouth. British Medical Journal 298:1222–1223

World Health Organization 1990 Cancer pain relief and palliative care. WHO, Geneva

FURTHER READING AND RESOURCES

Kinghorn S, Gamlin R (eds) 2001 Palliative nursing: bringing comfort and hope. Bailliere Tindall, Edinburgh, in conjunction with the Royal College of Nursing, London

Montgomery F 2002 Pain management in palliative care. Pharmaceutical Journal 268:254–256

Scottish Intercollegiate Guidelines Network 2000 Control of pain in patients with cancer. No. 44. SIGN, Edinburgh

Serpell M 2006 Recognising and treating neuropathic pain. Progress in Neurology and Psychiatry 10:15–20

GLOSSARY, APPENDICES AND ANSWERS TO SELF-ASSESSMENT QUESTIONS

Glossary

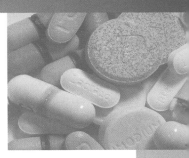

A

Absorption. Process by which a drug reaches the general circulation and becomes biologically available.

ACE inhibitors. Drugs that act on the renin–angiotensin–aldosterone system, inhibiting the angiotensin-converting enzyme.

Active immunisation. Injection of an antigen in the form of live or attenuated organisms or their products to provide protection against certain infections.

Active transport. Cellular activity that transfers a drug from an area of low concentration to one of higher concentration.

Addiction. Inability to control craving for a drug.

Additive. Substance added to, for example, an existing solution.

Adjuvant therapy. The simultaneous use of different forms of treatment (e.g. drugs with other types of drugs, drugs with radiotherapy and/or surgery).

Adjuvant. Substance included in the formulation of a medicine to improve stability of the dosage form.

Adsorption. The taking up of a liquid or vapour on the surface of a solid.

Adverse drug reaction. Any response to a drug that is noxious or unintended and occurs at doses used for prophylaxis, diagnosis or therapy (see also *Side effect*).

Aerobe. An organism that can live and reproduce only in the presence of free oxygen.

Agonist. Drug with an affinity for a receptor, resulting in stimulation of the receptor's functional properties.

Alkylating drugs. Cytotoxic agents that act by providing an unbreakable link between the strands of DNA, thus blocking cell replication.

Allergy. Hypersensitivity reaction to an intrinsically harmful substance, varying from a mild form to severe and life-threatening.

Ampoule. A sterile glass or plastic container that usually contains a single dose of a solution to be administered parenterally.

Anaerobe. An organism that can live and reproduce only in the absence of oxygen.

Analogue. A drug that resembles another in structure and constituents but has different effects.

Anaphylaxis. Life-threatening reaction to a foreign protein or other substance.

Antagonist. An agent that exerts an opposite action to an agonist.

Antibacterial. A chemical compound that kills or prevents the growth of bacteria.

Antibiotic. A chemical compound derived from natural sources that kills or prevents the growth of bacteria or fungi.

Anticholinergic drug. Substance that competes with the neurotransmitter acetylcholine for its receptor sites at synaptic junctions.

Anticoagulant. Substance that delays or prevents clotting of the blood.

Antimetabolites. Cytotoxic agents that mimic the respective partners for purines and pyrimidines and because of imperfect pairing arrest the development of new DNA.

Antimicrobial. A chemical compound that kills or prevents the growth of microorganisms (viruses, bacteria, or fungi).

Antimuscarinic drug. Substance that inhibits the stimulation of postganglionic fibres.

Apoptosis. Programmed cell death.

Attenuated. Reduction of virulence of a micro-organism with retention of antigenic properties.

B

Bactericidal. Destroying bacteria.

Bacteriostatic. Inhibiting growth or multiplication of bacteria.

Beta-blocker. Agent that inhibits the action of catecholamines at beta-adrenergic receptor sites.

Bioavailability. Amount and rate of appearance of a drug in the blood after administration of the dosage form.

Biocide. Chemical agent such as a pesticide that is capable of destroying living organisms.

Buccal. Between the gum and the cheek.

C

Calcineurin. A phosphatase that is activated by a calcium complex which in turn activates elements of the immune system.

Chemotherapy. Treatment using drugs – generally used when referring to cytotoxic therapy.

Clinical pharmacy. Discipline concerned with application of pharmaceutical expertise to help maximise drug efficacy and minimise drug toxicity in individual patients and patient populations.

Colloid. Microscopic insoluble particles.

Compliance. The extent to which the patient's behaviour coincides with medical or health advice.

Concordance. Partnership between prescriber and patient in which there are shared objectives aimed at achieving a therapeutic outcome.

Controlled dosage system. Sealed compartmentalised tray presentation normally based on a week's supply.

Controlled drug. Drug of addiction subject to strict regulatory control.

Crystalloid. An electrolyte in solution.

Cycloplegic. An agent that causes paralysis of the ciliary muscle of the eye, used prior to ophthalmic examination or surgery.

Cytotoxic. Capable of destroying cells.

D

Diuretic. A drug that increases the manufacture of urine by the kidneys.

Drug. Substance used to prevent, diagnose or treat disease.

Dyspnoea. Shortness of breath or difficulty in breathing.

E

Enteral. Via the intestine.

Enteric coating. An acid-resistant coating of tablets or compounds that prevents release of active ingredient(s) until the dosage form reaches the alkaline medium of the small intestine, where release and absorption take place.

Excipient. Substance mixed with a medicine to provide consistency, bulk or stability of a formulation.

Extemporaneous. One-off production of a preparation to meet an individual patient's requirement.

Extravasation. Escape of a fluid from a blood vessel into surrounding tissues.

F

Femtolitre. A thousand-million-millionth of a litre (10^{-15}).

Fingertip unit. Amount of cream or ointment (steroid preparations) expressed from a tube with a standard 5-mm diameter nozzle, applied from the distal crease to the tip of the adult index finger.

First-pass effect. Effect caused by metabolism of a drug mainly by the liver, resulting in only part of the drug reaching the systemic circulation.

Formulary. Approved list of pharmaceutical items for routine use together with information to assist in rational prescribing.

Formulation. Form in which a medicine is made up (e.g. tablet, capsule, solution, suspension).

G

Gene therapy. Treatment of diseases by insertion into the body of genetic material.

H

Half-life. Time taken for a drug to lose 50% of its effect in a person's body.

Hickman catheter. Example of a device used to access a central vein for the infusion of large amounts of fluid and irritant substances and for obtaining blood samples.

Hydrophilic. Associating freely with water and readily entering into aqueous solution.

Hygroscopic. Absorbing moisture from the air.

Hypercalcaemia. Abnormal increase of calcium in the blood.

Hyperglycaemia. Abnormal increase in blood glucose level.

Hyperinflation. The inability to fully exhale, leading to air being trapped in the lungs, such as happens in those who have chronic obstructive pulmonary disease or are chronic smokers.

Hyperkalaemia. Abnormal increase of potassium in the blood.

Hypernatraemia. Abnormal increase of sodium in the blood.

Hypersensitivity reaction. Exaggerated response to a drug.

Hypertonic. Of a solution, having a higher osmotic pressure than a specified solution.

Hypocalcaemia. Abnormally low blood calcium level.

Hypoglycaemia. Abnormally low blood glucose level.

Hypokalaemia. Abnormally low blood potassium level.

Hyponatraemia. Abnormally low blood sodium level.

Hypotonic. Of a solution, having a lower osmotic pressure than a specified solution.

I

Iatrogenic. Of a condition, caused by treatment.

Idiosyncracy. An individual's unique hypersensitivity to a particular drug.

Immunoglobulin. Humoral antibody produced by the blood.

Inotropic. Controlling muscular contraction, especially in the heart.

Intrathecal. Within the subarachnoid space.

L

Loading dose. Initial dose of a drug that is twice the maintenance dose given, to allow the effective blood concentration to be reached promptly.

M

Medicine. Formulation of a drug into a suitable preparation for administration.

Microgram. One-thousandth of a milligram.

Milligram. One-thousandth of a gram.

Monoclonal. Pertaining to a group of cells derived from a single cell.

Monoclonal antibody. An antibody that is biologically engineered to target specific cells.

Monomer. The simplest of any series of compounds having the same empirical formula (opposite of polymer).

Mydriatic. A drug that dilates the pupil of the eye by contraction of the muscle of the iris.

N

Nanogram. One-thousandth of a microgram.

Nosocomial infection. Hospital-acquired infection.

O

Orphan drugs. Drugs used to treat very rare conditions which may be difficult to source via normal channels.

Over-the-counter medicines. Medicines available without a prescription.

P

Palliative. Providing relief as opposed to a cure.

Parenteral. Other than the alimentary canal; by injection.

Passive immunisation. Injection of antibodies from immunised animals against the invading organism.

Pharmaceutical care. Direct pharmaceutical contribution to patient care.

Pharmacodynamics. Process by which specific drug dosages produce biochemical or physiological changes in the body.

Pharmacokinetics. Study of actions of drugs within the body.

Pharmacology. The science of drugs.

Pharmacy. Concerned with supplying, preparing, compounding, dispensing and safe use of medicines.

Picogram. A million-millionth of a gram.

Piggyback technique. Method of administering intermittent intravenous medication via a small secondary container attached by tubing to a primary infusion line.

Placebo. Inactive substance prescribed as if it were an effective medication dose (e.g. in clinical trials).

Polymer. One of a series of substances alike in composition but differing in molecular weight.

Polypharmacy. Use of many different drugs in treatment of disease.

Polysaccharide. A carbohydrate that hydrolyses into more than one molecule of simple sugars.

Potency. Of a drug, the relative amount of a drug required to produce the desired response.

Prion. Microscopic mutant protein particle similar to a virus but lacking nucleic acid; thought to be the infectious agent responsible for certain degenerative disorders of the nervous system such as bovine spongiform encephalitis.

Prophylaxis. Disease prevention.

Proprietary drug. Any pharmaceutical preparation protected from commercial competition by trademark and/or patent.

R

Recreational drug. One that is used for its stimulating psychological or physical effects with no therapeutic intent.

S

Scheduled drugs. Drugs classified by legislation into categories known as schedules (of which there are five) according to their potential to cause harm if abused.

Shared-care protocol. Signed agreement between hospital specialist and GP that clearly defines roles and responsibilities when a patient requires care from both hospital and primary care.

Side effect. Undesirable, unwanted or unexpected effect of a drug administered within the therapeutic range (see also *Adverse drug reaction*).

Subcutaneous. Fatty layer beneath the dermis of the skin.

Sublingual. Under the tongue.

Sympathomimetic. Mimicking the sympathetic nervous system by producing similar effects.

Systemic. Pertaining to the whole body.

T

Tolerance. Ability to endure a substance without it causing physiological or psychological harm.

Topical. For local effect; often used to refer to a drug applied to the skin.

V

Vasoconstriction. Narrowing of the lumen of blood vessels.

Vial. Small glass rubber-capped container holding a drug either as a liquid or as a powder for reconstitution.

X

Xanthine. Nitrogenous by-product of metabolism of nucleoproteins, normally found in muscles, liver, spleen, pancreas and the urine.

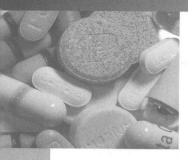

Appendix 1 - Abbreviations

ABVD	adriamycin, bleomycin, vinblastine, dacarbazine
ACAG	acute closed-angle glaucoma
ACBS	Advisory Committee on Borderline Substances
ACE	angiotensin-converting enzyme
ACTH	adrenocorticotrophic hormone
AIDS	acquired immune deficiency syndrome
APTT	activated partial thromboplastin time
ART	assisted reproduction therapy
AZT	zidovudine (azidothymidine)
BCG	bacille Calmette–Guérin
BEAM	BCNU, etoposide, cytarabine, melphalan
BEP	bleomycin, etoposide, cisplatin
BMI	basal metabolic index
BM-test	Boehringer–Mannheim reagent strips for blood glucose monitoring
BNF	British National Formulary
BP	British Pharmacopoeia
BPC	British Pharmaceutical Codex
CAM	Complementary and alternative medicine
CAP	capsule
CAPD	continuous ambulatory peritoneal dialysis
CAV	cyclophosphamide, adriamycin, vincristine
CCK-PZ	cholecystokinin-pancreozymin
CD	controlled drug
CFCs	chlorofluorocarbons
ChlVPP	chlorambucil, vinblastine, procarbazine, prednisolone
CHOP	cyclophosphamide, adriamycin, vincristine, prednisolone
CIVAS	central intravenous additive service
CMF	cyclophosphamide, methotrexate, fluorouracil
CMV	cytomegalovirus
COC	combined oral contraception
COPD	chronic obstructive pulmonary disease
COSHH	control of substances hazardous to health
COX	cyclo-oxygenase
CSM	Committee on Safety of Medicines
CTZ	chemoreceptor trigger zone
CVP	cyclophosphamide, vincristine, prednisolone
D&TC	Drug and Therapeutics Committee
DdATP	dideoxyadenosine triphosphate
ddCTP	dideoxycytidine-5-triphosphate
ddI	didanosine
DDI	didanosine
dL	decilitre(s)
DMARD	disease-modifying antirheumatic drug
DMSO	dimethylsulphoxide
DNA	deoxyribonucleic acid
DT	diphtheria, tetanus
DTP	diphtheria, tetanus, pertussis
DUMP	disposal of unwanted medicines and pills
e/c	enteric-coated
FBC	full blood count
FEV_1	forced expiratory volume in 1 second
fL	femtolitre(s)
FTU	fingertip unit (adult)
g	gram(s)
G6PD	glucose-6-phosphate dehydrogenase
GABA	gamma-aminobutyric acid
G-CSF	granulocyte-colony stimulating factor
GFR	glomerular filtration rate
GP10	GP prescription
GSL	General sale list
HBP(A)	hospital-based prescribers' form for addicts (Scotland)
HDCV	human diploid cell vaccine
HDL	high-density lipoprotein
HFAs	hydrofluoroalkanes
Hib	*Haemophilus influenzae* type b
HIV	human immunodeficiency virus
HRT	hormone replacement therapy
HT	hydroxytryptamine
HTBS	Health Technology Board for Scotland
ID	intradermal
IDDM	insulin-dependent diabetes mellitus
IM	intramuscular
INHAL	inhalational
INR	international normalised ratio
IOP	intraocular pressure
IPV	inactivated poliomyelitis vaccine
ISA	intrinsic sympathomimetic activity
IV	intravenous
kg	kilogram(s)
L	litre(s)
LDL	low-density lipoprotein
LFTs	liver function tests
m/r	modified-release
MAOI	monoamine-oxidase inhibitor
MBC	minimum bactericidal concentration
MCA	Medicines Control Agency
mg	milligram(s)
MHRA	Medicines and Healthcare products Regulatory Agency
MIC	minimum inhibitory concentration
MIMS	Monthly Index of Medical Specialities
mL	millilitre(s)
MMR	mumps, measles, rubella
MOPP	chlormethine (mustine), vincristine, procarbazine, prednisolone
MRSA	methicillin-resistant *Staphylococcus aureus*

MST	morphine sulphate tablets
NEFA	non-esterified fatty acid
ng	nanogram(s)
NG	nasogastric
NHS	National Health Service
NICE	National Institute for Health and Clinical Excellence
NIDDM	non-insulin-dependent diabetes mellitus
nm	nanometre
NMC	Nursing and Midwifery Council
NNRTIs	non-nucleoside reverse transcriptase inhibitors
NPF	Nurse Prescribers' Formulary
NSAID	non-steroidal anti-inflammatory drug
OGTT	oral glucose tolerance test
ORS	oral rehydration salts
ORT	oral rehydration therapy
OTC	over the counter
PACG	primary angle-closure glaucoma
PCA	patient-controlled analgesia
PEFR	peak expiratory flow rate (maximal flow) – expressed as L/min – after a full inhalation
PEG	percutaneous endoscopic gastrostomy
pg	picogram(s)
PGD	patient group direction
POAG	primary open-angle glaucoma
PODs	patients' own drugs
POM	prescription-only medicine
POP	progestogen-only pill
PPD	purified protein derivative

PPI	proton pump inhibitor
PR	per rectum
PTT	partial thromboplastin time
PUVA	psoralen. A combination of long-wave ultraviolet (UVA) with a psoralen (P).
PV	per vaginam
PVA	polyvinyl alcohol
RCV	rubber-capped vial
RIMA	reversible inhibitor of monoamine oxidase A
rINN	recommended international non-proprietary name
RNA	ribonucleic acid
RT	reverse transcriptase
s/c	sugar-coated
SC	subcutaneous
SI units	Système International
SIGN	Scottish Intercollegiate Guidelines Network
SL	sublingual
SPF	sun protection factor
SSRI	selective serotonin re-uptake inhibitor
Tab	tablet
TENS	transcutaneous electrical nerve stimulation
TIVA	total intravenous anaesthetic
TPN	total parenteral nutrition
U and Es	urea and electrolytes
UVA	ultraviolet radiation (long wavelength)
UVB	ultraviolet radiation (medium wavelength)
WBC	white blood count

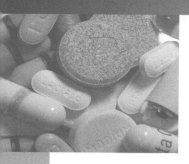

Appendix 2 - Normal values

BIOCHEMICAL

VENOUS BLOOD: APPROXIMATE ADULT REFERENCE VALUES

Acid phosphatase	
Total	up to 12 IU/L
Prostatic	up to 4 IU/L
Alkaline phosphatase	30–120 IU/L
Bicarbonate	22–30 mmol/L
Bilirubin	0–17 micromoles/L
Calcium	2.26–2.60 mmol/L
Chloride	95–105 mmol/L
Cholesterol	
Male	2.5–7.9 mmol/L
Female	2.5–8.8 mmol/L
Copper	12–26 micromoles/L
Creatinine	
Male	50–100 micromoles/L
Female	50–80 micromoles/L
Glucose (fasting)	2.9–6.4 mmol/L
Iron	
Male	14–32 mmol/L
Female	10–28 mmol/L
Iron-binding capacity	45–72 mmol/L
Lactate dehydrogenase (LDH)	100–300 IU/mL
Magnesium	0.70–1.20 mmol/L
pH	7.36–7.44
Phosphate	0.80–1.45 mmol/L
Potassium	3.4–5.2 mmol/L

Proteins	
Total	60–80 g/L
Albumin	35–58 g/L
Sodium	133–144 mmol/L
Urea	2.5–7.5 mmol/L
Uric acid	
Male	0.15–0.42 mmol/L
Female	0.10–0.36 mmol/L

HAEMATOLOGICAL

VENOUS BLOOD: APPROXIMATE ADULT REFERENCE VALUES

Erythrocyte sedimentation rate (ESR)	0–6 mm in 1 h
Fibrinogen	150–400 mg/dL
Folate	2.1–21 micrograms/L
Haemoglobin (Hb)	
Male	13–18 g/dL
Female	11.5–16.5 g/dL
Leucocytes: differential count	
Neutrophils	$2.5–7.5 \times 10^9$/L
Lymphocytes	$1.5–3.5 \times 10^9$/L
Monocytes	$0.2–0.8 \times 10^9$/L
Eosinophils	$0.015–0.1 \times 10^9$/L
Basophils	$0.04–0.44 \times 10^9$/L
Mean cell haemoglobin (MCH)	27–32 pg (1.7–2.0 pg/cell)

Mean cell haemoglobin concentration (MCHC) — 30–35 g/dL

Mean cell volume (MCV) — 78–98 fL

Packed cell volume (PCV)
- Male — 0.40–0.54
- Female — 0.35–0.47

Platelet count — $150–400 \times 10^9$/L

Prothrombin time (PT) — 10–14 s

Reticulocytes — 0.2–2.0% of red blood cells

Vitamin B_{12} — 120–600 micrograms/L

ARTERIAL BLOOD: APPROXIMATE ADULT REFERENCE VALUES

Carbon dioxide ($P_a CO_2$) — 4.8–6.0 kPa (36–45 mmHg)

Oxygen ($P_a O_2$) — 11–13 kPa (83–98 mmHg)

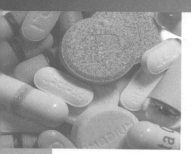

Answers to self-assessment questions

CHAPTER 2   CONTROL OF MEDICINES IN HOSPITAL AND COMMUNITY

SECTION A

1. b.
2. b.
3. c.
4. c.

SECTION B

1. Go to the medicine cupboard with the doctor, open the cupboard to allow access and then lock the cupboard. Keep the keys on your person.
2a. Write in the controlled drugs record book, on the appropriate page, after the last entry: 'Stock checked. One tablet missing. Stock balance 17 tablets. [Signatures of both nurses.] [Date.]'
2b. Report discrepancy to ward manager and clinical pharmacist. At the next routine check, it should be especially noted that all stock is correct.
3. The Nursing and Midwifery Council's statement on transcribing is that it is not illegal. However, registrants, because they are accountable, should check the local policy before transcribing.
4. Two years.
5. Remove the backing, fold it over (so that it sticks to itself) and place in a colour-coded medicines waste disposal bin or return to pharmacy with other medicines waste.
6. During transportation and distribution; careless custody of keys; inadequate storage.
7. That the label on a medicine dispensed by a pharmacist is clearly written and unambiguous, and that the expiry date has not passed.
8. Yes, as long as there is a registered nurse to check the controlled drug with.

CHAPTER 3   THE ROLE OF THE NURSE IN DRUG THERAPY

SECTION A

1. The person administering the medicine.
2. Safety and security; to the correct patient, at the correct time, on the correct date, by the correct route, in the correct dose; signed for by the prescriber.
3. Exceptionally, yes, although not a controlled drug in schedules 2 and 3. Should ideally get a second person to listen to and confirm the telephone instruction. Must be followed up by written prescription within 24 h.
4. Address patient by name, read bedside chart, read wristband, ask patient to state name, ask another member of staff, ask relative.
5. The very old and the very young.
6. What it is being given for; the strength, dose, route, time(s) or frequency; if known, how long the course will last; any side effects to expect; any special considerations.
7. Eyesight; literacy, language, intelligence; dexterity; motivation.
8. Returned to the pharmacy.
9. Temperature, pulse, respirations, blood pressure; blood gases, blood glucose, international normalised ratio, white blood count.
10. In the absence of any authorised variation from the original prescription, the prescriber should be consulted.

CHAPTER 4   ADMINISTRATION OF MEDICINES

SECTION A

1. Date, name of drug dose, route, time or frequency of administration and prescriber's signature.
2. Address patient by name, read bedside chart, read wristband, ask patient to state name, ask another member of staff, ask relative.

3. Encourage into sitting position, if possible; give suitable drink to start process; ensure plenty to drink; encourage to place tablet at back of tongue; consider whether tablet can be divided or crushed, or available in liquid form. Ask pharmacist's advice.

4. Shake bottle to mix contents, hold bottle with label uppermost, pour at eye level in a good light, wipe bottle after use.

5. Only when it is uncoated and scored.

6. Using a tablet splitter or seeking help from the pharmacist.

7. Internal medicines cupboard, external medicines cupboard, patient's own cabinet, drug refrigerator, controlled drugs cupboard, disinfectants cupboard, clinical reagents cupboard, resuscitation trolley, open shelving for intravenous or irrigation fluids, pharmacy box.

8. Return container and contents to pharmacy.

9. British National Formulary, MIMS, Data Sheet Compendium, medicine information service.

10. Place medicine in trolley or cupboard and lock, and attend to patient OR ask another nurse to attend to patient, place medicine in trolley or cupboard, label it and arrange to give when patient available.

SECTION B

	Paracetamol	Prednisolone	Diamorphine
Class of drug	Pharmacy medicine or general sale list, depending on pack size	Prescription-only medicine	Controlled drug
Storage	Internal medicines cupboard	Internal medicines cupboard	Controlled drugs cupboard
Formulations available	Tablet, soluble tablet, capsule, oral suspension, suppository, IV infusion	Tablet, enteric-coated tablet, soluble tablet, injection	Tablet, injection
Indications for use	Mild to moderate pain, pyrexia	Suppression of inflammatory and allergic disorders	Severe pain, acute pulmonary oedema
Contraindications	None; caution in liver or renal disease and in alcohol dependence	Systemic infection; avoid live vaccines	Acute respiratory depression, acute alcoholism, raised intracranial pressure or head injury
Normal dose range	500mg–1 g every 4–6 h to a maximum of 4 g daily	By mouth, up to 10–20 mg daily, 60 mg in severe cases; by IM injection, 25–100 mg once or twice a week	5 mg every 4 h if necessary
Common side-effects	Rare; rash, blood disorders	Gastrointestinal, musculoskeletal, endocrine, neuropsychiatric, ophthalmic and numerous other effects	Nausea and vomiting, constipation, drowsiness; larger doses produce respiratory depression, hypotension

SECTION C

1. If swallowed, the drug passes to the liver, where it is metabolised, and only a small amount enters the bloodstream. Taken sublingually, the drug enters the bloodstream immediately, thus bypassing the liver and first-pass effect.
2. Taken by mouth, insulin would be destroyed in the stomach.
3. Drugs given directly into a vein are immediately transported to the heart, from where they are pumped to their site of action.
4. Blood should always be preceded by sodium chloride 0.9% solution. Any other substance would cause the blood to coagulate.
5. Potassium is a highly toxic substance that, if infused too rapidly, can cause cardiac arrest.
6. There is an increased risk of bruising.
7. Drugs given intrathecally come into direct contact with the brain and nervous tissue. Drugs intended for intravenous use have been given intrathecally in error and have caused fatalities.
8. Unless a tablet or capsule is swallowed with a drink, there is a danger of it sticking in the oesophagus, in some cases leading to ulceration of the oesophagus.
9. The validity of the test may be destroyed by the alcohol in the swab.
10. Muscles are highly vascular; leukaemia patients are at risk of bleeding. There is therefore too great a risk of a large bleed into the site of the injection.

SECTION D

1. d.
2. b.

3. e, a, d, c, b.
4. b.
5. c.

SECTION E

In all cases, the nurse in charge would be informed. The following personnel would be specifically informed.

1. Doctor (urgently).
2. Technician from medical physics department.
3. Pharmacist.
4. Nurse in charge, ?doctor.
5. Occupational therapist, pharmacist.
6. Patient.

SECTION F

1. The buttock.
2. Into the subarachnoid space of the spinal cord.
3. High up between the gum and cheek.
4. Abdomen, front of thighs, upper arm, renal angle.
5. Antecubital fossa, back of hand.
6. In a refrigerator.
7. A different hairless site normally on the chest wall.
8. On the forearm.
9. Pharmacy department.
10. In the patient's case notes in the medical records department.

SECTION G

1. Fig. 14.17 20 mL of syrup.
2. Fig. 14.18 6.25 mL of oral suspension.
3. Fig. 14.19 0.2 mL intravenous injection.

SECTION H

Dose prescribed	Dose available	What would you give?
1.5 g	300 mg/5 mL	25 mL
75 mg	25 mg/mL	3 mL
0.1 mg	0.05 mg	2 tablets
500 000 units	300 000 units/mL	1.7 mL
12 mg	4 mg	3 tablets
1 g	500 mg	2 tablets
60 mg	5 mg	12 tablets
15 mg	5 mg	3 tablets

Continued

Dose prescribed	Dose available	What would you give?
24 mg	8 mg	3 tablets
125 micrograms	62.5 micrograms	2 tablets
100 mg	50 mg/mL	2 mL
0.5 g	250 mg	2 tablets
100 mg	25 mg/mL	4 mL
0.4 mg	0.6 mg/mL	0.7 mL
62.5 mg	250 mg/mL	0.25 mL
175 micrograms	50 micrograms/mL	3.5 mL
1 g	250 mg/mL	4 mL
20 000 units	5000 units/mL	4 mL
500 mg	250 mg/mL	2 tablets
1.6 g	800 mg/3 mL	6 mL
3 mg	0.6 mg/mL	5 mL
125 micrograms	50 micrograms/mL	2.5 mL
12.5 mg	12.5 mg/2 mL	2 mL
50 micrograms	100 micrograms/mL	0.5 mL
1 million units	10 million units/mL	0.1 mL
0.5 g	500 mg	1 tablet
50 micrograms	100 micrograms/mL	0.5 mL
12 mg	15 mg/mL	0.8 mL
40 mg	80 mg/mL	0.5 mL
2.5 mg	10 mg/2 mL	0.5 mL

CHAPTER 5   NURSE PRESCRIBING

1. The CMP must contain information to ensure the safety and efficacy of treatment. It must contain:

- the name of the patient and consent, preferably signed
- the illnesses or conditions that may be treated by the supplementary prescriber, in this case hypertension
- the date on which the plan is to start and the date when it is to be reviewed by the doctor; this may be set at a year as a maximum or could be sooner

- the name of the medicine(s) and the class of medicine that you may wish to prescribe under the plan, for example angiotensin-converting enzyme inhibitors (class) or ramipril (medicine-specific)
- any restrictions or limitations as to the strength or dose of any product that may be prescribed or administered under the plan, and any period of administration or use of any medicinal product that may be prescribed or administered under the plan (e.g. bendroflumethiazide dose not greater than 2.5 mg daily)

- relevant warnings about the known sensitivities of the patient to, or known difficulties of the patient with, particular medicinal products (e.g. ankle oedema with amlodipine)
- the arrangements for notification of adverse reactions to any medicines and the circumstances in which the supplementary prescriber should refer to the doctor (e.g. not achieving blood pressure target within 3 months of therapy)
- the plan must be agreed by both you, as the supplementary prescriber, and the doctor as the independent prescriber.

Additional points include the following.

- Consider the patient; all patients are individuals and response to treatment can vary.
- Decide which treatment strategy to use; non-drug treatments may be included. Consider choice of product, e.g. potential side-effects, interactions, dose.
- Negotiate contract with patient (concordance). Remember drug can only work if patient takes it.
- Review – is the treatment working? Are there side-effects? Can therapy be discontinued?
- Record keeping – can someone else find out diagnosis, decision and therapy patient received when I am not about?
- Reflect – as a prescriber, what have I learned? Could I have managed this patient better? What areas do I need to improve upon? do I need further training?

CHAPTER 6 CLINICAL GOVERNANCE AND SAFETY IN THE USE OF MEDICINES

1. Failure to learn and prevent the likelihood of an actual error.
2. Standard terminology; error reduction.

CHAPTER 7 THE ROLE OF PATIENTS AND CARERS IN MEDICINES MANAGEMENT

SECTION A

1. Being able to instil drops during school hours. Suitable location close to handwashing facilities to instil drops. Drops sting and patient may therefore decide to skip dose. For life, and therefore tedious. Smudging of make-up.
2. Understanding condition. Taking blood glucose samples. Ensuring cleanliness.

Measuring dose.
Injecting insulin: correct technique, correct times.
Security and disposal of syringes and needles.

3. Remembering to take medicines and at correct times. Reading labels.
Difficulty with packages and closures and with handling tablets.
Understanding importance of taking.
Remembering he has taken the medicines.
4. Getting breaks from meetings to take tablets. Lack of motivation.
Too stressed, deadlines to meet, to take at correct intervals.
5. Not wanting peers to know she is on medication. Difficulty taking tablets on time when on shifts. Not wanting to develop cushingoid features. May increase dose because of belief that this may help.
6. Interfering with travel.
Forgetting when visiting, holidaying.
Feeling well and therefore 'out of mind'.
If diuretic, restricting going out and fearing accidents.
7. Not wanting to smell.
Not having enough time to cleanse and apply.
Having to keep skin covered.
Fear of staining clothes, etc.
8. He needs to be encouraged to take his medication. Drugs are bought in bulk and may not be as expensive as they might seem. If he neglects to take his medication, he may end up in hospital with worsening of his original condition, i.e. stricture, ulceration or haemorrhage, and that would waste a much greater amount of money.

CHAPTER 8 PHARMACOKINETICS AND PHARMACODYNAMICS

Absorption changes include the following.

- Reduced amount of saliva can reduce the *rate* of absorption of buccally absorbed drugs (e.g. glyceryl trinitrate). It does not decrease the total amount absorbed.
- Increasing gastric pH, reduced gastric acid secretion and delayed gastric emptying, as peristalsis is weakened and may delay the dissolution of orally administered drugs.
- Increasing atrophy of the intestinal epithelium, leading to a decrease in surface area for drug absorption. Decreased blood flow in the splanchnic area and decreased mesenteric blood flow will often result in a slower absorption rate. This leads to an increased time to reach peak drug levels.
- Changes in absorption rate in the elderly do not usually require changes in dose.

CHAPTER 9 AUTONOMIC NERVOUS SYSTEM

Non-selective beta blockers such as propranolol and sotalol have an effect on both β_1 and β_2 receptors. They therefore have an effect on the heart and also on bronchial muscle. Their effect on β_2 receptors causes bronchoconstriction, and their use is contraindicated in asthmatic patients. Their effect on the heart causes it to slow and reduces cardiac output. The vasodilatory effects on skeletal muscle allow them to be used in the management of hypertension and angina, although β_1-receptor-specific antagonists are preferred.

CHAPTER 10 ADVERSE DRUG REACTIONS AND DRUG INTERACTIONS

1. The term *anaphylaxis* is commonly used for hypersensitivity reactions typically mediated by immunoglobulin E. Anaphylactoid reactions are similar but do not depend on hypersensitivity. The symptoms and management are similar. Both may present clinically with angioedema, urticaria, dyspnoea and hypotension. Some patients may die from acute irreversible asthma or laryngeal oedema, with few more generalised manifestations. Other symptoms include rhinitis, conjunctivitis, abdominal pain, vomiting, diarrhoea and a sense of impending doom. The skin colour usually changes: the patient may appear either flushed or pale. Cardiovascular collapse is a common manifestation, especially in response to intravenous drugs or stings, and is caused by vasodilatation and loss of plasma from the blood compartment. Any cardiac dysfunction is due principally to hypotension, or rarely to an underlying disease or to adrenaline (epinephrine) that has been administered intravenously.

   Anaphylactic reactions vary in severity, and progress may be rapid, slow or (unusually) biphasic. Rarely, manifestations may be delayed by a few hours (adding to diagnostic difficulty) or persist for more than 24 h.

2. Key areas include the following.

   - Ensuring patients receive patient information leaflets and counselling on correct use of their medicines and side-effects to watch out for.
   - Indentifying drugs known to produce predictable dose-related adverse effects and avoiding their use where an equally effective and safer alternative is available.
   - Checking patients are not unnecessarily exposed to risk through use of unrequired drugs, disregard for warnings, special precautions or contra-indications.
   - Recognising where a patient has had a previous allergic reaction or known allergy, e.g. peanut, and ensuring no exposure to the allergen.
   - Identifying early signs of adverse effects, e.g. rash, linking signs and symptoms to a possible adverse drug reaction.
   - Knowing signs and symptoms of anaphylactic reaction and how to treat it.

CHAPTER 11 DRUG TREATMENT OF GASTROINTESTINAL DISORDERS

1. The investigations are:

   - history, including family, dietary, social, occupational and medication
   - physical examination
   - weight recording
   - visual examination of faeces for blood, mucus, consistency
   - stool recording
   - stool for faecal occult blood testing
   - stool for culture and sensitivity testing
   - barium studies
   - ultrasound
   - endoscopy
   - computerised scanning.

2. Drugs matched with their mode of action.

Ranitidine	Suppresses gastric acid production by blocking the action of histamine of receptors in the stomach.
Omeprazole	Inhibits gastric acid by blocking the hydrogen potassium ATP enzyme system of the gastric parietal cell.
Misoprostol	Inhibits acid secretion and protects gastric mucosa.
Magnesium trisilicate	Neutralises gastric acid.

3a. ii.
3b. iii.
3c. Breath test.
3d. vi.
4. Inform the doctor. The patient may have an underlying gastrointestinal condition of a serious nature that is being overlooked.
5. b.
6. a, e, f, g and h are constipating. The rest are laxative in nature. Colestyramine is both.
7. A laxative – an agent used to evacuate the bowel by increasing the bulk of the faeces, stimulating

intestinal motility, softening the stool, lubricating the intestinal wall or having an osmotic effect by drawing water from the body into the large bowel.

8. Loss of potassium, leading to hypokalaemia; damage to the bowel known as atonic colon.

9. Prolonged or enforced immobility, regular use of opioids, angina, haemorrhoids.

10. The following are important when administering rectal medicines.
   Minimising risk:

   - ensure correct patient, medicine(in date), dose, route, time
   - leave call bell within reach.

   Respect:

   - promote and protect the patient's interests and dignity
   - maintain appropriate professional boundaries
   - encourage self-administration where appropriate.

   Rights:

   - provide information
   - obtain patient's consent.

   Privacy:

   - ensure curtains drawn and close bathroom door
   - ask permission to enter cubicle or bathroom.

11. Much more specific; less side-effects; more effective.

12. Because of the antimuscarinic effects of the antidepressant.

CHAPTER 12   DRUG TREATMENT OF CARDIOVASCULAR DISORDERS

1. In general health and lifestyle, advice should address diet, exercise and smoking.

- Encourage patients to eat a healthy diet. This may be achieved by:
  — increasing the amount of fruit and vegetables eaten to at least five portions a day
  — reducing the amount of fat eaten, particularly saturated fat
  — combining healthy eating with regular physical exercise
  — encouraging and enabling patients to develop skills and knowledge that will help them to improve their diet
  — reinforcing the message that eating a balanced diet is a positive step that can be taken towards improving health.

- Encourage patient to stop smoking. Key messages are:
  — it is harmful to health to use tobacco products or be around tobacco smoke
  — everyone has the right not to be exposed to tobacco smoke
  — smokers should be encouraged and supported to stop smoking
  — young people should be encouraged and supported not to start smoking, or to stop
  — young people who smoke should be encouraged to look at why they started
  — discourage patients from using tobacco around pregnant women or children and young people.

- Advise on undertaking regular exercise. Key messages are:
  — 30 min of moderate-intensity physical activity a day can make a real difference to health
  — try to be physically active on at least 5 days of the week
  — don't work too hard, but make sure you are breathing more heavily and getting a bit sweaty
  — do 30 min of activity each day; if a 30-min session is too long, try doing 2×15 min or 3×10 min of activity instead
  — encourage weight loss if appropriate.

2. Increase in heart rate; increase in blood pressure.

3. Use of beta-blockers.

4. With noradrenaline (norepinephrene).

5. Vasoconstrictor sympathomimetic

CHAPTER 13   DRUG TREATMENT OF RESPIRATORY DISORDERS

A.

1. Sit the patient upright, well supported with pillows. Act calmly and try to reassure him and his wife. Discourage him from trying to talk.

2. Ensure that oxygen is flowing unimpeded at the prescribed rate using the correct appliance. Ensure that no matches or cigarettes are in use. Reduce friction in the vicinity of the oxygen. Avoid the use of paraffin-based lubricants.

3. Colour; conscious level; temperature; pulse; rate, depth and sound of respirations; blood pressure.

4. Medical history, physical examination, blood gas estimation, chest X-ray, pulmonary function tests, ?lung scan, sputum for bacteriology and cytology.

5. Irritation of the bronchioles, damage to the cilia, inflammation of the bronchial mucosa, hypersecretion of the ciliary glands, tenacious bronchial secretions, infected sputum.

6. Intravenous, inhalation.

7. In COPD, the sensitivity to carbon dioxide as the main drive for breathing is lost. The second stimulus for breathing, i.e. oxygen lack, becomes essential. If too high, a concentration of oxygen is given; this stimulus is also lost, which results in the patient developing respiratory failure.

8. Bronchodilator, corticosteroid, antibiotic, mucolytic.

9. Beta agonist (e.g. salbutamol) or an antimuscarinic (e.g. ipratropium) beclometasone, benzylpenicillin, carbocisteine.

10. After each use, the nebuliser and mask should be washed in hot, soapy water and dried using a paper towel. Inner tubing should be similarly treated once a week. A complete change of equipment should be made each week if the patient has a chest infection.

11. Oxygen has a drying effect. Inhaled corticosteroids can cause a fungal infection of the mouth (thrush).

12. Pharmacist, physiotherapist, ?occupational therapist, ?social worker.

13. She should:
    — keep house at even temperature and well ventilated
    — discourage her husband from smoking
    — encourage concordance with all medication
    — encourage him to have annual flu vaccination
    — ensure that he has had pneumoccocal vaccine
    — encourage healthy diet and good fluid intake
    — encourage exercise within limits of condition
    — prevent contact with infection, if possible
    — report change in colour or tenacity of sputum promptly.

B.

1. Salbutamol; terbutaline.

2. Ipratropium.

3. Short action of beta$_2$ agonist; longer 'protective' action of corticosteroid.

4. Cause bronchoconstriction.

CHAPTER 14   DRUGS ACTING ON THE CENTRAL NERVOUS SYSTEM

1. Drowsiness and confusion next day.

2. Antidepressants, hypotension; opioid analgesics, potentiation.

3. Diazepam.

4. True.

5. Fewer side-effects; more specific action.

6. Hyoscine.

7. Drowsiness, dry mouth, vision disturbed.

8. Difficult to adjust doses; source of side effects may be difficult to identify.

9. Constipation, nausea and vomiting, cardiac side effects.

10. More potent; more soluble.

11. Status epilepticus.

12. Self-help group, focus on strengths rather than weaknesses, acetylcholinesterase inhibitors.

13. a. Bupropion^T(amfebutamone), nicotine replacement.
    b. Methadone, lofexidine, buprenorphine.
    c. Disulfiram, chlordiazepoxide, diazepam, acamprosate.

14. Encouragement of a healthy low-fat, low-calorie, low-sugar, high-fibre, fruit and vegetable diet; increased and regular exercise; counselling if required; appetite suppressant (e.g. orlistat, sibutramine, rimonabant).

15. Failing to take their tablets.

16. End of dose: fluctuations in motor response after 5 years of levodopa therapy. On–off effects: sudden fluctuations in disability lasting minutes to hours.

17. Slowly.

18. Avoid caffeine, take milky drink at bedtime, do something to unwind (e.g. read; talk over worries if necessary or possible), create a comfortable environment if possible (e.g. quiet, blacked-out room, suitable temperature), seek doctor's advice as final resort.

19. In the medulla oblongata in the brain stem.

20. A common condition characterised by episodes of photophobia, headache, nausea and vomiting. Simple analgesics, over-the-counter migraine preparations, antiemetics, 5HT$_1$ agonists, triptans.

CHAPTER 15   DRUG TREATMENT OF INFECTIONS

A.

1. Frequency of micturition, dysuria, fishy smelling urine, pyrexia, loin pain, vomiting.

2. Obtain midstream specimen of urine and wait for result to administer antibiotic prescribed, pending result; analgesic as required; fluids.

3. Midstream specimen of urine sent to bacteriology laboratory for culture and sensitivity.

4. A violent attack of shivering, which may be associated with fever or reaction to a drug. Followed by feeling of intense heat and then sweating.

5. Symptomatically:
    — when cold, take action to warm him up
    — when hot, take action to cool him down
    — when sweating, take action to freshen him up.

B.
1. Tetracycline.
2. Chlorhexidine.
3. Vancomycin.
4. Bacterial resistance.
5. Mantoux.
6. Anaerobes.
7. Intravenous.
8. Culture.
9. Phagocytes.
10. E. Coli.
11. Threadworms.
12. Anaphylaxis.
13. Antifungals.
14. Oral thrush.
15. Benzylpenicillin.
16. Athlete's foot.
17. Urinary tract infection.
18. Gram.
19. HIV.
20. MRSA.
21. Sensitivity.
22. Bactericidal.
23. Parasite.

CHAPTER 16   DRUG TREATMENT OF ENDOCRINE DISORDERS

SECTION A

It is essential to stress that, because this drug is replacing a naturally occurring hormone, it must be continued for life.

SECTION B

1. Polydipsia, polyuria, weight loss.
2. Type 1 results from a total absence of insulin from the pancreas and a high blood sugar, and it must be treated with insulin. Type 2 is associated with the ageing process and those who are overweight, and is usually controlled by either diet alone or diet and an oral hypoglycaemic agent.
3. Corticosteroids.
4. Approximately 4–7 mol/L.
5. Acting out of character. Sweating profusely, especially on the forehead and upper lip.
6. Just before a meal is due or during the night.
7. Give the patient, at once, two digestive biscuits and a glass of milk OR glucose 25 g in warm water BEFORE calling a doctor to administer intravenous glucose.

8. Low-carbohydrate, low-fat, sugar-free, high-fibre diet.
9. True.
10. Soluble insulin, intravenously.
11. It is stored in the refrigerator at a temperature between 2 and 8°C.
12. Retinopathy, nephropathy, neuropathy.

SECTION C

Diabetes <u>mellitus</u> is a <u>complex</u> disorder of carbohydrate, fat and <u>protein</u> metabolism caused by a <u>relative</u> or complete lack of <u>insulin</u> secretion by the β cells situated in the islets of Langerhans in the <u>pancreas</u>.

SECTION D

Hyperglycaemia	Hypoglycaemia
Slow onset	Rapid onset
Thirst	Slurred speech
Polyuria	Change in behaviour
Dehydration	Facial sweating
Smell of ketones on breath	Lack of food
Glycosuria	Tachycardia
Raised blood glucose	Low blood glucose
Treat with insulin	Treat with glucose

SECTION F

Contributing factors: increased availability of fast carbohydrate and sugary foods and drinks with soaring numbers who are grossly obese. Nurses should take every opportunity to spread the word about healthy eating and exercise. The opportunity to carry out diabetic urinalysis should never be missed.

SECTION G

See British National Formulary.

CHAPTER 17 DRUGS USED IN OBSTETRICS, GYNAECOLOGY AND URINARY TRACT DISORDERS

1.

Pituitary hormone	Ovarian hormone	Uses in obstetrics and gynaecology
Follicle-stimulating hormone	Oestrogen	Hormonal contraception (plus progestogen-only pill) Hormone replacement therapy Prevention of osteoporosis
Luteinising hormone	Progesterone	Dysmenorrhoea Endometriosis Hormonal contraception Hormone replacement therapy

2. Because of its hypotensive effect, it is advisable to take alfuzocin before bedtime.
   Warn patient of possible effects and to lie down if symptoms such as dizziness, fatigue or sweating develop.
   Ensure that course of ciprofloxacin is completed.
   Ensure adequate fluid intake.
   Change from day bag to overnight bag every 24 h.
   Attend follow-up clinic as directed.
3. a. Muscarinic side-effects, e.g. bronchoconstriction, gastrointestinal disturbances.
   b. Alfuzocin; doxazocin.
   c. Salbutamol; ritodrine.
   d. Suby G; Solution R.
   e. Absorption of sodium leading to hypertension.
   f. Impotence and decreased libido.
   g. Depot injections; transdermal injections.

CHAPTER 18 DRUGS USED IN KIDNEY DISEASES

SECTION A

1. The passage of water and small molecules through the walls of the glomerulus and glomerular capsule.
2. Removal of certain elements from the blood by virtue of the difference in their rate of diffusion through an external semipermeable membrane or, in the case of peritoneal dialysis, the peritoneum.
3. Pain and spasm in the ureter, caused by the presence of a stone (calculus).
4. An element that when dissolved in water dissociates into ions and is able to conduct an electric current.

SECTION B

1. True.
2. True.
3. False.
4. False.
5. True.

SECTION C

1. A solution of higher osmotic pressure than plasma; drugs increasing the excretion of water and sodium chloride.
2. Vitamin D is produced in the kidney.
3. High blood pressure; infection; diabetes mellitus.
4. True.
5. Erythropoetin is produced in the kidneys.
6. Azathioprine; ciclosporin.
7. Renal transplantation; hypertension.

CHAPTER 19 DRUG TREATMENT OF MALIGNANT DISEASE

SECTION A

Chemotherapy protocols include clear and unambiguous statements on the following:

- definition of the clinical condition being treated
- all chemotherapy medicines to be given
- dosing schedule for each medicine
- route, method and duration over which the chemotherapy is to be administered
- maximum cumulative doses when applicable
- any premedication required
- diluents AND appropriate infusion volumes
- hydration schedules (if required)

- supportive therapy
- relevant haematology and biochemistry results
- any other tests that need to be performed before chemotherapy starts and during treatment
- special precautions and contraindications to treatment
- potential interactions and medications to be avoided
- recommendations for treatment delays or dose reductions
- expected toxicities
- when relevant, reference should be made to policies for the management of side effects
- advice on when patients should be referred for review by the consultant
- reference source(s).

SECTION B

1. d.
2. a.
3. c.
4. b.
5. d.
6. a.

SECTION C

1. e: omeprazole is a proton pump inhibitor, the others are antiemetics.
2. d: ciclosporin is an immunosuppressant, the others are cytotoxics.
3. c: vigabatrin is used in epilepsy, the others are cytotoxics.
4. Mesna is not a cytotoxic drug, it is an adjunct used to treat malignant disease.

CHAPTER 20   DRUGS AFFECTING THE IMMUNE RESPONSE

1. Passive immunity can be provided by the injection of human immunoglobulin that contains antibody to the target infection. This will temporarily increase the patient's antibody level to the infection. Protection occurs within a couple of days but may last only a few weeks. Human normal immunoglobulin is derived from the pooled plasma of donors and contains antibodies to infections that are currently prevalent in the general population. Human normal immunoglobulin is used for the protection of immunocompromised children exposed to measles and protection of individuals after exposure to hepatitis A.

   Specific immunoglobulins are available for tetanus, hepatitis B, rabies and varicella zoster. Specific immunoglobulins are obtained from the pooled blood of donors who are convalescing from the target infectious disease, or have been recently immunised with the relevant vaccine or are found on screening to have sufficiently high antibody titres.

2. Immunity produced by the natural mechanisms of the body which is long-lasting.
3. Short-life immunity conferred by the administration of an antitoxin.
4. They prevent organ rejection in cases of severe illness where transplantation is the only option for the patient.
5. Malignant disease; skin disease; organ transplantation; autoimmune disease.

CHAPTER 21   NUTRITION AND BLOOD, FLUID AND ELECTROLYTES

SECTION A

1. They add fibre to the diet and help to prevent constipation and disorders of the bowel. They are rich in vitamins; vitamins cannot be stored and therefore have to be taken on a regular and frequent basis.
2. Fat and carbohydrate.
3. Bananas.
4. It stands for body mass index and is used to assist in identifying those patients who require nutritional supplementation:

$$BMI = \frac{weight~(kg)}{height~(m^2)}.$$

5. To treat diarrhoea and provide nutritional supplements.
6. Aspiration pneumonia from inhaling the feed.
7. Attaching a 50-mL syringe to the tube, aspirate a small quantity of gastric contents. Test the aspirate using pH-indicating paper (pH should be in range 1–4). Alternatively, syringe a small amount of air down the tube and at same time, using a stethoscope, listen for a gurgling sound over the epigastrium. Radiological confirmation is reserved for the unconscious patient or when there is doubt about the tube's position.
8. Has to be prepared in a rigorously sterile environment, as bacteria readily grow in the foodstuff.
9. Colour and respirations: not inhaling feed. Temperature and pulse: no infection. Blood pressure: no cardiac embarrassment. Blood glucose: to ensure not developing hyperglycaemia.
10. Danger of blocking the tube.

SECTION B

- Charlie should have a healthy meal: any starter, meat or fish, plenty of green vegetables, fresh fruit or biscuits and cheese. Avoid pure sugars.
- Lou can have anything from the food menu. She should avoid cranberry juice.
- Dorothy should choose lentil soup and any main course, with plenty of green vegetables (especially broccoli); she should ask for a café latte to finish.
- Alfred could have any starter. He must avoid pastry and fried fish. He could have any sweet and he should avoid alcohol totally.
- Reg can eat whatever he fancies as a starter or main course. On no account should he take mature cheese, and he would be well advised to stick to a soft drink.

SECTION C

1. Fatigue, breathless, feeling the cold.
2. Iron deficiency.
3. Erythropoietin.
4. Neutrophils.
5. Schilling test.
6. Hydroxocobalamin (vitamin B_{12}).
7. Folate.
8. Granulocyte-colony stimulating factor.
9. Desferrioxamine.
10. Z-track technique.
11. Milk.
12. Intrinsic.

SECTION D

1. 1500–2000 mL.
2. Approximately the same as above.
3. 1500 mL.
4. 71 mL/kg of body weight.
5. Food and fluid.
6. Thiazide, loop, potassium sparing, aldosterone antagonists.
7. Removal of certain elements from the blood by virtue of the difference in their rate of diffusion through an external semipermeable membrane or in the case of peritoneal dialysis the peritoneum.
8. An element that when dissolved in water dissociates into ions and is able to conduct an electric current.
9. Level of potassium in the blood below 3.4 mmol/L, resulting in clinical symptoms.
10. Level of sodium in the blood above 144 mmol/L, resulting in clinical symptoms.

CHAPTER 22   DRUG TREATMENT OF MUSCULOSKELETAL AND JOINT DISEASES

1. Suggest initiate treatment with an NSAID taken after food. Suggest use of long-acting formulation (e.g. diclofenac modified release) to cover morning stiffness. Also include paracetamol initially as required, which can be increased to 1 g four times daily regularly if required to control pain. In view of high erythrocyte sedimentation rate and C-reactive protein, would initiate a DMARD early on. Exclude pregnancy and ensure that effective contraceptive methods are employed. First choice would probably be methotrexate, initial dose 7.5 mg ONCE weekly, increased according to response. Carry out baseline chest X-ray, full blood count, urea and electrolytes, liver function tests and urinalysis. Full blood count, urea and electrolytes and liver function tests every week until 6 weeks after the last dose increase, and then monitoring increased to monthly thereafter.

   Miss D. should be advised to report any new or increasing fever, especially sore throat, cough or the presence of rash or oral ulceration. If Miss D. is sexually active, she should be advised to seek advice on contraception.
2a. 10mg test dose followed by 50mg injection weekly
3. - inhibits gastric acid secretion
    - relaxes bronchi
    - dilates blood vessels and reduces blood pressure
    - mediates some aspects of inflammation

CHAPTER 23   DRUG TREATMENT OF EYE CONDITIONS

1. The meanings are as follow.
   a. A mydriatic dilates the pupil by contraction of the muscles of the iris.
   b. A cycloplegic paralyses the ocular muscles of accommodation.
   c. A parasympathomimetic constricts the pupil.
   d. A sympathomimetic dilates the pupil.
2. Drugs matched with their mode of action.

Aciclovir	Antiviral
Sodium chloride	Irrigation
Oxybuprocaine	Local anaesthetic
Fluorescein	Diagnostic stain
Betamethasone	Anti-inflammatory
Chloramphenicol	Antibacterial
Timolol	Reduces intraocular pressure
Tropicamide	Mydriatic

Ketoconazole   Antifungal

Hypromellose   Artificial tears

3. Water, salts and lysozyme plus oil from the meibomian glands.

4. Keep the eye moist.

   Help to reduce infection.

   Protect the eye by removing grit.

5. Handwashing prior to administration.

   Utilising clean technique.

   Eye bathing prior to administration if required.

   Using single-use containers (especially in surgery).

   Ensuring that eye drops are in date.

   Avoiding touching eye with dropper.

6. When multiple-dose container in use, discarding after 1 week in hospital and 28 days at home.

7. Remove the lenses.

   Store in sterile container containing sodium chloride 0.9% solution.

   Label container with patient's name, ward and unit number.

   Store in safe place.

8. Intraocular pressure would otherwise increase, leading to loss of vision.

CHAPTER 24 DRUG TREATMENT OF EAR, NOSE AND THROAT DISORDERS

1. Chemotherapy can interfere with growth of healthy cells as well as cancer cells. When the healthy cells in the lining of the mouth are affected, this can lead to a number of side effects. Chemotherapy can cause the lining of the mouth to become very sore, and small ulcers may form (mucositis). If the patient is immunocompromised, then infections of the mouth are more likely. Thrush is the most common mouth infection. Chemotherapy sometimes leads to a dry mouth. Occasionally, some bleeding or ulceration of the gums may develop. Damage to the cells lining the mouth is usually temporary, and most side effects will disappear once the treatment has finished and the white blood cell count returns to normal. The likelihood of developing a sore mouth varies from treatment to treatment.

   It is a good idea for the patient to visit a dentist prior to starting chemotherapy. Dentists can advise on any problems and can help to get the teeth and gums into good condition before treatment begins. It is important to inspect the mouth daily for any signs of redness, swelling, sores, white patches or bleeding.

Patients should be advised to:

- clean teeth or dentures gently every morning and evening, and also after each meal, using a soft-bristled or child's toothbrush
- gently use dental tape or floss daily, but only after checking that the level of platelets is high enough (a low platelet count can cause bleeding in the mouth even with very gentle flossing)
- keep lips moist by using Vaseline or a lip balm
- avoid neat spirits, tobacco, hot spices, garlic, onion, vinegar and salty food
- keep mouth and food moist; add gravies and sauces to food to help swallowing
- try to drink at least 1.5 L (3 pints) of fluid a day
- avoid acidic drinks such as orange and grapefruit juice; warm herbal teas may be more soothing
- let the doctor know if mouth ulcers appear
- keep the mouth fresh and moist.

2. Perforation of the tympanic membrane.

3. Ear, between room and body temperature; nose, room temperature if previously stored in fridge.

4. Radiotherapy to head or neck, reduced salivary flow, certain drugs, infection of a salivary gland, dental or oral surgery, debilitation or immunosuppression, fungal and viral infections of the mouth.

5. White plaques on the mucous membrane that cannot be easily removed.

6. Nystatin oral suspension or pastilles, *or* amphotericin suspension or lozenges *or* miconozole gel.

7. Phenytoin.

8. Some drugs used to treat osteoporosis can cause osteonecrosis of the jaw.

9. Bronchoconstriction; gastrointestinal disturbances; cardiovascular side-effects.

10. Desmopressin.

11. Yes; there are dangers of absorption and systemic side-effects in prolonged use.

12. Yes; administering a topical microbial.

CHAPTER 25 DRUG TREATMENT OF SKIN DISORDERS

1a. Eczema is an inflammatory reaction in the skin that may be either endogenous (atopic, e.g. allergy) with a hereditary tendency or exogenous (contact dermatitis) associated with an irritant (hypersensitivity to nickel, rubber, etc.); psoriasis is a chronic skin disorder characterised by dry, flaky plaques especially on elbows and knees.

1b. Creams are water-based; ointments are greasy and anhydrous.

1c. Acne vulgaris involves inflamed spots and comedones; rosacea may be an inflammatory condition that leads to facial erythema but is non-comedonal.

1d. Hydrogel dressings provide a moist environment to assist wound healing; hydrocolloid dressings are gel-forming when in contact with a wound, providing a moist environment.

2a. Paper-thin skin, viral infections.

2b. Eczema, psoriasis, body lice, scabies, fungal infections, haemorrhoids; obstructive jaundice, uraemic frost, lymphomas, diabetes mellitus, viral illnesses in childhood.

2c. Chlorhexidine, mupirocin; ketoconazole, miconazole; aciclovir, formaldehyde.

2d. Wash hands before and after applying skin preparations and wear gloves.

3a. Location, cause, form, aetiology, tissue type, size, exudate, pain, overall condition of adjacent tissues.

3b. A hydrogel, hydrocolloid or alginate dressing.

3c. Dandruff, scabies.

3d. Skin protection factor. It is needed to keep out the damaging rays of the sun.

3e. Psoralen ultraviolet A. Used in the treatment of psoriasis.

3f. Difficult to apply, messy on hands and clothes, dangerous to eyes.

3g. Methotrexate.

4. You would want to establish (tactfully) if she is using the cream for her children. This could be highly dangerous for them. If she is a worrier, she may appreciate someone who will listen to her. Referral to a doctor may also be indicated.

CHAPTER 26   PALLIATIVE CARE

1. Dexamethasone.
2. Amitriptyline.
3. Hyoscine, glycopyrronium.
4. No injections, long-term control.
5. Gastric distension, hiccup.
6. Methadone is long-acting and may accumulate.
7. Hyoscine, glycopyrronium.
8. Antimuscarinic
9. Metoclopramide; rashes, pruritus, oedema, central nervous system disturbances.
10. Nausea, bowel obstruction, patient's wishes.
11. Transdermal patch.
12a. Paracetamol.
12b. Dihydrocodeine.
12c. Morphine.
13. Dexamethasone, diazepam.
14. Palliative care incorporates symptom control, support for the patient and support for the family. It includes the palliation of physical symptoms; maintenance of independence; alleviation of isolation, anxiety and fear; and provision for a dignified death.
15. See British National Formulary.

Index

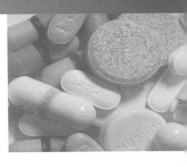